国家卫生和计划生育委员会"十三五"规划教材

全国高等学校教材

供本科护理学类专业用

老年护理学（双语）

Gerontological Nursing

第 **2** 版

U0284769

主　编　郭桂芳　黄　金

副主编　谷岩梅　郭　宏

编　者（按姓氏笔画排序）

于　放	▶	（美国亚利桑那州立大学埃德森护理和创新学院）
刘　宇	▶	（中国医科大学护理学院）
刘红霞	▶	（北京中医药大学护理学院）
吴丽华	▶	（英国哈德斯菲尔德大学护理助产学院）
谷岩梅	▶	（河北中医学院护理学院）
张　静	▶	（中国人民解放军海军军医大学护理学院）
陈　茜	▶	（四川大学华西护理学院/四川大学华西医院）
胡　洁	▶	（美国俄亥俄州立大学护理学院）
晋溶辰	▶	（湖南中医药大学护理学院）
郭　宏	▶	（沈阳医学院护理学院）
郭桂芳	▶	（北京大学护理学院）
黄　金	▶	（中南大学湘雅二医院）
奚　兴	▶	（江苏卫生健康职业学院）
梁　涛	▶	（北京协和医学院护理学院）
曾　慧	▶	（中南大学湘雅护理学院）
穆晓云	▶	（中国医科大学护理学院）
Deborah Lekan	▶	（美国北卡罗来纳大学格林斯伯勒分校护理学院）
Linda Phillips	▶	（美国加州大学洛杉矶分校护理学院）

编写秘书　晋溶辰　奚　兴

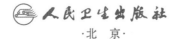人民卫生出版社

·北　京·

图书在版编目（CIP）数据

老年护理学：英汉对照 / 郭桂芳，黄金主编. —2
版. —北京：人民卫生出版社，2022.8
ISBN 978-7-117-32534-9

Ⅰ. ①老… Ⅱ. ①郭… ②黄… Ⅲ. ①老年医学－护
理学－医学院校－教材－英、汉 Ⅳ. ①R473

中国版本图书馆 CIP 数据核字（2021）第 242321 号

人卫智网　www.ipmph.com　医学教育、学术、考试、健康，
　　　　　　　　　　　　　　购书智慧智能综合服务平台
人卫官网　www.pmph.com　人卫官方资讯发布平台

老年护理学（双语）

Laonian Hulixue (Shuangyu)

第 2 版

主　　编：郭桂芳　黄　金
出版发行：人民卫生出版社（中继线 010-59780011）
地　　址：北京市朝阳区潘家园南里 19 号
邮　　编：100021
E - mail：pmph @ pmph.com
购书热线：010-59787592　010-59787584　010-65264830
印　　刷：三河市宏达印刷有限公司（胜利）
经　　销：新华书店
开　　本：850×1168　1/16　印张：37
字　　数：900 千字
版　　次：2012 年 8 月第 1 版　　2022 年 8 月第 2 版
印　　次：2022 年 9 月第 1 次印刷
标准书号：ISBN 978-7-117-32534-9
定　　价：118.00 元

打击盗版举报电话：010-59787491　E-mail：WQ @ pmph.com
质量问题联系电话：010-59787234　E-mail：zhiliang @ pmph.com

国家卫生和计划生育委员会"十三五"规划教材
全国高等学校本科护理学类专业规划教材

第六轮修订说明

为了在"十三五"期间，持续深化医药卫生体制改革，贯彻落实《"健康中国2030"规划纲要》，全面践行《全国护理事业发展规划（2016—2020年）》，顺应全国高等护理学类专业教育发展与改革的需要，培养能够满足人民群众多样化、多层次健康需求的护理人才。在对第五轮教材进行全面、充分调研的基础上，在国家卫生和计划生育委员会领导下，经第三届全国高等学校护理学专业教材评审委员会的审议和规划，人民卫生出版社于2016年1月进行了全国高等学校护理学类专业教材评审委员会的换届工作，同时启动全国高等学校本科护理学类专业第六轮规划教材的修订工作。

本轮教材修订得到全国百余所本科院校的积极响应和大力支持，在结合调研结果和我国护理学高等教育的特点及发展趋势的基础上，第四届全国高等学校护理学类专业教材建设指导委员会确定第六轮教材修订的指导思想为：坚持"规范化、精品化、创新化、国际化、数字化"战略，紧扣培养目标，遵循教学规律，围绕提升学生能力，创新编写模式，体现专业特色；构筑学习平台，丰富教学资源，打造一流的、核心的、经典的具有国际影响力的护理学本科教材体系。

第六轮教材的编写原则为：

1. 明确目标性与系统性 本套教材的编写要求定位准确，符合本科教育特点与规律，满足护理学类专业本科学生的培养目标。注重多学科内容的有机融合，减少内容交叉重复，避免某些内容疏漏。在保证单本教材知识完整性的基础上，兼顾各教材之间有序衔接，有机联系，使全套教材整体优化，具有良好的系统性。

2. 坚持科学性与专业性 本套教材编写应坚持"三基五性"的原则，教材编写内容科学、准确，名称、术语规范，体例、体系具有逻辑性。教材须符合护理学专业思想，具有鲜明的护理学专业特色，满足护理学专业学生的教学要求。同时继续加强对学生人文素质的培养。

3. 兼具传承性与创新性 本套教材主要是修订，是在传承上一轮教材优点的基础上，结合上一轮教材调研的反馈意见，进行修改及完善，而不是对原教材进行彻底推翻，以保证教材的生命力和教学活动的延续性。教材编写中根据本学科和相关学科的发展，补充更新学科理论与实践发展的新成果，以使经典教材的传统性和精品教材的时代性完美结合。

4. **体现多元性与统一性**　为适应全国二百余所开办本科护理教育院校的多样化教学需要，本套教材在遵循本科教育基本标准的基础上，既包括有经典的临床学科体系教材，也有生命周期体系教材、中医特色课程教材和双语教材，以供各院校根据自身教学模式的特点选用。本套教材在编写过程中，一方面，扩大了参编院校范围，使教材编写团队更具多元性的特点；另一方面，明确要求，审慎把关，力求各章内容详略一致，整书编写风格统一。

5. **注重理论性与实践性**　本套教材在强化理论知识的同时注重对实践应用的思考，通过教材中的思考题、网络增值服务中的练习题，以及引入案例与问题的教材编写形式等，努力构建理论与实践联系的桥梁，以利于培养学生应用知识、分析问题、解决问题的能力。

全套教材采取新型编写模式，借助扫描二维码形式，帮助教材使用者在移动终端共享与教材配套的优质数字资源，实现纸媒教材与富媒体资源的融合。

全套教材共 50 种，于 2017 年 7 月前由人民卫生出版社出版，供各院校本科护理学类专业使用。

人民卫生出版社

2017 年 5 月

获取图书网络增值服务的步骤说明

❶ —— 扫描封底圆形图标中的二维码，登录图书增值服务激活平台。

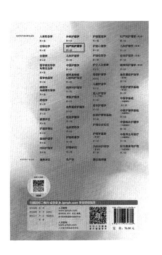

❷ —— 刮开并输入激活码，激活增值服务。

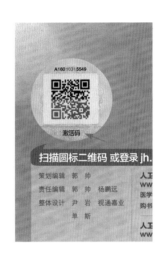

❸ —— 下载"人卫图书增值"客户端。

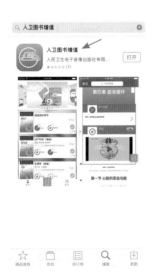

❹ —— 使用客户端"扫码"功能，扫描图书中二维码即可快速查看网络增值服务内容。

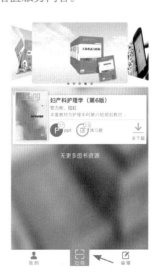

国家卫生和计划生育委员会"十三五"规划教材

全国高等学校本科护理学类专业规划教材

第六轮教材目录

1. 本科护理学类专业教材目录

序号	教材	版次	主审	主编	副主编
1	人体形态学	第4版		周瑞祥 杨桂姣	王海杰 郝立宏 周劲松
2	生物化学	第4版		高国全	解 军 方定志 刘 彬
3	生理学	第4版		唐四元	曲丽辉 张翠英 邢德刚
4	医学微生物学与寄生虫学	第4版		黄 敏 吴松泉	廖 力 王海河
5	医学免疫学	第4版	安云庆	司传平	任云青 王 炜 张 艳 胡 洁
6	病理学与病理生理学	第4版		步 宏	王 雯 李连宏
7	药理学	第4版		董 志	弥 曼 陶 剑 王金红
8	预防医学	第4版		凌文华 许能锋	袁 晶 龙鼎新 宋爱芹
9	健康评估	第4版	吕探云	孙玉梅 张立力	朱大乔 施齐芳 张彩虹 陈利群
10	护理学导论	第4版		李小妹 冯先琼	王爱敏 隋树杰
11	基础护理学	第6版		李小寒 尚少梅	王春梅 郑一宁 丁亚萍 吕冬梅
12	内科护理学	第6版		尤黎明 吴 瑛	孙国珍 王君俏 袁 丽 胡 荣
13	外科护理学	第6版		李乐之 路 潜	张美芬 汪 晖 李惠萍 许 勤
14	妇产科护理学	第6版	郑修霞	安力彬 陆 虹	顾 炜 丁 焱 罗碧如
15	儿科护理学	第6版		崔 焱 仰曙芬	张玉侠 刘晓丹 林素兰
16	中医护理学	第4版		孙秋华	段亚平 李明今 陆静波
17	眼耳鼻咽喉口腔科护理学	第4版		席淑新 赵佛容	肖惠明 李秀娥
18	精神科护理学	第4版		刘哲宁 杨芳宇	许冬梅 贾守梅
19	康复护理学	第4版		燕铁斌 尹安春	鲍秀芹 马素慧
20	急危重症护理学	第4版		张 波 桂 莉	金静芬 李文涛 黄素芳
21	社区护理学	第4版		李春玉 姜丽萍	陈长香
22	临床营养学	第4版	张爱珍	周 芸	胡 雯 赵雅宁
23	护理教育学	第4版		姜安丽 段志光	范秀珍 张 艳
24	护理研究	第5版		胡 雁 王志稳	刘均娥 颜巧元

序号	教材	版次	主审	主编		副主编			
25	护理管理学	第4版	李继平	吴欣娟	王艳梅	翟惠敏	张俊娥		
26	护理心理学	第4版		杨艳杰	曹枫林	冯正直	周 英		
27	护理伦理学	第2版		姜小鹰	刘俊荣	韩 琳	范宇莹		
28	护士人文修养	第2版		史瑞芬	刘义兰	刘桂瑛	王继红		
29	母婴护理学	第3版		王玉琼	莫洁玲	崔仁善	罗 阳		
30	儿童护理学	第3版		范 玲		崔文香	陈 华	张 瑛	
31	成人护理学（上、下册）	第3版		郭爱敏	周兰姝	王艳玲	陈 红	何朝珠	牟绍玉
32	老年护理学	第4版		化前珍	胡秀英	肖惠敏	张 静		
33	新编护理学基础	第3版		姜安丽	钱晓路	曹梅娟	王克芳	郭瑜洁	李春卉
34	护理综合实训	第1版		李映兰	王爱平	李玉红	蓝宇涛	高 睿	靳永萍
35	护理学基础（双语）	第2版	姜安丽	王红红	沈 洁	陈晓莉	尼春萍	吕爱莉	周 洁
36	内外科护理学（双语）	第2版	刘华平 李 峥	李 津	张静平	李 卡	李素云	史铁英	张 清
37	妇产科护理学（双语）	第2版		张银萍	单伟颖	张 静	周英凤	谢日华	
38	儿科护理学（双语）	第2版	胡 雁	蒋文慧	赵秀芳	高 燕	张 莹	蒋小平	
39	老年护理学（双语）	第2版		郭桂芳	黄 金	谷岩梅	郭 宏		
40	精神科护理学（双语）	第2版		雷 慧	李小麟	杨 敏	王再超	王小琴	
41	急危重症护理学（双语）	第2版		钟清玲	许 虹	关 青	曹宝花		
42	中医护理学基础（双语）	第2版		郝玉芳	王诗源	杨 柳	王春艳	徐冬英	
43	中医学基础（中医特色）	第2版		陈莉军	刘兴山	高 静	裴秀月	韩新荣	
44	中医护理学基础（中医特色）	第2版		陈佩仪		王俊杰	杨晓玮	郑方遒	
45	中医临床护理学（中医特色）	第2版		徐桂华	张先庚	于春光	张雅丽	闫 力	马秋平
46	中医养生与食疗（中医特色）	第2版		于 睿	姚 新	聂 宏	宋 阳		
47	针灸推拿与护理（中医特色）	第2版		刘明军		卢咏梅	董 博		

2. 本科助产学专业教材目录

序号	教材	版次	主审	主编		副主编		
1	健康评估	第1版		罗碧如	李 宁	王 跃	邹海欧	李 玲
2	助产学	第1版	杨慧霞	余艳红	陈 叙	丁 焱	侯 睿	顾 炜
3	围生期保健	第1版		夏海鸥	徐鑫芬	蔡文智	张银萍	

刘华平	‣	北京协和医学院护理学院
陆　虹	‣	北京大学护理学院
孙宏玉	‣	北京大学护理学院
孙秋华	‣	浙江中医药大学
吴　瑛	‣	首都医科大学护理学院
徐桂华	‣	南京中医药大学
殷　磊	‣	澳门理工学院
章雅青	‣	上海交通大学护理学院
赵　岳	‣	天津医科大学护理学院

常务委员

（按姓氏拼音排序）

曹枫林	‣	山东大学护理学院
郭桂芳	‣	北京大学护理学院
郝玉芳	‣	北京中医药大学护理学院
罗碧如	‣	四川大学华西护理学院
尚少梅	‣	北京大学护理学院
唐四元	‣	中南大学湘雅护理学院
夏海鸥	‣	复旦大学护理学院
熊云新	‣	广西广播电视大学
仰曙芬	‣	哈尔滨医科大学护理学院
于　睿	‣	辽宁中医药大学护理学院
张先庚	‣	成都中医药大学护理学院

第四届全国高等学校护理学类专业教材建设指导委员会

本科教材评审委员会名单

指导主委	尤黎明	‣	中山大学护理学院
主任委员	李小妹	‣	西安交通大学护理学院
	崔焱	‣	南京医科大学护理学院
副主任委员	郭桂芳	‣	北京大学护理学院
	吴瑛	‣	首都医科大学护理学院
	唐四元	‣	中南大学湘雅护理学院
委 员	陈垦	‣	广东药科大学护理学院
（按姓氏拼音排序）	陈京立	‣	北京协和医学院护理学院
	范玲	‣	中国医科大学附属盛京医院
	付菊芳	‣	第四军医大学西京医院
	桂莉	‣	第二军医大学护理学院
	何朝珠	‣	南昌大学护理学院
	何桂娟	‣	浙江中医药大学护理学院
	胡荣	‣	福建医科大学护理学院
	江智霞	‣	遵义医学院护理学院
	李伟	‣	潍坊医学院护理学院
	李春玉	‣	延边大学护理学院
	李惠玲	‣	苏州大学护理学院

李惠萍	‣	安徽医科大学护理学院
廖　力	‣	南华大学护理学院
林素兰	‣	新疆医科大学护理学院
刘桂瑛	‣	广西医科大学护理学院
刘义兰	‣	华中科技大学同济医学院附属协和医院
刘志燕	‣	贵州医科大学护理学院
龙　霖	‣	川北医学院护理学院
卢东民	‣	湖州师范学院
牟绍玉	‣	重庆医科大学护理学院
任海燕	‣	内蒙古医科大学护理学院
隋树杰	‣	哈尔滨医科大学护理学院
王　军	‣	山西医科大学汾阳学院
王　强	‣	河南大学护理学院
王爱敏	‣	青岛大学护理学院
王春梅	‣	天津医科大学护理学院
王君俏	‣	复旦大学护理学院
王克芳	‣	山东大学护理学院
王绍锋	‣	九江学院护理学院
王玉琼	‣	成都市妇女儿童中心医院
徐月清	‣	河北大学护理学院
许　虹	‣	杭州师范大学护理学院
许燕玲	‣	上海市第六人民医院
杨立群	‣	齐齐哈尔医学院护理学院
张　瑛	‣	长治医学院护理学院
张彩虹	‣	海南医学院国际护理学院
张会君	‣	锦州医科大学护理学院
张美芬	‣	中山大学护理学院
章泾萍	‣	皖南医学院护理学院
赵佛容	‣	四川大学华西口腔医院
赵红佳	‣	福建中医药大学护理学院
周　英	‣	广州医科大学护理学院

秘　书	王　婧	‣	西安交通大学护理学院
	丁亚萍	‣	南京医科大学护理学院

数字教材评审委员会名单

指导主委	段志光	‣	山西医科大学

主任委员	孙宏玉	‣	北京大学护理学院
	章雅青	‣	上海交通大学护理学院

副主任委员	仰曙芬	‣	哈尔滨医科大学护理学院
	熊云新	‣	广西广播电视大学
	曹枫林	‣	山东大学护理学院

委　员 （按姓氏拼音排序）	柏亚妹	‣	南京中医药大学护理学院
	陈　嘉	‣	中南大学湘雅护理学院
	陈　燕	‣	湖南中医药大学护理学院
	陈晓莉	‣	武汉大学 HOPE 护理学院
	郭爱敏	‣	北京协和医学院护理学院
	洪芳芳	‣	桂林医学院护理学院
	鞠　梅	‣	西南医科大学护理学院
	蓝宇涛	‣	广东药科大学护理学院
	李　峰	‣	吉林大学护理学院
	李　强	‣	齐齐哈尔医学院护理学院
	李彩福	‣	延边大学护理学院
	李春卉	‣	吉林医药学院

李芳芳 ‣ 第二军医大学护理学院

李文涛 ‣ 大连大学护理学院

李小萍 ‣ 四川大学护理学院

孟庆慧 ‣ 潍坊医学院护理学院

商临萍 ‣ 山西医科大学护理学院

史铁英 ‣ 大连医科大学附属第一医院

万丽红 ‣ 中山大学护理学院

王桂云 ‣ 山东协和学院护理学院

谢　晖 ‣ 蚌埠医学院护理学系

许　勤 ‣ 南京医科大学护理学院

颜巧元 ‣ 华中科技大学护理学院

张　艳 ‣ 郑州大学护理学院

周　洁 ‣ 上海中医药大学护理学院

庄嘉元 ‣ 福建医科大学护理学院

秘　　书

杨　萍 ‣ 北京大学护理学院

范宇莹 ‣ 哈尔滨医科大学护理学院

吴觉敏 ‣ 上海交通大学护理学院

数字内容编者名单

主　编　郭桂芳　黄　金

副主编　谷岩梅　郭　宏

编　者　（按姓氏笔画排序）

于　放	▸	（美国亚利桑那州立大学埃德森护理和创新学院）
刘　宇	▸	（中国医科大学护理学院）
刘红霞	▸	（北京中医药大学护理学院）
吴丽华	▸	（英国哈德斯菲尔德大学护理助产学院）
谷岩梅	▸	（河北中医学院护理学院）
张　静	▸	（中国人民解放军海军军医大学护理学院）
陈　茜	▸	（四川大学华西护理学院 / 四川大学华西医院）
胡　洁	▸	（美国俄亥俄州立大学护理学院）
晋溶辰	▸	（湖南中医药大学护理学院）
郭　宏	▸	（沈阳医学院护理学院）
郭桂芳	▸	（北京大学护理学院）
黄　金	▸	（中南大学湘雅二医院）
奚　兴	▸	（江苏卫生健康职业学院）
梁　涛	▸	（北京协和医学院护理学院）
曾　慧	▸	（中南大学湘雅护理学院）
穆晓云	▸	（中国医科大学护理学院）
Deborah Lekan	▸	（美国北卡罗来纳大学格林斯伯勒分校护理学院）
Linda Phillips	▸	（美国加州大学洛杉矶分校护理学院）

编写秘书　晋溶辰　奚　兴

主编简介

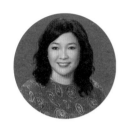

郭桂芳

郭桂芳，博士，现任北京大学护理学院教授，博士生导师，美国护理科学院院士；任中国老年学和老年医学学会常务理事兼护理和照护分会主任委员，中国心理卫生协会常委兼护理心理专委会主任委员，国内外多家护理专业杂志的编委会委员；2007年在亚利桑那大学获护理学博士学位；2007～2010年在美国加州大学洛杉矶分校护理学院做博士后研究员和老年护理研究项目主任，2011～2016年被美国宾夕法尼亚大学护理学院聘为兼职教授，2014～2016年被英国伦敦国王学院南丁格尔护理学院聘为国际顾问委员会委员；曾任中华护理学会第23届理事会副理事长，1990～2000年任中国国家艾滋病专家委员会委员，1992～2001年间担任世界卫生组织护理专家顾问委员会委员，2010～2015年任北京大学护理学院院长，全国高等学校护理学类专业本科教材评审委员会副主任委员；2005年获得美国老龄学会杰出研究生科研论文奖，2007年和2011年获亚利桑那大学护理学院杰出校友奖和全球成就奖，2011年获美国宾夕法尼亚大学全球基金杰出国际学者奖。主编的《老年护理学（双语）》教材获2013年北京高等教育精品教材奖。主要研究方向涉及老年人群的健康促进和功能维护，重点关注老年人衰弱的护理理论和干预的研究。

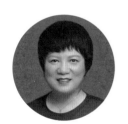

黄　金

黄金，主任护师，教授，医学博士，硕士导师，中南大学湘雅二医院临床护理学教研室主任。美国耶鲁大学访问学者，先后赴美国、荷兰、比利时、丹麦、西班牙、泰国等地学习和交流。其主编教材及著作17部、副主编6部及参编22部；主持国家自然科学基金面上、省重点研发、其他省级及国际合作科研课题20项；发表论文170余篇，其中SCI论文15篇；曾获湖南省自然科学优秀学术论文奖及湖南省护理学会优秀护理专著奖多项。主要研究方向为老年护理学及慢性疾病管理，目前主要承担内科护理学、老年护理学（双语）、高级临床护理实践、护理管理学等主干课程教学，其中老年护理学（双语）获批"中南大学精品示范课堂"；兼任中国老年学和老年医学会护理与照护分会常委、中国研究型医院学会医疗质量管理与评价专业委员会委员、中华护理学会糖尿病专业委员会委员、湖南省护理学会糖尿病专业委员会主任委员及湖南省糖尿病专科护士培训负责人等职；兼任《中华护理教育杂志》《护理学》《当代护士》等期刊编委。

副主编简介

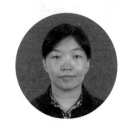

谷岩梅

谷岩梅，教授，硕士研究生导师，多伦多大学访问学者，河北中医学院护理学院副院长。1996年毕业于上海第二军医大学护理系，获得医学学士学位；2002年毕业于解放军军医进修学院（解放军301医院），获得重症监护专业硕士学位。她兼任中国红十字会培训师培训讲师（ToT），世界中医药学会联合会翻译委员会常务理事，世界中医药学会联合会护理专委会委员、河北省老年医学会常务理事。

从事护理专业30年，护理学专业负责人，护理学导论、护理学研究方法课程负责人。主要研究方向为老年人慢性疾病管理和高等护理教育。从业以来发表专业论文80余篇，其中SCI 4篇；主编《护理专业英语》，参编《老年护理学》等教材10余部；主持省级及以上课题6项，获得河北医学科技奖一等奖1项、二等奖1项；获得河北省教学成果奖一等奖1项。

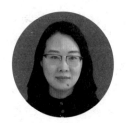

郭　宏

郭宏，三级教授，沈阳医学院护理学院院长，沈阳市拔尖人才、辽宁省高校教学名师、沈阳市名教师、沈阳市优秀教师。1991年毕业于中国医科大学护理学专业，获医学学士学位，同年任职中国医科大学附属第二临床学院从事临床护理、临床教学、护理管理等工作。1999年、2009年于泰国清迈大学分别获得护理学硕士及博士学位，主要研究方向为护理教育学及老年护理学。其目前主要讲授护理学导论及老年护理学课程，其中老年护理学课程被评为辽宁省精品资源共享课程；主编、副主编规划教材10余部，主持或参与省部级、市级科研及教改课题20余项，发表科研及教改论文40余篇；任全国医学高职高专教育研究会护理教育分会委员、东北三省护理教育学会常务理事、辽宁省高等教育护理专业教学指导委员会副主任委员等社会职务。

前　言

人口老龄化已成为全世界共同面临的人口发展趋势。老年护理学是在健康服务体系面临老龄化社会带来的巨大挑战的环境下应运而生的一门学科。编写本教材对我国实施健康中国战略、积极应对人口老龄化具有重要意义。《老年护理学》双语教材第 2 版是本科生教学的规划教材，亦可用作研究生层次教学的参考教材。编者期望本教材能够帮助学生和临床护理人员增强对于老年护理学的认识，明确老年护理的原则和要点，了解国际老年护理发展动态，提高对老年护理领域中常见问题的理解和有效护理方法的选择，为正在发展中的老年护理专业学科建设和课程建设提供支持和参考。

本教材针对老年护理涉及面广的特点，从老年人带病生存、功能状态、精神健康以及社会经济体制、医疗体制、养老政策法规保障、社会文化和伦理对老年护理的影响等角度探讨老年护理中的重点问题。全书共 21 章，前 8 章为老年护理学基础，主要介绍老年护理过程中的基础知识和共性问题；后 13 章为老年护理学实践，主要介绍临床常见的护理问题。

本教材关注当今社会高龄老人的特有护理需求，基于世界卫生组织关注老年人的功能维护的理念，以老年人功能维护、失能风险防控等为重点，突出老年人群护理的重要知识点和实用性，重点介绍对临床、社区、居家及长期照顾机构中的老年人护理有指导意义的概念、理论和技能；除介绍患病老年人的护理之外，亦包括健康老年人的护理内容。教材内容的可操作性强，如老年人功能评估方法、针对痴呆老人的护理措施等。另外，本教材还为从事临床实践、护理教学和研究的同行们提供老年学理论和近年来老年护理新概念等前沿知识及其应用的介绍。本书在内容组织上尽量减少与内外科护理学、社区护理学及基础护理学重复的内容，适当引入国际上老年护理经验和养老模式介绍。

本教材编写人员均为活跃在国内外老年护理领域的学者和临床护理专家，他们有较为丰富的临床或社区老年护理经验，并有各自擅长的老年护理研究领域。本教材第 1 版在 2013 年被北京市教育委员会评为北京高等教育精品教材。由于老年护理学涉及诸多的医学护理领域，因此在编写过程中难免有疏漏和错误之处，敬请广大师生和读者不吝赐教和指正。本书在编写过程中得到编委的大力帮助，在此表示诚挚的谢意。

郭桂芳　黄　金

2022 年 2 月

目 录

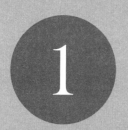

Chapter 1 Introduction of Gerontological Nursing

第一章　老年护理学绪论

Learning Objectives

On completion of this chapter, the reader will be able to:

- Define aging related concepts;

- Discuss challenges of population aging to the healthcare system and nursing;
- Describe the development of gerontological nursing in the context of population aging;
- Discuss basic features of gerontological nursing in relation to the characteristics of aging population;
- Identify general goals and principles of gerontological nursing;
- Discuss recommended competency requirements for baccalaureate-educated nursing graduates.

学习目标

学完本章节，应完成以下目标：

- 解释老龄化相关的概念；

- 讨论人口老龄化对医疗体系和护理的挑战；

- 描述人口老龄化背景下老年护理学的发展趋势；

- 讨论老年护理学的基本特征；

- 确定老年护理的总体目标和原则；

- 讨论本科学历护理毕业生在老年护理中的基本能力要求。

"Good health adds life to years" was the major theme of the WHO World Health Day 2012, which emphasized the importance of development and maintenance of optimal mental, social and physical well-being and function of older adults. Population aging is a global phenomenon which brings both challenges and opportunities to our society. Healthy aging has become a major concern to the elderly, their families and the society. To help the elderly to maintain their ideal health status and to postpone the onset of disease or dependency, it is very important that health professionals in all settings should be familiar with geriatric health problems and demonstrate proficiency in providing care to ensure optimal health outcomes for the elderly. It is the internationally recognized goal of action.

Gerontological nursing has emerged to meet these challenges and needs. This chapter discusses challenges of population aging to the healthcare and nursing systems and provides an overview of gerontological nursing.

"老龄化与健康：健康有益长寿"是 2012 年世界卫生日的主题。这个主题强调了发展和保持老年人身体、心理、社会适应及功能完好状态的重要性。人口老龄化是人类社会共同面临的问题，为我们带来了机遇与挑战。"健康老龄化"已成为现代社会关注的要点。为了帮助老年人保持理想的健康状态，推迟疾病或依赖的发生，所有卫生专业人员都应熟悉老年人的健康问题，并熟练地提供护理，以确保老年人的最佳健康结果。这是国际社会普遍认同的行动目标。

医疗卫生系统正面临老龄化社会带来的巨大挑战，老年护理学应运而生，该专业旨在为提高老年人的生命质量做出积极贡献。本章将介绍人口老龄化与社会发展给护理学发展带来的机遇和挑战，以及老年护理学的发展状况、老年护理的基本目标和原则，老年护理专业人员的核心能力要求和发展趋势等。

Section 1　Population Aging and Challenges to Healthcare System

Population aging is now a predominant demographic issue in almost all countries in the world. While global aging is viewed as the triumph of health care, social and economic advances, it also proposes a series challenges in many aspects of the global economic development, social stability, and health care.

第一节　人口老龄化对保健系统的挑战

人口老龄化对世界各国经济发展、社会稳定、医疗与卫生保障等诸多方面提出一系列严峻的挑战。除老年人自身的变化外，老年人的问题还涉及多种社会关系，比如老年人的亲属和社会上的其他团体和个人。老龄化社会的建设和政策制定所涉及的问题除了社会代际关系问题外，还有全社会的资源和利益分配，照顾负担等问题。

I. Aging Related Concepts

i. Different Definition of Age

Older adults' perceptions of age may be different from each other due to their different life experience, physical conditions and psychosocial status. Age is defined

一、人口老龄化的相关概念

（一）年龄

由于老年人的生活经历、身体状况和心理社会状况的不同，他们对年龄的感知可能会有所不同。在文献中，年龄有不同的定义，

in several ways in the literature. There are chronological age, biological age, psychological age, and social age. Chronological age represents actual number of years that a person has been alive, or real age. Biological age is inferred based on the developmental status of human physiology and anatomy. It indicates a person's body organizational structure and physical function, for example, loss of muscle strength and endurance, the loss of ability to resist diseases, and change in appearance; from biological perspective, aging is associated with the accumulation of a wide variety of molecular and cellular damage, and these changes lead to a gradual decrease in physiological reserves, an increased risk of many diseases and a general decline in the intrinsic capacity of the individual. Psychological age is used to indicate the level of psychological development. For example, how elder people feel and think about themselves. Social age related to people's interaction with the environment. For example, how elder people are treated and categorized by society, how they shift in roles and social positions, need to deal with the loss of close relationships.

ii. The Elderly / The Aged

There is no standard numerical criterion for older age. Many developed countries have accepted the chronological age of 65 as criterion of older age, while other countries or regions, most of them are developing countries, use the age of 60. Currently the United Nation agreed cutoff point is the age of 60 and above. China adopted this criterion and use the age of 60 referred the older population.

iii. Young-aged Elderly/Middle-aged Elderly/Advanced-aged Elderly

Population aging is the process of rising proportion of elderly population in total population. Aging society, according to the United Nation, refers to a place where people aged 65 and older account for more than 7% of the total population or the proportion of people aged 60 and overmakes up 10% or more.

iv. Population Aging and Aging Society

There are other categories of the elderly people in the literature. People who are in 60-69 year-old group are called the young-aged elderly, who are in 70−79 year-old group are called the middle-aged elderly, and people who are 80 years old and above are the real elderly, known as the oldest old.

包括实足年龄、生物学年龄、心理年龄、社会年龄。实足年龄是指一个人已经度过的年份，又称真实年龄。生物学年龄是根据正常人体生理学和解剖学的发育状态所推断出来的年龄，表明人体的组织结构和生理功能的实际状态。例如，肌肉力量和耐力的损失，失去抵抗疾病的能力，及在外貌上的变化等。从生物学角度看，衰老与多种分子和细胞损伤的积累有关，这些变化导致生理储备逐渐减少，许多疾病的风险增加，个体内在能力下降。心理学年龄用来表示心理发展的水平。例如，一个人对自己年龄的感知。社会学年龄是指一个人在其所处的环境中，被其他人在心理上所认为处在的年龄状态。例如，老年人如何被社会对待和分类，他们如何在角色和社会地位上转变，面临失去亲密关系等问题。

（二）老年人

目前对于老年人的年龄还没有标准的定义。在许多发达国家将实足年龄 65 岁及以上定义为老年；而在其他国家和地区，以发展中国家居多，将实足年龄 60 岁及以上定义为老年。中国将 60 岁及以上的人群定义为老年人。

（三）人口老龄化和老龄社会

人口老龄化是指老年人口占总人口的比例不断上升的过程。按照联合国公布的年龄构成标准，当 65 岁以上老年人口与总人口的比例上升到 7% 以上，或 60 岁以上人口占人口总数 10% 以上称为老年型人口，达到这个标准的社会称之为老龄化社会。

（四）年轻老年人 / 中年老年人 / 高龄老年人

现在，60 岁和 65 岁都是国际通用的老年划分标准。中华医学会老年分会于 1982 年建议：中国 60 岁以上为老年人。一些专家将 60～69 岁称为年轻老人，70～79 岁称为中年老人，80 岁以上为真正的老年人，称高龄老人。

v. Healthy Aging

Healthy aging is a process to promote well-being of the elderly through a series of positive measures to reduce the risks of disease and related disabilities, and assist the elderly function well physically and mentally, and be actively engaged in life. The term of "healthy aging" first appeared at the World Health Assembly in May 1987. In 1990, at the World Assembly on Aging in Copenhagen, the World Health Organization proposed "healthy aging" as a developmental strategy in response to the global population aging. This proposal significantly influenced health and quality of life of the elderly and the development of society as well. Promoting healthy aging is not only a great significance to the healthy development of the national health in China, but also has a far-reaching impact on the social development.

II. Perception of Aging and Health

Developing a comprehensive response to population aging is a challenge because many common perceptions and assumptions about older people are based on outdated stereotypes. Life course has been framed as the stages like early childhood, studenthood, working age and retirement. It is assumed when people live longer their extra years are simply added to the end of life and allow a more extended retirement. Ageist stereotype views older people as dependent, a burden, or a drain on economies.

Older age does not imply dependence. More and more elderly people still contribute to family and society. They rethink their frame of lives, involve in further education, and shift in new career or pursuing a long neglected passion. To optimize the opportunity from longevity, health plays a key role. Despite of presences of frailty and co-mobidity of acute or chronic health conditions, the impacts of these conditions are having on an elderly person's functioning and well-being are the key factors. Genetic inheritance, physical and social environment we inhabit affects health directly or through barriers or incentives that influence our opportunities, decisions and behaviors toward a healthy aging.

（五）健康老龄化

健康老龄化指在实足年龄增长的同时，通过一系列积极的措施来推迟生物性老化（身体功能的受损）和社会性老化（社会参与的活力退化）。"健康老龄化"的概念最早出现于 1987 年 5 月召开的世界卫生大会，1990 年世界卫生组织在哥本哈根世界老龄大会上把"健康老龄化"作为应对人口老龄化的一项发展战略。健康老龄化不仅仅保证老年人的健康，而且更注重生活质量和价值的提高。健康老龄化观点的提出不仅对我国全民健康的发展具有重要意义，同时对社会的发展也具有深远影响。

二、对人口老龄化和健康的认识

全面认识人口老龄化是一个挑战，因为许多关于老年人的看法和假设都是基于过时的定型观念。通常人生被定义为几个特定的阶段，如幼儿期、学生期、工作期和退休期。当人们寿命更长时，往往被认为他们的额外时间只是添加到生命的终点，及更长的退休期。传统观念中对老年人刻板印象认为老年人是依赖或负担，是经济消耗。

事实上，老年并不意味着依赖。越来越多的老年人仍然对家庭和社会做出着贡献。他们重新思考生活安排，参与继续教育，寻求新的职业或追求长期被忽视的爱好。健康在达到长寿的目标过程中发挥着关键作用。在老年阶段常伴随急性或慢性健康问题和衰弱，这些健康问题对老年人的功能和健康的影响是更为关键的因素。遗传、物理和社会环境直接地影响老年人的健康状态，成为我们走向健康老龄化过程中的机会、决定和行为产生影响的障碍或激励因素。

Box 1-1 Global Strategy and Action Plan on Ageing and Health 2016—2020

On May 26 in 2016, the Global Strategy and Action Plan on Ageing and Health 2016—2020 were adapted by the member states at the 69th World Health Assembly. The Strategy outlines a set of goals and strategic objectives to move towards a decade of Healthy Ageing beginning in 2020, and an action plan to achieve those goals.

According to WHO report, healthy aging is the process of developing and maintaining the functional ability that enables wellbeing in older age. Functional ability has two important parts, intrinsic capacity and environment. Intrinsic capacity is referred as all the physical and mental capacities that an individual can draw on at any point in time. Environment we inhabit and interact provide a range of resources or barriers that will ultimately decide whether people with a given level of capacity can do things they feel important. The goal of healthy aging is to maximize functional ability. Although people's intrinsic capacity or functional capacity tend to decline with increasing of age, having access to affordable health care and supportive environment can optimize their capacity. According to WHO framework (figure 1-1), there are three subpopulations of the elderly including elderly with high and stable capacity, elderly with declining capacity and elderly with significant losses of capacity. To enhance elder's functional capacity, four areas of actions are needed: a. aligning health systems to the aging population they now serve by addressing multidimensional demands of older age in an integrated way, ensuring access to services and comprehensive assessment, focusing on intrinsic capacity building, developing home and community care services; b. developing systems of long-term care by establishing the foundations necessary for a system of long-term care, building and maintaining a sustainable and appropriately trained workforce, and ensuring the quality of long term care; c. creating age-friendly environments that facilitate their continuing development of personality, to contribute to their communities and to retain their autonomy and health, including transportation, housing, labor, social protection, information, communication, and health care services; d. improving measurement, monitoring and understanding of the health status and needs of older populations and how well their needs are being met.

Box 1-1 2016—2020 年老龄化和健康全球战略和行动计划

2016 年 5 月 26 日，世界卫生组织在第 69 届世界卫生大会上通过了"2016—2020 年老龄化和健康全球战略和行动计划"。该战略概述了一系列目标和战略目标，以便从 2020 年开始实现"健康老龄化"，并制订了实现这些目标的行动计划。

世界卫生组织的报告中指出健康老龄化是发展和维持老年人健康功能的过程。人体健康功能有两个重要的部分，内在的能力和环境。内在能力是指个人在任何时间点可以利用的所有身体和精神上的能力。我们所居住和相互作用的环境为我们提供了一系列资源或屏障，且最终决定我们是否可以做我们认为重要的事情。健康老龄化的目标是促进综合能力。虽然人们的内在能力或功能有随着年龄的增长而下降的趋势，但是可获得的医疗保健和支持性的环境可以提高人的能力。根据世界卫生组织框架（图 1-1），老年人分为三个类型：具有稳定且较高能力的老年人，能力下降的老年人和能力显著丧失的老年人。提高老年人的功能可以从以下四个领域着手：①通过综合处理老年人的多层面需求，使卫生系统与他们现在服务的老年人相一致，确保获得服务和综合评估，促进能力提升，发展家庭和社区护理服务；②通过建立长期护理制度，培养和保持可持续和适当的受过培训的护理人力资源，确保长期护理的质量，建立长期护理制度；③创建促进积极老龄化的适老环境以利于他们维持个体化，支持他们为社区做出贡献，并保持其自主能力和健康，包括交通、住房、劳动、社会保护、信息、通信和保健服务；④改善对老年人口的健康状况的评估、了解并监测其需求及需求的满足。

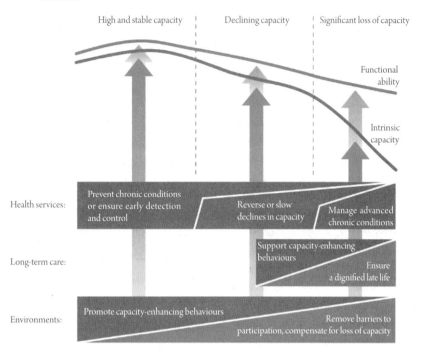

A public-health framework for *Healthy Ageing*: opportunities for public-health action across the life course

Figure 1-1   WHO a public health framework for healthy aging

III. Developmental Trends of Population Aging

The aging of the world's population is related to the continuous rising life expectancy (longevity) and low fertility. With the continuous improvement of medical technology and living conditions, the life span of human beings is prolonged, which leads to the increase of the number of elderly people. Almost all countries in the world have gradually begun to enter the aging society. The speed of global aging is compelling.

i. Development Trend of World Population Aging

The proportion and absolute number of elderly people in the world are increasing dramatically. About 9% of the world's population is over 65. It is expected that by 2050, the global population aged 60 and over will increase from 900 million to 2 billion, the proportion of the total aging population will increase from 12% to 22%, and people aged 60 and above will outnumber 10-to 24-year-old. The oldest old population will be a fast growing group. The population aged 80 and over will increase from 125 million to 434 million, 80% of elder people will be living in the lower middle income countries. Although population aging began in high-income countries, but

三、人口老龄化的发展趋势

世界人口的老龄化与人类寿命不断延长、生育率持续较低有关。不断进步的医学技术、持续改善的生活条件使人类寿命延长，进而导致老年人口数量增长。几乎世界上所有国家都已经逐渐进入老龄化社会。全球老龄化速度快得惊人。

（一）世界人口老龄化发展趋势

世界老年人口的比例和绝对数量正在急剧增加。世界上 65 岁以上的老年人超过总人口的 9%。预计到 2050 年，全球 60 岁及以上的人口将由 9 亿增长到 20 亿，占总人口的比例将从 12% 增长到 22%，60 岁及以上人口数将超过 10 至 24 岁人口数。高龄老人将是一个快速增长的群体。80 岁及以上的人口数将由 1.25 亿增长到 4.34 亿；而且，80% 的老年人将生活在中低收入水平国家。虽然人口老龄化开始于高收入水平国家，但现在经历最大变化的

now the biggest change is in the lower income countries. Although the level of medical technology and living conditions have been greatly improved in recent years, the health of elder people has not been significantly improved.

ii. Current Situation and Development Trend of Population Aging in China

China entered the aging society in 1999, and the aging process is accelerating. As of the end of 2019, China's average life expectancy has reached 76.34 years; The results of the seventh national census show that the population aged 60 and over is 260 million, accounting for 18.70% of the total population in China, including 190 million people aged 65 and over, accounting for 73.08% of the elderly population, and 35.8 million people aged 80 and over, accounting for 13.56% of the elderly population. The dependency ratio of the elderly population in China is 19.70%. According to the prediction of *The National Strategic Research on Population Aging*, China's elderly population will increase by an average of 10 million per year, about 54 million during "the 14th Five Year Plan" period, and the total elderly population will exceed 300 million by 2025. It is estimated that by 2050, China's elderly population will reach 438 million, the proportion of the elderly population will reach 1/3, over the age of 80 will reach up to 108 million. This means that China will long remain the world's largest elderly population in this century.

China's population aging process has its similarities with and differences to other countries. Unlike some economically developed countries where population aging took place gradually, population aging is more rapid in China and is occurring on a relatively larger population bases. Population aging process took decades to hundred years in Western countries. For example, it took 115 years in France, 85 years in Switzerland, 80 years in United Kingdom, and 60 years in the US. It took only 18 years in China. As a consequence of this accelerated aging, China has entered a premature stage of aging society. At present, there are 44 million elderly with partial or total disability in China, accounting for 16.7% of the elderly population. The fourth national survey on the living conditions of the elderly in urban and rural areas shows that there are a large number of poor and low-income seniors in China. This feature is described as aging ahead of industrialization, and "getting old before getting rich".

是中低收入水平国家。尽管医疗技术水平和生活条件比过去有很大提高，但是目前老年人的健康状况却并没有明显改善。

（二）中国人口老龄化现状和发展趋势

中国已于 1999 年进入老龄化社会，而且老龄化进程正在加快。截至 2019 年底，我国人均预期寿命已达 76.34 岁。第七次全国人口普查结果显示，60 岁及以上人口为 2.6 亿人，占全国总人口的 18.70%（其中，65 岁及以上人口为 1.9 亿人，占老年人口的 73.08%，80 岁及以上老年人口 3 580 万人，占老年人口的 13.56%）。全国老年人口抚养比为 19.70%。根据《国际上应对人口老龄化战略研究》的预测，我国老龄人口将以平均每年新增 1 000 万持续增长，在"十四五"期间新增约 5 400 万，到 2025 年老年人口总量将超过 3 亿。据估计，到 2050 年，中国老年人口将达 4.38 亿，老年人口比重将达 1/3，80 岁以上老人将达 1.08 亿。这意味着在 21 世纪中国将一直是拥有世界上最多老年人的国家。

中国人口老龄化的发展既有与经济发达国家类似的方面，也有不同的特点。我国人口老龄化速度明显快于经济发达国家，法国 60 岁以上人口比例从 10% 增长到 20% 经历了约 115 年的时间，瑞士 85 年，英国 80 年，美国 60 年，而中国仅仅 18 年的时间。此外，中国老龄化先于工业化，呈现出"未富先老"的特点，而且困难老人数量多。第四次中国城乡老年人生活状况抽样调查结果显示，我国贫困和低收入老年人口数量较多，失能、半失能老年人口数量较大，目前全国失能、半失能老年人约 4 400 万，占老年人口的 16.7%。

IV. Challenges of Population Aging

Aging issues are social issues involving multiple systems such as political and public policy, social economy, environment construction, community resources, and healthcare services. How elderly people are treated in a society reflects its social value and norms. In places with strong traditional influence, elder people are cared by family at home until they die; in other places, elder people are sent to nursing homes. Influenced by Confucianism, many Asian countries highly value filial piety, obedience and respect to elderly people. At the same time, ageism or age discrimination exists in this world. Social value, policy and image of elder people have direct effects on elder's personal beliefs in itself, their selection of action, and further influence their health and quality of life. So, gerontological nursing practice and studies should have a social perspective.

i. Increasing Needs for Gerontological Care

Although old age is not a disease and many elder people are leading to a well functional life, morbidity, mortality, and social problems rise rapidly among elder population, resulting in substantial strains on the health care system and social security nets. Many people exhibit some degree of frailty and chronic illness by age 75 and above. Non-communicable diseases (NCDs) such as heart disease, cancer and diabetes are problems typically encountered in the elder population in both rich and poor countries. The risk of dementia rises sharply with age. Many people aged 85 or older have some degree of cognitive decline. Society need to invest substantial resources to the care of the increasing elder population, especially gerontological care for the oldest, sickest, and most frail patients with multiple medical problems and fewer social supports.

ii. Increasing Needs for Long-term Care and Transitional Care

Many elder people lose their ability to live independently because of limited mobility, frailty or other physical or mental health problems. There are about 30 million elder people need different forms of long-term care in China. It is expected that the number of elder people with partial loss of self-care ability will reach 40 million. However, current elder care facilities are far from being

四、人口老龄化带来的挑战

老龄化问题同时也是社会问题，涉及国家政策、社会经济、环境建设、社区资源以及医疗卫生服务等。社会如何对待老年人反映了这个社会的价值和准则。在传统儒家思想的影响下，许多亚洲国家尊崇孝道，尊重并顺从长辈。在固守我国传统的家庭养老方式的一些地方，老年人在家中由亲人照料直至离世；而在其他地方，老年人则被送到养老院照顾。与此同时，虐待老年人的现象依旧存在。社会价值观、政策和对老年人的认识直接影响了老年人的自我认知和行为的选择，进而影响他们的健康和生活质量。因此，老年护理实践和研究也应该从社会的角度开展。

（一）老年护理需求增多

尽管老化本身不是疾病，很多老年人依旧功能健全，能过上功能良好的生活，但老年人的发病率、死亡率和社会问题迅速上升，导致医疗系统和社会保障系统承受巨大压力，最终导致了医疗卫生资源和社会保障资源的紧张。许多75岁及以上的老年人呈现出不同程度的衰弱和慢性疾病状态。无论在发达国家还是发展中国家，非传染性疾病，如心脏病、肿瘤、糖尿病在老年人群中发病率极高。另外，随着年龄的增长，痴呆的发病危险也显著增长。许多85岁及以上的老年人都有不同程度的认知下降。全社会投入了大量资源用于老年人的照护，特别是高龄、疾病、极度衰弱并伴有多个健康问题、缺乏社会支持的老年人群。

（二）长期照护和过渡性护理的需求增加

大量老年人由于行动受限、衰弱或其他躯体和精神疾病导致功能障碍，生活不能自理。我国大约有三千万的老年人需要不同形式的长期照护，预计今后存在不同程度自理缺陷的老年人将达到四千万。然而，现在的老年照护机构远远不能满足老龄社会的需求，

able to meet the need of society. The serious shortage of elder care facilities creates great challenges.

With the shrinking of family size and job related migration, many elder people live alone. Empty nest phenomenon becomes common in both urban and rural areas. Needs are rising for nursing home, community care, assisted living, residential care and long stays in hospitals, as well as transitional care between hospitals and home or long term care facilities.

iii. Increasing Needs for Protecting from Mistreatment

With the increased prevalence of disability and dementia among elderly people, there are increasing risks for mistreatment. Mistreatment includes many forms such as ignorance of elder people's basic needs, physical restraining, depriving dignity, and intentionally providing insufficient care. Mistreatment among elder people, especially those frail or cognitive impaired elderly, may result in serious physical injuries and psychological harm.

Section 2　Overview of Gerontological Nursing

The growing needs for gerontological nursing provide nurses with important roles in health promotion and disease prevention. No matter where they work, most nurses will have the opportunity to take care of elder adults in their career. It is important for all nurses to have a better understanding of gerontological nursing so they can actively participate in promotion of healthy aging.

Gerontological nursing is a nursing specialty which applies a body of knowledge and skills to elder adults to meet the unique bio-psycho-social and spiritual needs related to aging process. The theoretical basis of gerontological nursing lies on the existing nursing theories and theories from other disciplines such as clinical medicine, biology, sociology, psychology, and health policy. For the purposes of providing evidence-based and individual centered high-quality nursing services for the elderly and promoting, maintaining or reshaping their physical and mental health, gerontological nursing studies the impacts of nature, society, culture and education as well

老年照护机构的严重不足给我们提出了巨大挑战。

随着家庭结构的改变和劳动人口迁移，越来越多的老年人独居家中，空巢老人现象在城市和农村地区已非常普遍。社会对于护理院、社区照护机构、生活协助照料机构的需求日益增加。过渡性护理是连接医院与家庭或长期照护机构之间的一种护理模式，已越来越受到关注。

（三）保护老年人免于受虐待的需求增加

随着老年人中残障和痴呆的发生率不断增加，老年人受虐待的危险也在增高。虐待包括多种形式，诸如无视老年人的基础需求、身体约束、尊严剥夺以及故意不提供足够的照料等。对老年人，尤其是衰弱或是认知受损的老年人进行的虐待最终将导致严重的身体和心理伤害。

第二节　老年护理学概论

对老年护理需求的日益增长，使护士在促进健康和预防疾病方面发挥着重要作用，赋予了护士更重要的使命。无论在哪里工作，大部分护士在职业生涯中都有机会参与老年人护理。提高对老年护理学的认识，有助于所有护士更有效地参与促进健康老龄化的过程。

老年护理学是护理学中的一个专业方向，它是运用老年护理的知识与技能来满足衰老过程中特有的生理、心理、精神需要。老年护理学以护理学理论和临床医学、生物学、社会学、心理学、健康政策等学科理论为基础，遵循人类生命发展的规律，从老年人的生理、心理、社会文化以及发展的角度出发，研究自然、社会、文化教育以及生理和心理因素对老年人及其家庭健康的影响，从而为老年人提供以循证为基础，以个体为中心的

as physiological and psychological factors on the health of the elderly and their families from life-span perspective.

Gerontological nurses work with the elderly and their families for the purposes of maximizing their functional ability, promoting, maintaining and restoring their physical and mental health. They are also dedicated to the exploring strategies of promoting a health care environment that reflects accessibility, evidence-based practice and high quality, person centered care for elder adults.

I. Development of Gerontological Nursing

i. Gerontological Nursing in America

The history of gerontological nursing can be traced back to as early as 1900s and it has gone through four stages. (a) 1900-1955: there was no theory as the basis for implementation of care during this time. The milestone of this stage was the recognition of gerontological nursing as a special area of nursing practice, which laid the basis for the future development of gerontological nursing. (b) 1955-1965: this is a period of rapid development of theory and research in nursing. The researches on gerontological care were promoted, and the first edition of gerontological nursing book was published, as well as the geriatric nurse specialty group was established by the recommendation of American Nurses Association (ANA). All these achievements indicated that gerontological nursing moved a big step towards professionalization. (c) 1965-1981: this is a period that gerontological nursing moved towards professionalization. During this time, the first gerontological clinical nurse specialist (GCNS) program was developed in 1966 at Duke University in the US. Geriatric Nursing Division of ANA was formed in 1966 and the *Standards of Geriatric Nursing Practice* was first published in 1970. A statement on the scope of gerontological nursing practice was published and had several revisions since 1981. This is a very important document that reflects the comprehensive concepts and dimensions of practice for the nurses working with elder adults. Also, in this period, ANA promoted gerontological nursing education. Care of the elderly became an important part in nursing curriculum, at the same time certifications were awarded to nurses who specialized in the care of elder adults. Gerontological nursing also became an important area of study at graduate education. (d) 1985 to present: gerontological nursing moved to a rapid growth and fruitful stage with progresses in clinical

高质量护理服务，达到促进、维持或重塑老年人身心健康的目标。

老年专业护士与老年人及其家属合作，最大限度地发挥他们的功能能力，促进、维持和恢复他们的身心健康。他们还致力于促进健康环境的战略探索，使老年护理的可及性，循证实践和高质量、以人为本的护理理念得以实现。

一、老年护理学的发展历程

（一）美国老年护理学的发展历程

老年护理学的历史可以追溯到 1900 年，至今共经历了 4 个时期。1900—1955 年为理论前期：虽然在这一时期尚无任何理论作为实施专业护理活动的基础，但在 1900 年，老年护理学被确认为独立的护理专业，这奠定了日后老年护理学发展的基础。1955—1965 年为理论基础初期：在这一时期，护理理论和科研快速发展，推动了整个护理学科的进步，有关老年护理的研究随之展开，出版了第一部老年护理教材；1961 年，美国护理学会设立了第一个老年护理专业小组，标志着老年护理学在专业化的道路上前进了一大步。1965—1985 年为专业发展期：这一时期是老年护理走向专业化的时期；1966 年美国杜克大学成立了第一个老年护理专家项目；与此同时，美国护理学会成立老年病护理分会以及在 1970 年出版了第一本《老年护理实践标准》；并在 1981 年发表了一份关于老年护理实践范围的声明，之后进行了多次修订，这是一份非常重要的文件，反映了护士与老年人一起工作的综合概念和实践维度；1976 年美国护理学会提出发展老年护理学教育，不仅推动了许多国家的护理学院将老年护理纳入大学护理课程体系，而且许多学校还设立了老年护理学硕士和博士学位。1985 年至今是全面完善和发展时期：这个时期有关老年护理的临床实践、教育和科研都在迅速发展并取得丰硕成果；各种老年护理专业机构和项目的设立促

practice, education and research. Many professional organizations and programs with a gerontological nursing focus were established; for example, in the US, there are the American Academy of Nursing's Expert Panel on Aging, the Hartford Institute for Geriatric Nursing, the American Assisted Living Nurse Association, the National Association of Directors of Nursing in Long Term Care, and the Gerontological Advanced Practice Nurse Association established. ANA proposed replacing the term of "Geriatric Nursing" with "Gerontological Nursing" in 1987. The change of term gave a broader scope of practice in care of the elderly. In response to the increasing health care needs of the elderly, many countries provide continuing education opportunities to facilitate nurses to improve gerontological nursing knowledge and skills, including web-based courses, distance learning, and certification programs for gerontological clinical nurse specialist (GCNS) or gerontological nurse practitioner (GNP). In 2008, the American Nurse Certification Center included the qualification certification of elderly clinical nursing experts in the content of specialty certificate registration examination, which means that the elderly clinical nursing experts have been officially recognized.

ii. Gerontological Nursing in China

In 1987, China first hospice hospital was established in Beijing, called "Beijing Songtang Caring Hospital". In 1988, Tianjin Medical College established the first Hospice Care Research Center in China. Inspired by the Chinese Nursing Association (CNA) proposal of Improving Community-based Elderly Care, Shanghai, Shenzhen and other regions have successively developed community service projects such as elderly care center and nursing institutions.

Although specialized gerontological nursing programs are emerging in mainland China, gerontological nursing education is still seriously lagging behind the fast growth of aging population. At present, the Gerontological Nursing education in China is in the exploratory stage, and faculties still lack of systimitic training in the elderly care. The Higher Education Steering Committee of the Ministry of Education published *The National Standard for Undergraduate Education* in 2018, and gerontological nursing courses have listed in the National Standard for Nursing Education. Since then, the gerontological course has been popularized in the undergraduate and graduate curricula in the country. Gerontological clinical nurse specialist program was installed in mainland of China in 2005. Some southern provinces started

进了老年护理学在教学、临床实践和研究方面的快速发展。例如，在美国成立了美国护理科学院老龄问题专家小组、哈特福德基金会老年护理研究所、美国辅助生活护士协会、全国长期护理主任协会和老年高级实践护士协会。由于老年护理学涉及的护理范畴日益扩展，美国护理学会在 1987 年提出用"老年护理学（Gerontological Nursing）"概念代替"老年病护理（Geriatric Nursing）"的概念。另外，为应对老年人的医疗保健需求，越来越多的国家为护士提供继续教育机会，帮助护士提高老年护理的专科知识与技能，其中包括以网络为基础的课程、远程教学、老年护理专业网站等。2008 年美国护士认证中心将老年临床护理专家的资格认证列入专科证书注册考试内容之中，这意味着老年临床护理专家得到了正式的认可。

（二）我国老年护理学的发展历程

1987 年，我国首家临终关怀医院"北京松堂关怀院"在北京成立。1988 年天津医学院创建了中国第一家临终关怀研究中心。在中华护理学会倡导发展和完善我国社区老年护理的影响下，上海、深圳等地区相继开展老年护理和养老院等社区服务项目。

目前，我国老年护理教育正在探索阶段，学校和临床仍缺乏接受过老年护理系统培训的师资。自 1998 年起，老年护理学课程开始在几所高等护理学院开设。2018 年老年护理学被教育部高等学校护理学专业教学指导委员会列入本科《护理学类教学质量国家标准》，老年护理学本科教学在全国范围内得到普及。中国内地的老年护理专科护士培训项目于 2005 年启动，由广东省卫生厅委托南方医科大学和香港理工大学联合培养老年护理专科护士。这是中国内地通过研究生教育培养老年护理专科护士的初步尝试。目前全国

program in cooperation with universities in Hong Kong and have achieved very good outcomes. Currently, many gerontological nurse training programs have been established in many places over the country.

II. Scope and Feature of Gerontological Nursing

Scope of gerontological nursing: Scope of gerontological nursing has broad range from health promotion aspects that enable people to optimize health, well-being and independence in later life; to curative and rehabilitative dimensions that focus on functional or psychological recovery from illness or injury; facilitating self-care and enabling effective management of long-term conditions; providing care for those who become frail or with limited and/or declining self-care capacity, and need palliative and end-of-life care.

Features of Gerontological Nursing: Gerontological nursing is a theoretical based practice with a multidisciplinary approach. It is social and family context embedded.

Characteristics of the elderly, as individuals and groups, determined the feature of gerontological nursing. The elderly have accumulated a lot of life experiences from the aging process. Due to age related changes as well as extended exposure to environmental risks, many elders experience physical and mental function decline, which results in decreased adaptability and resistance to diseases and function impairment. Living with co-morbidity is a common phenomenon in the elderly population, especially among the oldest old group. Suffering from different chronic diseases at the same time leads to polypharmacy, which has been identified as a major concern by the health professionals. Atypical symptom presentation and serious complications are common phenomena among elder patients. These characters add the complexity in the care of elderly. All the factors discussed above need to be considered in theory building and competence development.

Multidisciplinary approach is another feature of gerontological nursing. Elder care involves a wide range of knowledge and resources. Gerontological nursing is embedded in the social context. Nurses need to deal with not only the complex health conditions, but also issues of cultural, social welfare, legal, and relationship in the health care and social systems. So, it is essential to involve experts from clinical medicine, sociology, psychology, economics,

各地护理学会等机构在积极开展老年护理专科护士培训项目。

二、老年护理学的范畴和特点

老年护理学的范畴广泛：从健康促进方面，帮助老年人在生活中优化健康、促进和维护独立功能、感知幸福；在治疗和康复方面，注重从疾病或伤害中恢复身体功能和心理康复；在促进自我护理和有效管理长期疾病方面，协助自理和慢性病管理；以及为衰弱和自理能力缺失的人提供护理服务、姑息治疗和临终关怀等。

老年护理的特点：参与及引领多学科合作，在多种场所服务，强调合作关系，需要社会家庭的共同努力。

老年护理学具有较强的理论性、实践性和多学科性。老年人的个体和群体特点决定了老年护理学的特点。随着年龄的增长，老年人积累了大量的生活经验；同时暴露于各种环境危险之下，老年人的机体各组织器官生理功能出现衰退，导致调节功能不足，抗病能力减退，适应力下降，心理状态也随着老年人内外环境的变化而改变。带病生存是老年人群中的一个普遍现象，在高龄老年人中尤为常见，多种慢性疾病共存进而导致了多重用药，这也成为健康学者所担心的重要问题。另外，高龄老年人患病后临床症状不典型，疾病并发症多且较严重，这提示了老年护理的复杂性。在老年护理学科的理论构建与能力培养中，必须考虑到上述特点。

多学科合作是老年护理的另一个特点。老年护理牵扯面广，涉及疾病、功能状态、精神健康、社会经济体制、医疗体制、养老政策和法规、社会文化、伦理等，因而决定了老年护理必须与多学科进行合作，建立老年护理专业综合的教育系统，才能满足老年

religion, and ethics in the solution of the problem.

III. General Goals and Basic Principles in Gerontological Nursing

Gerontological nursing contributes to the interdisciplinary and multi-agency care of elder people. Gerontological nurses practice in a variety of settings where services are dedicated to the care of elder people. Gerontological nursing takes a relationship-centered approach that promotes healthy ageing and the achievement of well-being in the elder person and their families by enabling them to adapt to the elder's health and life changes and to face ongoing life challenges.

i. General Goal of the Gerontological Nursing

The general goal of the gerontological nursing is to optimize health and well-being among older population. Gerontology nurses provide effective nursing activities to help the elderly maintain optimal mental, social and physical well-being and function, postpone the onset of diseases and disabilities to the final stage of life journey, and prepare for a peaceful death.

Although aging is an inevitable nature process for everyone, how well people endure this process are different, some are very healthy, and some are very frail. For many elder adults, especially the oldest old people, cure is not the main purpose of treatment and nursing activities. The emphasis is on protecting the quality of life by preventing deterioration of diseases and disease induced disabilities.

ii. Basic Principles in Gerontological Nursing.

Basic principles in gerontological nursing that facilitate optimizing health and well-being of the elderly are to address their basic needs, maintain daily life functions, support independence, minimize suffering, promote social and civic engagement, and protect dignity. Although the elderly have many constrain that affect their daily living, application of these basic principles will help the elderly enjoy life with compensation and maintain their quality of life.

人多方面需求。在预防疾病、治疗护理、社会福利方面，与医学、护理学、社会学、心理学、经济学、宗教和伦理学等专家探讨问题的解决途径是至关重要的。

三、老年护理的目标和原则

老年护理在学科内合作和多机构间照护中起到了沟通作用。护士主要在服务于老年人的多种机构中进行实践。老年护理的目标在于促进健康老龄化，通过帮助老年人及其家庭适应衰老所带来的健康挑战，最终实现老年人及其家庭的幸福。

（一）老年护理的目标

老年护理的总目标是实现"健康老龄化"，即通过有效的护理活动帮助老年人在晚年保持身体、心理和社会功能的完好状态，将疾病或生活不能自理推迟到生命的最后阶段，使其有尊严地走完人生旅程。

衰老是人类必须经历的自然过程，但是每个人在这一过程的表现截然不同，有的老年人相对健康，有的则非常虚弱。对于大多数老年人，特别是高龄老人而言，治愈疾病并非医疗和护理的最终目的，取而代之的是通过控制疾病和残障的进一步发展恶化，保证老年人的生活质量，尽可能延长老年人的生活自理期，让老年人病而不残、伤而不残、残而不废。

（二）老年护理的基本原则

老年护理的基本原则是满足老年人基本需要，维护日常生活功能，促进和保持最大程度的独立性，预防和减轻残障的发生，减轻痛苦，促进社会生活的参与以及保证尊严。尽管衰老限制了老年人的日常生活，但通过遵循上述原则，可以帮助老年人最大限度地维持生活质量。

IV. Competency for Baccalaureate-educated Nursing Graduates

Nursing professionals have been working dedicately to strengthen quality of care for the elderly. In 2010, American Association of Colleges of Nursing (AACN) and Hartford Institute for Geriatric Nursing published the *Recommended Baccalaureate Competencies and Curricular Guidelines* for the Nursing Care of Older Adults. This document provides the necessary information and guidance to assist nurse educators to incorporate gerontological nursing content into the baccalaureate nursing curriculum. Following 19 gerontological nursing competency statements are included in this recommendation.

1. Incorporate professional attitudes, values, and expectations about physical and mental aging in the provision of patient-centered care for older adults and their families.

2. Assess barriers for older adults in receiving, understanding, and giving of information.

3. Use valid and reliable assessment tools to guide nursing practice for older adults.

4. Assess the living environment as it relates to functional, physical, cognitive, psychological, and social needs of older adults.

5. Intervene to assist older adults and their support network to achieve personal goals, based on the analysis of the living environment and availability of community resources.

6. Identify actual or potential mistreatment (physical, mental or financial abuse, and/or self neglect) in older adults and refer appropriately.

7. Implement strategies and use online guidelines to prevent and/or identify and manage geriatric syndromes.

8. Recognize and respect the variations of care, the increased complexity, and the increased use of healthcare resources inherent in caring for older adults.

9. Recognize the complex interaction of acute and chronic co-morbid physical and mental conditions and associated treatments common to older adults.

10. Compare models of care that promote safe, quality physical and mental health care for older adults such as The Program of All-Inclusive Care for the Elderly (PACE), The Nurses Improving Care to Health System (NICHE), Guided Care, Culture Change, and Transitional Care Models.

四、从事老年护理的本科护士应具备的基本核心能力

护理专业人员一直致力于提高老年人的护理质量。2010 年，美国护理院校委员会和哈特福德基金会老年护理研究所发布了《护理本科教育老年护理的核心能力标准和课程指南》。该建议为协助老年护理教育者制订本科护理课程中老年护理相关内容，提供了必要的信息和指导。十九项老年护理的核心能力如下：

1. 在为老年人和家庭提供以患者为中心护理时，以专业化的态度、价值观和期望值对待老年人的身体和精神老化现象。

2. 评估老年人接受、理解和提供信息过程中的障碍。

3. 应用有效和可靠的评估工具指导老年护理实践。

4. 评估影响老年人的功能、身体、认知、心理和社会需要的相关生活环境。

5. 根据对居住环境和社区资源的可利用性分析，提供帮助老年人及其支持体系实现个体目标的干预措施。

6. 识别现存的或潜在的虐待老年人问题（包括身体、心理或经济上的虐待，和／或自我忽视），并转介给适当的机构。

7. 应用有效措施和网上指导资源预防、识别和管理老年综合征。

8. 承认和尊重老年护理中不断增加的变异性、复杂性及对医疗资源的消耗。

9. 认识老年人身体和精神方面急、慢性病共同存在的共病状况以及相关治疗的复杂性。

10. 比较促进安全和身心健康的护理模式，如老年人全人护理模式，促进老年人健康模式，护士改善医疗保健系统、指导性护理、文化变迁和过渡护理模式等。

11. Facilitate ethical, non-coercive decision making by older adults and families/caregivers for maintaining everyday living, receiving treatment, initiating advance directives, and implementing end-of-life care.

12. Promote adherence to the evidence-based practice of providing restraint-free care (both physical and chemical restraints).

13. Integrate leadership and communication techniques that foster discussion and reflection on the extent to which diversity (among nurses, nurse assistive personnel, therapists, physicians, and patients) has the potential to impact the care of older adults.

14. Facilitate safe and effective transitions across levels of care, including acute, community-based, and long-term care (e. g. , home, assisted living, hospice, nursing homes) for older adults and their families.

15. Plan patient-centered care with consideration for mental and physical health and well-being of informal and formal caregivers of older adults.

16. Advocate for timely and appropriate palliative and hospice care for older adults with physical and cognitive impairments.

17. Implement and monitor strategies to prevent risk and promote quality and safety (e. g. , falls, medication mismanagement, pressure ulcers) in the nursing care of older adults with physical and cognitive needs.

18. Utilize resources/programs to promote functional, physical, and mental wellness in older adults.

19. Integrate relevant theories and concepts included in a liberal education into the delivery of patient-centered care for older adults.

V. Trends for Gerontological Nursing Development in China

China's aging population has brought opportunities and challenges to the development of elderly care. According to national policies, the future trends of gerontological nursing in China will be the development of the national strategic plan for gerontological nursing; setting up clear goals for gerontological nursing as a discipline and competency requirements for specialist; establishment of scientific assessment system for needs of elderly care; enhancement of the leadership of the gerotological nursing specialist and facilitation of their active participation in research and policy making; improvement of the primary health care and service extension to the young elderly population; promotion of

11. 鼓励老年人、家庭和照顾者对有关维持日常生活、接受治疗、预立遗嘱和临终关怀等问题做出符合伦理道德的，非强迫性的决定。

12. 促进在循证的基础上提供无（物理性和化学性的）约束的护理。

13. 在护士、护理辅助人员、治疗师、医生和患者这样多样化的团队中应用领导艺术和沟通技巧，促进针对可能影响到老年人护理问题的讨论和反思。

14. 协助老年人和家庭在不同机构之间安全和有效的过渡，包括医院、社区、长期护理机构之间的转诊和过渡（例如从家庭到长期照顾机构、临终关怀医院、养老院）。

15. 在计划以患者为中心的护理时，考虑到正式和非正式的照顾者的身心健康。

16. 倡导为有生理和认知残障的老年人提供及时和适当的姑息治疗和临终关怀。

17. 实施和监测风险防范的措施，促进老年人躯体和精神需要的护理质量和安全性（如预防跌倒、用药管理不善和压力性损伤）。

18. 有效利用资源／项目，促进老年人的功能，保持身体和精神健康。

19. 在为老年人提供护理过程中应用通识教育中的相关理论和概念。

五、中国老年护理发展趋势

中国人口老龄化给老年护理的发展带来了机遇和挑战。为实现促进健康老龄化的目标，我们要依据国家政策，制订我国老年护理学的学科定位和发展策略；明确人才培养目标和能力标准，加快培养老年护理专科人才，促进老年护理学实践专科化发展；建立科学的养老服务需求评估体系和组织机构；提升老年专科护士的领导力，积极参与老年护理政策研究和制订；加强老年人群初级卫生保健工作，拓展服务对象至老年前期人群；

evidence-based gerontological care and implement the continuity of care; and integration of Chinese culture into gerotological nursing while promotion of international academic communication.

大力开展老年护理实践中的循证护理，积极开展延续性护理；同时开展国际间学术交流，发展具有中国文化特色的老年护理。

Box 1-2 Learning Resource

Administration on Aging: http: //www. aoa. gov

Alliance for Aging Research: http: //www. agingresearch. org

American Geriatrics Society: http: //www. Americangeriatrics. org

American Society on Aging: http: //www. asaging. org

Agency for Health Care Policy and Research(AHCPR): http//www. ahcpr. gov

American Association of Colleges of Nursing(AACN): http: //www. aacn. nche. edu

Centers for Disease Control and Prevention: http: //www. cdc. gov/aging

Exercise Assessment and Screening for You Tool: http: /www. easyforyou. info

eHow: About Depression in the Elderly: http: //www. ehow. com/about_5124659_depression-elderly. html

Geriatric Nursing Resources for Care of Older Adults: http: //consultgerirn. org

Hartford Institute of Geriatric Nursing: http: //www. hartfordign. org/

Healthy People 2020 documents online: http: //www. health. gov/healthpeople/

National Institute on Aging: http: //www. nih. gov/nia/

National Cancer Institute: http: //www. cancer. gov

National Institutes of Health: http: //www. nih. gov

National Institute of Mental Health: http: //www. nimh. nih. gov/

National Guideline Clearinghouse: http//guideline. gov

National Pressure Ulcer Advisory Panel(NPUAP): http//www. npuap. gov

UCSF Memory and Aging Center: http: //memory. ucsf. edu

U. S. Department of Health and Human Services: http: //www. os. dhhs. gov

WHO: http: //www. who. int/ageing/en/

Box 1-2 学习资源

(GUO Guifang)   （郭桂芳）

Key Points

1. Healthy aging is a process to promote well-being of the elderly through a series of positive measures to reduce the risks for disease and related disabilities, and assist the elderly function well physically and mentally, and be actively engaged in life.

本章要点

1. 健康老龄化是通过一系列积极的措施来促进老年人的福祉，减少疾病和相关残疾的风险，促进老年人身心健康，积极参与生活。

2. Challenges of population aging to healthcare system are increased the needs for grontoloical care, long-term care, transitional care, and protecting elder people from mistreatment.

3. Gerontological nursing is a theoretical based specialty with a multidisciplinary approach. It applies theories from existing nursing theories and theories from other disciplines such as clinical medicine, biology, sociology, psychology, and health policy.

4. Gerontological nurse apply a body of knowledge and skills to elder adults to meets the unique biopsychosocial and spiritual needs related to aging process.

5. Scope of gerontological Nursing has broad range from health promoting aspects that enable people to optimize health, well-being and independence in later life; to curative and rehabilitative dimensions that focus on functional or psychological recovery from illness or injury; facilitating self-care and enabling effective management of long-term conditions; providing care for those who become frail or with limited and/or declining self-care capacity and palliative and end-of-life care.

6. Roles of gerontological nurses are to work with the elderly and their families for the purposes of maximizing their functional ability, promoting, maintaining and restoring their physical and mental health.

7. Gerontological nursing practice is dedicated to exploring strategies of promoting a health care environment that reflects accessibility, evidence-based practice and high quality, person centered care for elder adults.

8. Gerontological nursing researches focus on the impacts of social, cultural, physical, psychological, and environmental factors on the health of the elderly and their families.

9. The general goal of gerontological nursing is to optimize health and well-being among elder adult population. Gerontology nurses provide effective nursing activities to help the elderlymaintain optimal mental, social and physical well-being and function, postpone the onset of diseases and disabilities to the final stage of life journey, and prepare for a peaceful death.

10. The basic principles of gerontological nursing that facilitate optimizing health and well-being of the elderly are to address their basic needs, support independence, minimize suffering, promote social and civic engagement, and protect dignity.

11. Competencies of baccalaureate nursing graduates range from abilities to incorporate professional attitudes

2. 人口老龄化对医疗保健系统的挑战是增加了老年护理、长期护理、过渡性照顾和保护老年人免受虐待的需求。

3. 老年护理学是基于理论的专业性护理实践。应用的理论包括现有的护理理论和相关学科理论，如临床医学、生物学、社会学、心理学等学科、卫生政策。

4. 老年科护士应用有关老化和护理的知识和技能，通过多学科合作来满足老年人独特的生理、心理、社会和精神需求。

5. 老年护理学的范畴包括健康促进、治疗和康复、协助自理和慢性病管理、为衰弱和自理能力缺失的人提供护理服务、姑息治疗和临终关怀等。

6. 老年护士的角色与功能是帮助老年人和他们的家庭最大限度地发挥他们的能力，促进、维护和恢复他们的身体和心理健康。

7. 老年护理学重点在于探索促进健康的策略，建立可获得的、基于循证实践的、高质量的、以人为中心的老年护理环境。

8. 老年护理研究的重点是社会、文化、生理、心理和环境因素对老年人及其家庭的健康的影响。

9. 老年护理的总目标是实现"健康老龄化"，即通过有效的护理活动帮助老年人在晚年保持身体、心理和社会功能的完好状态，将疾病或生活不能自理推迟到生命的最后阶段，使其有尊严地走完人生旅程。

10. 老年护理的基本原则是满足老年人基本需要，促进和保持最大程度的独立性，预防和减轻残障的发生，减轻痛苦，促进社会生活的参与以及保证尊严。

11. 护理本科毕业生老年护理能力要求涵盖较广，从老年护理实践中的职业态度，到运

toward the elderly in practice, to apply knowledge and skills in providing person centered-care for the elderly and their families.

Critical Thinking Exercise

1. The general goal of nursing practice is to improve quality of life through accessible, person-centered, and evidence-based high quality nursing care to everyone. Please discuss how this goal can be met when working with older population.

2. Please discuss the basic principles of gerontological nursing, and how to apply them during nursing practice.

3. Please discuss how to incorporate gerontological nursing competencies into nursing curriculum and how to reinforce them through clinical practice.

用知识和技能为老人和他们的家庭提供以人为本的照顾。

批判性思维练习

1. 衡量老年人健康的最佳指标是其功能状态，请讨论在老年护理中如何通过可获得的、以人为本的和以证据为基础的高质量护理达到维护老年人基本功能的目标。

2. 请讨论如何在护理实践中应用老年护理的基本原则。

3. 请讨论如何将老年护理能力纳入护理课程设置，如何通过临床实践强化这些能力。

Chapter 2　Concepts and Theories of Aging

第二章　衰老的相关概念和理论

Learning Objectives

On completion of this chapter, the reader will be able to:

- Describe the process of aging using selected aging theories;

- Identify types of biological theories of aging, types of psychological development theories of aging and types of sociological theories of aging;
- Discuss nursing implications of biological, psychological and sociological aging theories;
- Apply selected aging theories in clinical nursing practice.

学习目标

学完本章节，应完成以下目标：

- 能够运用不同的衰老理论来描述衰老的过程；

- 能够识别不同衰老相关的生物学、心理学和社会学理论；

- 能够讨论衰老相关的生物学、心理学和社会学理论对护理的启示；

- 能够将不同的衰老理论应用于临床护理实践。

Aging is a gradual continuous process of change that begins in early adulthood and is characterized by a decline in physical capacity and physiological functions. Although aging is a normal developmental process, people do not become old at any specific age. Senescence means "to grow old", is not inevitable and may be delayed.

The demographics of aging are changing dramatically globally, with steady increases not only in the numbers of older persons but also in longevity. China currently has the world's largest elderly population and Chinese older adults constitutes one-fifth of the world's elderly population and growth will continue to accelerate. By the end of 2015, China's elderly population (aged 60 and above) totaled 222 million, accounted for 16.1% of the population. In addition, the proportion of persons aged ≥ 80 years has increased more rapidly than any other age group among older Chinese people, a phenomenon referred to as super-aging.

With these compelling demographic developments comes increasing diversity and heterogeneity in how people age. Distinctions are often made between chronologic aging, which is the number of years lived, and biological aging, which refers to changes in the body that commonly occur with age and are the result of lifestyle, behaviors, and the effects of disease. Some older adults seem "young" at the age of 90, while others seem "old" at 65 years of age. For example, changes in muscle mass, strength, and endurance that is a part of usual aging contributes to gradual functional decline and this may be negatively impacted and accelerated by lifestyle factors such as sedentary behavior, obesity, and smoking, leading to earlier development of chronic disease and disability.

Human aging is influenced by biologic, psychological, social, functional and spiritual factors. Aging is a bio-psychosocial process that involves biological influences, such as inflammation and oxidative damage of cells and metabolic hormones; the social structure and demographic factors, such as gender, socioeconomic status, age and cultural context; and individual influences, such as psychosocial and behavioral factors. Health and social disparities influence the aging process. In China, disparities in morbidity and mortality are also found in geographic location (urban versus rural), education attainment, and socioeconomic status. Indeed, many studies have found that morbidity, disability and mortality are associated with biology, age, and gender socioeconomic status and health behaviors and disparities.

老化是起源于成年早期的渐进性、持续性的改变，躯体和生理功能下降是老化的标志。虽然衰老是有机体发育的正常过程，但有机体并不是在某个特定年龄才变老的。老化不可避免，但有可能被延缓。

全球范围内，老年人口的统计学特征存在较大差异性，不仅老年人的数量在逐渐增加，老年人的寿命也在逐渐延长。目前中国的老年人口数量居世界首位，占全球老年人口总数的五分之一，而这一数字还在持续增长。截至 2015 年底，中国老年人口（即 60 岁及以上老年人）总数为 2.22 亿，占中国总人口的 16.1%。此外，在中国，80 岁及以上的高龄老年人增长速度远快于其他年龄段的老年人群，这一现象被称为"超速老化"。

伴随着这些引人注目的人口发展，人口老化呈现出越来越多的多样性和异质性。人口老化的差异性主要在于年代性老化即实际生存的周期和生物性老化即随着年龄的增长和生活方式、行为、疾病影响下而发生的身体变化。有些老年人在 90 岁还能活动自如，而有些老年人则从 65 岁开始就已经衰弱。例如，由于正常老化造成的肌肉含量、力量和耐力的变化可引起功能的逐渐下降，但这种功能下降，也可能是由于不良的生活方式，如久坐、肥胖、吸烟造成的。同时这些不良生活方式还会进一步导致慢性疾病和残疾的早期发展。

人类的衰老过程受生物、心理和社会的影响。衰老的生物学理论强调的是有机体的生理过程，人的衰老过程可受生理、躯体功能、信仰和社会文化等的影响，是一个涉及生物、心理和社会等方面的综合过程。生物-心理老化强调老化过程不仅受到炎症、细胞氧化性损伤、代谢激素等生物因素的影响，也可受到人生各阶段的应激及适应等心理因素的影响。社会性老化则强调性别、健康行为、社会经济状况及文化因素对老化过程的影响。研究表明，老年人疾病的发病率、残疾率及死亡率与生理状况、年龄、性别、经

The heterogeneity in biological and chronological age and aging-associated conditions have been attributed to different lifestyle, genetic, and environmental factors (e. g., diet, pollution, stress) that are linked to socioeconomic factors. It is important to consider these factors in the aging process as they are important targets for intervention that can potentially improve quality of life in the aging experience. Understanding the aging process and healthy or successful aging can potentially lessen burdens by promoting health behaviors that may reduce or delay illness and dependency and increase wellbeing and quality of life.

Numerous theories have been proposed to explain the aging process from biological, psychological, and sociological perspectives, but there is no single definition or theory that adequately explains all aspects of aging. Biologic theories of aging focus on physiologic processes that occur in living organism over time. Psychological theories of aging address the individual's response or adjustment to the developmental tasks of aging. Sociological theories of aging focus on roles and relationships in late life.

This chapter provides an overview of prominent theories of aging from biological, psychological and sociological perspectives. Theories of aging can provide guidance to nurses in understanding the aging process and delivering high quality care to older adults. When providing care to older adults, nurses should consider the older adults' individual differences and their interaction with their environment from these multiple perspectives.

Section 1　Biological Theories

Biological theories explain aging from the point of view of physiologic processes that occur over time. Biological aging is a complex dynamic process of gradual deterioration in basic structures of the cells and organs beginning in adulthood and ending with death. Aging is also influenced by the interaction between organisms and their environment resulting in changes in cells, molecules, and body systems. Healthy aging refers to postponing or reducing the undesired effects of aging and maintaining physical and mental health, avoiding or minimizing the impact of chronic conditions, and remaining active and

济状况及健康行为有关。衰老的个体差异和生活方式，遗传和环境因素（例如饮食、污染、压力）相关。在衰老过程中考虑这些因素很重要，因为它们可干预，并且可以改善生活质量。了解衰老过程，可通过促进健康行为来减轻老化带来的机体影响、减少或延迟疾病、提高自理能力，并改善生活质量。

目前学术界已经提出许多衰老理论，从生物学、心理学和社会学的角度来解释衰老综合过程。然而目前，老年学领域仍无一个衰老理论可以系统地解释衰老的全面过程。衰老的生物学理论侧重于生物体随着时间推移所发生的生理过程。衰老的心理学理论重点解释个人对衰老的阶段的反应或适应。衰老的社会心理学理论则关注老年人对衰老过程的适应及调整。

本章将从生物学、心理学和社会学三个方面介绍目前较为认可的衰老理论。护士应从生物学、心理学和社会学的角度综合考虑所遇到的护理问题，并结合患者的个体差异以及他们对环境的适应能力提供高质量护理。

第一节　衰老的生物学理论

生物学理论主要从生理角度揭示随着时间推移而产生的老化过程。生物学老化是指细胞和器官的基本结构从人的中年开始逐渐衰退直至人体死亡的复杂动态过程。生物学老化理论认为衰老是有机体与环境相互作用的结果，构成人体组织和器官的细胞、分子的改变导致了老化。健康老龄化指的是延缓或减少老化所造成的影响，保持身体和心理健康，避免或降低慢性疾病的影响，同时维

independent.

Longevity continues to increase as a result of social and medical advancements, although how long a person may expect to live varies considerably. Life expectancy is a measure of the average time a person is expected to live based on year of birth, current age, and demographic factors such as sex, race, and socioeconomic status. In addition, multiple factors affect individual life expectancy including heredity, lifestyle, exposure to toxins and radiation, life stress, and health care. Life expectancy has increased globally; for example, in China, life expectancy has risen from 40 years in 1950 to 76 years in 2016. In contrast, the maximum life span, which refers to the maximum amount of time that one or more members of a population have survived between birth and death, has not increased in humans and is estimated at about 120 years. For example, the oldest person documented in recent times wasa French woman named Jeanne Louise Calment (1875-1997) and represents the near-maximum human life span. In general, despite an optimal genetic makeup and healthy lifestyle, the chance of living to be 120 years old is small.

Aging has been conceptualized as the result of two interactive, overlapping processes known as primary and secondary aging. Primary aging is the progressive deterioration in organ structure and function that occurs with advancing age alone, independent of other factors, such as decreased bone mineral density, muscle mass, and decline in cardiac, pulmonary, renal, and immune function. Secondary aging is the accelerated decline in organ structure and function due to disease, such as diabetes and hypertension, or by harmful environmental factors (pollution, chemical or radiation exposures) and lifestyle factors (sedentary, obesity, smoking). Numerous mechanisms have been proposed for these aging processes such as oxidative stress and inadequate DNA repair, accumulation of advanced glycation end products, amyloid, and proteins, alterations in the neuroendocrine system, and chronic inflammation. A number of biological theories of aging have been proposed, including error theory, free radical theory, cross-linkage theory, wear and tear theory, programmed theory, immunity theory, and genetics. In this chapter, four theories will be examined: free radical theory, immunological theory, chronic inflammation, and genomics.

持老年人的积极性和独立性。

由于社会和医疗的进步，长寿老年人不断增加，然而人类预期寿命的长短因人而异。预期寿命是衡量一个人平均生存周期的指标，预期寿命取决于出生年份、当前年龄和人口因素（如性别、种族和社会经济地位）。此外，包括遗传、生活方式、毒素暴露和辐射、生活压力和健康保健在内的多种因素会影响一个人的预期寿命。在全球范围内，人类的预期寿命都有所增加，如在中国，人均预期寿命已从 1950 年的 40 岁延长到了 2016 年的 76 岁。与之相反，人类的最高寿命（人群中一个或多个成员在出生和死亡之间存活的时间）并没有增加，估计在 120 岁左右。例如，在最近的几次记录中，最长寿的人是法国的一个名叫 Jeanne Louise Calment 的女性（1875—1997 年），她的记录代表了人类的最高寿命。在一般情况下，即便有最佳的遗传结构和健康的生活方式，存活到 120 岁的概率也是很小的。

老化被定义为两个交互的、重叠的过程，这两个过程称为原发性和继发性老化。原发性老化是指随年龄增长而发生的器官结构和功能的逐步退化，例如骨密度降低，肌肉质量下降以及心脏、肺、肾和免疫功能下降。继发性老化是指由于疾病（例如糖尿病和高血压），有害环境因素（污染、化学或辐射暴露），生活方式因素（龋齿、肥胖、吸烟）而导致的器官结构和功能的加速下降。对于这些衰老过程，已经提出了许多机制，例如氧化应激和 DNA 修复不足，糖基化终产物增多，淀粉样蛋白和蛋白质的积累，神经内分泌系统的改变以及慢性炎症。衰老的生物学理论包括误差理论、自由基学说、交叉连接理论、磨损理论、程序学说、免疫理论和遗传学。本章介绍自由基学说和免疫理论。

I. Free Radical Theory of Aging

The free radical theory proposed by Harman (1956) suggested that aging and death were caused by free radicals produced during physiological processes causing cumulative oxidative damage to cells. Free radicals are created when a molecule either gains or loses an electron (a small negatively charged particle found in atoms). Free radicals are formed naturally in the body and are a component of normal cellular processes. Free radicals can damage the major components of cells, including deoxyribonucleic acid (DNA), proteins, and cell membranes, and this damage may play a role in the development of cancer and other health conditions.

Excessive production of free radicals is associated with the progression of numerous pathological conditions. Free radicals that contain the element oxygen are the most common type of free radicals produced in living tissue. Another name for them is "reactive oxygen species" or ROS. The oxygen molecule (O_2) is electrically charged and attracts electrons from other molecules, which causes damage to DNA. Free radicals react with proteins, lipids, DNA, and ribonucleic acid (RNA) to cause damage through various reactive oxygen species. Free radicals arise during metabolism, but environmental factors such as air pollution, radiation, cigarette smoke, pesticides, and ozone can also cause free radicals. When antioxidants in the body are unable to manage free radicals, damage occurs and accumulates with age. The oxidative damage to mitochondrial DNA results in breaks to nuclear DNA strands causing gene modulation or deletions. These oxidative lesions can lead to abnormal cellular processes such as uncontrolled cell proliferation or mutations in specific genes or reduced DNA repair capability as found in cancer. Free radicals may also accelerate aging when lipid peroxidation damages phospholipid molecules in cell membranes, leading to structural modifications. Cumulative oxidative damage is responsible for aging and death. Harman (2006) extended the free radical theory and proposed that the life span is determined by the rate of oxidative damage to the mitochondrial DNA, which contributes to development of disease and malignancy and accelerated aging.

Application of the Free Radical Theory

Strategies to reduce free radicals and delay mitochondrial DNA damage and therefore to prolong the life span have been suggested. One approach is caloric

一、自由基学说

Harman 在 1956 年提出了自由基学说。自由基学说认为老化和死亡主要是由机体生理过程中所产生的自由基所致。当分子获得或失去一个电子（在原子中发现的一个带负电荷的小粒子）时，就产生了自由基。自由基在体内自然形成，是正常细胞代谢过程的一个组成部分。自由基会损害细胞的主要成分，包括脱氧核糖核酸（DNA）、蛋白质和细胞膜，而这种损害可能会在癌症和其他疾病的发展中发挥作用。

自由基的过量产生与许多病理状况的发展有关。含有氧元素的自由基是活体组织中最常见的自由基类型。自由基的另一个名称是"活性氧类"或 ROS。氧分子（O_2）带电并吸引其他分子产生的电子，因此损坏脱氧核糖核酸（DNA）。自由基与蛋白质、脂质、DNA 和核糖核酸（RNA）反应，通过各种活性氧类造成损害。自由基在新陈代谢过程中产生，但是，诸如空气污染、辐射、香烟烟雾、农药和臭氧等环境因素也会导致自由基的生成。当体内的抗氧化剂无法控制自由基时，会随着年龄的增长而受损并累积。线粒体 DNA 的氧化损伤导致核 DNA 链断裂，进而导致基因调节或缺失。这些氧化损伤会导致异常的细胞过程，例如不受控制的细胞增殖或特定基因的突变或癌症中 DNA 修复能力降低。当脂质过氧化作用破坏细胞膜中的磷脂分子，导致结构改变时，自由基也可能加速衰老。累积的氧化损伤导致衰老和死亡。Harman（2006）扩展了自由基学说，并提出寿命由线粒体 DNA 的氧化损伤速率决定，线粒体 DNA 的氧化损伤可促使疾病和恶性肿瘤的发展并加速衰老。

自由基学说的应用

有假说提出减少自由基并延缓 DNA 损伤从而延长寿命的策略。方法是限制热量摄入。研究者假设，在营养充足的情况下，限制热

restriction. Calorie restriction or the reduction of food intake without causing under-nutrition is hypothesized to slow the aging process, prolong youthfulness, postpone the onset of age-associated disease, and extend the life span by reducing the production of free radicals and oxidative damage. A reduction of 30%-50% in calories in early life in animals has been associated with a positive effect on age-related disease, and aging with an increase in lifespan of 30%-50% by improving insulin sensitivity and metabolic function and lowering body temperature, rate of metabolism, and oxidant production. Critiques of calorie restriction note that in some studies, animals fed a liberal diet compared to the restricted diet tended to over-eat and develop obesity, which may have contributed to a shorter lifespan. In recent research, the CALERIE (comprehensive assessment of long term effects of reducing intake of energy), findings from a study to determine the effects of two years of 25% caloric restriction in young and middle-aged non-obese men and women in the U. S. indicate that caloric restriction was associated with weight loss, reduced stress, and improved general health, mood, vigor, sleep quality, and sexual functioning compared to the control group. Caloric restriction has also been associated with reduction of abdominal fat mass, increased insulin sensitivity, reduced levels of pro-inflammatory cytokines, reactive oxygen species ROS and atherosclerotic lipids in the blood, lowered body temperature and metabolic rate, and improved cognitive performance. However, caloric restriction can lead to decreased bone density and anemia. Although calorie restriction with adequate nutrients may not prolong the maximum life span, it could increase life expectancy and quality of life by reducing chronic disease. However, compliance with a caloric restricted diet is difficult to sustain and malnutrition is a common problem in older persons. The caloric intake needed for optimal health varies for each individual based on genetics, age, and activity and diet pattern, and the ideal caloric intake to slow the aging process is not known. In addition, determining a safe threshold of caloric restriction for all persons may be difficult due to the influence of factors such as body composition, daily energy expenditure, and duration of restriction. Also, certain calorie reductions will benefit some organ systems (e. g. , cardiovascular) and potentially harm others (e. g. , bone density). Finally, caloric restriction could be harmful in some populations such as lean persons with low body weight (e. g. , BMI $<18.5 \text{ kg/m}^2$)and those who are malnourished. More research is needed in humans to determine the benefits and outcomes of this approach.

量或减少食物摄入，通过减少自由基的产生和脂质过氧化损伤，可以延缓衰老及衰老相关疾病，延长寿命。如研究表明，早期限制30%~50%的能量摄入，可以改善胰岛素敏感性和代谢功能，降低体温、代谢率，减少氧化剂的产生，从而延长30%~50%的寿命。对于热量限制呈相反意见的学者，则指出，在一些研究中，相比限制饮食的动物，那些不限制饮食的动物反而会出现食物的过量摄入，发生肥胖，从而导致寿命缩短。在最近的研究中，CALERIE（一项对减少能量摄取长期效果的综合评价研究）的某项研究结果显示，在美国非肥胖的中青年男性和女性中，进行为期两年的25%热量限制后。相比对照组，干预组出现了体重减轻，压力减少，整体健康、情绪、活力、睡眠质量和性功能改善。此外，限制热量的摄入还与腹部脂肪量降低、胰岛素敏感性增加、炎症细胞因子水平降低、血液中的活性氧自由基和动脉粥样硬化的血脂降低、体温和代谢率降低、认知能力改善有关。然而，限制热量也会导致骨密度降低和贫血。在有足够的营养素的情况下，进行热量限制，可能不会延长最高寿命，但可以减少慢性病，从而增加预期寿命，提高生活质量。但是限制热量的饮食是很难坚持的，此外营养不良又是老年人的一个常见问题。不同的个体在遗传学、年龄、活动和饮食模式上存在差异，因而实现个体最佳健康所需的热量摄入不同，可延缓老化过程的最佳热量摄入量也不明确。此外，由于一些因素的限制，如体成分、每日能量消耗和热量限制的持续时间，很难确定一个适用于所有人的热量限制安全阈值。热量限制对某些器官系统有益（如心血管），而对其他器官系统则有害（如骨密度）。最后，热量限制可能在某些人群中是有害的，如低体重人群（例如，体重指数小于 18.5kg/m^2）和营养不良人群。因此，需要更多的人类研究来确定这种方法的有效性和结果。

Another approach examines antioxidants. Antioxidants may delay the aging process through their interaction with free radicals. Antioxidants are enzymes that make up the body's defense system to prevent the damage caused by free radicals, but integrity of the defense system depends on sufficient intake of antioxidant-rich foods. For example, vitamins C, E, and A, beta-carotene, and lycopene are major sources of antioxidants and are found in orange and red fruits and dark leafy green vegetables. Polyphenols such as resveratrol are antioxidants that are synthesized in many plants, such as peanuts, blueberries, pine nuts, and grapes. Research on resveratrol in red wine for examplefinds reduction in inflammation and damage tothe linings of blood vessels and decreased low-density lipoprotein (LDL) cholesterol (the "bad" cholesterol), which may prevent blood clots to prevent or delay cardiovascular disease and mortality. Resveratrol comes from the skin of grapes and eating grapes and drinking grape juice is a way to get resveratrol without drinking alcohol. Moderate ingestion of alcohol, not only red wine, may also yield benefits, but there is no evidence that drinking alcohol can replace other heart-healthy measures such as physical activity, weight control, and lowering cholesterol and blood pressure. Curcumin (turmeric), a popular Indian spice used in curry, is a polyphenol with strong antioxidant effects. Green tea has strong antioxidant, anti-inflammatory, anticancer, and immunomodulatory properties. The epicatechins in green tea have been shown to be more effective antioxidants than vitamins C and E and are powerful scavengers of free radicals.

Critical nutrients in the elderly include vitamins B_{12} and D. About 6% of elderly have a vitamin B_{12} deficiency, which is mainly due to vitamin B_{12} malabsorption resulting from atrophic gastritis. This deficiency is associated with neurodegenerative diseases and bone loss. In addition, about half of community-living elderly living is deficient in vitamin D which is primarily due to reduced endogenous biosynthesis, low UVB exposure, and diet insufficient in vitamin D. A vitamin D deficiency increases the risks for falls and fractures and neurodegenerative diseases, and increased mortality.

High-dose supplements of antioxidants may be linked to health risks and increased mortality. For example, high doses of beta-carotene may increase the risk of lung cancer in smokers, high doses of beta-carotene and vitamin E may increase risks of prostate cancer and stroke, and supplements may also interact with some medicines.

抗氧化剂是有机体的一种保护酶，可以防止自由基对细胞的损伤而延长生命，水果和蔬菜中所含的维生素 C、维生素 E、维生素 A、β- 胡萝卜素及茄红素是抗氧化剂的主要来源。多酚类，如白藜芦醇，是常见的抗氧化剂，可由许多植物合成，如花生、蓝莓、松树和葡萄等。以红酒中白藜芦醇为例，研究发现，其可以降低炎症和血管内皮的损害，降低低密度脂蛋白（LDL）和胆固醇（"坏"胆固醇），进而可预防血液凝集，防止或延缓心血管疾病和死亡。白藜芦醇来自葡萄皮，吃葡萄和喝葡萄汁是在非饮酒的情况下摄入白藜芦醇的方法。除了红酒，适量摄入酒精，还可以产生有益的作用，但没有证据表明饮酒可以取代其他有益心脏健康的措施，如体力活动、体重控制和降低胆固醇和血压。姜黄素（姜黄）是一种用于咖喱的印度香料，它也是一种具有较强抗氧化作用的多酚。绿茶具有较强的抗氧化、抗炎、抗肿瘤、免疫调节作用。绿茶中的儿茶素已被证明是比维生素 C 和维生素 E 更有效的抗氧化剂，具有较强的自由基清除作用。

在老年人中，重要营养物质包括维生素 B_{12} 和维生素 D。大约 6% 的老年人有维生素 B_{12} 缺乏症，这主要是由于萎缩性胃炎导致的维生素 B_{12} 吸收不良。维生素 B_{12} 缺乏与神经退行性疾病和骨质流失有关。此外，约一半在社区生活的老年人缺乏维生素 D，主要是由于内源性合成不足，紫外线照射不足和含维生素 D 的食物摄入不足。而维生素 D 缺乏会增加跌倒、骨折和神经退行性疾病的风险，并增加死亡率。

高剂量的抗氧化剂补充可能与健康风险和死亡率增加有关。例如，高剂量的 β- 胡萝卜素可能会增加吸烟者患肺癌的风险，高剂量的 β- 胡萝卜素和维生素 E 可能会增加前列腺癌和脑卒中的风险，补充剂也可能与一些

In sum, there is insufficient research to support antioxidant supplementation and caloric restriction for increased survival. The optimal source of antioxidants is from the diet and not from supplements. More research is needed to understand the role of nutrients and their interactions (e. g. , protein/amino acids, fatty acids, vitamins, phytochemicals, and minerals), caloric restriction methods, and the mechanisms that influence anti-aging biologic pathways and age-associated diseases.

II. Immunological Theory of Aging

The immunological theory, proposed by Walford (1961) hypothesized that normal aging was pathogenically associated with faulty immunological process. Aging is generally associated with declines in the immune system, also termed immuno-senescence. The immune system consists of cells, tissues and organs that interact between internal and external environment and play an important role in protection of body against pathogens throughout life. Innate and adaptive immunities are two components in the immune system. Essential immune system components include T lymphocytes and B lymphocytes; B lymphocytes produce antibodies that can neutralize pathogens, and T lymphocytes recognize and kill infected cells. With advancing age, the T lymphocytes deteriorate and the functioning capabilities of B lymphocytes decline.

The thymus, which is the organ in the body whose functions include the selection and maturation of T cells, shrinks and reduces its production of mature T cells and hormones after age 30. After the age of 60 years, the thymus is undetectable. These immunological changes lead to impaired immune function and impaired capacity to respond to new antigens, both vaccines and new infections. Resistance to infections and infectious disease increases and there is decreased protection against cancer and heightened production of auto-antigens which may lead to an increase in autoimmune-related and other chronic diseases. For example, systematic inflammation caused by infections may contribute to the development of cardiovascular disease as evidence by the presence of T cells in atherosclerotic lesions, and the interactions of T cells with vascular endothelial cells. In addition to promotion of a pro-inflammatory state by the aging immune system is the contribution of obesity. Adipose

药物相互作用。总之，尚无充足研究支持抗氧化剂补充和热量限制对于延长生命的作用。抗氧化剂的最佳来源是饮食，而不是补充剂。营养的作用和它们之间的相互作用（例如，蛋白质、氨基酸、脂肪酸、维生素、植物化学物质和矿物质）、限制热量的方法、影响衰老的生物学通路和年龄相关性疾病的发病机制等问题，还需通过更多的研究来解释。

二、免疫理论

免疫理论由 Walford 于 1961 年提出。该理论指出老化与病理性免疫功能下降有关。老化通常与免疫系统的衰退有关，也被称为免疫衰老。人体免疫系统包括所有参与免疫的细胞、组织和器官。免疫系统可与内外环境相互作用，保护人体免受致病物质的侵袭。免疫系统包括先天性免疫系统和获得性免疫系统，它们对保护人体免受细菌、病毒和寄生虫的侵袭有重要作用。获得性免疫系统中的免疫细胞包括 B 淋巴细胞和 T 淋巴细胞，可以识别和消灭外来微生物。其中，B 淋巴细胞产生的抗体可以中和病原体，而 T 淋巴细胞可以识别和吞噬受感染的细胞。

免疫系统的功能会随着年龄增加出现衰退，T 淋巴细胞和 B 淋巴细胞的功能也随之减弱。胸腺是 T 淋巴细胞分化和成熟的场所，胸腺于 30 岁时开始萎缩，T 细胞的生成随之减少；60 岁时已触摸不到胸腺，从而导致老年人免疫功能受损，其对新抗原、新疫苗和新感染的应答能力下降。老年人免疫系统的改变可以导致身体免疫监视功能下降，不能识别外来病原，对于感染和传染性疾病的抵抗力减弱，预防癌症的能力下降和自身抗原的提高，从而可能导致自身免疫相关疾病及其他慢性病的增加。例如，由感染引起的全身炎症可能会导致心血管疾病的发展，比如动脉粥样硬化病变时，可发现 T 细胞的存在，T 细胞可与血管内皮细胞发生相互作用。老化

tissue produces a great amount of pro-inflammatory cytokines, thus contributing to chronic, low-grade systemic inflammation. Such inflammation contributes to obesity-related diseases such as metabolic syndrome and Type 2 diabetes and this inflammageing is associated with increased mortality. A depressed immune system is also associated with the accrual of DNA damage with age which contributes to inflammation through increased secretion of pro-inflammatory cytokines. Overall, the biologic mechanisms of inflammageing are complex and further research is needed to more fully elucidate this process.

i. Telomere Length and Aging

Due to the wide variation and heterogeneity in how people age and the loose association between chronologic and biologic age, there has been interest in looking at the DNA structures for signs that might better characterize aging. The shortening of telomeres, which are DNA protein structures located at the ends of chromosomes, has been proposed as a biomarker of aging. Emerging research has found that the shortening of telomeres is associated with an accelerated rate of aging, development of age-associated conditions such as cardiovascular disease, cancer, and dementia, decline in physical function, and earlier mortality. However, study methodologies and populations vary and confirmative implications cannot be made. Findings from a recent review indicate that the evidence that telomere length is a biomarker of aging and is a better predictor of life span, of physical and cognitive function decline associated with normal aging, or with mortality than chronological age is so far inconclusive. Further research is needed in longitudinal studies to examine life-long effects that include influences such as infections, lifestyle behaviors such as smoking, BMI, alcohol ingestion, and environmental exposures.

ii. Chronic Inflammation and Inflammageing

A common feature of aging cells and organs and age-related diseases is chronic inflammation. Chronic low-grade systemic, unresolved inflammation, and termed inflammageing, have been implicated as a significant risk factor for morbidity and mortality in older people. Acute inflammation serves an important purpose in the repair of injured tissues, but inflammageing occurs without infection and leads to widespread tissue damage and degeneration. Inflammageing is associated with a reduction in the body's ability to cope with various stressors which leads to a pro-inflammatory state

免疫系统将促进炎症状态，此外还会引起肥胖。脂肪组织产生大量的炎症细胞因子，从而导致慢性、低度全身炎症。这种炎症促进了肥胖相关的疾病，如代谢综合征和2型糖尿病，因此这种炎性衰老与死亡率增加有关。受损的免疫系统与DNA损伤相关，其通过增加炎症细胞因子的分泌来促进炎症发生。总而言之，炎性衰老的生物学机制非常复杂，需要进一步的研究来更充分地阐明这一过程。

（一）端粒长度与衰老

个体在衰老过程、实足年龄和生物年龄之间的差距等方面具有广泛变化性和异质性，因此研究者一直对寻找DNA结构以更好地了解衰老过程充满兴趣。端粒的缩短是指位于染色体末端的DNA蛋白质结构缩短，已被提议作为老化的生物标志物。新兴的研究发现端粒缩短与加速老化、年龄相关性疾病（如心血管疾病、癌症和痴呆）的发展、身体功能下降和早期死亡有关。然而，研究方法和种群差异性使得研究结果尚无法验证。最近的综述结果表明，端粒长度被证明是衰老的生物标志物，相比实足年龄，端粒长度是预测寿命、预测与正常老化相关的躯体和认知功能下降，或死亡率的较好指标，但上述结论迄今为止尚不确切。未来还需要进一步进行纵向研究，以探讨端粒长度缩短的终身作用，以及包括感染，生活方式的行为，如吸烟、体重指数、酒精摄入和环境风险在内的影响因素。

（二）慢性炎症和炎性衰老

衰老的细胞和器官与年龄有关疾病的共同特征是慢性炎症。慢性、低度、系统性的不可控炎症，被称为炎性衰老，已被认为是一个重要的中老年人疾病发病率和死亡率的危险因素。急性炎症是组织修复的一个重要目的，而炎性衰老虽没有发生感染，却可以导致广泛的组织损伤和变性。正常情况下，当机体应对各种压力时，会由于应激反应而产生抗体，形成促炎状态，而炎性衰老和机

due to buildup of antigens from the stress response. Inflammageing is a determinant of the rate of the aging process and the lifespan and is highly related to Alzheimer's disease, Parkinson's disease, acute lateral sclerosis, multiple sclerosis, atherosclerosis, heart disease, age-related macular degeneration, insulin resistance, type 2 diabetes, osteoporosis, cancer, and other diseases, and increases morbidity and mortality.

There are two primary features of inflammageing that it not only is associated with decreased immune function but also increases the auto-reactivity of the body. Thus, the immune function is both weakened in response to infections or trauma, and over-reactive, which is associated with development of immune-related conditions. There are several proposed mechanisms of inflammageing. Stress theory suggests that stress is a strong component of immune function where in older persons, the immune response is decreased as a result of immuno-senescence, compared to the more robust immune response in younger persons, which is accompanied by a shift to a chronic pro-inflammatory state. Chronic, cumulative stress (physiological and psychosocial) and persistent activation of the stress response and numerous neuroendocrine and metabolic pathways leads to inflammageing. Oxidative stress and damage from free radicals are also processes that contribute to inflammageing. Pro-inflammatory cytokines play an important role in inflammageing, where elevate levels pro-inflammatory cytokines such as TNF-alpha, IL-1 IL-6, CD 4 and CD8 are associated with immune-inflammatory diseases and mortality. Another proposed mechanisms are a persistent DNA damage response caused by telomere shortening that contributes to senescence and inflammageing. Other mechanisms include failure of autophagy or the removal of harmful substances in cells in order to maintain homeostasis, and stem cell aging and dysfunctional differentiation of stem cells. Taken together, these mechanisms indicate that inflammageing is a complex biologic process that results from the combined effects of many factors.

iii. Application of the Inflammageing Theory

Lifestyle factors that may contribute to inflammageing include high fat, high carbohydrate, high calorie diet, excessive consumption of processed and fast foods, trans fatty acids, saturated fatty acids, omega-6 polyunsaturated fatty acids, inadequate sleep, low physical activity, and chronic psychosocial stress. Addressing these modifiable issues to reduce the systemic inflammatory response may alleviate or attenuate inflammation. The

体的这一能力下降有关。炎性衰老是老化进程和寿命的决定因素，同时和多种疾病高度相关，如阿尔茨海默病、帕金森病、急性侧索硬化症、多发性硬化症、动脉硬化、心脏病、老年性黄斑变性、胰岛素抵抗、2型糖尿病、骨质疏松症、癌症等，可增加这些疾病的发病率和死亡率。

免疫衰老有两个主要特点：免疫衰老与免疫功能下降有关，但也增加了身体的自动反应。因此，在对抗感染或创伤的反应中，人体的免疫功能减弱，而过度反应则与免疫相关疾病的发展相关。关于免疫衰老的机制有几种假设。应激理论提出，应激是免疫功能的一个重要组成部分，相比年轻人的免疫应答，老年人由于免疫衰老，免疫应答降低，同时伴有向慢性促炎症状态转变的过程。慢性累积压力（包括生理和心理）、压力应对的持续激活，以及众多的神经内分泌和代谢途径，最终导致了免疫衰老。氧化应激和自由基损伤是导致免疫衰老的过程。促炎细胞因子在免疫衰老中起着重要的作用，高水平的促炎细胞因子，如TNF-α、IL-1、IL-6、CD4细胞，与免疫炎症性疾病和死亡率相关。另一种机制是持续的DNA损伤反应造成端粒缩短，进而导致衰老和免疫功能衰弱。其他机制包括自噬障碍或细胞内有害物质的清除障碍，从而难以维持细胞内平衡，干细胞衰老和干细胞的分化功能失调。总之，这些机制表明，免疫衰老是一个由多种因素综合作用的复杂生物学过程。

（三）免疫衰老理论的应用

生活方式的因素，包括高脂肪、高碳水化合物、高热量饮食，加工食品和快餐食品的过度消费，反式脂肪酸、饱和脂肪酸、ω-6多不饱和脂肪酸，睡眠不足，低体力活动和慢性心理社会压力，可能促进免疫衰老。解决这些可纠正问题，可降低全身炎症反应，从而缓解或减轻炎症反应。如前所述，研究

Mediterranean diet, green tea, and resveratrol, as described previously, have been studied for their antioxidant and inhibitory effects on inflammageing. Zinc is an important mineral that regulates the immune-inflammatory reaction. Moderate zinc supplementation in addition to the diet may impact inflammageing and increase the lifespan. Metformin, a hypoglycemic drug that is prescribed to treat type 2 diabetes and metabolic syndrome has been studied as an antiaging drug to increase the health span. The mechanisms underlying the antiaging effects remain unclear but there is some evidence that metformin may induce metabolism associated with dietary restriction to increase lifespan and limit the onset of diseases. The Chinese traditional medicines, epimedium total flavonoids (EF) and icariin (Ica), were able to reduce inflammation and regulate immunity and inflammageing by establishing new equilibrium in the network of pro-and anti-inflammatory cytokines and receptors in animal studies. Research is ongoing to determine the implications of these approaches in diverse human populations.

者已研究了地中海饮食、绿茶、白藜芦醇等物质在免疫衰老中的抗氧化和抑制作用。锌是调节免疫炎症反应的重要矿物质。除了饮食外，补充适量的锌会影响免疫衰老，并增加寿命。用于治疗2型糖尿病和代谢综合征的降糖药物——二甲双胍，已被作为一种可延长寿命的抗衰老药物研究。二甲双胍抗衰老作用的机制尚不清楚，但有一些证据表明，该药物可引起与代谢相关的饮食限制，从而增加寿命，限制疾病的发生。动物实验显示，中国传统药材淫羊藿总黄酮（EF）和淫羊藿苷（Ica）通过在促炎因子、抗炎因子以及受体的网络中建立新的平衡，能够减少炎症、调节免疫和免疫衰老。研究还在持续以确定这些方法在不同人群中的影响。

Section 2 Psychological Development Theories

Psychological development theories of aging have explained the aging process in terms of behavior, personality, and attitude change. These theories view aging as a lifelong developmental process accompanied by transitions and adaptations to changes in health status and in the physical and social environment from middle to late life. The theories focus on personality or ego development, memory, learning capacity, mental process, emotions, intellectual functioning, and adaptation to physical and social environments. This chapter describes five psychological theories of aging.

I. The Psychological Theory of Personality Development

Erik Erikson in 1950 proposed a theory of personality development, with a focus on the individual's ego structure. This theory provides an overview of personality development over time and the types of crises an individual encounters at each stage of development. Erickson describes the development of human personality through eight stages. Each stage is characterized by a crisis that affects the development

第二节　衰老的心理学理论

衰老的心理学理论从人的行为、态度等方面解释老化过程。这些理论认为衰老是一个终身的发展过程，从中年到晚年，始终伴随着对健康状况、物理和社会环境变化的过渡和适应。老年心理学理论关注老年人的人格、自我意识、记忆力、学习能力、思维过程、情绪、智力以及社会适应能力。本节介绍衰老的心理学理论中广为认可的五个理论。

一、人格发展理论

Erik Erikson在1950年提出了人格发展阶段论。该理论强调个体的自我意识结构，描述人格的形成和发展过程以及个体在人格发展的各个阶段所遇到的危机和需要解决的心理冲突。Erikson将人格发展过程分为8个阶段，只有解决前一个阶段的心理冲突、顺利完成该阶段的发展任务，才能解决现阶段所出现

of the individual's ego and requires that tasks in prior stages be completed successfully in order to resolve the present stage's crisis. According to Erikson, at each stage of life one encounters developmental tasks pertaining to biological, psychological and cultural factors. Successful achievement of these tasks leads to happiness and success in later tasks whereas failure to achieve these tasks leads to unhappiness, disapproval by society and difficulty with later tasks. The final stage of development, called maturity, refers to older adulthood (age 65 and up). At this stage, developmental tasks of maturity include adjusting to declines in physical function and health, adjusting to retirement and reduced income, coping with the death of a spouse, friends, and family, and facing death. Erikson refers to the crisis in this stage as ego-integrity versus despair, which is characterized by evaluating one's life and accomplishments. During this stage, older adults reflect on their lives and accomplishments as they move toward death. They reconcile conflict and accept the life they have lived and adapt to changing physical functioning.

Erickson uses the term integrity to refer to older adults' feeling of well-being or satisfaction with their life, even they have failures and limitations in their life, and they reconciled their regrets and reflected on their positive aspects of life. Individuals, who successfully resolve this stage of crisis achieve ego integrity, look back on life with satisfaction and face death without fear. The term despair refers to holding on to negativity and a deep sense of regret for the past or a lack of accomplishment. Older adults that do not resolve the crisis of despair look back at life in desperation, and are bitter because that they will not have time to accomplish their goals.

In 1997, Erikson added stage nine to the theory of personality development, called 'gero-transcendence', to address those who are aged 80 or older. At this stage, an older person develops high motivation to overcome difficulties in the past and prepare for death. With gero-transcendence, there develops a feeling of worth and a sense of peace and harmony. Gero-transcendence provides a new concept for understanding the process of aging and the transition into very old age.

Peck (1968), who expanded Erikson's eight stages of personality development theory earlier, categorized ego-integrity versus despair in three stages for older adults: ego differentiation versus work role preoccupation, body transcendence versus body preoccupation, and ego transcendence versus ego preoccupation. During the stage of ego differentiation versus work role preoccupation,

的危机。如果顺利完成人格发展各个阶段的任务，个体就会在下一阶段体验到幸福和成就感；如果未完成某阶段的任务，则会导致个体的不幸福感，并会出现不被社会认同的行为和心理体验，造成下一阶段人格发展的障碍。人格发展的最后一阶段是指老年期（65岁及以上）。在这一阶段，老年人的生理、心理以及社交方面发生很大变化。老年阶段的人格发展任务包括适应身体功能的衰退和健康问题，适应退休以及收入减少的生活，应对丧偶，面对死亡。Erikson 将这一阶段的人格发展冲突描述为自我完整与失望。人格发展最后阶段的特征是回顾及评价个人的经历和成就。老年人需要接受自己的经历并适应身体功能的改变。

Erikson 用自我完整来形容老年人体验到的幸福和满足感。即使人生存有失败和遗憾，也能接受并关注积极的方面，成功地解决此阶段的危机，可达到自我完整。此阶段出现的失望源于老年人对人生的消极态度，感到遗憾或缺乏成就感。由于老年人觉得自己已经没有时间去弥补或达成自己的人生目标，因此他们会充满绝望和苦涩。如此，则认为其没有很好地完成此阶段的人格发展任务。

1997 年，Erikson 进一步完善了人格发展理论，增加了人格发展的第 9 个阶段，称为超越老年阶段。这一阶段指 80 岁及以上的老年期，是人生最后的阶段，老年人会运用人格发展动力来克服人生所经历的困难，从而坦然面对死亡。高龄老年人在超越老年阶段会发展出平静和谐的心态。超越老年阶段提供给我们一个理解衰老过程的新概念。

Peck（1968）较早地扩展了 Erikson 的人格发展理论的八个阶段，将老年人的自我完整与绝望分为三个阶段：自我分化与工作角色的专注，身体超越与身体的专注，自我超越与自我的关注。在自我分化与工作角色的专注之间，老年人通过退休后有意义的生活活

older adults achieve identity and a feeling of worth from meaningful life activities after retirement, instead of from work. The stage of body transcendence versus body preoccupation refers to older adults' perception of physical changes in the aging process. At this stage, the task is to cope with the functional decline of aging and to maintain physical and psychological well-being. In the last stage, ego transcendence versus ego preoccupation, older adults accept and prepare for death. Later, Tornstam (1989-2011) elaborated gero-transcendence theory which described a series of changes or developments that include a redefinition of the self and of relationships with others and new understandings of existential questions. Gero-transcendence theory suggests that aging includes a potential to mature into a new outlook and understanding of life and a shift from a materialistic and rational view of the world to a more transcendent one along with increased life satisfaction. This theory is differentiated from activity and disengagement theory by focusing on new growth based on introspection and a shift in perspective that increasingly values a sense of meaning or purpose in life, self-acceptance, altruism, connectedness to self and others in a deeper less superficial way, a greater feeling of connection to the universe, appreciation for the sacred and rejoicing in simple pleasures, generativity or living on through one's contributions and to influence future generations and decreased fear of death. This theory balances the challenges and losses associated with aging with greater opportunities for solitude and increased wisdom and knowledge gained from life experience. In China, the concept of transcendence is relevant to Confucianism, Daoism, and similar belief systems in Chinese culture.

Application of Personality Development Theory

Erikson's theory has been widely used as a framework for examining the challenges at each developmental stage. Research has shown that successful resolution of psychosocial crises at each stage leads to life satisfaction in late life. In a study that examined Erikson's resolution of Stage 8 (ego-integrity versus despair) and Stage 9 (gero-transcendence) in older (60-70 years) and very old adults (80-90 years), Brown and Lewis (2003) found a correlation between very older age and resolution of Stage 9 (gero-transcendence), suggesting the potential for psychological and spiritual growth during the entire life span.

According to traditional Chinese culture, persons aged 60 years and older should focus on achieving

动而不是工作来获得认同感和价值感。身体超越与专注于身体的阶段是指老年人对衰老过程中身体变化的感知。在这一阶段，任务是应对衰老的功能下降，并保持身心健康。在最后阶段，自我超越与自我专注，老年人接受并为死亡做准备。后来，Tornstam（1989—2011年）详细说明了超越老年理论的应用，他描述了这一阶段一系列的变化和发展，包括对自我与他人关系进行重新定义，以及对人类存在主义问题的新理解。超越老年理论认为老化包括从潜在的成熟到一个新的展望，对生活的理解，以及从唯物主义的理性世界观到随着生活满意度提高而来的更超越的世界观。不同于活动和脱离理论，这一理论以反思和转变的角度为基础，更加着眼于生命的价值感和意义或目的、自我接纳、利他主义、深化自我和他人的表面关系、深化个体与宇宙之间的关联性、通过简单的方式欣赏快乐和神圣、繁衍生息或通过个人贡献生存、影响后世和减少对死亡的恐惧。这个理论平衡了与衰老相关的挑战和损失，带来了更多的独处机会，并且增加了从生活经验中获得的智慧和知识。在中国，超越的概念与儒家、道教，以及中国文化中相似的信仰系统有关。

人格发展理论的应用

Erikson的理论已被广泛用作应对各发展阶段挑战的理论框架。研究表明，在每个阶段成功解决社会心理危机都会改善晚年生活满意度。Brown和Lewis（2003）的一项在老年人（60~70岁）和高龄老年人（80~90岁）的研究中发现（Erikson理论的第8阶段和第9阶段），高龄组与第9阶段的决断力之间存在相关性，表明整个生命周期内心理和精神成长的持续性。

根据中国的传统文化，年过六十，老年人可着眼于实现和谐、智慧，将知识传授给

harmony and wisdom, passing knowledge on to the next generation, Along these lines, suggestions to promote gero-transcendence include the following aspects:

a. Understand and respect that older persons can have different perceptions of time;

b. Encourage older persons to talk about their past and how they developed through their life experiences;

c. Let older people decide whether to be alone or participate in activities.

II. Maslow's Hierarchy of Human Needs

According to the hierarchy of human needs theory generated by Maslow (1943), human needs are ordered based on priorities which are graphically depicted in a triangle. Maslow's theory suggests that the most basic needs must be met before a person will be motivated to focus on the next higher level needs and implies that psychological growth is a linear, stepwise process. At the base of the triangle are basic human needs which are essential for life in the biological and physiological realm. These needs include food, water, air, sleep, and appropriate ambient temperature for survival. When these needs are met, safety and security needs emerge at the next higher level followed by feelings of belongingness and affection, esteem for self and respect from others, and finally, self-actualization or the process of a person becoming what he or she really and uniquely is, at the peak of the pyramid. Questions have arisen about the hierarchy of needs and suggest that it may be possible to achieve higher order needs despite deficits in lower order needs. For example, can self-actualization occur in the context of poverty and inadequate food? In recent research that operationalized and tested Maslow's theory using modified definitions for each of the needs in a Chinese population, the hierarchy of the needs was validated, whereas, the attainment of the higher need was predicted by achievement of the preceding need. In addition, family support, traditional values, and life satisfaction were significantly correlated with satisfaction of all five needs, and anxiety and worry were negatively correlated with satisfaction of all of the needs. Although some critiques of Maslow's theory assert that the hierarchy of needs was based on Western culture, this study supports the generality of the theory in an Eastern culture.

下一代，沿着这些思路，建议促进超越老年的方法包括：

a. 理解和尊重老年人可以有不同的时间观；

b. 鼓励老年人谈论他们的过去和他们如何通过自己的生活经验取得发展；

c. 让老年人决定是否独处或参与活动。

二、马斯洛的人类需要层次

根据马斯洛在 1943 年提出的人类需要层次理论，人的需要是基于一个三角形图形化的优先顺序进行排序的。马斯洛的理论认为，只有最基本的需要得到满足之后，一个人才会被激励专注于下一个更高层次的需要，该理论暗示，心理需要增长是一个线性的、逐步的过程。在三角形的底层是人类最基本的需要，也是生物和生理方面最重要的需要。这些需要包括食物、水、空气、睡眠和适宜的环境温度，以供生存。当这些需要得到满足时，下一个更高水平上的安全需要才会出现，之后是对归属感和爱、自我尊重和来自他人的尊重的需要，最后是自我实现的需要，这也是一个人成为真正的和唯一的个体的需要，是最高层次的需要。需要层次的结构并不绝对，可能低层次的需要尚未满足，个体就实现了更高层次的需要。例如，个体是否能在贫穷和缺少食物的状况下，获得自我实现。一项最近的研究是在中国人群中使用每个需要的修改定义进行调查，从而对马斯洛理论的可操作性进行验证。该研究显示需要层次论被证实，同时，可通过上一层次的需求满足情况来预测更高层次的需求。此外，家庭支持、传统的价值观、生活满意度和所有五个需求的满意度显著相关，而焦虑、担心和所有五个需求的满意度呈负相关。尽管一些马斯洛理论的批评者认为，需求层次理论是基于西方文化建立的，但这项研究支持了马斯洛理论在东方文化中的推广性。

Application of Maslow's Hierarchy of Needs

It is important for nurses to consider the older person's current level of need and unmet needs when considering different types of behavioral changes for maximizing self-care and outcomes. In the context of hospice care, Maslow's hierarchy was modified to include (a) distressing symptoms such as pain and dyspnea; (b) fears for physical safety, of dying or abandonment; (c) affection, love, and acceptance in the face of devastating illness; (d) esteem, respect, and appreciation for the person; and (e) self-actualization and transcendence. Maslow's hierarchy of needs theory has been used in nursing to plan care for older adults; however, older adult heterogeneity and personal preferences and desires may result in nonlinear and iterative movement along the hierarchy. For example, the desire for autonomy, which is a component of self-actualization, may take precedence over lower level needs such as safety and security, as in the situation whereby an older person may choose to be independent and autonomous in daily activities and accept a higher fall risk at the expense of safety needs in order to resist dependence. Helping older adults maintain autonomy and self-esteem as dependency needs increase is important to support motivations for self-actualization.

III. Selective Optimization with Compensation Model

Baltes (1990) developed a model of successful aging, the selective optimization with compensation model (SOC), which describes changes in resources and goals in the life course in older adults. In early adulthood, the individual usually focuses on personal gain and growth as major goals in life. However, as we age, the focus of life shifts toward minimizing declines and maximizing resources.

The theory proposes that aging is a psychological process through which older adults cope with the changes associated with aging and achieve successful aging. In the successful aging model, older adults confront declining function and limited resources and select the most important and realistic goals within their limited resources. Older adults' mental, physical, and environmental resources are limited; for example, age-related functioning declines occur which require older adults to allocate these limited resources to activities that seem most important

马斯洛需要层次论的应用

当考虑通过不同类型的行为改变以达到最大化自我护理和结果时，护士要关注老年人当前的需求水平和未满足的需求。在临终关怀的过程中，马斯洛需要层次论的内容可进行调整，即第一层次为痛苦症状，如疼痛和呼吸困难；第二层次为对身体安全的担心和对死亡、遗弃的恐惧；第三层次为面对绝症时的情感、爱和接受度；第四层次为自尊、尊重和对人的欣赏；第五层次为自我实现和超越。马斯洛的层次结构已被用于照顾老年人的护理计划中，然而，老年人的异质性和个人喜好以及愿望可能会导致沿层次结构的非线性和迭代运动。例如，对自主性的需要，是自我实现的一个组成部分，其可能优先于较低层次的需要，如安全性。在这种情况下，老年人可能选择独立和自主的日常活动，并以牺牲安全需要为代价，接受更高的跌倒风险，从而避免独立性的丧失。在老年人依赖他人的需要增加的同时，帮助老年人保持自主性和自尊，从而支持自我实现的动机是非常重要的。

三、SOC模式——选择、资源利用和补偿模式

Baltes 提出了一个成功衰老的模式：选择、资源利用和补偿模式。这一模式描述了老年人在整个人生中资源利用和人生目标的变化。在成年早期，个体通常将成就和成长作为人生的主要目标。随着年龄的增加，人生目标转向减慢身体功能衰退和充分利用资源。

这一理论认为老化是一个心理变化的过程。在这个过程中，老年人要应对衰老所带来的身心改变，并顺利地度过老年。该模式指出，老年人面临身体功能下降和有限的资源，要选择最主要且最实际的目标努力。老年人的生理、心理、精神及其他资源往往有限，如老年人的身体功能下降，因而需要重新分配有限的资源去做一些对老年人来说相

and within their capability like performing daily activities of living, remembering taking medication instead of participating social activities. The model proposed three strategies to successfully cope with these changes or losses. Baltes and Dickson (2001) defined successful development as "the maximization of desirable outcomes and the minimization of undesirable outcomes".

Older adults are more selective in the activities and roles that fit with their function and capability because their physical, mental and social resources and some of their activities and roles are limited. They change their focus and goals to cope with the changes related to aging. For example, older adults change their life goals from completing education and job promotion to mastering hobbies, engaging in cultural activities, or increasing their volume of exercise. Attention and memory decline in older adults, as thus the selection of tasks may change to daily living tasks, such as performing self-care activities instead of pursuing income opportunities.

Optimization refers to the use of strategies to achieve goals to enrich life. For example, if an older adult has a heart attack, he or she may not be able to perform daily activities or maintain an optimal level of functioning and may require help from another person, such as hiring a sitter to have their basic needs being taken care. The older adult is optimizing his or her existing functional ability to maintain its best-possible functioning.

Compensation refers to the use of strategies to achieve a goal or maintain status when functional decline occurs in late life. Older adults perform more activities in order to maintain health and independence. For example, such as monitoring tools to remember to take medications if they have mild memory problems.

Lang, Rieckmann, and Baltes (2002) used the SOC model to examine adaptation to aging loss in everyday functioning in older adults. Their study examined selection, compensation, and optimization in everyday activities over a 4-year period among older adults with more resources and those with fewer resources.

Selection was defined as reduced activities, goals or domains with focus on important areas in everyday life. Selection also included leisure activities, such as playing sports, reading, helping others by visiting or talking to others. When older adults faced aging loss, they coped with the situation by reducing activities and concentrating on those activities that were more meaningful to them and most relevant to their goals. The authors found that this

对重要且力所能及的事情，如放弃参与社交活动而重点关注个人的日常生活，记住每日服药。为此，该模式提出了应对老化过程中的改变与衰退的 3 种策略，即选择、资源利用和补偿。Baltes 和 Dickson（2001）将成功的发展定义为"期望结果的最大化和不期望结果的最小化"。

由于生理、心理、社会资源受到限制，老年人应该选择与自身功能及能力相适应的活动，通过改变努力的目标来适应老化。例如，老年人改变过去要完成大学学位或工作晋升的人生目标，而是参加文娱活动，增加体育锻炼。由于注意力和记忆力的衰退，老年人可放弃工作，而选择居家进行自我照料。

资源利用是指运用恰当的方法达到目标以丰富生活。例如，患有心脏病的老年人在日常生活中可能无法自理，也无法维持最佳的身体功能状态，需要他人的照顾及协助才能维持其功能，在这种情况下，老年人可选择利用周围的资源来维持最佳的身体状态。

补偿是指在身体功能逐渐衰退时恰当地使用各种资源达到目标或维持现有的状态。例如，老年人通过锻炼来维持健康和自立；健忘的老年人通过使用服药计时器帮助按时服药并促进记忆。

Lang，Rieckmann 和 Baltes（2002）使用 SOC 模型考察了老年人在日常生活中的应对情况，调查了资源丰富和资源匮乏的老年人在 4 年内的日常活动。

研究发现老年人会通过减少活动并专注于对他们而言更有意义的活动来应对衰老后活动减少的状况。例如减少休闲时间，有助于老年人维持必需的日常活动并维持健康。补偿是指老年人更加集中精力于维持健康的基本活动。例如，老年人可以通过增加休息或睡眠来补充体力。日常功能的优化被定义为最大化利用老年人选择的资源。如老年人

type of selection, say limiting leisure time activities, helped older adults to maintain resources for daily activities and maintain health. Compensation referred to the use of new strategies to focus on essential activities to maintain health when older adults lost a level of functioning. For example, older adults might compensate for aging losses in everyday life with more rest or sleep to enhance their resources. Optimization in everyday functioning was defined as strategies to maximize the resources that older adults selected. Older adults engaged more in physical activities, cultural, intellectual and social leisure activities, and when older adults chose the activities, spending time with friends, gardening or playing sports, or reading were more satisfying (optimization).

This study found that participants with more resources were more likely to use more strategies in selection, compensation, and optimization in everyday activities, and they were more likely to survive after 4 years than those with fewer resources. Older adults with rich resources showed more selectivity in everyday activities, more contact with family members during the day and less diversity in leisure time activities than those with poor resources. Older adults in the resources-rich group showed an increased number and duration of sleep periods during the day. Survivors after four years reported that they had more housekeeping activities, as well as intellectual, cultural, physical, social leisure activities. Older adults in the non-survivor group with poor resources reported that they spent more time in passive activities, less time on work, but had greater variety in leisure activities. The authors concluded that older adults with rich resources showed greater use of strategies of selection, compensation and optimization in everyday functioning than older adults with poor resources.

IV. Cognitive Plasticity Theory

Recently, cognitive plasticity has become an area of interest in both developmental psychology and neuropsychology. Plasticity refers to an individual's ability to acquire cognitive skills. The theory of cognitive plasticity proposes that an individual has latent cognitive potential for adaptation and change, in order to learn cognitive skills and maintain cognitive functions. This theory is linked to life span developmental psychology theory, in which development at all stages of life is considered as modifiable or plastic.

更乐于参加体育活动和社会活动，当老年人选择这些活动时，可与朋友共度时光；园艺、阅读等活动也会使老年人更愉悦。

这项研究发现，拥有更多资源的参与者更有可能在选择，补偿和优化日常活动中使用更多策略，并且与那些拥有较少资源的参与者相比，他们在4年后生存的可能性更高。与资源贫乏的人相比，资源富裕组在日常活动中表现出更大的选择性，在白天与家人的接触更多，闲暇活动更少。资源丰富组白天的睡眠次数和持续时间增加。四年后的幸存者报告说，他们进行了更多的家政活动，以及智力、文化、身体、社交休闲活动。非幸存者群体中资源贫乏的老年人报告说，他们在消极活动上花费的时间更多，在工作上花费的时间更少，但休闲活动的种类更多。作者得出的结论是，资源丰富的老年人比资源贫乏的老年人在日常工作中显示出更多的选择、补偿和优化策略。

四、弹性认知理论

弹性认知理论是目前老年发展心理学和老年神经心理学的研究重点。这里的"弹性"是指个体依靠自身的能力去获得认知的技能。弹性认知理论提出每个人都有适应环境改变的认知潜力。弹性认知的基本假设是，人的一生在维持基本认知能力的基础上不断学习新的认知技能。这一假设与心理学中的人格发展理论相一致。人格发展理论认为人生的每一个发展阶段都是可调整的或有弹性的。

Life span theory views biological development as it occurs in early life and decreases with age. According to the theory, an individual's development depends more on culture in early and middle adulthood. However, due to biological aging, the influence of culture on one's development diminishes. From cognitive plasticity perspective, individuals are able to improve their cognition through learning and practice. An individual's current level of cognitive functioning and potential ability or capacity is affected by both social interactions and training exercises. The theory of cognitive plasticity proposes that cognitive aging reflects the modifiability or development of an individual's cognition through life conditions and experiences. Cognitive functions require strong neural networks. Exposure to external stimuli, for example, environmental opportunities can stimulate neural networks in the brain and improve cognitive functioning. Vance and Crowe (2006) proposed several strategies to maintain cognitive function or decrease age-related cognitive loss. These strategies include living a healthy life-style, engaging in mentally stimulating activities such as educational pursuits, novel experiences, and participating in cognitive remediation. A healthy lifestyle provides the physiological foundation to support neuronal health and therefore to improve cognitive functioning. Chronic diseases such as hypertension and diabetes may increase cognitive decline. Maintaining a healthy diet with a high intake of antioxidants and physical exercise have been associated with improved cognitive functioning in older adults.

Vance and colleagues (2008) suggested that mental stimulation can help maintain or improve cognitive functioning, and education has been associated with cognitive functioning in older adults. Older individuals with advanced education show less or a lower rate of cognitive impairment and dementia in late life because of neural connections that occurred while learning what could improve cognitive functioning or decrease age-related cognitive decline.

Nurses play an important role in education and interventions for older adults who are at risk of cognitive impairment. Nurses can teach adults about how to promote successful cognitive aging. For example, they can provide information on performing regular exercise and maintaining a healthy diet with more vegetables and fruits. They also can encourage older adults to use mental stimulation activities, such as continuing education pursuits, learning a second language, playing a musical instrument or working on a word or math puzzle.

人格发展理论认为个体的人格发展开始于早年并随着年龄增长而变化，这是由于个体发展受到了文化的影响。然而随着年龄的增长，文化对人格发展的影响逐渐减退。弹性认知理论认为每个人都有通过学习与实践提高自身认知水平的能力，社会互动和训练可以影响一个人现有的和潜在的认知水平。弹性认知理论认为，老化即个体通过生活条件和经验调整或发展个人认知能力的过程。大脑是认知功能发展的基础，外界环境的刺激可以提高大脑的认知功能。Vance 和 Crowe（2006）提出了维持认知功能、减缓衰老所致的认知衰退的策略，其中包括健康的生活方式、接受教育、体验新经历和参加认知功能锻炼活动等。健康的生活方式能够从生理上维持神经系统的健康、改善认知功能。如高血压、糖尿病等慢性疾病会加速认知功能衰退，而保持健康的饮食结构以及摄入足量的抗氧化剂可以提高老年人的认知功能。

Vance（2008）和他的同事认为对大脑的刺激能够帮助维持或提高认知功能。研究显示，受过教育的老年人在晚年出现认知功能障碍或老年痴呆的可能性较未受教育的人群低。这是因为学习可促使大脑神经元之间建立起联系，从而提高了认知功能。

护士对患有认知障碍的高危老年人的教育和干预起重要作用。护士可以对成年人进行如何促进正确认知衰老的宣教。例如，护士可以提供有关进行定期运动及多吃蔬菜和水果以保持健康饮食的信息。护士还可以鼓励老年人做刺激大脑的活动，如继续教育、学习第二种语言、弹奏乐器或拼单词或解数学难题。

Section 3　Sociological Theories

Sociological theories explain older adults' behavior in the context of society and view changing roles, relationships and aging from a cultural or societal perspective. Early theories focused on the losses in later life and more recent theories focus on social structure as the major factor influencing an individual's life course. Social structures include family, religion, cultural traditions, norms, and expectations, ethics, morals, economics, income, education, social expectations, social status and social support systems. Five major sociological theories of aging include disengagement theory, activity theory, continuity theory, socioemotional selectivity theory, and person-environment fit theory. The first three theories focus on the role changes as we age and adjust to the changes. Person-environment fit theory emphasizes an individual's personal interactions with the society or environment. Socioemotional selectivity theory refers to how personal and social relationships and goals are determined based on the person's perception of time remaining to be lived in the future.

I. Disengagement Theory

Disengagement theory was the earliest and considered the most controversial theory of aging. Cumming and Henry (1961) proposed in disengagement theory that aging is characterized by a natural withdrawal from society and a greater focus on personal meaning. Withdrawal behavior is desired by older adults and the society. Individuals change their role from society-centered to self-centered for maintenance of social equilibrium. According to this theory, the disengagement process is mutual and beneficial to both older individuals and society. However, many gerontologists have argued that engagement in meaningful relationships and activities is important for the satisfaction with life and well-being of older adults. This theory has been criticized for lack of consideration of individual differences in sociocultural settings and environmental factors. Withdrawal from society varies in older individuals, indeed, many older adults remain active and involved in society. Therefore, there is little research evidence to support the theory.

第三节　衰老的社会学理论

社会发展理论从文化和社会的角度来诠释老年人的角色转变及其对社会环境变化的适应，而衰老的社会学理论即在社会背景下解释老年人的行为。早期的理论着重于晚年的损失，而最新的理论则着重于社会结构，社会学理论认为社会结构是影响人一生的主要因素。社会结构包括家庭、信仰、文化传统、文化价值、社区文化传统和价值、道德、伦理、经济、收入、教育、社会期望、社会地位及社会家庭支持系统。五个主要的衰老社会学理论有隐退理论（角色退出理论）、活动理论、持续理论、人 - 环境适应理论和社会情绪选择理论。前三个理论主要描述老年人的角色转换与调整，而人 - 环境适应理论则强调人与社会环境的相互作用。社会情绪选择理论指的是基于个人对未来寿命的预期，个人与社会的关系和目标是如何确定的。

一、隐退理论

隐退理论是最早提出的，同时也是最具争议的衰老社会学理论。该理论由 Cumming 和 Henry 提出，认为老年的特征就是从社会中退出并把精力集中于个人。这种隐退的行为也是老年人和整个社会所期望的。老年人的个体角色从以社会为中心转变为以自我为中心，以此维持社会平衡。根据这一理论，从社会中退出对老年人和社会都有益处。但是，许多老年学专家认为，老年人从事有意义的社会活动和由此带来的幸福满足感有助于老年人保持身心健康，因此这一理论遭到了许多学者的批判，认为此理论未考虑到社会文化环境对个体的影响。老年人是否完全从社会角色中退出也取决于不同个体，事实上许多老年人退休之后仍活跃在社会活动当中。目前，支持该理论的研究证据依然不足。

II. Activity Theory

Unlike disengagement theory, activity theory posits that activity is important in maintaining life satisfaction and a positive self-concept in older adults. Activity may be physical or intellectual. Older adults who are actively engaged in social activities stay young, and they do not withdraw from society. According to activity theory, activity is associated with psychosocial well-being and it delays the negative effects of aging. This theory suggests that even when older individuals suffer from illness, they can maintain their activity and be satisfied with life. Many studies have supported activity theory. One study showed cultural activities and interacting with children and grandchildren were associated with well-being among older adults, while watching television and listening to the radio were negatively associated with well-being. Active engagement in social activities is considered a healthy way of coping with stress for older adults. Critics of activity theory state that it overlooks iniquities in health and socioeconomics that impede the ability for older people to engage in activities and disregards personal preferences of older adults and the fact that some do not wish to participate in new activities.

III. Continuity Theory

Continuity theory was developed by Havighurst, Neugarten and Tobin (1963) to reconcile the contrasting disengagement and activity theories. A central premise of continuity theory is that old age is not a final or separate part of life, but that the later years of life are an integral component of the life cycle. From this perspective, adults maintain the same personalities, values, morals, preferences, role activity, behaviors, and relationships across the life span regardless of life change. Older adults maintain continuity by applying strategies used in middle life to adapt to changes associated with normal aging. Later life is simply a continuation of earlier adulthood. Atchley (1989) later advanced continuity theory, proposing that individuals maintain both internal psychological structure and external structure in the social and physical environment and use adaptive choices to cope with changes, producing a sense of continuity between life in the past and current life.

Havighurst and colleagues (1963) described four types of personality in older adults: integrated, armored-defended, passive dependent, and un-integrated. A person with an integrated personality engages in activities and

二、活跃理论

与隐退理论相反，活跃理论认为活动对维持老年人的生活满意度和自我认可非常重要。理论中提到的活动是指体力或脑力活动。根据活跃理论，老年人并未从社会退出，而是通过积极参加社会活动来保持年轻。另外，活跃理论还认为老年人即使患有疾病也可以继续参加社会活动，保持对生活的满意度。很多研究均支持活跃理论，认为老年人积极参加社会活动是一种缓解压力的方式。研究表明，文娱活动、与家人相聚等活动可以让老年人有幸福感，而看电视、听广播则对幸福感具有负面影响。活动理论的批评者表示，该理论忽视了健康和社会经济状况的不公平性，这种不公平会阻碍老年人参与活动，使老年人忽视个人喜好，此外还有一些老年人不愿意参加新的活动。

三、持续理论

持续理论是 Havighurst，Neugarten 和 Tobin 于 1963 年提出，调和了活跃理论和隐退理论的对立局面。持续理论的重要前提是人不论遇到什么样的人生变化，都应维持一致的人格、价值、道德、喜好、角色活动、行为和关系。晚期生活是对早期生活的持续，老年人可采取中年时期所用的方式适应衰老带来的正常变化，从而维持生活方式的连续性。研究表明，个体早年的休闲活动可以预测晚年的生活活动方式。1989 年，Atchley 发展了持续理论，指出个体应维持生理、心理、社会等内外环境的平衡，并且可运用恰当的应对方式来适应各种变化，从而联系现在与过去的生活，保持其连续性。

Havighurst 以及他的同事（1963）描述了老年人的 4 种人格类型，即完善型、防卫型、被动依赖型和非完善型。完善型的老年人积极

adjusts well to aging. Armored-defended individuals continue the activities and roles they used in middle adulthood, and passive-dependent persons are usually highly dependent or have less interest in the external world. Older individuals with un-integrated personalities have difficulty in adjusting with changes and coping with aging. This theory allows us to study aging in relation to an individual's behavior or personality in the past. What a person becomes in late life is a product of a lifetime of personal choices.

Efklides and colleagues (2003) examined the effects of demographics, health status, attitude, and adaptation to older age on quality of life among older adults. The findings showed that older adults who had a more positive attitude and adapted to aging perceived better quality of life. In another study, Agahi and colleagues (2006) used continuity theory as a framework for examining continuity of participation in leisure activities from middle age to old age. Congruent with the continuity theory, as well as disengagement and activity theories, active participation in leisure activities declined over time. Participation in leisure activities generally predicted activity patterns in late life.

IV. Person-Environment Fit Theory

Lawton's (1982) Person-Environment Fit Theory (P-E Fit) refers to the relationships between an older individual's competencies and the society or environment that leads to an individual's psychological well-being. Lawton's person-environment fit theory defines an individual's functional competence in the areas of biological health, sensation and perception, motor skills, and cognitive capacity. Individuals use these skills and competencies to interact with environment in which they live. Lawton states that individual competencies are reflected by their daily performance, such as breathing, walking, and ability to solve problems (intelligence). Individuals' competencies decrease with aging, and then influence their ability to interact with the environment. For example, if an individual suffers from chronic disease, his or her functional competencies will be affected, and this will lead to difficulties in adjusting to the environment. The model has been modified and personal resources, such as personality, have been added in recent years.

The P-E fit theory has been used in research to examine the interactions between person and environment as determinants of the satisfaction and well-being of older adults. Phillips and colleagues (2009) used person-environment fit theory to identify the perceptions

参加活动，能很好地适应衰老。防卫型的老年人会持续中年时的活动与角色。被动依赖型的老年人依赖性强，对外部世界缺乏兴趣。非完善型的老年人则难以适应和应对衰老所带来的变化。研究表明，态度积极的老年人生活质量较高。

Efklides 及其同事（2003）研究了人口统计学、健康状况、态度以及适应力对老年人生活质量的影响。调查结果表明，态度更积极、适应力更好的老年人的生活质量更高。在另一项研究中，Agahi 及其同事（2006）使用连续性理论作为框架来研究中老年到老年休闲活动的连续性。与连续性理论、脱节和活动理论相一致，休闲活动的积极参与随着时间的流逝而下降。参加休闲活动通常可以预测晚年的活动方式。

四、人－环境适应理论

Lawton（1982）的"人与环境适应"理论（P–E Fit）指老年人的能力与社会环境之间的关系，认为两者的良好关系可以促进老年人的幸福感和满足感。个体的功能性能力包括生理健康、感知觉、认知力和活动能力等，表现于呼吸、走路和解决问题（智力活动）等日常活动。个体可运用这些能力适应生活环境。然而个体的能力可随着衰老而降低，从而影响其与社会环境的相互作用。例如，老年人的功能性能力可受到慢性疾病的影响，患者则难以适应环境的变化。该模型已被修改，并且近年来增加了诸如个性之类的个人资源。

人－环境适应理论已广泛用于研究人与环境的相互作用对老年人满意度和幸福感的影响。Phillips 及其同事（2009）使用人与环境适应理论来研究中国香港老年人对生活环境

of older adults in Hong Kong on their fit with their living environment in regard to psychological well-being. In their study, characteristics of the person, environment and P-E fit were important predictors of satisfaction and psychological well-being among community-dwelling elders. Personal factors were conceptualized as age, education, health, and living arrangements; environmental factors were defined as housing type, age of housing area, housing structures, and environmental hazards; and cultural factors were filial piety and life stressors. The model proposes that personal and environmental factors, as well as cultural determinants, affect the residential satisfaction and psychological well-being of the older adults. The study showed that a model based on person-environment fit theory significantly predicted psychological well-being in older adults.

V. Socioemotional Selectivity Theory

Socioemotional selectivity theory (SST), proposed by Cartensen (1999), suggests that the perception of time plays a fundamental role in the selection and pursuit of social goals. SST is a lifespan theory of motivation that is grounded in the human ability to monitor time, to adjust time horizons with increasing age, and to appreciate that time eventually runs out. SST maintains that time horizons play a key role in motivation. When time is perceived as open-ended, knowledge-related goals such as acquiring new learning experiences, pursuit of employment, and building a careerare prioritized. In contrast, when time is perceived as limited, emotional goals become a priority and efforts to spend quality time with selected individuals increase. This is particularly salient in older persons who anticipate a shortened future than younger persons, and there is a shift from focusing on career and new life experiences to eliminating negative and less gratifying social relationships and focusing on closer, more meaningful relationships. The theory has also been applied to younger persons who have experienced life changing events and may face a different future than anticipated, either by shorter-than expected life expectancy, or changed circumstances such as disability or chronic illness, or traumatic experiences such as war or violence. According to the theory, diverse social goals, ranging from seeking the answer to a question to seeking emotional comfort, can be classified into one of two categories: those related to the acquisition of knowledge and those related to the regulation of emotion. As people age they become more aware of time and having more social contacts begins

的心理适应度。在他们的研究中，个体因素、环境和体育锻炼是社区老年人满意度和心理健康的重要预测指标。个体因素指年龄、教育程度、健康状况和生活方式；环境因素被定义为房屋类型、房屋面积、房屋结构和环境危害；文化因素是孝道和生活压力。该模型提出，个体因素、环境因素和文化因素都会影响到老年居民的满意度和心理健康，而应用人–环境适应理论可以预测老年人的心理健康。

五、社会情绪选择理论

社会情绪选择理论（SST）是 Cartensen 于 1999 年提出的，该理论指出个体对时间的感知对于其在选择和追求社会目标中起基础作用。社会情绪选择理论是一个和动机相关的寿命理论，其根据是人类随着年龄的增长，是具备管理时间、调整时间跨度的能力，并敬畏时间的流逝。社会情绪选择理论坚持时间跨度在动机中有重要作用。当时间被看作是开放式的，与知识相关的目标，如获得新的学习经验、追求就业、建立职业生涯，将被列为优先级。相反，当时间被认为是有限的，情感目标则成为一个优先选项。这一现象在老年人中特别突出，当老年人未来的预期寿命短于年轻人，就会有一个转变，即关注点从职业生涯、减少消极和不佳社会关系的生活经验，转向建立更密切、更有意义的关系。该理论也被应用到经历了生活事件改变的年轻人身上，其可能会面临和预期不同的未来，可能是预期寿命缩短，或是改变了环境（如残疾或慢性疾病），或是经历创伤（如战争或暴力）。根据该理论，不同的社会目标，可以从寻求问题的答案到寻求情感的舒适，因而目标可以分为两大类：与知识获取相关的目标和与情绪调节相关的目标。随

to feel superficial and less gratifying in contrast to the deepening ties of existing close relationships. As a result, older people elect to focus on fewer but more emotionally meaningful relationships and goals and not focus on or let go of the negative ones. Research has also found that older persons tend to prefer and remember emotionally positive information more than emotionally negative information.

Socioemotional selective theory may help explain reasons why the number of interpersonal relationships in older adults decreases more than the decrease in relationships caused by illness or death. The theory emphasizes the importance of supporting and promoting closer and meaningful relationships among older adults. The quality of interpersonal relationships is perceived more important than quantity. The older adults are more inclined to positive social information rather than negative one. When assisting the older adults to making plans and decisions, nurses should focus on positive and emotionally satisfying stimulus activities. However, the preference for positive stimuli may make the older adults vulnerable to fraud, exploitation and abuse. Therefore, nursing care for older adults should pay attention on information management and decision making to provide education with focus on positive outcomes.

Section 4　Implications for Nursing

Nurses can integrate theories of aging into practice when taking care of older adults. Using biological concepts, nurses can help older adults avoid risk factors, such as smoking, excessive consumption of alcohol or high fat high calorie diets, and exposure to air pollution and other environmental toxins to prevent the adverse effects of free radicals, cytokines, and inflammageing. Nurses can advise older adults to consume a balanced and healthy diet rich in antioxidants including fruits and vegetables, green tea, and omega fatty acids. They can encourage daily exercise, such as walking, swimming, chair-based activities, and tai chi for promotion of balance, physical function, falls prevention, and mental cognition. Managing stressors

着人们年龄的增长，他们越来越意识到时间有限，越来越觉得更多的社会交往开始变得肤浅和令人失望，同时会对现有亲密关系进一步加深。因此，老年人选择专注于较少，但情感上更有意义的关系和目标，而不是专注于负面的人际关系和目标，或是忘记这些负面人际关系。研究还发现，老年人倾向于喜爱和记住情感上积极的信息，而非情感上负面的信息。

社会情绪选择理论可能有助于解释为何老年期人际关系数量的减少比由于生病或死亡而造成的关系减少要多，该理论强调了支持和促进老年人亲密关系的重要性，关系的质量比数量具有更重要的意义。老年人更加倾向于积极的社会信息而非消极的社会信息，这表明在协助老年人制订计划和决策时，应着眼于积极的和情感上令老年人满意的刺激。然而，对积极刺激的偏好可能使老年人容易受到欺诈、剥削和虐待的影响，因此老年护理时应注意老年人如何进行信息管理和决策，以及如何制订患者教育以专注于积极及正面的效果。

第四节　衰老理论在护理工作中的应用

护士可以结合各种老化理论开展老年护理的工作。衰老的生物学理论可以提示护士自由基损伤细胞可导致老化。因此，护士可通过健康教育，让老年人学会避免一些危险因素，如吸烟、过量饮酒或高脂肪高热量饮食、暴露于空气污染和其他环境毒素，从而减少自由基、细胞因子和炎症的不利影响。另外，建议老年人保持健康平衡的饮食结构，摄入富含抗氧化剂的食物，包括水果和蔬菜、绿茶和 ω 脂肪酸等。鼓励老年人参加散步、座椅运动、放松训练、太极拳等日常锻炼，

in life can be facilitated by mindfulness meditation, stress reduction activities, spiritual or religious practices, and cultivating meaningful social networks. Applying the immune theory of aging, nurses can recognize that immune systems decrease with age, and encourage older adults to obtain influenza, pneumococcal, and herpes zoster vaccine, use good hand hygiene, and avoid infections.

Psychological theories of aging help nurses consider the developmental tasks and challenges faced by older adults. Learning new things, such as drawing Chinese pictures, practicing Chinese calligraphy, reading books, playing cards and board games and doing puzzles are important to preserve cognitive function. Exploring how to access resources and social networks on the internet can alleviate social isolation and boredom. Nurses can assist older adults to accept the meaning in their life and promote positive thinking and attitudes toward life through life review, reminiscence, and photo journaling. An important role of nurses is to help older adults feel satisfaction with the life they have lived and assist very old adults to successfully achieve gero-transcendence so they can accept and face death and have harmony in late life.

Using sociological theories of aging, nurses can assess older adults' social and cultural values and beliefs, economic status, life experiences and social support system, which may influence their adjustment to stresses encountered. Working with older adults in reviewing their life, nurses can use these adults' life experiences to understand their current health behaviors. Older adults who withdraw or disengage from society may have symptoms of depression. Nurses can encourage these older adults to attend social activities and physical activities to improve life satisfaction.

China has the largest and fastest growing aging population in the world. Providing high quality care to older adults in China presents challenges to nurses, who play an important role in promoting health and providing care to the aging population. Theories of aging can help nurses understand the aging process, older individuals' physiological, psychological, and social functions and needs, and the behaviors associated with aging. Biological theories help nurses to recognize physiological changes within the body as individual ages. Nurses can use knowledge to educate older adults to prevent or delay disease. By applying psychological theories of aging, nurses can help older adults and their family members

从而提高身体平衡性、保持躯体功能、促进精神健康和认知功能。通过正念冥想、压力减轻活动、精神或宗教实践，以及培养有意义的社交网络等方式，管理生活中的压力源。基于老化免疫的理论，人的免疫功能可随着年龄的增加而降低，因此，应鼓励老年人及时注射流行性感冒疫苗、肺炎球菌疫苗和带状疱疹疫苗，进行良好的手卫生，从而预防感染。

衰老的心理学理论提示在护理工作中应考虑到老年人可能面临的发展危机和挑战。鼓励老年人学习新事物，如书画、阅读、下棋、玩纸牌和下棋以及拼图等，以保持或促进老年人的认知功能。探索如何在互联网上访问资源和社交网络，从而缓解老年人的社会隔离和生活乏味。通过回顾人生、怀旧和照片日志等方式，帮助老年人接受他们的过去，积极面对生活。协助高龄老年人顺利度过超越老年阶段，使其能坦然地面对死亡，平静和谐地度过生命最后的日子。

衰老的社会学理论可指导护士对影响老年人适应能力的因素进行评估，这些因素包括社会文化价值、经济状况、生活经历和社会支持等。护士可与老年人一起回顾他们的人生经历，了解老年人目前的健康状况和健康行为。护士也应考虑到从社会隐退的老年人可能出现的抑郁问题，鼓励老年人参加力所能及的社会活动，坚持锻炼，从而提高其对生活的满意度。

中国是世界上老年人口增长最快的国家。在中国为老年人提供高质量的护理给护士带来了挑战，护士在促进健康和为老龄化人口提供护理方面发挥着重要作用。衰老理论可以帮助护士了解衰老过程，老年人的生理，心理和社会功能与需求以及与衰老相关的行为。生物学理论可帮助护士认识到个体年龄段的生理变化。护士可以利用知识来教育老年人预防或延迟疾病。通过应用衰老的心理学理论，护士可以帮助老年人及其家人了解

understand the life they have lived and the challenges they face and promote ego-integrity that contributes to the psychological well-being of older adults. They can assist older individuals who are at the developmental stage of despair to accept their life in the past and work with family members to reduce psychological stress and help the older adults move to a stage where they have a sense of satisfaction with life and feel peace and harmony. When providing patient care, nurses could apply sociological theories of aging to take into consideration the effects of culture, socioeconomic, spirit and social resources on older adults. Nurses are in a unique position to contribute to holistic care and promote quality of life among individuals in their last journey of life.

(HU, Jie, Deborah LEKAN)

Key Points

1. The aging process involves biological, psychological and sociological perspectives and there is no single theory explaining complex phenomena of aging process.

2. Biological theories focus on factors such as free radicals in the cells, senescencece and the immune system, DNA damage, and inflammageing as influential in the aging process.

3. Psychological theories address the aging process from developmental stages of growth and motivation, crisis, and resolution that each individual faces throughout their entire life.

4. Human development is a process that occurs over the life span. Older adults who successfully resolve each developmental stage can have a sense of psychological well-being and life satisfaction in late life.

5. Cognitive plasticity is a psychological theory of aging that emphasizes that the individual's cognitive function can be improved and preserved through physical exercise, and cognitive training and stimulation.

6. Social development theories view changing roles, relationships and aging from cultural and societal perspectives.

7. Social structure is the major factor influencing an individual's life course including family, religion, cultural traditions and expectations, neighborhood traditions, ethics, morals, norms, economics, income, education, social expectations, social status and social support systems.

8. The continuity theory proposes that older people age in ways that are consistent with prior lifestyle and preferences

他们的生活和面临的挑战，并促进自我完善，这有助于老年人的心理健康。他们可以帮助处于绝望发展阶段的老年人面对过往的生活，并与家人一起减轻心理压力，帮助老年人迈向对生活感到满意并感到安宁的阶段。在为患者提供护理时，护士可以运用衰老的社会学理论来考虑文化，社会经济，精神和社会资源对老年人的影响。护士处于独特的位置，可以为他们的生命的最后旅程提供整体护理并提高个人的生活质量。

（胡　洁，Deborah LEKAN）

本章要点

1. 衰老的过程涉及生物学、心理学和社会学等方面，没有单一的理论可以解释衰老过程中的复杂现象。

2. 衰老过程中的影响因素较多，如细胞中自由基、老化和免疫系统、DNA 损伤、炎性衰老等，都是生物学理论所关注的因素。

3. 衰老相关的心理学理论涉及成长的各个阶段，每个人在其一生中所面临的动机、危机和问题解决等问题。

4. 人类发展是一个跨越生命周期的过程。能够成功解决每个发展阶段发展任务的老年人在晚年会有较好的心理幸福感和生活满意度。

5. 认知可塑性是一种心理老化理论，其强调通过体育锻炼、认知训练和刺激来改善和保持个体的认知功能。

6. 社会发展理论是从文化和社会的角度来看待角色、关系和老化的。

7. 社会结构是影响个体生命历程的主要因素，包括家庭、宗教、文化传统和期望、邻里传统、伦理、道德、规范、经济、收入、教育、社会期望、社会地位和社会支持系统。

8. 持续理论认为，老年人的生活方式、偏好和价值观与既往相一致，老年人会保留熟悉

and value retaining familiar patterns and activities.

9. An individual can adapt, accept or cope with changes occurred with biological aging and achieve a successful aging.

10. Nurses play an important role in understanding and educating older adults, family members and communities to assist them in achieving psychological well-being and life satisfaction to successfully pass their last journey of life.

Critical Thinking Exercise

1. Discuss how biological theories of aging may cause aging process.

2. Make a nursing plan using biological theories of aging to provide education to older adults.

3. What health promotion strategies would you recommend to encourage a successful aging?

4. Identify strategies for older adults who feel regret about their life in the past and assist them to move to a stage of feeling a sense of life satisfaction.

5. When an older adult has difficulties in walking, remembering things and begin to withdraw from family and social activities, how could you use psychological and sociological theories to guide your care to this old adult?

6. As a person ages, one's ability to adaptive to changes in the environment may decrease, for example, when an older adult moves from home to assistant living or nursing home he or she may have difficulties in adjusting to the new environment. How would you help older adults cope with these changes that they may encounter in later life?

7. What biological, psychological and sociological factors you would consider when you take care of older adults in the hospital or community settings?

8. Imagine yourself at age of 80. Describe your physical function, psychosocial and social function, health problems and your lifestyle using biological, psychological and sociological theories. How will you set the stage for your vision of aging?

的模式和活动。

9. 个体能够适应、接受或应对生物老化所发生的变化，并实现成功老龄化。

10. 护士在理解和教育老年人、家庭成员和社区中发挥重要作用，帮助他们实现心理健康和生活满意，成功地度过他们最后的人生旅程。

批判性思维练习

1. 通过生物学衰老理论，讨论个体如何衰老。

2. 使用生物学理论为老年人教育制订护理计划。

3. 为了促进成功老龄化，你建议使用哪些健康促进策略？

4. 对于那些对过去生活存在遗憾的老年人，有哪些方法可以帮助他们在今后提高生活满意度。

5. 当老年人出现行走不便，记忆开始衰退，逐渐退出家庭和社会活动时，你如何在心理学和社会学理论的指导下，照顾这样的老年人？

6. 随着一个人衰老，其适应环境变化的能力可能会降低。例如，当一个老年人从家里搬到护理院时，他（她）可能会因适应新环境而产生困难。你将如何帮助老年人应对这些他们可能在晚年生活中会遇到的变化？

7. 当你在医院或社区护理老年人时，你会考虑哪些生物学、心理学和社会学的因素？

8. 假设你现在是80岁，你将如何描绘你的老年？请用生物学、心理学和社会学理论描述你的身体功能、心理社会功能、健康问题和生活方式。

Chapter 3 Normal Aging and Care
第三章　正常老化特点与老年保健

<table>
<tr><td>

Learning Objectives

On completion of this chapter, the reader will be able to:

- List normal aging-related psychosocial changes and physiologic changes that occur in different systems;

- Analyze normal aging-related changes to distinguish abnormal findings in each organ system;

- Describe characteristics of health promotion for elders;

- Identify models of health promotion;

- Describe barriers to health promotion activities;

- List nurse's role in health promotion.

</td><td>

学习目标

学完本章节，应完成以下目标：

- 列出正常老化相关的不同系统的生理变化和心理变化；

- 分析正常的老化相关变化，以区分每个器官系统的异常改变；

- 描述老年人健康促进的特点；

- 确认健康促进模式；

- 描述健康促进活动的阻碍因素；

- 列出护士在老年人健康促进中的作用。

</td></tr>
</table>

There are normal biological, psychological, and social changes in the process of aging, resulting in decline of older adults' abilities to maintain homeostasis and regulate organ systems. There is a large variability in the timing and rate of the decline among older adults because the bio-psycho decline and reserves are also modified by environmental and lifestyle factors. This chapter focuses on three topics including normal aging-related changes in each organ systems, major age-related psychosocial changes, and needs of health care with highlights on interventions to promote healthy aging.

人的老化过程伴随着生物、心理和社会老化改变，导致老年人维持体内平衡和调节器官系统的能力下降。老年人衰退的时间和速率有很大的变异性，因为个体生理、心理功能的下降和储备也受环境和生活方式因素影响。本章重点讨论三个主题：各个器官系统的正常老化改变，主要的老化相关的心理社会变化，以及卫生保健的需求和促进健康老龄化的干预重点。

Section 1　Age-related Physiological Change

第一节　老年人生理变化

Age-related physiologic decline is a near-universal phenomenon among body systems but varies markedly from system to system. Major age-related changes of the clinically vital systems are reviewed in this section.

生理衰退在身体各系统中普遍存在，但各系统的老化程度不一。主要的生理老化改变如下：

I. Age-related Changes in Pulmonary System

一、呼吸系统

The specific age-related changes in pulmonary system include loss of elasticity resulting in stiffening of the chest wall, inefficiency in gas exchange, and increased resistance to air flow (figure 3-1).

呼吸系统特别的老化改变主要包括丧失弹性导致胸壁变硬、气体交换效能降低以及气流阻力增加（图 3-1）。

1. Increased stiffness of thoracic cage　Stiffness of thoracic cage increases due to osteoporosis and calcification of costal cartilage. Kyphosis and degeneration of the intervertebral disks result in a shorter thorax with an increased anterior and posterior diameter, the barrel chest. These may limit the scope of activity of the thorax, which is, increased thoracic elastic resistance or decreased compliant. The combination of increased stiffer skeletal structure and weaker respiratory muscles result in additional effort and energy to breathe, so that the lung ventilation and respiratory capacity decrease.

1. **胸壁变硬**　由于骨质疏松症和肋软骨钙化，胸廓变硬。脊柱后凸和椎间盘变性导致胸腔前后径增宽，出现桶状胸。这些老化结构改变使胸廓活动幅度受限，即胸廓弹性阻力增大或顺应性降低。骨骼结构的僵硬化和呼吸肌肌力的减弱导致呼吸需要额外费力和耗能，从而使肺通气和呼吸容量降低。

2. Decreased gas exchange capacity　With age, the number of alveoli and alveolar wall elastic fibers decrease gradually, leading to the thinner alveolar septal walls and decreased alveolar elasticity, as well as the lack of pulmonary ventilation. The increase in ventilation is achieved by increased respiratory rates rather than more depth during exertion. As a result, the vital capacity

2. **气体交换能力降低**　随着老化，肺泡数量和肺泡壁弹性纤维逐渐减少，导致肺泡间壁变薄，肺泡弹性下降，以及肺通气不足。通气量的增加是通过增加呼吸频率而不是增加运动时的深度来实现的，从而导致肺活量减少、残气量增加。最大呼气量和有效肺容

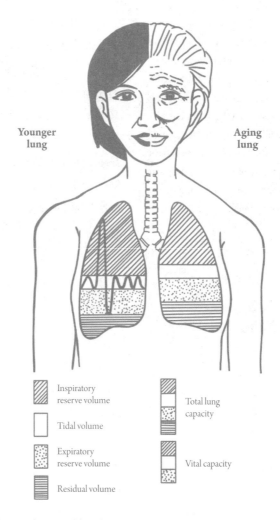

Younger lung

Aging lung

	Inspiratory reserve volume
	Tidal volume
	Expiratory reserve volume
	Residual volume

	Total lung capacity
	Vital capacity

Figure 3-1　Changes in lung volumes with aging

decreases, but residual volume increases. There is a progressive decline in maximal expiratory volume and lung volume reserve with aging as well. The alveoli enlarge because of dilation of the terminal bronchioles. Due to the diminished capillary structures surrounding the alveoli and age-related reduction of pulmonary perfusion flow, the available surface area for gas exchange is decreased, which contributes to the systematic reduction in partial pressure of arterial oxygen (PaO_2).

3. Increased airway resistance　Bronchial mucosa atrophy and increased mucus secretion lead to stenosis resulting in airway resistance. At the same time, the decrease of elasticity of bronchiole wall and the decrease of elastic traction of surrounding lung tissue make the resistance increase during breathing.

4. Easy to develop respiratory infection　In addition, decreased immunoglobulin A (IgA) found in the nasal respiratory mucosal surface results in declined

量随着增龄也逐渐下降。终末细支气管因失去弹性而扩张，肺泡扩大。由于围绕肺泡的毛细血管表面积减少和老化引起的肺灌注流量减少，可用于气体交换的表面积减少，从而导致系统动脉氧分压（PaO_2）降低。

3. 气道阻力增加　细支气管黏膜萎缩、黏液分泌物增加，可导致管腔狭窄，增加气道内在阻力。同时，细支气管壁弹性减退及其周围肺组织弹性牵引力减弱，使呼吸时阻力增高。

4. 容易发生呼吸道感染　分布于鼻黏膜表面的免疫球蛋白（IgA）减少，导致中和病毒的能力下降。气管和支气管黏膜上皮和黏

capability of neutralizes viruses. The number and effectiveness of cilia in the tracheobronchial tree also decrease, which increases difficulty clearing secretions. Together these place older adults at high risk of potentially life-threatening infections.

II. Age-related Changes in Cardiovascular System

The aging heart has decreased the numbers of myocytes and pacemaker cells as well as reduced sensitivity to beta-receptor, baroreceptor, and chemoreceptor stimulations. Myocardium is infiltrated with interstitial fibrosis. The connective tissues of heart experience calcifications. The normal aging-related changes in heart collectively result in increased systolic blood pressure, left ventricular after load, hypertrophy, and prolonged diastolic relaxation.

Resting heart rate remains relatively unchanged throughout the adulthood, whereas resting stroke volume decreases, the net result is decreased resting cardiac output. Maximal cardiac output decreases with aging, which is attributable to both decreased maximal stroke volume and maximal attainable heart rate (predicted maximal heart rate = 220 – age in years).

Meanwhile, arterial stiffness and increased peripheral vascular resistance occur with aging as a result of collagen infiltration and elastin deteriorations in the vessel walls. The overall effects are increased systolic blood pressure and mean arterial pressure. Isolated systolic hypertension (ISH), which occurs when the systolic pressure is high and the diastolic pressure is within the normal range, is often seen in elderly persons. In addition, reduced sensitivity of the blood pressure-regulating baroreceptors increases problems with postural hypotension.

Overall, older adults have sufficient cardiac output at rest. They are, however, at increased risk for cardiac dysfunction when the cardiovascular reserve is stretched.

III. Age-related Changes in Gastrointestinal System

Many essential aspects of the digestive system are preserved with aging and physiological changes are minor. Many of the gastrointestinal disorders prevalent in older adults are caused by the superimposed effects of chronic conditions, environmental insults, and lifestyle factors.

Dental decay, tooth loss, and mild loss of saliva production occur with aging, affecting the efficiency and completeness of mastication, thus affecting the absorption

液腺退行性病变，气管支气管内膜上的纤毛数量减少，纤毛运动减弱，防御和清除分泌物能力下降。这些都增加了老年人发生有可能危及生命的感染风险。

二、循环系统

老年人心肌细胞和心肌起搏细胞数量减少，对β-受体、压力感受器和化学感受器刺激的敏感性降低。心肌间质纤维化，心脏的结缔组织钙化。心脏的正常老化相关变化共同导致收缩压增加，左心室后负荷增大，左心室肥大和舒张期延长。

老年人静息心率保持相对不变，而静息心排血量减少。最大心排血量减少，这归因于最大心排血量和最大可达到的心率减小（预测的最大心率 = 220 – 年龄）。

同时，老年人血管壁因弹性蛋白减少、胶原蛋白增加，导致动脉硬化，外周血管阻力增加。总体效果是收缩压增加，平均动脉压增大。单纯性收缩压升高在老年人中常见，即收缩压升高，舒张压处于正常范围。另外，降低血压的压力感受器的敏感性增加容易发生直立性低血压。

总的来说，老年人在休息时有足够的心排血量。然而，当应激发生、心血管储备不足时，就有心功能障碍发生的危险。

三、消化系统

消化系统的许多重要方面尚能保持，与衰老相关的生理变化不大。老年人中常见的许多胃肠道疾病是由慢性病症、环境污染和生活方式因素的叠加效应引起的。

随着年龄的增长，会发生龋齿、牙齿脱落和唾液分泌轻微减少，影响咀嚼的效率和完整性，从而影响营养的吸收，容易发生营

of nutrition, prone to malnutrition. Xerostomia increases in prevalence and impairs chewing and swallowing. The risk for aspiration increases in older adults because aging gradually decreases upper esophageal sphincter pressure and reduces the ability to clear food from pharynx. Lower esophageal sphincter relaxation isprone to result in spontaneous reflux gastroduodenal contents, leaving the elderly reflux esophagitis, esophageal cancer incidence increased.

In the stomach, aging-related changes include delayed gastric emptying, increased colonization of gastric autoantibodies and Helicobacter pylori, and reduced gastric mucosal cytoprotective factors such as mucosal prostaglandins. As a result, older adults are prone to atrophic gastritis (shrinking and inflammation of the inner lining of the stomach), achlorhydria (insufficient production of stomach acid), and ulcerations (an area of the stomach that is eroded by digestive juices and stomach acid).

Aging does not affect food transport through the intestines in general except for decreased update of lactose, calcium, folic acid, vitamin B_{12}, copper, zinc, fatty acids, and cholesterol. The muscle or connective tissue of the colonic wall become thinner, combined with reduced activity of the elderly, so that intestinal contents go through the extended time, water re-absorption increases, the elderly people are prone to constipation. The prevalence of diverticulosis increases with aging because intestinal pressure tends to increase due to aging-related intestinal muscle weakness and wall thinness.

The major functional changes in the liver are reduced liver size, blood flow, and perfusion. The liver has reduced ability to clear medications that are metabolized via the cytochrome P450 system. As a result, older adults are at increased risks for drug side effects and drug-drug interactions. Therefore, the long-term use of certain drugs in the elderly should take into account the changes in pharmacokinetics of the elderly, and the dosage of drugs should generally be reduced.

There is little evidence that aging is associated with clinically significant decreases in the pancreatic exocrine function. The size and weight of the pancreas decreases after 70 years of age with ductal epithelial hyperplasia, interlobular fibrosis, and acinar cell degranulation.

养不良。口干燥症的发生率增加，损害咀嚼和吞咽。老年人食管上端括约肌松弛，从咽部清除食物的能力降低，误吸风险增加。食管下端括约肌松弛，容易发生胃十二指肠内容物自发性反流，而使老年人反流性食管炎、食管癌的发病率增高。

在胃中与衰老相关的变化包括胃排空时间延长，胃自身抗体和幽门螺杆菌的增殖，以及胃黏膜细胞保护因子（如黏膜前列腺素）的减少，导致老年人容易发生萎缩性胃炎（胃内层的收缩和炎症）、胃酸缺乏（胃酸产生不足）和溃疡（由消化液和胃酸侵蚀的胃部区域破溃）。

衰老一般不会影响通过肠道的食物运输，除了肠道对乳糖、钙、叶酸、维生素 B_{12}、铜、锌、脂肪酸和胆固醇的吸收降低。结肠壁的肌肉或结缔组织变薄，加之老年人活动减少，使肠内容物通过时间延长，水分重吸收增加，粪便坚硬，向前推进粪便的动力不足，直肠对扩张的敏感性降低，故老年人易发生便秘。老年人结肠壁的肌肉或结缔组织变薄，加上结肠内压上升，易形成结肠憩室病。

肝脏的主要变化是肝脏变小、血流量和灌注减少。肝脏清除通过细胞色素 P450 系统代谢药物的能力降低，因此，老年人的药物副作用和药物之间相互作用的风险增加。故老年人长期服用某些药物应考虑到老年人药物代谢动力学的改变，用药剂量一般应减少。

很少有证据表明，衰老与临床上胰腺外分泌功能显著下降有关。老年人 70 岁后胰腺的大小和重量减少，伴有导管上皮增生、小叶间纤维化和腺泡细胞脱颗粒，影响胰腺功能。

IV. Age-related Changes in Urinary System

Substantial changes in the urinary system occur with aging. The kidneys undergo three clinically significant changes, although they can function more than adequately under normal circumstances. The first change is reduced intrarenal vasculature with renal blood flow decreasing 10% per decade. The second change shows both decreasing numbers and sizes of the nephrons. Older adults lose a quarter to a third of their kidney mass with the total number of glomeruli falling 30% to 40%, while another 30% of the glomeruli may become nonfunctional or sclerotic. The third change is the reduced ability for the kidneys to regulate hormones in response to dehydration, conserve salt, concentrate urine, and eliminate wastes from the blood circulation. Between 30 and 70 years of age, renal function declines about 30% to 50% which is accompanied by reduced acid-base control, glucose tolerance, and drug clearance. The total body water declines 10%-50% compared to that in younger adults. In addition, the bladder experiences decreased capacity and flow, increased sense of urinary urgency, and increasing residual urine, which contributes to increased nocturia (increased urinary frequency at night time) and risks for urinary tract infection.

V. Age-related Changes in Endocrine System

Although the pancreas continues to produce adequate amount of insulin with aging, the aging muscles are less responsive to the effect of insulin, resulting increased blood glucose level. Fasting glucose level is estimated to rise after 50 years of age at a rate of 0.6-1.4 milligrams per deciliter per decade. Decreased insulin responses, along with increasing physical inactivity and obesity, contribute to increasing incidences of type 2 (or adult-onset) diabetes mellitus in older adults. In addition, aldosterone level decreases by 30% by the seventh decade of life, which predisposes older adults to orthostatic hypotension.

VI. Age-related Changes in Neurologic System

Modest decline in brain weight happens with aging, which is primarily due to loss of the gray matter in healthy older adults. Reduced neuron dendrites and synapses are observed with aging. Although the loss of neurons and brain function is previously portrayed as irreversible,

四、泌尿系统

随着年龄的增长，泌尿系统会发生老化变化。尽管在正常情况下老年人的泌尿系统可以充分地发挥功能，肾脏在老年期所发生的三个临床变化对泌尿系统的功能还是有一定影响。第一，肾内脉管系统减少，肾血流量每十年减少10%。第二，肾单位的数量和体积都在减少，肾实质减少四分之一到三分之一，肾小球总数下降30%~40%，而另外30%的肾小球可能丧失功能或硬化。第三，肾脏调节激素以减轻脱水、保钠、浓缩尿液和消除血液循环中的废物的能力降低。从30~70岁，肾功能下降约30%~50%，并伴随着酸碱控制能力、葡萄糖耐量和药物清除率的降低。与成年早期相比，身体水的总量减少了10%~50%。此外，膀胱功能和流量降低，尿急感增加、残留尿增多，促使夜尿增多（夜间尿频率增加）和尿路感染的风险增多。

五、内分泌系统

虽然老年人的胰腺继续分泌足够量的胰岛素，但老化使组织对胰岛素的敏感性降低，导致对葡萄糖的耐受性下降，血糖水平升高。空腹血糖水平在50岁后估计以每十年0.6~1.4mg/L的速率上升。对胰岛素的敏感性减低，以及身体活动减少和肥胖，促使老年人2型（或成人发病）糖尿病的发病率增加。此外，醛固酮水平在70岁时降低30%，使得老年人容易发生直立性低血压。

六、神经系统

脑重量随老化稍下降，这主要是由于灰质的损失造成的。随着老化，神经元树突和突触减少。虽然以前认为神经元和脑功能的损失不可逆，但现在越来越多的证据支持大

increasing evidence support that the brain is remarkably plastic and neurons do regenerate.

Vibration perception in the lower extremities decreases with aging. The position sense is affected as well, but to a lesser degree, which often manifests as a mild swaying during the Romberg test. Pain and temperature sensation diminish with aging. A depression or loss of the Achilles tendon reflex is the most common aging-related changes, although other reflexes remain either intact or are diminished.

Because of the changes in the neurologic and musculoskeletal systems, it is more difficult for older adults to tandem, toe, and heel walk for an extended period of time. However, older adult does have adequate postural righting reflexes and are not prone to spontaneous falls.

VII. Age-related Changes in Musculoskeletal System

With aging, the muscle bulk and strength progressively decline. The loss of muscle mass and strength associated with aging is called sarcopenia, which results from decreased muscle fibers, motor unit size, protein synthesis, growth factor alterations, and capillarization. The loss of muscle mass is primarily responsible for the loss of muscle strength while other factors such as neural factors also contribute to the loss of strength and functional limitations. The speed and coordination of movements decreases with advancing age. Weakening abdominal muscle results in accentuated lordosis and contributes to back pain.

Degenerations of joints, especially the spine, occur with aging due to multifaceted factors such as diseases, progressive loss of collagen fibers, and deterioration of joint structures that begin in early adulthood. Furthermore, bone mineral density decreases with aging. Bone senescence generally begins at the sixth decade of life and is characterized by predominantly osteoclastic activity (bone reabsorption). It is estimated that women begin to lose bone mass between 30 and 35 years of ages at a rate of 0.75 % to 1% per year and men start to lose bone mass between 50 to 55 years of age at a rate of 0.4% per year. The gender difference in bone mass loss is because women have less initial bone mass compared to men and experience decreased calcium intake during menopause. However, the gender difference in bone mass loss is reversed somewhat by 80 years of age where women drop 40% of their peak bone mineral contents and men lose 55%.

The overall aging effect on the musculoskeletal

脑的可塑性和神经元确实可再生。

下肢的振动感知随着老化而减弱。位置觉也受到影响，但程度较小，在 Romberg 测试期间经常表现为轻微的摇摆。疼痛和温度觉也随老化而减弱。虽然其他反射尚能保持完整或减弱，但是跟腱反射的降低或缺失是最常见的老化改变。

由于神经系统和肌肉骨骼系统的老化，老年人很难在较长的时间内保持双脚一前一后脚趾到脚跟地发力走路。然而，老年人在一般情况下仍有足够的姿势纠正反射，不会轻易自发跌倒。

七、运动系统

随着老化，肌肉体积和力量逐渐下降。与衰老相关的肌肉质量和强度的损失称为肌少症。其由肌纤维减少、活动度降低、蛋白质合成减少、生长因子改变和肝窦毛细血管化导致。肌肉质量的丧失是肌力丧失的主要原因，而神经因素等其他因素也会导致肌力丧失和功能受限。运动的速度和协调性随着年龄的增长而降低。腹部肌肉减弱导致脊柱前凸加重，并导致背部疼痛。

随着老化，多种因素可导致关节的退化（特别是脊柱的退化，如疾病、胶原纤维的进行性丧失和在成年早期开始的关节结构恶化）。此外，骨矿物质密度随着老化而降低。骨老化通常在六十多岁开始，并且主要表现为破骨细胞活性（骨再吸收）改变。据估计，女性在 30～35 岁之间开始以每年 0.75%～1% 的比例失去骨量，男性在 50～55 岁之间开始每年以 0.4% 的比率失去骨量。骨量损失的性别差异是因为与男性相比，女性初始骨量较少，并且在绝经期钙吸收减少。然而，骨量损失中的性别差异在 80 岁时有所逆转，其中女性降低其峰值骨矿物质含量的 40%，男性损失 55%。

肌肉骨骼系统的整体老化效应包括到 60

system includes decreased height averaged 5.08 cm, increased weight until 60 years of age, decreased weight after 60 years of age, doubled body fat mass, decreased lean muscle mass, and decreased bone density. Together, sarcopenia, joint degeneration, and reduced bone mass and mineral contents predispose older adults to fractures, falls, injuries, slower gait speed, functional limitations, and disability.

VIII. Age-related Changes in Reproductive System

After menopause that occurs between 45 and 52 years of age, women experience a 95% drop in estrogen level, while the follicle stimulating hormone and luteinizing hormones increase greatly and slowly level off over 30 years. Those hormonal changes cause the relaxation of the ligaments and loss of the muscular tone that alters the breast contour. Depleting estrogen places women at higher risks for osteoporosis, heart attack, stroke, and possibly Alzheimer's disease. In contrast, men experience a gradual 35% decline in testosterone by 85 years of age. Further, aging is associated with a decrease in sex drive and slower and less intense sexual response.

IX. Age-related Changes in Immunologic System

Aging and environmental factors such as smoking and environmental pollutants contribute to decreased immunologic function to various degrees. Over the life span, the immunologic function declines 5% to 30% which are mainly attributable to impaired suppressor T-cell function. The thymus gland shrinks with aging, resulting in decreased production of the thymic hormones. Thymic hormones can transform stem cells from bone marrow into T lymphocytes, thus enhancing cellular immune function. Thymic hormones decrease to such a level that they cannot be detected in the blood by 60 years of age. The productions of antibodies are also reduced and their responses to foreign pathogens are less potent. As a result, older adults are less resistant to pathogens, more likely to die from infections, and prone to incidence of both tumor and autoimmune disorders.

X. Age-related Changes in Sensory Organs

1. Eyes and vision Due to decreased muscle elasticity of the eye, fat reduction around the orbits, the

岁时身高平均减少 5.08cm、体重增加；60 岁后则体重减轻，体脂肪量增加到两倍，瘦肌肉质量减少和骨密度降低。肌少症、关节退化、骨量和矿物质含量减少一起导致老年人易于发生骨折、跌倒、受伤、步态速度减慢、功能受限和残障。

八、生殖系统

女性在 45～52 岁之间发生绝经后，雌激素水平下降 95%，而促卵泡激素和黄体生成素显著增加并在之后 30 年内缓慢地达到平衡。这些激素变化引起韧带的松弛和肌张力下降，从而导致乳房轮廓改变。雌激素的缺乏使女性成为患骨质疏松症、心脏病发作、卒中和阿尔茨海默病的高危人群。相比之下，男性到 85 岁后睾酮逐渐下降 35%。此外，衰老与性欲减退、性反应较慢、不强烈有关。

九、免疫系统

老化和环境因素如吸烟和环境污染导致免疫功能出现不同程度的降低。在整个生命过程中，免疫功能下降 5%～30%，这主要归因于抑制性 T 细胞功能受损。胸腺随老化而萎缩，导致胸腺激素的产生减少。胸腺激素可使由骨髓产生的干细胞转变为 T 淋巴细胞，因而可增强细胞免疫功能。60 岁以后胸腺激素水平会降到在血液中难于检测得到。抗体的产生也减少，并且它们对外来病原体的反应不敏感。结果，老年人对病原体的抵抗力较低，更可能死于感染，并且易于发生肿瘤和自身免疫性疾病。

十、感觉器官

1. 眼和视觉 由于眼部肌肉弹性减弱，眼眶周围脂肪减少，老年人可出现眼睑皮肤

elderly may appear eyelid skin relaxation, the upper eyelid ptosis, and lower eyelid can occur fat bag-shaped bags bulged. Lacrimal gland secretion of tear reduces, making the conjunctiva dry, dull, and the elderly thus are susceptible to dry eye discomfort.

Changes in intraocular structure:

(1) The diameter of the cornea is slightly smaller or flattened, so that the refractive power of the cornea is reduced which results in hyperopia and astigmatism. Corneal surface microvilli significantly reduce, leading to corneal dryness and corneal transparency decreased. After 60 years of age in the corneal stroma layer appears gray ring-like lipid deposition, known as "the elderly ring".

(2) With the lens aging regulation function decline, there may be presbyopia. Lens and ciliary muscle regulation function and focus function gradually decrease, the ability to see close things declines, hyperopia, also called "presbyopia", may occurs. Non-water-soluble protein in the lens gradually increases resulting in lens opacity, so that the transmittance of the lens becomes weakened, increasing the incidence of senile cataract. Lenticular ligament tension decreases, making the lens forward; it is possible to close the anterior chamber angle, affecting aqueous reflux, resulting in increased intraocular pressure. Pathological intraocular pressure can cause optic nerve damage and visual impairment, the occurrence of glaucoma.

(3) Vitreous aging is mainly manifested as liquefaction and vitreous detachment. With the increase of age, vitreous liquefaction area is expanding. Vitreous detachment can cause retinal detachment. Vitreous body loses liquid due to aging, and its color changes, inclusion bodies are increased, which can cause "floaters disease".

(4) Retinal aging is mainly around the retina with thinning, age-related macular degeneration. In addition, retinal blood vessels become narrow, hardening, and even occlusion, pigment epithelial cells and melanoma cells decrease, lipofuscin increases, so that visual acuity decreases significantly. Due to retinal pigment epithelium thinning and vitreous traction, the risk of retinal detachment in the elderly is increased.

(5) Due to the elderly pupil sphincter of the relative increase in tension and miosis become smaller, and the field of vision is narrowed. Therefore, the elderly is particularly sensitive to light, often feel dazzling to the outdoor, feel visual difficulties from the bright to the dark, and may complain the visual object is not bright.

松弛，上眼睑下垂；下眼睑可发生脂肪袋状膨出即眼袋。泪腺分泌泪液减少，使得结膜干涩，失去光泽，老年人因而易感到眼睛干燥不适。

眼内结构的改变为：

（1）角膜的直径稍小或呈扁平化，使角膜的屈光力减退引起远视及散光。角膜表面的微绒毛显著减少，导致角膜干燥及角膜透明度减低。60岁以后在角膜边缘基质层出现灰白色环状类脂质沉积，称"老人环"。

（2）随着晶状体老化调节功能减退，可出现老视。晶状体和睫状肌调节功能和聚焦功能逐渐减退，视近物能力下降，出现远视，即"老花眼"。晶状体中非水溶性蛋白逐渐增多而出现晶状体浑浊，使晶状体的透光度减弱，增加了老年性白内障的发病率。晶状体悬韧带张力降低，使晶状体前移，有可能使前房角关闭，影响房水回流，导致眼压升高。病理性眼压升高可引起视神经损害和视力障碍，发生青光眼。

（3）玻璃体的老化主要表现为液化和玻璃体后脱离。随着年龄的增长，玻璃体液化区不断扩大。玻璃体后脱离可引起视网膜脱离，同时玻璃体因衰老而失水，色泽改变，包涵体增多，可引起"飞蚊症"。

（4）视网膜的老化主要是视网膜周边带变薄，出现老年性黄斑变性。另外，视网膜血管变窄、硬化，甚至闭塞，色素上皮层细胞及其细胞内的黑色素减少，脂褐质增多，使视力显著下降。由于视网膜色素上皮层变薄和玻璃体的牵引，增加了老年人视网膜脱离的危险。

（5）由于老年期瞳孔括约肌的张力相对增强，瞳孔缩小，视野变窄。因此，老年人对强光特别敏感，到室外时往往感觉耀眼，由明到暗时感觉视物困难，并可能诉说视物不明亮。

2. Hearing

(1)Atrophy of the nerve endings in the external auditory canal leads to slow sensorineural. Auditory nerve function gradually subsides; dysfunction of sound waves transmitted from the inner ear to the brain occurs; the elderly gradually loss hearing, leading to senile deafness.

(2) Due to the thickening of the inner ear vascular wall, luminal narrowing, leading to inner ear ischemia, the function of the inner ear changes, to promote the occurrence and development of senile deafness. At the beginning, high-frequency hearing reduces, with the general decline in hearing sensitivity, often need to speak loudly, but at the same time the elderly will feel harsh discomfort, accompanied by tinnitus.

(3) Analysis on voice signal in the senior hearing centre becomes slow, unresponsive, and positioning dysfunction, resulting in hearing impairment in the noise environment significantly.

3. Taste With aging, taste buds become gradually shrinking, and the number gradually decreases, so taste function declines gradually. Oral mucosa cells and salivary gland atrophy, reduced saliva secretion, and dry mouth, can also cause the loss of taste function.

4. Olfactory Olfactory nerve reduces in the number, and becomes atrophy and degeneration. After the age of 50, the sense of smell gradually decreases and the sense of smell begins to be slow; at the same time, the ability to distinguish the smell goes down, especially in men. Loss of olfactory function can also cause lack of appetite, thus affecting the body's intake of nutrients.

XI. Age-related Changes in Skin

Aging-related changes in skin refers to the aging damage of skin function, include inability to retain moisture, thinning between dermis and epidermis by about 20%, and decreased elasticity and resilience due to decreased elastin and collagen. The subcutaneous fat dwindles with aging too.

With aging, hair follicles on the scalp become fewer and the hair growth rate decreases in the scalp, armpits, and pubic areas. Conversely, hair growth accelerates in nostrils, ear, and eyebrows, especially in men. Women experience more facial hair as the estrogen level drops with menopause and ceases with aging.

2. 听觉

（1）由于外耳道的神经末梢日趋萎缩而导致感音迟钝。听神经功能逐渐减退，声波从内耳传至脑部的功能障碍，使老年人听力逐渐丧失，导致老年性耳聋。

（2）由于内耳血管的管壁增厚、管腔缩小，导致内耳缺血，使内耳的功能发生改变，促使老年性耳聋的发生和发展。首先从高音频听力减弱开始，随着听力敏感度的普遍下降，常常需要说话者大声说话，但此时老年人又会感到刺耳不适，同时伴有耳鸣。

（3）听觉高级中枢对音信号的分析减慢，反应迟钝，定位功能减退，造成在噪声环境中听力障碍明显。

3. 味觉 随着年龄的增长，味蕾逐渐萎缩，数量逐渐减少，味觉功能逐渐减退。口腔黏膜细胞和唾液腺发生萎缩，唾液分泌减少，口腔较干燥，也会造成味觉功能的减退。

4. 嗅觉 嗅神经数量减少、萎缩、变性。50岁以后，嗅觉的敏感性逐渐减退，嗅觉开始迟钝，同时，对气味的分辨能力下降，男性尤为明显。嗅觉功能的减退，也可造成食欲缺乏，从而影响机体对营养物质的摄取。

十一、皮肤

皮肤的老化是指皮肤功能衰老性损伤，包括皮肤不能保湿，真皮和表皮之间变薄约20%，以及由于弹性蛋白和胶原减少而导致皮肤弹性和韧性降低。皮下脂肪也随着老化而减少。

随着年龄增长，头皮上的毛囊变少，并且头皮、腋窝和耻骨区域中的毛发生长速率降低。相反，鼻毛、耳毛和眉毛加速生长，特别是男性。女性则因绝经雌激素水平下降而出现面部多毛。

Section 2　Age-related Psychosocial Change

It is very important for nurses and caregivers to understand about the psychosocial changes of the elderly. Most healthy older adults experience the following mild psychosocial changes:

I. Aging Intelligence

Intelligence has been generally assumed to consist of crystallized intelligence and fluid intelligence. Crystallized intelligence involves knowledge that comes from prior learning and past experiences. As individuals age, crystallized intelligenceremains relatively stable, and with the accumulation of acquired learning and experience, some individuals' crystallized intelligence even becomes stronger, and then slowly decline until advanced age. Fluid intelligence involves our current ability to reason and process complex information around us. This type of intelligence tends to decline during late adulthood.

II. Aging Memory

Memory has three components containing immediate recall, short-term memory, and remote or long-term memory. Immediate recall and long-term memory of the elderly may remain intact, but short-term memory declines, and differentiating this "benign forgetfulness" from early dementia is often impossible (box 3-1). Normal older adults may not recall details of a situation but does remember the situation or experience. Unlike malignant memory loss, this type of impairment is not progressive, nor is it disabling, for the details not remembered at one time may be remembered later. And psycho-neuronal assessment may be helpful. It is found that nerve cell regeneration does occur in the hippocampus of the brain, where memory formation occurs. Through this plasticity, experience constantly changes the brain, which gives us good evidence to continue to learn and grow and experience the world around us even into very old age.

Box 3-1　Normal Aging vs Dementia

Dementia is not normal aging. It is characterized by multiple cognitive deficits with memory impairments

---

第二节　老年人心理社会变化

了解老年人的心理社会变化对照护老年人非常重要。老年人的心理社会变化特点主要表现在以下几方面：

一、智力的变化

智力分为晶体智力和流体智力两大类。晶体智力指从先前的学习和过去的经验中学到的知识。随着年龄增长，老年人的晶体智力保持相对稳定，随着后天的学习和经验积累，有的甚至还有所提高，到高龄后才缓慢下降。流体智力涉及我们当前推理和处理周围复杂信息的能力。流体智力在成年后随着增龄呈逐渐下降的趋势。

二、记忆的变化

记忆包括三种：瞬时记忆、短期记忆、长期记忆或远程记忆。老年人的瞬时记忆和长期记忆可保持不变；但短期记忆下降，并且通常难于将老年人的短期记忆下降这种"良性健忘"与老年痴呆早期的记忆损害区分开来（box 3-1）。与恶性记忆丧失不同，正常老化导致的记忆下降表现为老年人当时忘了细节，事后可能回忆起来，并且正常记忆老化不像病理性的记忆在短期内进行性衰退。心理 – 神经评估可能有助于区分"良性健忘"与早期痴呆。研究发现，神经细胞再生确实发生在脑的海马中，记忆形成发生于此。通过这种可塑的、经验不断增长促成的大脑结构改变，为人们的继续学习、成长和体验周围的世界提供良好的佐证，直至末年。

Box 3-1　正常老化与痴呆

痴呆不是正常老化，而是以记忆损害等多种认知缺陷作为常见早期症状为特征的病理改

as a frequent early symptom. Generally, there must be impairment in social functioning and independent living for a diagnosis of dementia to be given, while independent living should not be compromised during normal aging. It is important to receive regular medical checkups in order to monitor the extent and severity to which someone may be experiencing cognitive decline.

Symptoms to watch for:

- Getting lost in familiar places.
- Repetitive questioning.
- Odd or inappropriate behaviors.
- Forgetfulness of recent events.
- Repeated falls or loss of balance.
- Personality changes.
- Decline in planning and organization.
- Changes in diet/eating habits.
- Changes in hygiene.
- Increased apathy.
- Changes in language abilities, including comprehension.

III. Learning in Later Life

Spatial awareness, intuitive and creative thoughts may decline in the elderly. Older adults may have barriers to learning, including memory impairment, vision and hearing impairment, fatigue, and delayed cognitive processing. New learning must relate to what the elder already knows.

IV. Other Psychosocial Issues

Older adults, especially the years beyond age 80, often deal with disability, caregiving, bereavement, and loneliness. Sensory impairments particularly declined visuospatial abilities, hearing impairment, limit many individuals' abilities to make new friends. Invariably physical impairments not only limit the ability to travel outside the home, but they also influence on activities of daily living. Family and friends are sources of strength. It is a major source of concern to remain alive with major disabilities, particularly stroke and Alzheimer's disease, or to be a burden to others.

变。一般而言，正常老化过程中日常生活能力不受影响，而诊断为痴呆者其社会功能和独立生活能力一定是有损害的。及时发认知功能异常的重要手段是进行定期检查，以便监测某人可能发生认知衰退的范围和严重程度。

要注意的症状：

- 在熟悉的地方迷路。
- 重复提问。
- 奇怪或不当的行为。
- 忘记最近发生的事情。
- 重复跌倒或失去平衡。
- 人格变化。
- 计划和组织能力下降。
- 饮食/饮食习惯的变化。
- 卫生习惯变差。
- 变得冷漠。
- 语言能力减退，包括理解能力降低。

三、晚年学习的变化

老年人的空间意识、直觉和创造性思维可能有所下降，还有一些因素可妨碍老年人的学习，包括记忆障碍、视力和听力障碍、疲劳和延迟的认知处理。对新事物的学习必须联系老年人已有的知识经验来获取。

四、其他心理社会变化

老年人，特别是 80 岁以上的高龄老年人，常常面临残疾、需要照顾、丧偶、孤独等问题。感觉障碍特别是视觉空间能力下降，听力障碍，限制了许多人交新朋友的能力。不可避免的躯体功能衰退不仅限制了外出的能力，而且还可能影响日常生活活动，家人和朋友就成为支持老年人的主要资源。老年人特别担心失能，尤其害怕脑卒中或患阿尔茨海默病而成为家人亲友的负担，这是引起人们关注的主要因素。

Section 3　Aging and Health Promotion

Health promotion and disease prevention are very important to healthy aging. This section will introduce essentiality of health promotion for elders, model of health promotion, barriers and interventions of health promotion among elderly population.

I. Essentiality of Health Promotion for the Elderly

Health promotionis defined as the science and art of helping people change their lifestyle to move toward a state of optimum health. The purpose of health promotion is to reduce the potential years of life lost in premature mortality and ensure a higher quality of remaining life. As people live longer, health promotion activities are all the more important.

In general, the elder people suffer from more chronic conditions than younger adults; thereby, they have more complex health care needs, and take advantage of considerably more health care services. Health promotion programs are essential for preventing disease and disability, and improving functioning and quality of life of elders. However, elders as a group receive fewer prevention and screening services than other populations because of inaccurate perceptions that elders are less responsive to health promotion interventions. In fact, evidence suggests that elders benefit just as much from health promotion activities as those who are middle-aged. Many governmental and nonprofit organizations in the US such as Administration on Aging, American Society on Aging (ASA), and Centers for Disease Control and Prevention (CDC) are leading efforts to promote healthy aging and sponsoring national health promotion initiatives for elders.

II. Models of Health Promotion

There are a number of significant models that underpin the practice of health promotion. The commonly used models in the gerontological health care setting are health belief model, health promotion model and cross-theoretical model.

第三节　老年人健康促进

健康促进和疾病预防对健康老龄化非常重要。本节将介绍老年人健康促进的重要性，健康促进模式，老年人健康促进的障碍和干预。

一、老年人健康促进的必要性

健康促进的定义是帮助人们改变现有生活方式，向着最佳健康状态发展的科学和艺术。健康促进的目的是减少过早死亡导致的潜在寿命损失；确保存活者有较高的生活质量。随着人类寿命的延长，健康促进变得更加重要。

相对于年轻人来说，老年人受到更多慢性病的折磨，其健康需求更复杂，需要更全面广泛的健康照顾。因此，对老年人而言，健康促进项目在预防疾病、减少伤残和促进功能恢复、提高生活质量方面更加必不可少。然而，由于受一些错误观点的影响，如对健康促进措施不敏感等，老年人群所接受的疾病预防和筛查要比其他人群少。事实上，有充分的证据表明，老年人与中年人在健康促进措施中的获益程度相近。在美国，官方和非营利组织例如美国老龄化管理局，美国老龄化协会（ASA）和疾病控制与预防中心（CDC），都在致力于促进老年人健康老龄化的全民健康活动并发起了针对老年人的国家健康促进计划。

二、健康促进模式

有许多重要的模型支持健康促进实践，老年照护常用的模式有健康信念模式、健康促进模式和跨理论模式等。以下是在老年医学保健环境中经常使用的代表不同重点领域或健康组成部分的模型的简要概述。

i. Health Belief Model

The health belief model (HBM) was developed by a group of US Public Health Service social psychologists in 1950s. It is to determine the likelihood of an individual's participation in health promotion, health protection, and disease prevention. This model includes three basic components which are the individual's perception of susceptibility to and the severity of an illness or disease, modifying factors such as knowledge of the disease, personal demographic and psychosocial variables, and cues or triggers to action and a cost-benefit ratio that is acceptable to the individual. The health belief model addresses the relationship between an individual's beliefs and behaviors.

ii. Health Promotion Model

The health promotion model (HPM) proposed by Pender describes the multi-dimensional nature of persons as they interact within their environment to pursue health. The model focuses on following three areas including individual characteristics and experiences, behavior-specific cognitions and affect, and behavioral outcomes. Each person has unique personal characteristics and experiences that affect subsequent actions. Variables for behavioral specific knowledge and affects have important motivational significance and can be modified through nursing actions. Health promoting behavior is the desired behavioral outcome and is the end point in the HPM. Health promoting behaviors should lead to improved health, enhanced functional ability and better quality of life at all stages of development.

iii. Transtheoretical Model

The transtheoretical model (TTM), also called the "stages-of-change" model was developed by Prochaska and Diclemente. TTM has been widely used to explain stages of behavior change and has been used successfully in programs for smoking cessation, alcohol and drug cessation, medication compliance, diet and weight control, stress management, sun exposure, and screening for cancers. TTM describes five unique stages of change: precontemplation, contemplation, preparation, action and maintenance. Transition among stages results from the processes of change, which are the experiential and behavioral processes that the individual may experience. Each of these stages is characterized by changes in decisional balance; that is, the balance between benefits and costs related to engaging in a specific behavior.

Precontemplation is the first stage (Not Ready). In this stage, people have no intention of changing their behaviors within the next 6 months. They are unaware

（一）健康信念模式

健康信念模式（HBM）是20世纪50年代由美国公共卫生服务部的社会心理学家推出，旨在提高个体参与健康促进、健康保护和疾病预防活动的可能性。健康信念模式包括3个基本要素：①个体对疾病的易感性和疾病严重程度的认识；②制约因素，如人口统计学、社会心理学资料及对疾病的知识等；③促使个体采取应对措施的因素和人们可以接受的投资收益比。健康信念模式论述了个人信念和增进健康行为的关系。

（二）健康促进模式

健康促进模式（HPM）是由Pender提出的，它描述了人们在追求健康的过程中，与环境的相互作用的多维特性。此模式主要关注以下3个领域：①个体性格和经验；②对特定行为的认知和影响；③行为结果。人的性格和经验影响其行为；对特定行为的认识和情感可以促使个体采取一定的应对措施，而护理工作可以对其进行干预；健康促进行为是预期的行为结果，它可以在个体发展的所有阶段里起到促进健康、增强躯体功能并提高生活质量的作用。

（三）跨理论模式

跨理论模式（TTM）又称"改变阶段"模式，由Prochaska和Diclemente提出。改变阶段模式被广泛应用于解释个体行为改变的过程，并且已经成功应用于戒烟、戒酒和戒除毒品，提高服药依从性，节食、控制体重以及个体适应压力和癌症筛查等健康促进项目。此模式描述了5个行为改变的独特阶段：沉思前期、沉思期、准备期、行动期和维持期。阶段之间的转换缘于变化过程，即个体可能经历的体验和行为过程。每一个阶段的特征都是决策平衡的变化；也就是说，与采取某一特定行为有关的利益和成本之间的平衡。

沉思前期是第一阶段（未准备就绪）。在这一阶段，人们并没有在短期6个月内改变自己行为的打算。他们没有察觉到问题，否

of the problem, in denial of the need for change, or resistant to change. Contemplation, the second stage (Getting Ready), is characterized by an intention to change in the next 6 months. People recognize the negative consequences of current behaviors and positive consequences of different behaviors. People may ask questions and to seek information about the short-and long-term costs and benefits of various behaviors. The balance between the costs and benefits of changing can produce profound ambivalence that may keep people stuck in this stage for long periods of time. Preparation, the third stage (Ready), is characterized by a stronger inclination to change to healthier behaviors in the next month. People acknowledge the need for change and begin to identify strategies for implementing healthy behaviors. During this stage, people are encouraged to seek support from families and friends, state their plan to change and seek help from others in accomplishing their goals. Action is the fourth stage, in which people have changed their behavior within the last 6 months. At this stage, people need to work hard to keep moving ahead as they usually do not fully experience the benefits of the new behavior and are vulnerable to resuming prior unhealthy behaviors. People need to learn how to strengthen their commitments to change and to fight urges to relapse. Maintenance, the fifth stage, occurs when people have continued the healthy behaviors for 6 months or longer. In this stage, people are less tempted to relapse and increasingly more confident that they can maintain the healthier lifestyle.

Models mentioned above attempt to explain health behavior and health behavior change by focusing on the individual. There are some health promotion models that explain change in communities and community action for health such as the PRECEDE/PROCEED model. This model is developed based on multidisciplinary scientific designs and studies from educational, psychosocial, and epidemiologic sciences. The PRECEDE stands for predisposing, reinforcing, and enabling constructs in education/environmental diagnosis and evaluation. The PRECEDE phase examines health goals, health problems, and life quality. The PROCEED stands for policy, regulatory, and organizational constructs in educational and environmental development. The PROCEED phase examines implementation and evaluation. The PRECEDE/PROCEED model is particularly useful in planning health education programs.

认需要改变，或者拒绝改变。第二阶段是沉思期（准备就绪），本期的标志是个体在短期6个月内有改变的意图。人们意识到了当前行为的不良后果以及改变行为后可能带来的积极后果。但是，人们对于自身行为改变的效果存在疑虑，反复衡量自己的付出是否能带来预想的效果，需要相应的信息和帮助。第三阶段是准备阶段（准备就绪），此阶段的特征是个体有强烈的短期内1个月内开始改变行为的意图。人们意识到需要改变并做出具体的行动计划。此时，应鼓励个体宣布出自己的计划并寻求家人和朋友的支持，共同努力达到目标。行动阶段是第四阶段，个体的行为在6个月内有了改变。但是，在这个过程中，人们容易恢复到以前不健康的行为，需要强化健康行为、杜绝懒散。第五阶段是维持阶段，人们的健康行为能够维持6个月或更长时间。这一阶段，较少出现行为的反复，个体对于保持健康的生活方式更加自信。

上述健康促进模式关注对个体健康行为和健康行为的改变的描述。除此以外，还有应用一些模型用来解释在社区的健康行动，例如保健教育过程模式。这一模式是基于教育学、社会心理学、流行病学等多学科的设计和研究的基础上发展的，此模式在健康教育项目中应用广泛。保健教育过程模式中PRECEDE代表教育/环境诊断和评估中的倾向、强化和形成结构化，该阶段关注健康目标、健康问题和生活质量；PROCEED则代表教育和环境发展中的政策、法规和组织结构，本阶段检查实施和评价。保健教育过程模式在规划健康教育项目时特别有用。

III. Barriers to Health Promotion

Elders lack participation in health promotion activities such as exercise, healthy diets, and adherence to medications. A number of factors affect elders' willingness to engage in specific health-promoting activities. Functional impairment such as inability to see or hear adequately or inability to physically engage in a behavior can decrease willingness to participate in the health maintenance behaviors. Cognitive impairment of elders can result in a lack of understanding of the health behavior and rationale for engaging in the behavior. Lack of access to resources (e. g. inability to access health care providers due to transportation challenges, insufficient numbers of providers, inability to afford health food options), inadequate environment for physical activity, and financial limitations are socioeconomic barriers to health promotion in elders. Ethnic and cultural factors can have negative effects on health promotion behaviors. If the diversity among communities is not adequately considered by health policy makers, it will create barriers to health promotion programs. Elders vary with regard to their wiliness to engage in health-promoting activities. It is useful to use an individualized approach to encourage elders to engage in health promotion behaviors.

Health care professionals are also a contributing the cause of lacking participation in health promotion among elders. The guidelines around activities that identify and treat asymptomatic persons who have developed risk factors or preclinical disease are not clear. For example, US Preventive Services Task Force created evidence-based guidelines on the premise that screening will improve patient outcomes. However, screening for those 85 years or older seems contradictory as very little data provide evidence that cancer screening tests are benefit for this age group.

IV. Health Promotion Interventions for the Elderly

Nursing interventions are directed toward improved health, functioning, and quality of life for elders, with emphasis on teaching elders and their caregivers about health promoting activities. Types of interventions include screening programs, risk-reduction interventions,

三、开展健康促进的障碍

一些老年人缺乏参与健康促进活动的积极性，这些活动包括身体锻炼、健康饮食、遵医嘱服药等。其中的影响因素是多方面的。首先，衰老或疾病带来的一些功能损害（如失明、失聪等或者身体残疾），会降低老年人参与维护健康行为的能力和意愿，特别是认知障碍限制了老年人对于健康行为的理解以及从事该行为的理由。其次，缺乏获得资源的机会（例如资源缺乏、无法负担保健食品的选择，以及经费受限等）身体活动的环境不足以及财务限制，都是影响老年人健康促进的社会经济因素。另外，种族和文化也可能对健康促进产生消极的影响。阻碍老年人健康促进开展的另一方面因素还有，如果决策者在制订健康政策时没有充分考虑不同社区的差异，那么所制定的健康政策反而会阻碍某些社区的健康促进和维护。因此，老年人参与健康促进活动的意愿各不相同，应当采用个性化的方案以鼓励尽可能多的老年人积极参与健康促进活动。

如果医护人员针对有危险因素或临床前无症状人群的疾病预防和干预的指南尚不清楚，也会大大影响老年人健康促进活动的参与。关于识别和治疗已发展为危险因素或临床前疾病的无症状者活动的指导方针尚不明确。例如，美国预防服务工作组建了基于证据的保健指南，其前提是疾病筛查要有利于改善患者的预后。然而，对85岁或85岁以上的人进行癌症筛查似乎与改善预后相违背，因为很少有数据能证明癌症筛查对这个年龄组是有益的。

四、老年人健康促进的具体措施

护理干预能够直接提高老年人的健康水平、维持躯体功能，改善其生活质量，其重点在于教会老年人及其照顾者健康促进的具体措施和行为。干预的方法包括疾病筛查、

environmental modifications, and health education. Following reviews these types of programs in relation to promoting wellness for elders:

i. Screening Programs

As screening programs may detect serious and progressive conditions as early as possible, they have been an essential component of disease prevention. Recommendations for screening related to conditions such as diabetes, hypertension, hyperlipidemia, hypothyroidism, osteoporosis, glaucoma, and many types of cancer have been published by the National Guideline Clearinghouse in the US. These conditions usually can be accurately detected and effectively treated before they progress to a serious or fatal stage. Criteria for recommending a screening test include cost effectiveness of the screening test, its ability to detect a condition or risk factor at an early stage, and early intervention being superior to waiting until signs or symptoms of disease are present.

For older adults, screening recommendations such as screening for breast, colon, prostate, and cervical cancer are often based on predictions of life expectancy and health status, which is consistent with the focus on increasing years of healthy living rather than on simply extending the quantity of life. The intent of these recommendations is to target those who are most likely to benefit, not only the elders in poor health, but also those in good health. Health beliefs of the older adults need to be considered because the health beliefs are likely to influence their participation in the screening programs. Table 3-1 summarizes some guidelines for use when educating elders about health promotion interventions.

ii. Risk-reduction Intervention

The purpose of risk-reduction interventions is to reduce the chance of developing a particular condition. Risk-reduction interventions are based on an assessment of the risk for developing that condition. Some risk-reduction interventions such as vaccinations are applicable to all elders, and others vary according to specific risk factors and the health status of an older person. Risk assessment tools for various conditions (e. g., falls, incontinence, pressure ulcers, heart disease, and elder abuse and neglect) have been developed. These tools serve to identify risk factors and people who are most likely to develop a particular condition so that health care professionals can develop and implement preventive interventions for them. Risk factors that are most dominant or likely to have the most serious negative consequences are often addressed first.

降低危险因素的具体措施、改变环境和健康教育等。以下是与促进老年人健康有关的这类计划的评论：

（一）疾病筛查

疾病筛查可以尽早发现疾病或监测已有疾病的进展情况，它已成为疾病预防中必不可少的组成部分。在美国，已经发布了系统的疾病筛查推荐标准，包括糖尿病、高血压、高血脂、甲状腺功能减退、骨质疏松症、青光眼以及肿瘤的筛查。这样就可以在疾病发生和进一步发展之前及时发现，并做出相应的预防和治疗干预。疾病筛查推荐标准的内容包括筛查的经济效益、筛查的效度和灵敏度以及在疾病症状出现之前的早期干预措施的效果等。

针对老年人的疾病筛查推荐项目有乳腺癌、结肠癌、前列腺癌、宫颈癌等。这些项目是基于对预期寿命和健康状况的综合考虑，其重点在于延长老人的健康预期寿命，而不仅仅是延长其寿命。这些筛查针对的目标人群不仅仅是身体状况欠佳的老年人，还包括身体状况好的老年人。另外，在实施疾病筛查时，还应考虑到老年人的健康信念是否影响他们真正参与疾病的筛查。表 3-1 概括了一些老年人预防和健康促进指南。

（二）降低危险因素的具体措施

降低风险干预措施的目的是减少发生特定疾病的机会。降低危险因素的具体措施有赖于前期对危险因素的评估。一些具体措施，例如接种疫苗等，对所有老年人来说都适用；而另一些措施，只针对有特定的危险因素或特定的老年人群。现有的危险因素的评估工具（有跌倒、压疮、心脏疾病、老人虐待和忽视的危险评估量表）。这些工具是用来识别个体是否存在疾病的危险因素和筛查有危险倾向的人群，以便健康照顾专业人员采取预防措施，最主要或可能产生最严重负面后果的风险因素往往需要首先得到解决。

Table 3-1 Guidelines for Prevention and Health Promotion for Elders

Measures of prevention and health promotion	
	Immunizations
For All Elders	● Tetanus-diphtheria: booster shot every 10 years
	● Influenza: annually at beginning of influenza season
	● Pneumovax: once after age 65 years; booster after 5 years if initial vaccination was before age 65 years or if other risk factors are present
For At-Risk Elders	● Herpes zoster (shingles): once after the age of 60 years, regardless of prior status with exposure or infection
	● Hepatitis A and B
	● Measles, mumps, rubella: if evidence of lack of immunity and significant risk for exposure
	● Varicella: if evidence of lack of immunity and significant risk for exposure.
	Screening
For All Elders	● Blood pressure: checks at least annually, more frequently if range is 130–139 mmHg systolic or 85–90 mmHg diastolic or if with risk factors
	● Serum cholesterol: every 5 years, more frequently in people with risk such as personal or family history of cardiovascular disease
	● Fecal occult blood and rectal examination: annually
	● Sigmoidoscopy: every (3 to) 5 years after age 50 years and until age 85 years
	● Visual acuity and glaucoma screening: annually
For Women	● Breast examination: self-examination monthly, annually by primary care practitioner
	● Pap smear and pelvic examination: annually until three consecutive negative exams, then every 2–3 years; discontinue after 65 years of age if three consecutive negative exams
	● Mammogram: annually or biannually between 50 and 69 years, every 1–3 years between 70 and 85 years
For Men	● Digital rectal examination: annually
	● Prostate-specific antigen (PSA) blood test: if at risk.
	Health Promotion Counseling
For All Elders	● Exercise: at least 30 minutes of moderate-intensity physical activity daily
	● Nutrition: adequate intake of all vitamins and minerals, especially calcium and antioxidants
	● Dental care and prophylaxis: every 6 months
For Elders (if applicable)	● Protective measures: seat belts, sunscreens, smoke detectors, fall risk prevention
	● Smoking cessation, substance abuse cessation, weight loss, vitamin supplements or low-dose aspirin

表 3-1 老年人预防和健康促进指南

预防和健康促进措施	
	免疫接种
所有老年人	● 破伤风 – 白喉：每 10 年加强一次
	● 流行性感冒：每年流行性感冒季节之初接种
	● 肺炎：65 岁以后；如果初次接种是在 65 岁之前或如果存在其他危险因素，则 5 年后加强
对于高危老年人	● 带状疱疹（带状疱疹）：60 岁以后一次，无论是否有接触或感染的状况
	● 甲型和乙型肝炎
	● 麻疹、腮腺炎、风疹：如果存在缺乏免疫力和暴露风险大的证据
	● 水痘：如果存在缺乏免疫力和暴露风险大的证据

预防和健康促进措施	
筛查	
所有老年人	● 血压：至少每年检查一次，如果范围为收缩压 130～139mmHg 或舒张压 85～90mmHg，或如果有危险因素，则增加检查频率 ● 血清胆固醇：每 5 年检查一次，患有心血管疾病者或有家族史的人增加检查的频率 ● 粪便潜血和直肠检查：每年 ● 乙状结肠镜检查：50 岁至 85 岁间每 3～5 年检查一次
女性	● 视力和青光眼筛查：每年一次 ● 乳房检查：每月自我检查，每年由初级保健医生检查一次 ● 巴氏涂片和骨盆检查：每年检查直至连续 3 次阴性，然后每 2～3 年检查一次；65 岁后如果连续三次检查为阴性则停止检查 ● 乳房 X 光照片：在 50 和 69 岁之间每年或每半年检查一次，在 70 和 85 岁之间每 1～3 年检查一次
男性	● 数字直肠检查：每年检查一次 ● 前列腺特异性抗原（PSA）血液检测：如有风险检查
健康促进咨询	
所有老年人	● 运动：每天至少 30min 的中等强度身体活动 ● 营养：充分摄取所有维生素和矿物质，特别是钙和抗氧化剂 ● 牙科护理和预防：每 6 个月进行一次
老年人（如适用）	● 防护措施：安全带，防晒霜，烟雾探测器，防跌落风险 ● 戒烟，戒毒，减肥，维生素补充剂或低剂量阿司匹林

For all elders, risk-reduction interventions include lifestyle factors (e. g. , optimal nutrition, weight management, adequate physical activity, sufficient sleep, avoidance of secondhand smoke, and appropriate stress-relieving techniques) and vaccinations for influenza, pneumonia, tetanus, and herpes zoster. Health promotion interventions to reduce risk also include the use of over-the-counter medications such as low-dose aspirin, nutritional supplements such as vitamins and minerals, and complementary and alternative therapies such as yoga and Tai Qi.

iii. Environmental Modifications

Environmental modifications that reduce risks or improve an individual's level of functioning are health promotion interventions. Environmental modifications to reduce fall risks and to improve hearing and vision are examples of effective health promotion activities. Detailed information on these environmental modifications is discussed in related chapters.

iv. Health Education

Health education focuses on teaching elders to engage in self-care activities that are preventive and wellness enhancing. Health education has been an essential component of health promotion as its effectiveness on improving healthy behaviors has been supported by evidences. Health care professionals

适用于所有老年人的干预措施包括：①保持良好的生活方式（如最佳营养、控制体重、适当的体力活动、充足的睡眠、避免间接吸烟和采用适当的减压技术等）；②接种流行性感冒、肺炎、破伤风及带状疱疹的疫苗；③应用非处方药（如小剂量阿司匹林、多种维生素和矿物质等）营养补充剂；④补充和替代疗法（坚持身体锻炼，如进行瑜伽、太极等运动）。

（三）环境改善

健康促进的干预措施还包括改善环境，以便降低环境中的危险因素和调节个体生理功能，以适应环境。有效的环境改善还包括降低跌倒危险、提高老年人视力、听力功能等。有关改善环境的详细内容将在相关章节中讨论。

（四）健康教育

健康教育致力于教会老年人进行预防和增强健康的自我护理活动。证据表明，健康教育能有效地改进健康行为，是健康促进必不可少的一部分。护理人员针对影响老年人健康和功能的特定条件和生活方式因素进行

incorporate health education in relation to specific conditions and lifestyle factors that affect health and functioning of elders. Topics of health education that are important for older adults include physical activity, nutrition, dental care, and avoidance of smoking and secondhand smoke. Physical activity has emerged as the most widely recognized health promotion intervention because of the wealth of evidence about the beneficial effects of physical activity. However, less than one third of older people in the United States engage in physical activity regularly. Engaging in regular physical activity is a major focus of health education.

Health care professionals take many roles in promoting physical activity for elders, in particular, teaching elders about the health benefits of physical activity. It also is important to teach about recommendations for type, frequency, duration, and intensity of physical activity. Health care professionals also need to assess for and address factors that influence an elderly person to participate in regular physical activity.

Miller (2012) provided the following guide to teaching elders about recommended exercises:

1. Aerobic exercise Brisk walking, jogging, walking upstairs, etc.

Definition: Activity that requires the body to use oxygen to produce the energy necessary for the activity.

Benefits: Lowers blood pressure; diminishes blood glucose, strengthens heart muscle; improves lipids and triglycerides; decreases risk for cardiovascular disease; decreases intra-abdominal fat; improves self-esteem; and relieves symptoms of anxiety and depression.

Intensity: Identify your target heart rate by subtracting your age in years from 220 beats per minute (this is the maximum heart rate) and multiplying by 0.65.

Frequency: 2.5 hours weekly of moderate intensity OR 1.25 hours weekly of vigorous intensity (in episodes of at least 10 minutes).

2. Strength or resistance training exercises Stretch bands, weights, strap-on sandbags, bicep curls, bench presses.

Definition: Performance of muscle contractions against a resistance that is greater than usual for that muscle; slow and controlled movements of major muscled groups such as arms, back, hips, chest, and shoulders, with exhalation during exertion and inhalation during return to the starting position.

Benefits: Improves balance and diminishes risk for falls, strengthens musculoskeletal system,

健康教育。对老年人来说，重要的健康教育主题包括身体锻炼、营养、牙齿保健、避免直接吸烟和间接吸烟等。大量证据表明，身体锻炼是非常有益的，并得到广泛认可。然而，在美国，只有不到1/3的老年人进行规律的身体锻炼。因而，鼓励老年人进行规律的身体锻炼是健康教育一个非常重要的部分。

健康照顾专业人员在促进老年人进行身体锻炼上扮演着重要的角色，尤其是向老年人传授体育锻炼对健康的好处。健康照顾专业人员同样需要去评估和解决影响老年人参加规律的身体锻炼的因素，给予其有关锻炼的类型、频率、持续时间和强度等方面的建议。

Miller（2012）推荐的适合老年人锻炼的方式有：

1. 有氧运动 如快步走、慢跑、爬楼梯等。

定义：需要身体利用氧气来产生活动所需能量的活动。

益处：降低血压，降低血糖，增强心肌，改善血脂和甘油三酯，降低心血管疾病的风险，减少腹内脂肪，提高自尊，缓解焦虑和抑郁症状。

强度：确定你的目标心率，用220减去年龄（这是最大心率，次/min），再乘以0.65。

频率：每周2.5小时中等强度或每周1.25小时剧烈强度（至少10分钟）。

2. 力量或抗阻训练 如拉力计、举重、捆绑沙袋、举哑铃、仰卧推举等。

定义：肌肉收缩抵抗比一般肌肉活动阻力更大；主要肌群（手臂、背部、臀部、胸部和肩部等）缓慢而有控制地运动，在用力时呼气，在回到起始位置时吸气。

益处：改善平衡，降低跌倒风险，增强肌肉骨骼系统，改善功能和独立性，降低骨

improves function and independence, decreases risk for osteoporosis, favorably modifies risk factors for cardiovascular disease and type 2 diabetes.

Intensity: You should be able to repeat the movement 8 consecutive times, but not more than 12 times, before experiencing significant muscle fatigue.

Frequency: 8–10 different sets of exercises working all major muscle groups, each repeated 8–12 times, several days a week.

3. Stretching exercises Yoga, range-of-motion exercises, etc.

Definition: Activity that improves body flexibility.

Benefits: Increases flexibility, reduces muscle soreness, improves performance of daily activities.

Intensity: Stretch muscle groups, but not to the point of pain, and hold for 10–30 seconds.

Frequency: Repeat each stretch at least 4 times, a minimum of 2–4 times weekly.

The empowerment of elders to make their own health care decisions is also essential in health promotion for elders. Nurses should actively participate in encouraging elders to set health promotion goals aimed at maintaining the optimum level of health, function, and quality of life. Nurses should also learn about community resources and local, state, and federal programs that can provide services or information to elders and then disseminate the information to elders. Most important, nurses should use an individualized approach to health promotion for elders. Nurses provide appropriate health education both formally in health promotion classes and informally during health care visits. Nurses should provide current recommendations for health promotion activities and help elders decide what health behaviors they want to engage in. The individualized approach can increase adherence to positive health behaviors and help the elders to achieve their optimum health.

(ZENG Hui)

Key Points

1. Physiologic aging is universal, progressive, detrimental, intrinsic, and unavoidable.

2. Functionally significant aging changes are especially common in the urinary, musculoskeletal, and neurologic systems and in the special senses.

3. Lubrication of joints, elasticity, enzymatic processes, and cellular fluids gradually diminishes during aging.

质疏松的风险，有利于改善心血管疾病和 2 型糖尿病的危险因素。

强度：在出现明显的肌肉疲劳之前，需要连续重复 8 次，但不超过 12 次。

频率：8~10 次不同的锻炼，锻炼所有主要肌肉群，每次重复 8~12 次，每周几天。

3. 伸展训练 如瑜伽、关节活动度练习等。

定义：提高身体灵活性的活动。

益处：增加柔韧性，减少肌肉酸痛，改善日常活动表现。

强度：伸展肌肉群，但不要感到疼痛，保持 10~30 秒。

频率：每次伸展至少重复 4 遍，每周至少做 2~4 次。

增强老年人对自身健康照顾的决策能力是健康促进必不可少的一方面。应该积极鼓励老年人建立并维持较高的健康水平、机体功能和生活质量的目标。护士应该了解本地能够给老年人提供的健康服务和健康资源，然后向老年人传达这些信息。最重要的是护士应该为老年人制订个体化的健康促进方案。无论在课堂上，还是家庭访视中，都应该提供合适的健康教育。护士应该将最新的建议和指南提供给老年人，并帮助他们进行决策。个体化方案可以提高健康行为的依从性，帮助老年人达到最佳健康目标。

（曾　慧）

本章要点

1. 生理老化是普遍的、渐进的、衰退的、内在的和不可避免的。

2. 重要的功能老化在泌尿系统、肌肉骨骼和神经系统以及特殊感觉中尤其常见。

3. 在老化过程中，关节的润滑、弹性、酶促过程逐渐减低，基质逐渐减少。

4. Age-related changes in the cardiovascular system are most likely to progress toward a disease state.

5. Hormonal and endocrine changes influence more in the aging process.

6. Decreases in nervous system acuity and sensory acuity are significant.

7. Cognitive functions decline in older adults because of decreased number of neurons, decreased brain size, diminished brain weight, and changes in transmission of the chemical neurotransmitters.

8. Short-term memory, fluid intelligence, and learning speed in later life tend to decline with age.

9. Older adults, especially the years beyond age 80, often deal with disability, caregiving, bereavement, and loneliness.

10. People of all ages can benefit from health promoting activities.

11. There are a number of models of health promotion to guide the development of health promotion programs for older adults.

12. Functional and cognitive impairment, health beliefs and attitudes, psychosocial factors, economic factors, environmental factors, ethnic and cultural influences can be barriers to health promotion.

13. Interventions related to health promotion for older adults include screening programs, risk-reduction interventions, environmental modifications, and health education.

Critical Thinking Exercise

(Questions 1 to 2 share the same question stem)

In a clinic, you meet with an older woman. She reports that she gets up to the toilet four times every night and incontinence of urine occurs sometimes. She worries whether the condition is normal.

1. What recommendation is more appropriate for helping the old woman on incontinence of urine?

2. How to help the old woman to reduce her worry?

(Questions 3 to 4 share the same question stem)

Grandma Wang is 70 years old and lives alone. Her daughter comes back to see her twice a week and finds that her mother often forgets where the things she put some minutes ago and often repeats the words she talked several minutes before. But she can remember the things happened many years ago. Her daughter worries whether Grandma Wang' condition is normal.

4. 心血管系统的老化最有可能向疾病状态发展。

5. 激素和内分泌变化在衰老过程中影响更大。

6. 神经系统敏感度和感觉敏感度的降低明显。

7. 由于神经元数量减少、脑体积减小、脑重量减少以及化学性神经递质传递的变化，老年人的认知功能下降。

8. 短时记忆、流体智力和晚年的学习速度往往随着年龄的增长而下降。

9. 老年人，尤其是80岁以上老年人，常常面临失能、照顾老伴、丧偶、孤独等问题。

10. 所有年龄的人都可以从健康促进活动中受益。

11. 一些健康促进模式可指导老年人制订健康促进方案。

12. 功能和认知障碍、健康信念和态度、心理社会因素、经济因素、环境因素、种族和文化影响可妨碍健康促进。

13. 与老年人健康促进有关的干预措施包括筛查方案、减少风险干预措施、环境调适和健康教育。

批判性思维练习

（1～2题共用题干）

诊所里一位女性老人诉说她每天晚上要上4次厕所，有时会出现尿失禁。她担心自己的状况是否正常。

1. 如何帮助尿失禁的老年女性？

2. 如何减轻这个老人的担忧？

（3～4题共用题干）

王奶奶，70岁，独自生活。她的女儿每周回来看望她两次，发现她母亲经常忘记她几分钟前放东西的位置，经常重复她几分钟前所说过的话。但她可以记住许多年前发生的事情。女儿担心她母亲的状况是否正常。

3. What kind of memory has mainly decreased for Grandma Wang?

4. What measure is more appropriate for helping to differentiate benign forgetfulness from malignant memory loss?

(Question 5 to 6 share the same question stem)

Mr. Liu is 75 years old and lives by himself in a community near a park. However, he seldom goes out for a walk or meets with friends. He comes to see you to have his blood pressure checked once a month. Mr. Liu takes medications for hypertension and has expressed concern about heart disease. When you discuss risk factors for heart disease with Mr. Liu, he says that he would like to perform more physical activity as long as it doesn't worsen his arthritis.

5. What model is more appropriate for the practice of promoting Mr. Liu's health?

6. What change stage does Mr. Liu belong to?

3. 王奶奶主要是哪种记忆减退了？

4. 什么措施更适合帮助区分良性健忘与恶性的记忆丧失？

（5～6题共用题干）

刘先生，75岁，独自住在公园附近的社区。然而，他很少出去散步或与朋友会面。他每月来测一次血压。刘先生服用高血压药物，并表达了对自己心脏病的关注。当与刘先生讨论心脏病的危险因素时，他说，只要不使关节炎恶化，他就愿意进行更多的身体锻炼。

5. 什么模式更适合促进刘先生的健康？

6. 刘先生处于哪个变化阶段？

Chapter 4　Geriatric Assessment
第四章　老年人健康评估

Learning Objectives

On completion of this chapter, the reader will be able to:
- Describe the eight dimensions of geriatric assessment and their relationships;
- Define each dimension and its domains;
- Discuss the importance of geriatric assessment;
- Distinguish normal aging-related changes and abnormal findings;
- Apply health history, physical examination, and/or assessment tools to assess each domain of the eight dimensions of geriatric assessment;
- Analyze assessment findings to identify the status of each dimensions of geriatric assessment;
- Synthesize data from geriatric assessment to design interventions.

学习目标

学完本章节，应完成以下目标：
- 描述老年人健康评估的 8 个维度及其相互间的关系；
- 定义老年人健康评估的各个维度及其范畴；
- 讨论老年人健康评估的重要性；
- 区分正常老化和异常变化；
- 通过病史采集、体格检查及评估量表来筛查老年人健康评估的 8 个维度；
- 分析老年人健康评估 8 个维度的评估结果，从而明确相应的健康问题；
- 整合老年人健康评估的数据来制订干预措施。

Geriatric assessment is well established as the first step in providing high quality health care to the elderly people by generating comprehensive data to support individualized diagnoses, care plan, and outcome evaluation. Its critical role is heightened as health care shifts towards patient-centered care and precision medicine, gold standard practice for achieving the triple aims of geriatrics (healthcare safety, quality, and coordination) while improving quality of life. Patient-centered care refers to "Providing care is respectful of and responsive to individual patient preferences, needs, and values, and ensuring that patient values guide all clinical decisions." Clinicians elicit, support, and honor individuals' preferences guide all health care decisions. Precision medicine extends the patient-centered principles by taking into account individual differences in genes, environment, and lifestyle to prevent and treat diseases.

Section 1   Overview

I. Definition, Goals, and Practice Logistics of Geriatric Assessment

Geriatric assessment is a broad term that refers to a comprehensive, extensive, and multi-dimensional diagnostic and management process for evaluating and managing health in the elderly people. Geriatric assessment builds on but extends beyond conventional health assessment, recognizing that the elderly people often have multiple, chronic, and complex problems and their health status is frequently influenced by factors beyond their medical conditions.

Geriatric assessment has four major goals:

1) Generate comprehensive data to support nursing and medical diagnoses.

2) Inform patient-centered, holistic care planning within each older adult's unique context of health care goals, values, and preferences, genes, environment, and lifestyle.

3) Evaluate health care outcomes particularly important to the elderly people, e. g. , functional independence, wellbeing, quality of life, and survival.

老年人健康评估通过全面地搜集数据，从而辅助进行个体化诊断、护理计划制订和效果评价；老年人健康评估是为老年人提供高质量健康保健服务的第一步。近些年来，以患者为中心的护理模式和精准医疗模式成为健康照护领域关注的重点，这使得老年人健康评估的重要性提升到了新的高度。以患者为中心是指以患者的目标、价值观和意愿为中心，基于患者的价值观来指导临床决策。临床医护人员需支持、尊重患者的个人意愿。精准医疗模式是指进一步根据患者基因、环境和生活方式的差异给予有针对性地预防和治疗。

第一节   概述

一、老年人健康评估的概念、目标及实施方法

老年人健康评估是以临床诊断学为基础逐步发展和完善的一门综合学科，它适用于老年人复杂的诊疗过程，便于深入、全面地探讨老年人的健康问题。老年人的健康状况常受除疾病以外的多种因素影响以及长期而复杂的问题，临床诊断学局限于对躯体疾病的评估，不能对老年人健康状况进行全面描述。

老年人健康评估主要有4个目标：

1）为医疗和护理诊断提供综合、全面的初始数据。

2）指导符合老年人医疗保健目标、价值观、意愿、基因、环境和生活方式、以老年人为中心的全面医疗保健计划。

3）评价医疗保健服务的效果，尤其是老年人特别关注的结果，以达到促进老年人身心健康，增强功能独立性、幸福感，提高生活质量和生存能力及延长寿命的目的。

4) Realize the triple aims of health care in geriatrics: high care safety, quality, and coordination.

Geriatric assessment is flexible and adaptable. It usually connotes an interdisciplinary approach and is conducted by a team of nurses, physicians, pharmacists, physical/occupational/speech/recreational therapists, social workers, and/or chaplains. A nurse or social worker usually assumes the team leader or coordinator role. Depending on an older adult's unique context, geriatric assessment can be completed over multiple visits to serve a wide range of the elderly people in a variety of health care settings. It can occur in any settings such as community, clinic, nursing home, or hospital. A visit to the residence of the elderly people is a critical part of geriatric assessment, which augments the efficiency for health care resource mobilization, coordination, and utilization.

II. Dimensions of Geriatric Assessment

Historically, geriatric assessment has six traditional dimensions (medical conditions, geriatric syndromes, functional status, cognitive function, psychological status, and social status). Patient-centered care and precision medicine movements called for the addition of two more dimensions: health care goals, values, and preferences; and genes, environment, and lifestyle.

As figure 4-1 illustrates, health care goals, values, and preferences as well as genes, environment, and lifestyle provide the overall, intersecting context in which the other six dimensions operate. All eight dimensions interact with each other reciprocally. For example, functional status affects cognitive function in turn influences functional status. In addition, functional status occupies a central role in geriatric assessment, and reflects the collective impact of all other dimensions. It's a common wisdom in geriatrics that the elderly people's ability to function at a level consistent with their lifestyles should be an important consideration in all health care planning. It is likely that the dimensions of geriatric assessments will continue to evolve as research evidence accumulates.

4）实现为老年人提供安全、优质、协调的医疗保健服务的终极目标。

老年人健康评估的实施方法灵活多样，需考虑评估者、评估时机和评估地点。就评估者而言，强调跨学科合作，其团队包括护士、医生、康复治疗师、药剂师、社工等。团队领导通常由护士或社工承担。就评估时机而言，老年人健康评估一般在与老年人初次接触时即开始。根据评估目的的不同，可有侧重地选择评估内容。如针对社区老年人认知受损的筛查，可使用简明认知评估工具。通常老年人健康评估是由健康问题引出，可通过多次随访完成全部的评估内容。就评估场所而言，老年人健康评估的灵活性较高，可以在任何场合进行，也可根据需要随时调整。因而老年人健康评估并不局限于医院、门诊和社区，对家庭环境安全和老年人日常活动场所的实地考察也是必不可少的环节。

二、老年人健康评估的维度

老年人健康评估包括疾病，老年综合征，功能状态，认知功能，心理状态，社会状态，医疗保健目标及价值观和意愿，基因、环境和生活方式等八个维度。随着研究证据的积累，老年人健康评估的维度也将进一步演变。

如图4-1所示，医疗保健目标、价值观和意愿，基因、环境和生活方式为其他六个维度的实施提供整体背景。这八个维度彼此独立又互相影响。其中，功能状态在老年人健康评估中占主导地位，是其他七个维度的外在表现。

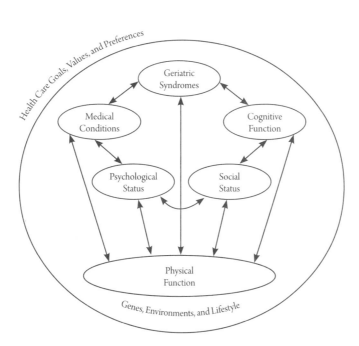

Figure 4-1　Dimensions of geriatric assessments and their relationships

Health care planning for the elderly people needs to emphasize whether the care will affect their functional status in a way that is consistent with their daily routine. Now let's review the definition and domains of each dimension:

i. Medical Conditions

Medical conditions refer to abnormal conditions in physiological structure and/or function. Geriatric assessment emphasizes the identification and management of acute and chronic conditions. While acute conditions are often short in duration and curable, chronic diseases cannot be cured and their trajectory is interspersed with episodes of acute exacerbation. The coexistence of multiple chronic conditions is known as multimorbidity. The elderly people are susceptible to chronic diseases and multimorbidity because of the progressive dysregulation of the biophysiological signals, reduced ability to maintain homeostasis, and presence of low grade, chronic proinflammatory state, which results in the gradual loss of physiological reserves and increased vulnerability to diseases.

ii. Geriatric Syndromes

Geriatric syndromes were coined to describe health conditions that disproportionately affected the elderly people but yet did not fit within a discrete disease category. Geriatric syndromes are defined as "the multi-factorial health conditions that occurs when the accumulated effects of impairments in multiple systems render an elderly person vulnerable to situational challenges" and include a host of conditions, e. g. , polypharmacy, falls,

老年医疗保健计划要重点考虑功能状态的影响是否符合老年人以往的生活方式。下面本节将逐一探讨这八个维度的定义及其评估方法：

（一）疾病状况

疾病指生理结构和／或功能的异常变化。在临床诊断学基础上，老年人健康评估更强调对急性和慢性病的识别和管理。急性病常在短期内急性发作，较易治愈；而慢性病是病理变化累积的结果，常伴有反复的急性发作，难以治愈。随着年龄增长，人体生理调节能力减弱，维持内在平衡能力降低，同时处于慢性炎症状态，因而易发生多病共存（即多种慢性病并发），生理储备逐渐降低，并对疾病的易感性增加。

（二）老年综合征

老年综合征是一种高发于老年人群中的健康问题，但不能归类于某一器官系统疾病。老年综合征指由多种原因造成的多个系统累积损伤，使老年人在遇到情境挑战时的易感性更强。常见的老年综合征有多重用药、跌倒、衰弱和痴呆等。不同的老年综合征往往具有某些共同的诱因和病理机制，涉及多个

fraily, and dementia. They also share some features such as common pathological pathways, multiple organ system involvement, treatments initiation without confirm the cause (s), and treatments targeting common etiological factors.

iii. Functional Status

Functional status refers to the ability to perform normal daily activities required to meet basic needs, fulfill usual role requirements, and maintain health and wellbeing and includes three domains: health-related physical fitness, physical function, and activities of daily living (ADLs). Physical fitness is composed of four domains: cardiorespiratory fitness, body composition, muscular strength, and flexibility. Physical function includes transfer, lower extremity strength, balance, gait speed, and mobility. ADLs have three domains including advanced ADLs (AADLs), instrumental ADLs (IADLs), and basic ADLs (BADLs).

iv. Cognitive Function

Cognitive function is defined as cerebral activities that acquire, process, and output information and accumulate knowledge by which a person becomes aware of, perceives, or comprehends ideas. Clinically, four discrete cognitive domains are typically assessed memory, executive functioning, visuospatial function, and language. It is not uncommon for clinicians to use more detailed domains such as orientation, abstraction, judgment, problem solving, and attention, or a broader term, global cognition which includes multiple, if not all, cognitive domains.

v. Psychological Status

Psychological status refers to one's mood states which are the display of emotions through body movements, facial expression, vocal tone, and self-description of own internal feeling. Mood disturbances are not a part of normal aging and occur in a wide variety of conditions such as dementia, schizophrenia, and Parkinson's disease. Although the entire spectrum of mood disorders can be represented in the elderly people, depression, anxiety disorder, and grief are the most common problems.

系统，在治疗时可能无明确病因，而是针对常见的共同病因进行治疗。

（三）功能状态

功能状态指老年人在生活中满足日常基本需要、社会角色需要以及维持健康和幸福感的能力，包括健康相关的体适能、躯体功能和日常生活活动能力（ADL）三个方面。健康相关的体适能包括四个部分，分别是有氧适能、体成分、肌肉力量及关节的灵活性；身体功能包括五个方面，分别是位置转移、下肢力量、平衡力、步速和移动能力；日常生活活动能力包括三个方面，即高级日常生活活动能力（AADLs）、工具性日常生活活动能力（IADLs）和基本日常生活活动能力（BADLs）。

（四）认知功能

认知功能指人脑通过收集、处理和传递信息而累积知识、灵活观察、理解和推理事物间复杂关系的能力。在临床上，通常会评估四个方面的认知情况：记忆、执行功能、视空间功能和语言功能。医护人员还会进一步具体地评估认知功能，如对定向力、抽象力、判断、解决问题能力和注意力进行评估，此外，总体认知功能是认知功能的另一个常用范畴。

（五）心理状态

心理状态指个体的情绪状态，可通过肢体动作、面部表情、语调和对自我内在情感的描述来反映。情绪障碍并不属于正常的老化改变，而是一些健康问题的症状，如痴呆、精神分裂症和帕金森病。尽管老年人会出现不同的情绪障碍，但最常见的是抑郁、焦虑和悲痛。

vi. Social Status

Social status refers to a person's standing and relationships within a society and is composed of six domains: social support, elder mistreatment, decisional capacity and competency, advance directives, financial situation, and spirituality. It goes beyond the social history collected about education, employment history, habits, hobbies etc. during a conventional health assessment.

vii. Health Care Goals, Values, and Preferences

Health care goals are defined as a person's perception of the aims or desired outcomes of health care. Values are a person's judgment of what is important in health care. Preferences refer to an individual's expression of desirability or selection of one course of health care actions and outcomes over others. A person's health care goals and values ultimately determine preferences. Understanding preferences is foundational to evidence-based practice and person-centered care and should guide health care decision-making. Eliciting preferences include three steps: identify a preference-sensitive situation; analyze the advantages and disadvantages of different health care options; and consult the elderly people's preferences for different options.

viii. Genes, Environment, and Lifestyle

Genes refer to loci or regions of DNA and are the molecular unit of heredity. Environment is the physical and cultural settings that an individual lives in. Lifestyle is defined as the way an individual lives. Currently, it is well established that there is tremendous heterogeneity in biological traits, disease susceptibility and treatment responses, which is heavily influenced by genes and their interactions with environment and lifestyle. Hence, precision medicine calls for the identification of subgroups based on genes, environment, and lifestyle to focus prevention and treatment efforts accordingly.

III. Importance of Geriatric Assessment

By now, you probably have a good idea why geriatric assessment is paramount to the care of the elderly people. Its first and utmost importance is the ability to overcome the following four limitations of conventional health assessment. Clinical diagnosis uses a single disease or system approach which defines a disease with unique

（六）社会状态

社会状态指个体在家庭、社区和社会中所处的位置及其社会关系。除了传统的教育水平、工作经历、习惯、爱好、烟酒嗜好等社会信息外，老年人的社会状态还包括了六个方面，即社会支持、虐待、决策力和决策胜任力、委托、经济状况和精神信仰。

（七）医疗保健目标、价值观和意愿

医疗保健目标指个体对医疗保健服务期望达到的目标或结果；价值观是指个体对医疗保健服务重要性的看法；偏好是指个人对医疗保健行动的期望或选择，以及对其他行动的选择的结果。一个人的医疗保健目标和价值观最终决定了他们的偏好。理解偏好是基于证据的实践和以人为本的护理的基础，并应指导医疗保健决策。产生偏好包括三个步骤：确定偏好敏感的情况；分析不同医疗保健选择的利弊；咨询老年人的偏好以选择其他选项。意愿指在有多个选择时，个体偏向的选择。医疗保健目标和价值观直接影响意愿，三者共同构成循证实践的基础，从而实现以患者为中心的照护。

（八）基因、环境和生活方式

基因是指 DNA（脱氧核糖核酸）分子上具有遗传信息的特定核苷酸序列；环境是个体生存的自然和社会环境的总称；生活方式指个体在衣、食、住、行、休息、娱乐等方面的选择。现在已广泛认可人与人之间对疾病的易感性和治疗效果存在较大差异，其主要源于每个人独特的基因、环境、生活方式和它们之间的协同作用。

三、老年人健康评估的重要性

到目前为止，您可能已经有了一个想法，为什么老年人健康评估对老年人的护理至关重要。它的首要任务是克服常规健康评估的以下四个限制。临床诊断学强调每个疾病的诱因、症状和病理过程。然而，在老年人中，

characteristics and its selective influences on particular aspects of homeostasis. The elderly people, however, often presents with atypical or vague chief complaints, signs, and symptoms that prohibits an easy identification of a disease. For example, the elderly people rarely show the typical heart attack symptoms of chest pain. Instead, they may report indigestion and nausea which in younger adults indicate an upset stomach or food poisoning. In addition, aging-related changes complicate the pathological processes of a single disease, which interacts with comorbid conditions in a complex way that are often not understood.

Functional status is critical to the elderly people, but is often unconsidered in conventional health assessment. With aging-related physiological changes and prevalent chronic conditions, outcomes are important to the elderly people including functional independence, wellbeing, quality of life, and survival. In elderly people, the number of medical conditions probably matter less than the strength of physiological reserves. The absence of medical diagnoses does not necessarily represent better health. An elderly person with low physiological reserve and functional status might not recover better than another person who has multiple medical conditions but higher physiological reserve and functional status.

Conventional health assessment emphasizes specialty care and lacks care integrity, coordination, and continuity. Although the elderly people often seek services from different medical specialties to meet different health care needs, each specialty focuses on own specialty area without adequate attentions to the treatments provided by other specialties, a well-known reason for polypharmacy in the elderly people.

The importance of geriatric assessment is further reflected in its grounding in interdisciplinary collaboration. Geriatric assessment employs an interdisciplinary team that includes nurses, physicians, pharmacists, rehabilitation professionals, nutritionists, psychologists, social workers, and/or community health workers. Each discipline brings its specific expertise to the care of the elderly people, coordinates care, and facilitates health care transitions. This approach prevents redundant care and ensures overall care safety, quality, completeness, and efficiency.

Geriatric assessment also lays the foundation for implementing patient-centered care and precision medicine to achieve the triple aims of health care safety, quality, and coordination. While many system-level approaches are needed to implement persons-centered or precision medicine, geriatric assessment provides the foundation for assessing the unique aspects of an elderly

疾病往往没有明确的诱因，且老年人主诉不典型或模棱两可，甚至临床表现跟疾病毫不相干。比如，心肌梗死的老年人并不会表现出压榨性心前区疼痛或胸闷，其反而会主诉消化不良、恶心。此外，在老化引起的生理变化的基础上，慢性病和多病共存使得各个器官、系统的互相影响机制更加复杂，当前尚无法通过医学知识进行解释。

对老年人至关重要的功能状态在临床诊断学中所占比重较轻。老年医疗保健的目的是促进功能独立，增强幸福感和生活质量，延长寿命。没有疾病并不一定代表健康。一个没有疾病，但生理储备低、功能差的老年人，其预后可能反而不如多病共存，但生理储备高且功能良好的老年人。

临床诊断学强调专科，因而其服务的整体性、协调性和连续性欠缺，不能满足老年人的需求。专科注重于一个系统疾病的治疗，也是造成老年人用药不当的原因之一。

老年人健康评估的优势还体现在跨学科合作上，跨学科团队往往由护士或社工领导，成员包括医生、药剂师、康复治疗师、营养师、心理治疗师、社区健康工作者等。每个学科都运用自己的专长来照护老年人，调动和协调医疗保健，共同实现过渡期服务。这一方法有助于防止过度照护，并保证了照护过程的安全、优质、完整和高效。

目前许多医疗体系都在寻求安全、优质、协调的医疗保健模式，以满足老年人群日益增长的健康需求。以患者为中心的照护和精准医疗是目前的黄金标准，老年人健康评估则为其进一步地开展和实施提供了良好的条件。

person which will inform the development of a patient-centered care plan tailored to each individual.

Finally, many health care systems have devoted extensive efforts to establish safe, high quality, coordinated, and cost-effective models of health care to meet the needs of the growing elderly people. Within this context, person-centered care and precision medicine have been established as the gold-standard care. Geriatric assessment empowers the elderly people to actively engage in their health care, and addresses their changing health care needs and preferences for care on an ongoing basis to adjust care accordingly in a timely fashion.

Section 2　Medical Condition

Medical conditions refer to abnormal conditions in physiological structure and/or function. The assessment of medical conditions is same as conventional health assessment of taking health history and conducting physical examination using an organ systems approach. A good history-taking is essential for focusing physical examination and increase the efficiency of assessment. However, aging contributes to various degrees of physiological changes in each organ system, which does not prevent the elderly people to function normally in ordinary circumstances, but induces normal aging-related changes. As a result, it's critical to distinguish abnormal signs and symptoms from normal aging-related changes albeit the fact that it not always possible to do so.

I. History-taking of Medical Condition

Health history for the elderly people spans decades of life, making history-taking challenging. Incomplete recall, impaired cognition, biased reports and interpretations by family members, and multiple providers often occur. The clinician should make every effort to collect data from multiple resources including the elderly people, families, other providers, and existing records. The reliability and objectivity of history sources must be continuously assessed to ensure accuracy and history data updated as new information becomes available.

Being a good listener, it should be having a detective mindset, focusing on critical historic points, and gathering information using both open- and close-ended questions

最后，老年人健康评估通过对医疗保健目标、价值观、意愿及基因、环境和生活方式的考虑，充分调动老年人的积极性和参与性，从而提高了老年人治疗依从性，并改善预后。此外老年人健康评估也满足了当前医疗环境背景下，老年人日益变化的照护需求和意愿。

第二节　疾病状况评估

疾病指生理结构和 / 或功能的异常变化。和传统的健康评估一样，老年人疾病的信息采集包含了基于器官系统的病史采集和体格检查。良好的病史采集有助于体格检查，提高信息采集的有效性。然而，由于衰老造成的各个器官系统不同程度的生理改变，使得机体出现老化相关的改变。因此，必须准确辨别正常的老化相关改变和异常的病理性变化。

一、病史采集

老年人病史较长，多达十几年甚至更久，这使得老年人的病史采集有一定难度。老年人回忆性错误、认知受损、家人陈述偏差等情况时有发生。为确保病史的全面和准确，医生需要从老年人、家人、专业和非专业医务人员及病历等多渠道进行资料采集。此外，评估资料来源的可靠性和客观性也是病史采集不可忽略的一个方面。

倾听、探究的心态、抓住关键点、开放和非开放问题相结合等方法，是病史采集的技巧。在进行老年人健康评估前，尤其需要

are central to becoming a skilled geriatric history taker. You may want to refresh your health assessment skills before you proceed.

Health history includes six domains that are demographic data, chief complaint, history of present illness, past medical history, family history, and review of systems. Social history will be covered under Section 7 Social Status. Table 4-1 summarizes the focus of each domain and its characteristics in the elderly people.

加强这些技巧。

病史采集涵盖传统病史的人口学资料、主诉、现病史、既往病史、家族史和系统评估等六个部分。社会状况的评估将在第七节中进行介绍。表4-1总结了各方面病史的重点和老年人的相关特点。

Table 4-1　Focus and Characteristics of Health History in Elderly People

Domain	Focus	Characteristics
Demographic data	Full name, age, gender, birthday, marital status, living situation, history source and reliability	Multiple sources (the elderly people, families, other clinicians, and medical records)
Chief complaint	Presenting symptom and its duration in own words	Atypical symptoms; disconnection between complaint and disease system
History of present illness	OLDCART for symptom (onset, location, duration, characteristics, aggravating factors, relieving factors, and treatment)	Atypical, unspecific, vague
Past medical history	Chronological list of all childhood and adult diseases, injuries, hospitalizations, and surgeries, immunizations, allergies, and medication review	Long life spans, multimorbidity, incomplete recalls, and family biases
Family History	Presence of diseases in first degree relatives	Similar chief complaint in family members

表4-1　老年人病史的重点和特点

项目	重点	特点
人口学资料	全名（及曾用名）、年龄、性别、生日、婚姻状态、民族、病史来源及可靠性	多重来源（老年人自身、家人、其他医务人员及病历）
主诉	老年人用自己的语言描述症状及持续时间	不典型症状、主诉和疾病间差异
现病史	始发时间、身体部位、特点、加重因素、减轻因素、治疗措施	不典型、不特定、模糊
既往病史	以年为主线，列举从儿童时期到现在的所有疾病、损伤、住院、手术、接种疫苗、过敏史和用药史	整个生命周期、多病共存、不完成回忆和家人偏见
家族史	直系亲属患有的疾病	家庭成员有相似主诉

i. Demographics

Demographic data include full name, age, gender, birthday, marital status, ethnicity/race, history source, and its reliability.

ii. Chief Complaint

Chief complaint describes the primary reason or symptom for the visit and the symptom duration in the elderly people's own words. Attention must be paid to

（一）人口学资料

人口学资料包括全名（及曾用名）、年龄、性别、生日、婚姻状态、民族、病史信息来源及可靠性。

（二）主诉

主诉是指老年人用自己的语言描述本次就诊的主要原因或症状（以及症状的持续时间）。需注意观察老年人在主诉时的语言和肢

both verbal and nonverbal language to evaluate if chief complaint matches body language. For example, an elderly person who reports no clear complaint but appears to be restless should raise suspicion of problems.

Eliciting chief complaint in the elderly people is not as straightforward as in younger people. The elderly people often report seemingly unrelated, atypical, trivial, or nonspecific complaints. Rarely will an elderly person give a clear chief complaint that leads to a recognizable problem due to five reasons:

(1) Atypical presentation of medical conditions is the rule in geriatrics. The elderly people often have chronic diseases and multimorbidity which result in complex patho-physiological changes. It is common that symptoms of one system may actually signal pathology in another system.

(2) The elderly people often attribute their symptoms or dysfunction to being "normal" signs of aging, so they do not seek medical attention timely.

(3) Fear and denial of serious problems may make an elderly person report no or irrelevant complaints.

(4) Communication barriers such as language and cultural differences, memory loss, depression, hearing and visual impairments may prevent the elderly people from receiving adequate attention from clinicians.

(5) The elderly people may minimize symptoms due to a lack of financial surpport means to pursue evaluations and treatments.

iii. History of Present Illness

History of present illness refers to the chronological narrative of chief complaint should be elicited using methods like OLDCART. OLDCART is the acronym for onset (When did the presenting symptoms start?), location (Where are the symptoms on your body?), duration (How long have you had those symptoms?), characteristics (How do the symptoms feel like?), aggravating factors (What makes your symptoms worse?), relieving factors (What makes your symptoms better?), and treatments (What have you done to relieve the symptoms and their effects?). The last one is especially important because the elderly people often self-prescribe, visit multiple providers, and take suggestions from others.

iv. Past Medical History

Past medical history gathers a chronological list of all childhood and adulthood diseases, injuries, hospitalizations, surgeries, immunizations, and allergies (to drugs, food, and environmental factors). A list of current medications (name, dosage, duration, and indications) is usually obtained here.

体语言，评估二者是否一致。例如，有的老年人没有明确的主诉，但是表现出坐立不安，就需要给予高度的关注。

老年人经常没有主诉或主诉不典型、不明确，甚至有模棱两可的主诉。主诉也可能与病理变化无关，从而增加诊断的难度。造成不典型和不明确主诉的原因有：

（1）老年疾病常常无典型的临床表现。老年人常患有慢性病或是多病共存。多种疾病互相影响，一个系统症状的主诉是另一个系统病变的结果。

（2）用老化改变来解释病理变化导致的症状，从而延误就诊。

（3）因为害怕患了严重的疾病，而否认症状或是主诉无关的内容。

（4）由于语言和文化差异等原因而造成沟通障碍。

（5）老年人可能会因为缺乏经济实力而轻化症状。

（三）现病史

现病史是记述患者病后的全过程，即发生、发展、演变和诊治经过。其包括症状的始发时间、身体部位、特点、持续时间、加重因素、减轻因素、采取的治疗措施及其效果。

（四）既往病史

既往病史应以年为主线，列举从儿童时期到现在的所有疾病、损伤、住院、手术、接种疫苗和过敏史（如药物、食物和环境因素）。另外要详细询问处方和非处方药物的使用情况（如药名、计量、用法、使用时间、

v. Family History

Family history identifies diseases in first degree relatives to estimate the elderly people's predisposition to medical conditions such as diabetes. It's also important to ask whether similar chief complaints have been presented in family members in case family members have not been diagnosed.

vi. Review of Systems

Review of systems follows the conventional approach. Table 4-2 displays the common symptoms and prevalent medical conditions in each organ system.

服用方法、适应证）。

（五）家族史

家族史是指直系亲属患有的疾病，从而预计老年人患病的可能性，如糖尿病。此外，询问家庭成员是否有类似主诉，也可避免对家庭成员疾病的漏诊。

（六）系统回顾

系统回顾全面收集各个器官系统的症状。表 4-2 列举了各个器官系统在老年人中的常见症状和疾病。

Table 4-2 Review of Systems in Elderly People

System	Common Symptoms	Prevalent Conditions
Visual	Changes in near, central, peripheral, night visions, pain, and glare	Cataracts, macular degeneration, glaucoma, diabetic retinopathy, and stroke
Auditory	Hearing loss and impaired high frequency range	Cerumen impaction, acoustic neuroma, and drug-induced ototoxicity
Pulmonary	Shortness of breath and cough	Chronic obstructive pulmonary disease
Cardiovascular	Shortness of breath, orthopnea, fatigue, indigestion, insomnia, and swelling ankles	Congestive heart failure, hypertension, arthrosclerosis, cardiac arrhythmia, aortic stenosis, carotid stenosi
Gastrointestinal	Constipation, fecal incontinence, diarrhea, acid reflex, upset stomach, obesity, and weight loss	Dehydration, constipation, fecal impaction, physical inactivity, colorectal cancer, and hypothyroidism
Musculoskeletal	Muscle pain or weakness, joint pain, and back pain	Osteoarthritis, rheumatoid arthritis, osteoporosis, systematic lupus, and cancer
Extremity	Leg pain, restless leg, leg and ankle swelling, sores, tingling, or numbness	Peripheral arterial disease, intermittent claudication, restless leg syndromes, venous insufficiency, and amputation
Neurologic	Dizziness, syncope, cognitive impairment, and headache	Transient ischemic attack, stroke, postural hypotension, seizure, Alzheimer's disease, Parkinson's disease, vascular dementia, and drugs-related
Endocrine	Eating, drinking, and elimination patterns	Diabetes mellitus and hypothyroidism
Psychiatric	Mood disorders, schizophrenia, depression, and anxiety	Depression, anxiety, and grief
Genitourinary	Urinary frequency, urgency, and leakage, and sexual function	Benign prostatic hyperplasia, estrogen deficiency, and detrusor instability

表 4-2 老年人各系统常见症状和疾病

系统	常见症状	常见疾病
视觉	近、中、远视觉的改变，夜间视觉、疼痛、眩晕等改变	白内障、老年黄斑变性、青光眼、糖尿病性视网膜病变、脑卒中
听觉	听力减弱、高频听力受损	耵聍堵塞、听神经瘤、药物性耳聋
肺	呼吸气促、咳嗽	慢性阻塞性肺疾病
心血管	气促、端坐呼吸、乏力、消化不良、失眠、脚踝水肿	充血性心力衰竭、高血压、动脉硬化、心律失常、主动脉瓣狭窄、颈动脉狭窄
胃肠道	便秘、大便失禁、腹泻、反酸、消化不良、肥胖、体重下降	脱水、便秘、大便失禁、活动力下降、结肠直肠癌、甲状腺功能减退
肌肉骨骼	肌肉疼痛或无力、关节疼痛、背部疼痛	骨关节炎、类风湿性关节炎、骨质疏松症、系统性红斑狼疮、肿瘤
肢体	肢体疼痛、无力、肢体关节水肿、压疮、麻木	周围动脉疾病、间歇性跛行、不宁腿综合征、静脉瓣功能不全、截肢
神经	头晕、晕厥、认知功能障碍、头痛	短暂性脑缺血发作、脑卒中、直立性低血压、失神发作、阿尔茨海默病、帕金森病、血管性痴呆、药物相关性痴呆
内分泌	饮食消化模式改变	糖尿病、甲状腺功能减退
精神	情绪障碍、精神分裂、抑郁、焦虑	抑郁、焦虑和悲痛
泌尿生殖	尿频、尿急、漏尿、性功能障碍	良性前列腺增生症、雌激素缺乏、逼尿肌功能障碍

II. Physical Examination of Medical Condition

Physical examination follows the conventional organ systems approach with a special emphasis on the distinction between normal aging-related changes from abnormal signs. Again, such a distinction is not always possible. Table 4-3 describes the focus of physical examination and common conditions in each organ system.

二、体格检查

体格检查遵循传统医学体格检查的方法和内容，但侧重于辨别异常病变和各器官、系统的常见疾病。表 4-3 列举了老年人体格检查的重点和常见疾病。传统体格检查的常规内容将不再一一列举。

Table 4-3　Foci of Physical Examination in Elderly People

Domain	Focus	Possible medical conditions
General appearance	General hygiene, age, state of health, nutritional status, alertness, and discomfort	Delirium, dementias, psychiatric conditions, Parkinson's disease, and malnutrition
Vital signs	Pulse rate and rhythm, respiratory rate and pattern, temperature, blood pressure, pain, and cognitive impairment	Bradycardia, orthostatic hypotension, infection, arthritis, mild cognitive impairment, Alzheimer's disease and other dementias
Height, weight, & nutrition	Height, weight, body mass index, and food intake	Malnutrition, weight loss, and failure to thrive
Lymph nodes	Size, consistency, mobility, and tenderness over the body	Cancers such as lymphoma, breast cancer, and prostate cancer

continued

Domain	Focus	Possible medical conditions
Head	Size, symmetry, tenderness, masses, and scalp	Stroke, temporal arteritis, and paralysis
Eyes	Visual acuity, corneal opacity, extraocular movements, and fundi abnormality	Visual impairment, cataracts, glaucoma, macular degeneration, and diabetic retinopathy
Ears	Hearing impairment, ear canals, and tympanic membranes	Hearing impairment, cerumen impaction, and hearing aids
Nose	Septal deviation, deformity, and mucous membrane	Septal deviation and sinusitis
Mouth and throat	Teeth, denture, and mucosa (remove denture before examination)	Denture, xerostomia, gingival and periodontal diseases, and precancerous and cancerous lesions
Neck	Thyroid enlargement and nodularity, carotid pulses, and bruits	Hyper-thyroidism, hypo-thyroidism, carotid stenosis, and cerebrovascular diseases
Chest and breasts	Tracheal position, chest shape and symmetry, and breast size, shape, symmetry, tenderness, and masses	Breast cancer
Lungs and back	Spine, breath sounds, bronchophony, and fremitus	Dorsal kyphosis, osteoporosis, and chronic obstructive lung disease
Heart	S4, irregular heart rate, and murmurs	Congestive heart failure, arrhythmia, and valvular stenosis and prolapse
Abdomen	Mass and bruits	Abdominal aortic aneurysm and cachexia
Pelvic and Rectal	Women: vaginal mucosa, uterine/rectal prolapse and Pap smear Men: prostate and inguinal hernias Both genders: incontinence and rectal masses	Uterine cancer, prostate cancer, colorectal cancer, urinary incontinence, constipation, fecal incontinence, and fecal impaction
Muscle and joints	Muscle strength, range of motion, joint mobility, pain, tenderness, effusion, erythema, deformity, and swelling, peripheral pulses and edema, cyanosis, clubbing, temperature, varicose veins, and hair loss	Muscle atrophy, malnutrition, arthritis, osteoporosis, diabetic neuropathy, peripheral arterial disease, and venous insufficiency
Neurologic	Cranial nerves, reflexes, gait, balance, and cognitive impairment	Balance, gait, diminished sensations, transient ischemic attacks, stroke, and cognitive impairment
Skin	Erythema, ulcerations, lesions, bruises, and tear	Pressure ulcers, actinic keratoses, squamous and basal cell carcinomas, melanoma, and elder abuse

表 4-3 老年人体格检查重点

项目	重点	可能存在的疾病
一般状况	整体卫生、年龄、健康状况、营养状况、反应、不适	谵妄、痴呆、精神疾病，帕金森病、营养不良
生命体征	脉率和脉律、呼吸速率和形态、体温、血压、疼痛、认知功能障碍	心动过缓、直立性低血压、感染、关节炎、轻度认知障碍、阿尔茨海默病和其他痴呆症
身高、体重和营养	身高、体重、BMI 指数和食物摄入	营养不良、体重减轻
淋巴结	大小、一致性、移动性和压痛	肿瘤，如淋巴瘤、乳腺癌和前列腺癌
头	大小、对称、压痛、肿块和头皮	脑卒中、颞动脉炎、瘫痪
眼	视力、角膜混浊、眼球运动和眼底异常	视觉障碍、白内障、青光眼、黄斑变性、糖尿病视网膜病变

项目	重点	可能存在的疾病
耳	听力减退、耳道和鼓膜	听力障碍、耵聍、助听器
鼻	鼻中隔偏曲、畸形和黏膜	鼻中隔偏曲、鼻窦炎
口腔和咽喉	牙齿、义齿和黏膜（在检查前需取下义齿）	义齿、口干、牙龈及牙周疾病、癌前病变
颈部	甲状腺肿大及结节、颈动脉搏动和杂音	甲状腺功能亢进、甲状腺功能降低、颈动脉狭窄、脑血管疾病
胸部和乳房	气管位置，胸部形状和对称性，乳房大小、形状、对称性、压痛和肿块	乳腺癌
肺和背部	脊柱、呼吸音、支气管呼吸音和震颤	脊柱后凸、骨质疏松症和慢性阻塞性肺疾病
心脏	第四心音、心律不齐和杂音	充血性心力衰竭、心律失常、瓣膜狭窄
腹部	肿块和杂音	腹主动脉瘤和恶病质
生殖器和直肠	女性：阴道黏膜、子宫和直肠脱垂、宫颈涂片 男性：前列腺和腹股沟疝 女性和男性：失禁和直肠肿块	子宫癌、前列腺癌、结直肠癌、尿失禁、便秘、大便失禁、粪便嵌塞
肌肉和关节	肌肉力量、活动范围、关节活动度、疼痛、压痛、积液、红斑、畸形、肿胀、周围脉搏、水肿、发绀、杵状指、皮温、静脉曲张、脱发	肌肉萎缩、营养不良、关节炎、骨质疏松、糖尿病神经病变、外周动脉疾病和静脉功能不全
神经	颅神经、反射、步态、平衡、认知障碍	平衡、步态、感觉减退、短暂性脑缺血发作、脑卒中、认知障碍
皮肤	红斑、溃疡、损伤、擦伤，撕裂	压力性溃疡、光化性角化病、鳞状上皮和基底细胞癌、黑色素瘤、老年人虐待

i. General Appearance

Acknowledging the general appearance in older adult is very important because unusual appearance raises the suspicion of medical conditions and geriatric syndromes. For example, a improper appearance might suggest dementia, delirium, or frontal lobe dysfunction. Stiff posture and lack of facial expressions may indicate Parkinson's disease.

ii. Vital Signs

In addition to traditional four vital signs, pain and cognitive impairment are considered two additional vital signs in the elderly people.

Bradycardia and atrial fibrillation are increasingly common in the elderly people and are often detected by palpating a radial or carotid artery.

Orthostatic hypotension affects about 30% of the elderly people who are 75 years old or older and predisposes them to falls. Orthostatic hypotension is demonstrated with a blood pressure drop of ≥ 20 mmHg when blood pressure is taking supine and then standing (take blood pressure after stand up for two minutes).

（一）一般状况

外表、穿着和姿势可以提供一个老年人是否有疾病或认知障碍的线索。例如，一位穿着不合适宜的老年人可能提示痴呆、谵妄或额叶功能障碍。老年人僵硬的姿势和缺乏面部表情可能提示帕金森病。

（二）生命体征

老年人的生命体征除了心率、血压、体温和呼吸外，还包括疼痛和认知。

在老年人中，心动过缓和心房颤动越来越常见，通常可以通过触诊桡动脉或颈动脉来决定。

直立性低血压常见于75岁及以上的老年人，并可导致跌倒。通常认为，站立后收缩压较平卧位时下降≥20mmHg即为直立性低血压（在站立2分钟后监测）。

Increased respiratory rate above 20-24 breaths/minute is clinically significant and could indicate infection of the lower respiratory system.

Afebrile state for younger adults could indicate fever in the elderly people because they their average core temperature is lower than younger adults. Several aging-related changes affect the elderly people's ability to thermo-regulate, including attenuated skin blood flow, so a 10%-50% decline in total body water, and reduced ability to regular core body temperature. Baseline temperature must be documented for every older adult to aid fever discernment.

Pain is prevalent but not part of normal aging. Pain can be effectively evaluated by simply asking "Do you have any pain or discomfort?" If, then use 0 (no pain)-10 (worst pain) visual analog or OLDCART to further evaluate pain characteristics.

Cognitive impairment needs to be evaluated at least annually, and discussed in detail in Section 5 Cognitive Function.

iii. Height and Weight

Anthropometric measurements of height and weight assist in detecting malnutrition, obesity, and weight loss, which are commonly caused by medical conditions, depression, inability to shop, cook, or eat, and financial hardship.

Height is measured using stadiometer. Measurement accuracy requires removing shoes, putting heels together, standing with head leveled, and taking and holding a deep breath.

Weight is measured by a calibrated scale, ideally with minimal clothes, and no shoes/accessories on the same scale every time. Weight should be measured at each visit to generate a weight trend. An unintentional 4.54 kg (10 pounds) or more weight gain or loss over a 6-month period demands further evaluation.

iv. Nutrition

Nutrition is assessed by body mass index and the mini-nutritional assessment (MNA).

Body mass index (BMI) is calculated as the ratio of weight in kg divided by squared height meter. The best practice is to measure height and weight at the same visit. Many electronic health records can automatically calculate BMI or a BMI table can derive BMI without mathematical calculations.

呼吸过速是指呼吸频率超过 20～24 次 /min，可提示下呼吸道感染。

对于年轻人而言不属于发热的温度，对于老年人可能预示发热，这主要是由于老年人的平均体核温度低于年轻人。多个老化相关改变会影响老年人体温调节的能力，如皮肤血流的下降、体液的减少和调节体核温度能力下降等。因此必须记录每位老年人的基础体温，以避免发热的漏诊。

在老年人中，疼痛很常见，但疼痛并不是正常老化的表现。疼痛可以通过直接询问"你是否感到疼痛或不舒服？"来评估。如果回答"是"，则需进一步询问始发时间、身体部位、特点、持续时间、加重因素、减轻因素、采取的治疗措施及其效果。

老年人每年都需要进行认知障碍的评估。认知障碍的评估方法将在本章第五节详细介绍。

（三）身高和体重

对身高体重的测量可用于发现由于疾病、抑郁、自理能力障碍而导致的营养不良、肥胖和体重降低。

身高可以用测距仪测量。老年人需要脱鞋、后跟并拢、眼睛平视、深吸一口气后量身高，这样才比较准确。

体重要用校准的体重仪，尽量让老年人穿单衣，并用同一个体重仪测量体重。应定期测量老年人体重，从而记录体重的变化趋势。在半年内，老年人的体重下降 4.54 kg 及以上时，提示其需要进一步的评估。

（四）营养

营养失调可以用体重指数（BMI）和微型营养评估量表（MNA）来筛查。

体重指数是用体重（kg）除以身高的平方（m²）而得的商。最佳做法是在同一次就诊时测量身高和体重。许多电子健康记录可以自动计算 BMI，或者通过 BMI 表也可以不用数学

For general adult population, BMI results are interpreted as follows:

BMI $<$ 18.5 kg/m^2: underweight;

BMI 18.5 -24.9 kg/m^2: normal weight;

BMI of 25 -29.9 kg/m^2: overweight;

BMI $\geq$ 30 kg/m^2: indicates obesity.

For the elderly people, the normal value of BMI is 20~26.9kg/m^2, which is recommended by the *Chinese Nutrition Society in the 2021 Dietary Guidelines* for Chinese residents.

Most weight gains in the elderly people are essentially excess body fat, making the BMI rather accurate for classifying nutritional status. However, BMI can misclassify nutritional status if the elderly people have recently done a vigorous resistance-training program or have a condition that results in excess fluid accumulation.

MNA is both a screening and an assessment tool for malnutrition in the elderly people. The screening portion has six questions about food intake, weight loss, mobility, psychological stress or acute disease, neuropsychological problems, and BMI over the past three months. Each question is scored 0-2 or 0-3 with a maximal score of 14. A MNA score $\leq$ 11 indicates possible malnutrition and the need to proceed for the assessment portion which has 12 items (living status, prescription drug use, pressure sores/skin ulcers, numbers of full meals daily, intakes of proteins, fruits/vegetables consumptions per day, daily fluid intake, mode of feeding, self-view of nutritional status, self-rated health compared to peers, mid-arm circumference, and calf circumference). Each item is scored 0-2 or 0-3 with a maximal score of 16. A final MNA score sums both screening and assessment scores and a score of 17 to 23.5 indicates at risk for malnutrition, while a score $<$ 17 suggests malnourishment.

v. Lymphatic and Immunologic System

Lymph nodes should be palpated for size, consistency, mobility, and tenderness in occipital, cervical, post-auricular, submandibular, supra-clavicular, epitrochlear, axillary, and inguinal regions. Enlarged lymph nodes could indicate metastasized cancer, lymphoma, breast cancer, prostate cancer, etc.

vi. Head

Head must be carefully examined to identify any asymmetrical facial, tongue, and extra-ocular muscle

计算就得出 BMI。对于一般成年人的 BMI 结果解释如下：

正常范围：18.5～24.9kg/m^2；

体重过低：低于 18.5kg/m^2；

超重：25～29.9kg/m^2；

肥胖：≥ 30kg/m^2。

中国营养学会发布的《2021 中国居民膳食指南》中推荐老年人 BMI 正常值为 20～26.9kg/m^2。

老年人大部分增加的体重实质上是身体多余的脂肪，这使得 BMI 对营养状况分类时相对准确。然而，如果老年人最近进行了剧烈的抗阻力训练，或出现了导致体液过多，产生积聚的情况，BMI 可能会对营养状况错误分类。

微型营养评估量表有筛查和评估两部分，先筛查出有营养失调危险的老年人，然后进一步评估营养状况。筛查量表部分共有六个问题，涉及食物摄入、体重下降、行动力、心理压力或急性病、神经精神问题和近三个月的 BMI 情况。每个问题得分为 0～2 分或 0～3 分，最后总分为 14 分。MNA 得分 ≤ 11 分提示可能存在营养不良，需要进一步评估其他十二个项目（居住状况、处方药使用、皮肤压疮、每日规律进食、蛋白质摄入、每日蔬菜水果摄入、液体摄入、进食方式、自评营养状况、自评健康状况、上臂臂围、小腿围）每个问题得分为 0～2 分或 0～3 分，最后总分为 16 分。MNA 的总分为筛查和评估两部分得分之和。得分在 17～23.5 分之间提示存在营养不良的风险，得分＜17 分提示存在营养不良。

（五）淋巴系统

触诊淋巴结时，需评估其大小、活动性、软硬度，一般触诊部位包括了枕后、颈后、耳后、颌下、锁骨上、滑车上、腋窝、腹股沟等。淋巴结增大提示可能存在转移癌、淋巴瘤、乳腺癌、前列腺癌等。

（六）头

头部检查重点是观察是否存在任何不对称的面部、舌和眼外肌的动作，这提示是

movements that suggest stroke or paralysis. Temporal artery tenderness hints temporal arteritis.

vii. Eyes

Visual acuity can be screened using Snellen eye chart has a positive predictive value of 0.75 and a negative predictive value of 0.89. It requires the elderly people to read letters on the chart with eyeglasses on while standing 6.67 meters (20 feet) away. Inability to read the 20/40 line is considered positive. Further examination focuses on ocular lens opacification for cataracts and funduscopic abnormalities for glaucoma, macular degeneration, arthrosclerosis, and diabetic retinopathy. Positive findings prompt referral to an ophthalmologist for further evaluation.

viii. Ears

The ear canals are inspected for cerumen impaction. Cerumen should be cleaned out before screening hearing impairment using the whisper test or Inventory for the Elderly U. S. National Health and Nutrition Examination Survey (NHANES) Battery.

The whisper test tests each ear separately by whispering 3-6 random numbers, words, or letters to an ear at a set distance (15-60cm) with clinician standing behind to prevent lip reading and the opposite ear covered or occluded. Inability to repeat half of the whispered words correctly suggests hearing impairment. The whisper test has a sensitivity of 80%-100% and a specificity of 82%-89%.

The NHANES Battery has six items with each positive item scored as 1 or 2: (a) age > 70 years = 1; (b) male gender = 1; (c) education of ≤ 12 years = 1; (d) previously saw an clinician about trouble hearing = 1; (e) without hearing aid, cannot hear whisper across the room = 1; and (f) without hearing aid, cannot hear normal voice across the room = 2. A score > 3 points suggests hearing impairment with 80% sensitivity and 80% specificity.

If the older adult wears hearing aids, the fitting and function of hearing aids need to be examined.

ix. Nose

The nose should be examined for deformities, septal deviation, and any obstructions. The mucous membrane is examined for redness, erythema, polyps, bleeding, and discharge.

x. Mouth and Throat

Dentures are common in the elderly people and must be removed and inspected for fitting because ill-fitted

否存在脑卒中或偏瘫。颞动脉触痛提示颞动脉炎。

（七）眼

斯内伦视力表可以用来检查视力。在检查时，要求老年人站在 6.67m 之外，佩戴眼镜阅读表格上的字母。若无法阅读第 20 行的字母，则提示存在视力障碍。进一步检查的重点为是否存在白内障和青光眼、晶状体混浊、黄斑变性、动脉粥样硬化和糖尿病视网膜病变。当存在视力检查结果的异常时，需进一步到眼科就诊。

（八）耳

检查耳道时，先观察是否有耵聍。在进行下一步的检查前，需清除耵聍。耳语实验及美国健康和营养老年人听力测试表可以检查听力。

耳语实验每次只能检查单侧耳朵听力。检查时，检查者在距离老年人 15～60cm 的位置，随机轻声念 3～6 个数字、单词或字母。检查人站在被检查者的身后或侧边，以防止读唇。若无法正确重复出一半的字母，就提示存在听力受损。耳语实验的灵敏度为 80%～100%，特异度为 82%～89%。

美国健康和营养老年人听力表共有六个条目，得分为 1～2 分，内容有年龄、性别、教育程度、听力减退史、远距离听力和戴助听器能否听到远距离的声音等。听力表得分＞3 分，提示可能存在听力受损，灵敏度和特异度均为 80%。

若老年人佩戴助听器，还需评估助听器的合适程度和性能。

（九）鼻

重点检查鼻腔结构是否有畸形、中隔偏曲和任何阻塞；鼻黏膜是否有充血、红肿、息肉、出血和分泌物。

（十）口腔和咽喉

老年人常由于牙齿脱落而戴义齿，而不合适的义齿往往会增加老年人营养不良和感

dentures increase the risk for malnutrition and infection. Because dentures are expensive, care must be taken when handling dentures. After removing dentures, the clinician checks for mucosal dryness for xerostomia, gingiva for gingival and periodontal diseases, and mucosal integrity for precancerous and cancerous lesions.

xi. Neck

Examination focuses on detecting thyroid enlargement and nodularity (hyper-or hypo-thyroidism). Carotid pulses and bruits are checked for carotid stenosis and cerebrovascular diseases.

xii. Chest and Breasts

Early detection of breast abnormality significantly improves survival in older women; however, the infiltration of fatty and fibrous tissues with aging makes it difficult to identify abnormal nodules. Although its value has been questioned, mammogram screening improves breast cancer detection, especially when palpation findings are inconclusive.

xiii. Lungs and Back

Dorsal kyphosis is a common posture change, especially in older women with osteoporosis. Kyphosis could resemble the barrel chest sign in emphysema.

xiv. Heart Key

Examination includes auscultation for S_4 (left ventricular thickening) and systolic ejection and regurgitation murmurs (valvar stenosis or prolapse).

xv. Abdomen

The presence of abdominal aortic aneurysm must be evaluated by palpating for a pulsatile mass. Any other abdominal masses are suspicious for cancer.

xvi. Genital and Rectal

Genital examination evaluates vaginal mucosa atrophy, uterine/rectal prolapse, and cervical cancer using Pap smear in older women, and prostate nodules in older men. All the elderly people should be evaluated for colorectal cancer by palpating rectal masses and testing occult blood.

xvii. Muscles and Joints

The appearance, temperature, skin color, form, and pulses of extremities need to be evaluated. Observation of muscle wasting further confirms nutritional status. Decreased range of motion, joint deformity, and pain suggest arthritis. Vertebral tenderness and dorsal kyphosis

染的风险。因此在检查口腔时，需要请老年人摘下义齿，评估义齿的合适程度。因为义齿昂贵，在处理义齿时必须小心。取下义齿后，医生需检查黏膜干燥程度和完整性、牙龈和牙周情况。

（十一）颈部

颈部检查的重点是甲状腺肿大和结节。此外通过颈动脉脉搏和杂音来评估是否存在颈动脉狭窄与脑血管疾病。

（十二）胸部和乳房

早期发现乳房异常有助于提高老年女性的生存率，然而由于年龄的增长，脂肪组织和纤维组织的浸润，使得异常结节难以识别。钼靶筛查检测有助于提高乳腺癌的发现，特别是当触诊检查结果不确定时。

（十三）肺和背部

脊柱后凸在老年人中很常见，常见于骨质疏松的老年女性。脊柱后凸与肺气肿的背部表现很像。

（十四）心脏

辨别第四心音和收缩期杂音是心脏体格检查的重点。

（十五）腹部

腹部检查应注重腹主动脉瘤和腹部肿瘤的评估。腹主动脉瘤的存在必须通过触诊到有搏动性肿块来判断。其他任何腹腔肿块都应怀疑是否存在癌症。

（十六）生殖器和直肠

生殖器检查评估阴道黏膜萎缩、子宫和直肠脱垂。可通过宫颈涂片评估老年女性是否存在宫颈癌，通过前列腺结节评估老年男性是否存在前列腺癌。所有的老年人都应进行直肠触诊，并做隐血试验，以检查是否存在结直肠癌。

（十七）肌肉和关节

四肢的温度、皮肤颜色、形状和脉搏可以提示有无静脉瓣膜功能不全、栓塞。肌肉萎缩预示营养不良。关节活动度改变、畸形提示可能有关节炎。脊柱侧弯和疼痛提示可

indicates osteoporosis. Heberden's nodes at distal interphalangeal joints signify osteoarthritis. Diminished or absent lower extremity pulses could suggest peripheral vascular disease and embolism. Pedal edema indicates possible venous insufficiency or congestive heart failure. Feet must be carefully inspected especially for the elderly people with diabetes.

xviii. Neurologic System

Neurologic examination focuses on the function of cranial nerves, tendon reflexes, gait, and balance. Gait and balance are detailed in Section 4 Functional Status.

xix. Skin

Skin abnormality such as ulceration and erythema should be checked, especially over bony prominences for immobilized the elderly people. Skin lesions could indicate actinic keratosis, squamous and basal cell carcinomas, and malignant melanoma, while unexplained bruises and skin tears suggest elder abuse.

Box 4-1　Case Study

Mrs. Liu is 78 years old, the Miao nationality and a widow. She lives in a small city. Her oldest daughter from out-of-town has been visiting and becomes concerned that mom seems to have declined quite a bit in function. Mrs. Liu feels she is doing just fine. The daughter insists for her mom to visit the clinic where you work. Her past medical history includes hypertension, diabetes, and arthritis. She takes metoprolol, metformin, Lipitor, amlodipine, and ibuprofen, and several traditional medicine recipes for health promotion. Mrs. Liu's parents were farmers and died from "old age".

Questions:

1. What components of health history will you particularly focus on for this patient?

2. What areas will you focus on during physical examination?

能有骨质疏松。足部水肿表示可能存在静脉回流障碍或充血性心力衰竭。对有糖尿病的老年人要定期进行足部检查。

（十八）神经

神经系统检查包括对中枢神经、反射、步态和平衡的评估。关于步态和平衡的具体评估内容见第四节功能状态。

（十九）皮肤

检查皮肤有无溃疡、红肿和皮肤缺损。对长期卧床和患糖尿病的老年人而言，皮肤评估尤为重要。皮肤病变可能表明光化性角化病、鳞状细胞癌、基底细胞癌和恶性黑色素瘤。另外，反复、无明确原因的瘀伤和皮肤撕裂提示老年人有被虐待的可能。

Box 4-1　案例

刘女士，78岁，苗族，丧偶，居住于一个三线城市。她的大女儿最近回家探亲，觉得母亲的健康状况下降了很多。而刘女士自我感觉还行。大女儿让母亲来你工作的诊所进行检查。刘女士的现病史包括高血压、糖尿病和关节炎，她通过药物来控制疾病，服用药物包括了美托洛尔、二甲双胍、立普妥、氨氯地平、布洛芬和几种促进健康的中药。刘女士的父母都是农民，是"老死的"。

问题：

1. 这个案例病史采集的重点是什么？

2. 体格检查的主要部分应该包括哪些？

Section 3　Geriatric Syndromes

I. Definition and Components of Geriatric Syndromes

Geriatric syndromes are defined as "The multifactorial health conditions that occur when the accumulated effects of impairments in multiple systems render an elderly person vulnerable to situational challenges." Geriatric syndromes are heterogeneous, including hearing loss, visual impairment, falls, polypharmacy, pain, sleep disorders, urinary incontinence, delirium, cognitive impairment, frailty, and substance abuse. They also share four common features:

- Multiple risk factors and organ systems are involved and work interactively and synergistically to produce the clinical manifestations.

- Geriatric syndromes share common etiological factors and pathological pathways. For example, four risk factors (older age, baseline functional impairment, cognitive impairment, and mobility impairment) are shared among pressure ulcers, falls, incontinence, functional decline, and delirium.

- Treatments are often implemented without a confirmation of the underlying cause (s).

- A unitary approach is likely efficient for managing multiple geriatric syndromes because of their shared risk factors and physiopathological pathways.

II. Assessment of Geriatric Syndromes

Assessment of geriatric syndromes relies on clinical interviews and assessment tools. Tests covered under Section 2 Medical Conditions will not be repeated here. One approach targets each geriatric syndrome one by one after completing the assessment of medical conditions. Another approach integrates geriatric syndromes into an organ system as part of medical conditions assessment, e. g., evaluating cognitive impairment in neurologic system, falls in musculoskeletal system, and malnutrition in gastrointestinal system. Either approach is effective depending on the clinician's preference and experiences. Table 4-4 summarizes the interview questions and assessment tools for geriatric syndromes.

第三节　老年综合征评估

一、老年综合征的概念和组成

由多种因素引起的多器官系统损伤导致老年人应激能力下降，出现老年综合征。老年综合征存在异质性，常见老年综合征包括失聪、视力障碍、跌倒、多重用药、疼痛、睡眠障碍、尿失禁、谵妄、认知障碍、衰弱和物质滥用。这些老年综合征有四个共同特点：

- 多种危险因素和器官系统参与，并相互作用，共同产生临床表现。

- 老年综合征有共同的病因和病理机制。例如，压疮、跌倒、失禁、功能下降和谵妄之间有四个共同的危险因素，即高龄、基础功能受损、认知障碍和行动障碍。

- 常在未明确潜在病因时进行治疗。

- 单一方法管理多个老年综合征有效，这可能是因为它们有共同的危险因素和病理生理途径。

二、老年综合征的评估

老年综合征的评估主要通过问诊和工具评估。在第二节中已介绍的测试方法，在本节不会再次介绍。在具体操作上，老年综合征的评估有两种方法。一是老年综合征的评估与各个器官、系统的疾病评估同时进行，比如在检查神经系统时评估认知功能；二是在疾病评估之后，集中评估老年综合征。这两种方法各有利弊，主要根据评估者习惯和经验来决定。表4-4总结了老年综合征评估时常用的问诊问题和评估量表。

Table 4-4 Interview Questions and Assessment Tools for Geriatric Syndromes

Geriatric syndrome	Interview questions	Assessment tools	Time for tool administration/ minutes
Hearing loss	"Do you feel you have a hearing loss?"	Whisper test; inventory for the Elderly NHANES Battery	1 2
Visual impairment	"Do you have difficulty watching television, reading, or doing any of your daily activities because of your eyesight?"	Hand-held Snellen chart	2
Malnutrition and weight loss	"Have you lost 4.54 kg or more over the past six months without trying to do so?"	Weight and BMI; MNA	1 5
Falls	"Have you had a fall before?" "Are you afraid of falling?" "Have you ever felt tripped over when walking?"	Timed up and go test; SPPB	1 5-10
Polypharmacy	"Are you prescribed more than four medications every day?" "Do you understand the reason for each of your medications?"	Dose, frequency, and indication of all prescription and nonprescription drugs and supplements	Depends on the kinds of medications
Pain	"Do you have any pain or discomfort?"	Visual analog scale	1
Sleep disorders	"Do you have trouble falling asleep, often fall into sleep during the day, or take naps during the day?"	PSQI	5-10
Urinary incontinence	"Have you ever lost your urine and gotten wet in the past year?"	3IQ	2
Delirium	Based on the interview with informants and clinical observations.	CAM	5
Dementia	"Do you have a concern about your memory?"		
Frailty	"Do you often feel you do not have the energy to carry out daily activities?"	Weight, grip strength, gait speed, exhaustion, and physical activity	10-15
Substance abuse	"Do you use any medications for recreation?" "Do you drink more than two drinks a day?"	MAST-G CAGE questionnaire for alcoholism	5-10 2

Note. BMI: Body Mass Index; CAM: The Confusion Assessment Method; MAST-G: The Michigan Alcoholism Screening Test – Geriatric; MNA: The Mini-Nutritional Assessment; NHANES: The National Health and Nutrition Examination Survey; PSQI: The Pittsburg Sleep Quality Index; SPPB: The Short Physical Performance Battery; and 3IQ: The Three Incontinence Questions.

表 4-4 评估老年综合征时的访谈问题和评估工具

老年综合征	访谈问题	评估工具	测试时间 /min
失聪	您是否感觉到有听力受损?	耳语测试; 老年人 NHANES Battery 量表	1 2
视力减弱	您感到视力改变影响到您看电视、阅读或者日常生活活动了吗?	手持 Snellen 视力表	2
营养失调	过去 6 个月内您有没有发生不明原因的体重增加或减少大于 4.54 kg?	体重和 BMI; 微型营养评估量表(MNA)	1 5

老年综合征	访谈问题	评估工具	测试时间 /min
跌倒	您有没有发生过跌倒？ 您害怕跌倒吗？ 您以往走路的时候，有没有过差点跌倒的经历？	计时站立行走试验； 简易躯体功能状况量表 SPPB	1 5~10
多重用药	您每天服用的处方药有无多于四种？ 您知晓您所服用的药物的作用和目的吗？	剂量、频率、处方药、非处方和保健药的使用说明	依据用药情况而定
疼痛	您身上有哪里疼痛或不适吗？	视觉模拟疼痛评估量表	1
睡眠障碍	您有无入睡困难、白天嗜睡或者打盹的情况出现？	匹兹堡睡眠质量指数量表（PSQI）	5~10
尿失禁	您有没有过漏尿的情况？	简易尿失禁评估 3IQ	2
谵妄	基于访谈和临床观察	谵妄评定量表（CAM）	5
老年性痴呆	您有无感到记忆减退		
衰弱	你经常觉得你没有精力进行日常活动吗？	体重、握力、步速、乏力、体力活动情况	10~15
物质滥用	您有服用药物消遣吗？ 您每天饮酒超过两杯吗？	密歇根酒精中毒筛查试验老年版（MAST-G），CAGE 酒精成瘾问卷	5~10 2

注：BMI，体重指数；CAM，谵妄评定量表；MAST-G，密歇根酒精中毒筛查试验老年版；MNA，微型营养评估量表；NHANES，国家健康和营养检查调查；PSQI，匹兹堡睡眠质量指数量表；SPPB，简易躯体功能状况量表；3IQ，简易尿失禁评估。

Since geriatric syndromes are not normal aging-related changes, important normal aging-related changes that have not been previously introduced are highlighted here to aid the identification of geriatric syndromes. It is also important to point out that many geriatric syndromes are under-reported, under-recognized, and under-treated despite of available, effective treatments. The content covered here focused on basic knowledge and tools for screening purpose only. Please refer to other chapters for detailed diagnosis and treatments of major geriatric syndromes.

i. Hearing Loss

The elderly people and clinicians often wrongly attribute hearing loss to normal aging and fail to report and assess it. It is true that the elderly people experience decreased ability to discriminate speech and lessening of hearing acuteness known as presbycusis. Nonetheless, hearing loss is not a part of normal aging, affects approximately one third of the elderly population, and relates to reduced cognitive, emotional, social, physical function, and satisfaction with life. Typically, hearing loss occurs to both ears and results in an inability to

老年综合征不是正常的衰老相关改变，在以往未被强调的正常衰老相关改变将在本节进行介绍，以帮助读者识别老年综合征。值得注意的是，尽管有行之有效的措施，许多老年综合征仍未被报道、识别或是治疗。本节内容侧重于老年综合征的基础知识，仅介绍筛查工具。老年综合征的具体诊断和治疗将在本书其他章节详细阐述。

（一）失聪

老年性耳聋特指正常老化引起的分辨语言能力的减弱和听力敏感力的下降。然而失聪是异常老化的表现。失聪通常影响双耳，导致老年人听不到高频率的声音进而无法理解别人说的话。失聪致使老年人感觉其他人说话模糊，尤其是在吵闹的环境里。大声喊对失聪没有帮助，但助听器可能有很大帮助。询问老年人是否感觉自己失聪及是否感觉听

hear high-frequency sounds, which makes it difficult to understand what is heard. They may report that people are mumbling and hearing in a loud environment is especially difficult. Shouting worsens the elderly people's ability to understand, but amplification devices like hearing aids help greatly. Simply asking if a person has hearing loss or trouble understanding what is said is an effective screening for hearing loss.

ii. Visual Impairment

Aging-related eye changes are almost universal, including changed lens shape and accommodation, smaller pupil sizes, and less reactive pupils to light. These changes make it harder for the elderly people to see things up close (loss of near vision known as presbyopia) and to the side (loss of peripheral vision). As a result, the majority of the elderly people require reading glasses. Four pathological conditions are prevalent in the elderly people to cause declined visual acuity, including cataracts, glaucoma, macular degeneration, and diabetic retinopathy. Although visual impairment contributes to cognitive and functional decline, falls, depression, reduced mobility, and social interactions, the elderly people usually do not realize the presence and extent of vision loss because visual impairment progresses slowly over years. Hence, screening should occur at least once a year by asking if they have difficulty watching television, reading, or doing any daily activities because of eyesight.

iii. Malnutrition

Malnutrition is an umbrella term that includes a range of nutritional disorders with obesity and weight loss most common in the elderly people, and predisposes them to functional decline, morbidity, and mortality. Obesity predominantly inflicts community-dwelling the elderly people, while weight loss and energy or protein under-nutrition mainly affects nursing home residents. Obesity indicates an accumulation of excess body fat and is different from overweight which is attributable to increased bone, muscle, and/or fat mass. Weight loss delineates the unintentional weight loss of ≥4.54 kilograms in the previous six months. Malnutrition is screened using a question "Have you lost or gained 4.54 kilograms or more over the past six months without trying to do so?"

iv. Falls

Falls are not a part of normal aging, but cause many poor outcomes (e. g. , institutionalization, poor quality of life, morbidity, mortality). At least one third of

懂别人的话有困难可以有效地筛选失聪。

（二）视力减弱

大多数老年人都会因晶状体、瞳孔和感光的老化而发生老花眼（近视力减弱）和周围视野变小。因此，大多数老年人需要佩戴眼镜进行阅读。造成老年人视力减弱的病理原因主要有白内障、青光眼、糖尿病眼病和黄斑变性。视觉障碍会导致认知和功能下降、跌倒、抑郁、行动能力降低、社会交往减少，但由于视力障碍进展缓慢，老年人往往估计不到视力下降及其严重程度。因此，视力筛查应至少每年进行一次，医护人员应询问老年人是否因为视力变化而使读书、看报和看电视变得困难。

（三）营养失调

营养失调包括肥胖和体重减轻，这些问题在老年人中非常常见，并会导致老年人出现功能下降、多病共存和死亡。肥胖常见于社区居住的老年人，而体重降低、能量或蛋白质不足主要见于护理院的老年人。肥胖提示身体脂肪过剩，其不同于超重，超重则是由于骨骼，肌肉和脂肪质量的增加。体重降低是指一个老年人在过去的 6 个月内，原因不明地体重减少至少 4.54kg。在进行营养失调筛查时，可询问老年人在过去的 6 个月内是否发生原因不明地体重增加或减少至少 4.54kg。若存在，则预示有潜在的病理问题。

（四）跌倒

跌倒在老年人中很普遍，但不属正常老化，跌倒可导致许多不良预后，如入住养老院、生活质量下降、多病共存，甚至死亡。

community-dwelling the elderly people fall every year and those who have fallen before are at a higher risk for another fall (recurrent falls). Screening questions include: "Have you ever felt tripped over when walking?" "Have you had a fall before?" and "Are you afraid of falling?"

v. Polypharmacy

Polypharmacy refers to simultaneous use of multiple medications. It is well documented that the use of ≥4 drugs significantly increases the elderly people's risk for adverse drug events, drug-drug interactions, non-compliance, and institutionalization. Polypharmacy screening should occur at every visit by asking the elderly people to bring all their medications, review the indication, dose, and usage of each drug, and reconcile or discontinue inappropriate medications that are duplicative, not effective, or no longer indicated.

vi. Pain

Acute pain has similar prevalence between older and younger adults, but chronic pain disproportionally afflicts 49% to 83% of the elderly people up to age 70s when the difference begins to taper and disappear. Chronic pain most commonly occurs in the joints, legs, back, and feet. Pain is frequently under reported, unrecognized, and under-treated despite its significant impact on function and quality of life, especially the oldest old (≥85 years old) and those with severe cognitive impairment. Pain can be screened with "Do you have any pain or discomfort?"

vii. Sleep Disorders

Aging increases sleep latency (time to fall asleep), nighttime awakenings, early wake-up, and daytime naps, and reduces sleep efficiency (actual time in sleep/time in bed). Whether the elderly people have reduced ability to sleep or if they need less sleep is still up for debate, but they do have reduced ability to sleep due to increased BMI (especially central adiposity), changes in airway anatomy, and decreased muscle tension, thyroid function, and lung volume. Common sleep disorders in the elderly people include sleep-disordered breathing, periodic limb movements in sleep and restless legs syndrome, circadian rhythms sleep disorders, rapid eye movement sleep behavior disorder, and insomnia, which contributes to poor health and depression. A sleep diary or the Pittsburgh sleep quality index (PSQI) can be used to screen sleep problems. Sleep diary tracks time to go to bed, fall asleep, wake up, and get up; number of nighttime awakenings; number and durations of daytime naps; use of sleeping aids; rating of quality and satisfaction with sleep; and energy level during the day. The PSQI has 10 self-reported

每年至少有 1/3 的社区老年人发生过跌倒，且有过跌倒史的老年人发生再次跌倒的风险大大增加。用于筛查的跌倒的问题包括了询问是否有过跌倒史和害怕跌倒。

（五）多重用药

老年人最常见的用药问题是用药种类过多或过量。老年人同时服用 4 种或 4 种以上药物将极大地增加药物不良反应、药物相互作用、不按时按量服药及其他老年综合征的风险。在老年人每一次就诊时，都应该进行多重用药筛查，如请老年人将其服用的所有药物都带来，检查用药原因、剂量和使用方法，核对停用不当的、重复的或无效的药物。

（六）疼痛

急性疼痛在老年人中的发生率和年轻人类似，但以关节、腿、背部和脚疼痛为主的慢性疼痛在老年人群中的发生率高达 49%～83%。疼痛往往被归类于正常老化而不被识别、报告或及时治疗，对老年人的生理、心理功能和生活质量造成严重的不良影响，尤其是高龄老年人和存在严重认知障碍的老年人。通过询问"你有没有哪里疼或者不舒服？"可以有效地筛查疼痛。

（七）睡眠障碍

衰老延长入睡期，增加夜间醒来、早醒和白天小睡的次数，并降低睡眠效率（实际睡眠时间/在床上的时间）。老年人睡眠减少还是老年人需要更少的睡眠尚有争议，但大多数研究结果显示睡眠能力随着年龄的增长而减弱。腰部肥胖、气道结构改变、肌肉的正常老化等是造成睡眠能力减弱的主要原因。老年人常见的睡眠障碍包括睡眠呼吸紊乱、睡眠中的周期性肢体运动和不宁腿综合征、昼夜节律性睡眠障碍、快速动眼睡眠行为障碍和失眠，这些睡眠障碍将进一步影响身体健康，导致抑郁发生。睡眠日记或匹兹堡睡眠质量量表（PSQI）可以用于筛查睡眠问题。睡眠日记可以记录就寝、入睡、醒来和起床的时间，夜间醒来的次数，白天小睡的次数和时间，是否服用安眠药，睡眠质量和

or interview-based questions about sleep duration, disturbance, latency, efficiency, quality, dysfunction during the day, and use of sleep medications. Each question is scored 0-3 with a total score of 0-21. A total score > 5 indicates poor sleep quality.

viii. Urinary Incontinence

Urinary incontinence is another under-reported syndrome and often wrongly attributed to aging. It is prevalent in the elderly people, especially older women, causes social isolation, depression, and poor quality of life, and can be screened using the three incontinence questions (3IQ):

(a) "Have you leaked an even small amount of urine during the past three months?" Proceed to the next questions if "yes".

(b) "Was the urine leakage associated with physical activity such as coughing, sneezing, lifting, or exercise, the feeling of urge to empty bladder but could not get to the toilet fast enough, or neither physical activity nor urge?"

(c) "Did you leak urine most often with physical activity, feeling of urge, both, or neither?" The response reveals the type of urinary incontinence.

ix. Delirium

Delirium represents a mental disturbance marked by confusion, inattention, acute onset, fluctuating course, disorganized thinking and/or altered level of consciousness. Delirium affects 14%-24% and 10%-30% the elderly people on admission to hospitals or in the emergency room, respectively, and carries 22%-76% mortality rate upon hospital discharge and 35%-40% mortality rate one year later. The confusion assessment method (CAM) assesses delirium with 94%-100% sensitivity and 90%-95% specificity:

(1) Acute onset and fluctuating course ascertained by an informant.

● There is an acute change in mental status from the person's baseline.

● The symptoms fluctuate during the day, e. g., come and go, increase or decrease in severity.

(2) Attention evidenced by being easily distracted or having difficulty keeping track of what is being said.

满意度，以及白天的精力。匹兹堡睡眠质量量表可以通过询问或老年人自填的方式筛查睡眠障碍，条目涉及睡眠持续时间、睡眠效率、睡眠质量、白天功能情况、安眠药的使用等。每个条目为 0～3 分，总分为 0～21 分，总分高于 5 分，提示睡眠障碍。

（八）尿失禁

尿失禁是另一种报告较少的综合征，往往被错误地归因于衰老。尿失禁在老年人中较为常见，特别是老年女性，可造成社交孤立、抑郁和生活质量不佳。尿失禁可通过 3-条目失禁量表（3IQ）进行筛查。

条目一："在过去的三个月里，你是否漏出少量的尿液？如果"是"的话，继续下一个问题。

条目二："漏尿是否与身体活动有关，例如咳嗽、打喷嚏、提举重物或运动？是否有急着排尿的感觉，但来不及如厕？"

条目三："你是否经常出现与身体活动有关的漏尿、尿急的感觉？或是两者都有，或两者都没有？"老年人的回答反映了尿失禁的类型。

（九）谵妄

谵妄是一种精神障碍，表现为意识混乱、注意力不集中、急性发作、病程波动、思维混乱和／或意识水平改变。谵妄可影响 14%～24% 的入院老年患者和 10%～30% 的入院或急诊老年患者，导致出院时老年人死亡率达 22%～76%，出院一年后老年人死亡率达 35%～40%。谵妄评估方法（CAM）评估谵妄的灵敏度为 94%～100%，特异度为 90%～95%。

（1）确定的急性起病和波动过程。

● 精神意识状态发生了急剧变化。

● 症状在一天中波动。

（2）注意力不集中。

(3) Disorganized thinking reflected by unpredictable switching from subject to subject, rambling or irrelevant conservations, and/or unclear or illogical flow of ideas.

(4) Altered level of consciousness.

x. Dementia

Dementia is not part of normal aging, and includes a variety of etiologies. Alzheimer's disease accounts for 60%-80% of all dementias, followed by vascular dementia (20%), dementia with Lewy bodies (10%-15%), frontotemporal dementia (5%), and others (5%). The latest, 2011 guidelines by the U. S. National Institute on Aging and the Alzheimer's Association updated dementia to three phases: asymptomatic, preclinical phase of Alzheimer's disease; symptomatic, pre-dementia phase of mild cognitive impairment; and dementia phase of probable or possible Alzheimer's disease. Cognitive screening is an important step in identifying dementia and will be discussed in Section 5 Cognitive Function.

xi. Frailty

Frailty refers to the increased vulnerability to adapt to stressors which results from aging-related decline in physiological function and reserves across multiple systems. Frailty is not disease specific, but leads to many poor outcomes such as falls, disability, institutionalization and death. The prevalence of frailty increases with advancing age, affecting 10%-25% of people 65 years old and 30%-45% of 85 years old; however, frailty is fluid where the elderly people can stay the same or transition to less or greater frailty. Screening for frailty focuses on evaluating its five cardinal symptoms:

○ Low strength: measured in kilograms by grip strength using a dynamometer. The following indicates low strength based on BMI for each gender:

- ■ Grip strength in men:
- ● < 29 kg for BMI ≤ 24 kg/m²;
- ● < 30 kg for BMI 24.1 – 28 kg/m²;
- ● < 32 kg for BMI > 28 kg/m².
- ■ Grip strength in women:
- ● < 17 kg for BMI ≤ 23 kg/m²;
- ● < 17.3 kg for BMI 23.1 – 26 kg/m²;

（3）思维混乱。

（4）意识水平改变。

（十）老年痴呆

老年痴呆并非衰老的正常表现，其包含多种病因。在各类型老年痴呆中，阿尔茨海默病占 60%～80%，其次是血管性痴呆（20%），路易体痴呆（10%～15%），额颞叶痴呆（5%）以及其他疾病（5%）。2011 年新颁布的诊断标准将老年痴呆分为 3 个阶段：临床前期（没有任何临床症状，但脑部已经有老年痴呆的病理性变化）、轻度认知障碍期（有一个或多个认知领域受损，但功能独立且不满足老年痴呆的诊断指标）和痴呆期（起病隐匿、多个认知领域受损、并引起功能受损、认知障碍不是继发于其他疾病）。前两者是老年痴呆的潜伏期。认知筛查是识别痴呆的重要步骤，认知功能相关内容将在第五节中讨论。

（十一）衰弱

衰弱是指对应激的易感性增加，导致多个系统的生理功能和储备下降。衰弱不同于疾病和残疾，是多器官系统失调的结果，可导致许多不良结局，如跌倒、残疾、入住机构和死亡。衰弱的发生率随年龄升高，在 65 岁及以上的老年人中，有 10%～25% 的老年人存在衰弱，在 85 岁及以上的老年人中有 30%～45% 的老年人存在衰弱。然而衰弱状态是动态变化的，不同程度的衰弱是可逆的。衰弱的五大临床表型包括：

（1）握力下降（通过握力计进行测量，单位为 kg，根据性别和身体质量指数判断）；

男性握力标准：

对于 BMI ≤ 24kg/m² 者，握力<29kg。

对于 BMI 为 24.1～28kg/m² 者，握力<30kg。

对于 BMI >28kg/m² 者，握力<32kg。

女性握力标准：

对于 BMI ≤ 23kg/m² 者，握力<17kg。

对于 BMI 为 23.1～26kg/m² 者，握力<17.3kg。

- $< 18\,kg$ for BMI $26.1 - 29\,kg/m^2$;
- $< 21\,kg$ for BMI $> 29\,kg/m^2$.

  ○ Low energy: "Everything I do was an effort." or "I could not get going."

  ○ Slowed motor performance: Takes $\geq$ 6-7 seconds to walk five meters.

  ○ Low physical activity: Expenses $< 383\,kcal/$week for men and $< 270\,kcal/week$ for women.

  ○ Unintentional weight loss: $> 4.54\,kg$ (10pounds) in the past year.

The Women's Health and Aging Study II suggests that frailty start with any of its five symptoms. Weakness tends to occur first, followed by slowness and low physical activity. Exhaustion usually appears the last. Early development of weight loss or exhaustion has been found to predict more rapid onset of frailty.

xii. Substance abuse

The elderly people are at risks for substance abuse just like younger populations, but largely use sedative-hypnotics like benzodiazepines and alcohol for sleep disturbances. They are prone to alcoholism and alcoholic complications because of decreased lean body mass, diminished efficiency of hepatic metabolism, increased brain sensitivity to alcohol, high incidence of alcohol-medication interactions, and prevalence of medical and psychosocial disorders. Hence, screening is important in the elderly people, especially those who live alone. Clinicians should ask the indication, dose, and duration of use about medications that have abuse potential. Alcohol abuse can be screening by asking the purpose, frequency, and amount of drinking and using a tool like the Michigan alcoholism screening test geriatric version (MAST-G) or the CAGE questionnaire for alcoholism. The MAST-G is a simple, self-scored test with 24 yes (1 point)/no (0 point) questions and a score $\geq$ 5 indicates alcohol problem. The CAGE includes four questions: cut down "Have you ever felt you should cut down on your drinking?"; annoyed "Have people annoyed you by criticizing your drinking?"; guilty "Have you ever felt bad or guilty about your drinking?"; and eye-opener: "Have you ever had a drink first thing in the morning to steady your nerves or get rid of a hangover?" A "yes" answer to any question suggests possible alcohol abuse.

对于 BMI 为 26.1～29kg/m² 者，握力<18kg。

对于 BMI >29kg/m² 者，握力<21kg。

（2）乏力（"做什么事都非常费力"或"我不能再继续坚持"）。

（3）步速慢（走 5m 需要用 6～7 秒或更长时间）。

（4）低体力活动（男性每周活动消耗量低于 383kcal；女性低于 270kcal）。

（5）体重减轻（过去 1 年内体重降低超过 4.54kg）。

《妇女健康与衰老研究Ⅱ》表明，衰弱是从其五个症状中的任何一个开始的。乏力往往首先发生，其次是低体力活动。疲劳通常出现在最后。体重减轻或疲劳的早期出现可以预测衰弱的进展加快。

（十二）物质滥用

老年人酒精和药物滥用情况往往是由于治疗其他健康问题导致的。例如：老年人用安眠药和酒精来解决睡眠障碍，时间久了，便对安眠药和酒精产生依赖。因此在老年人，特别是独居老年人中进行物质滥用的筛查非常重要。临床医生应该询问药物滥用的指征、剂量和持续时间。酗酒可以用密歇根酒精中毒筛查试验老年版或 CAGE 酒精成瘾问卷进行筛查。密歇根酒精中毒筛查试验老年版是一个简易的自评工具，共 24 道是非题，总分≥5 分就提示存在酗酒问题。CAGE 酒精成瘾问卷共包括了 4 个问题，分别是"你是否觉得自己应该减少喝酒？""是否有人批评你喝酒？""你是否曾因喝酒而感到内疚？""你是否会在早上喝酒以稳定神经或摆脱宿醉？"如果对任何一道题有肯定回答，则提示可能存在酗酒。

Box 4-2　Case Study

During health history interview, Mrs. Liu reported feeling dizzy, and stumbled to find balance when getting up at times, so she has stopped going to some routine gatherings in the neighborhood. She used to knit a lot, but she was upset for no remembering how to knit certain patters and stopped knitting altogether. She is also cutting down her social contacts because social conversations became boring, but she faithfully does evening square dances. She denies other abnormalities. Her blood pressure was 145/90 mmHg, heart rate 92 bpm, temperature 36.5 ℃ , respiratory rate 18, weight 45 kg, height152 cm. She has Heberden's nodes on both hands and a soft systolic murmur. Her right vision is 20/60 (Snellen chart) and left eye 20/40. Her MNA is 12 on screening and 6 on assessment. On the 3IQ, she reported leaking urine when she could not make to the bathroom quickly. Her PSQI is 18.

Questions:

1. What normal aging-related changes do you expect to find?

2. What geriatric syndromes is Mrs. Liu's at risk for?

3. What risk factors for geriatric syndromes do you need to target interventions?

Box 4-2　案例

刘女士主诉起床时头晕、腿脚不稳，所以除了广场舞，她不再参加社区活动，也不爱聊天了。她以前是编织能手，但现在记不得怎么织花样。经检查，刘女士血压145/90mmHg，心率92次/min，体温36.5℃，呼吸18次/min，身高152cm，体重45kg。刘女士双手都有Heberden结节，并有心脏收缩期杂音。她的右眼视力为20/60（斯内伦视力表），左眼视力为20/40。营养筛查量表12分。通过3IQ量表评分，刘女士得分为18分，存在漏尿，如果不能及时赶到洗手间，偶尔会小便失禁。

问题：

1. 你预测可能发现的正常老化改变有哪些？

2. 刘女士有哪些发生老年综合征的风险因素？

3. 你该如何针对老年综合征的危险因素制订干预方案？

Section 4　Functional Status

I. Definition and Domains of Functional Status

Functional status refers to the ability to perform normal daily activities required to meet basic needs, fulfill usual role requirements, and maintain health and wellbeing. It includes three domains: health-related physical fitness, physical function, and activities of daily living (ADLs). Although the ADLs are a useful marker for documenting functional decline, they are latent indicators compared to health-related physical fitness and physical function. Usually, the decline in health-related physical fitness precedes the decline in physical function which in turn occurs before impaired ADLs. Nonetheless, the three domains of physical function have reciprocal relationships with impairment in one domain negatively affecting the other two domains. Figure 4-2 presents the domains of functional status and their associated components.

第四节　老年人功能状态的评估

一、功能状态的概念和范畴

功能状态指老年人在生活中满足日常基本需要、社会角色需要以及维持健康和幸福感的能力。它包括健康相关的体适能、躯体功能和日常生活活动（ADL）能力三个范畴。临床中广泛使用日常生活活动能力作为功能状态的标志，但实际上，健康相关的体适能和躯体功能变化要先于日常生活活动能力下降。故而，日常生活活动能力变化是功能状态变化的晚期指标。这三个范畴的躯体功能相互关系，某一个范畴受损，就影响其他两个范畴。图4-2反映了功能状态及其相关组成。

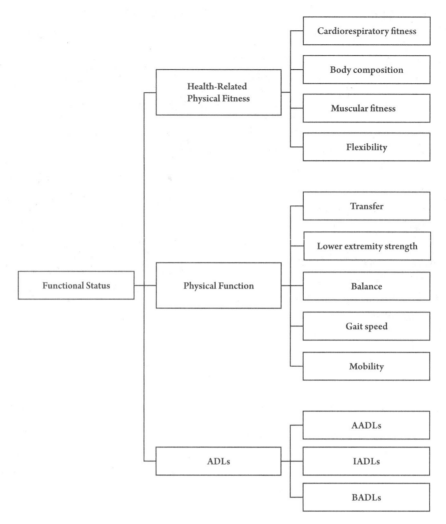

Figure 4-2　Domains of functional status

II. Assessment of Functional Status

The assessment of functional status requires the elderly people to wear proper shoes that are comfortable, flat, and hard-soled for safety, so any identified problems can be correctly classified as function-related instead of shoe-related. Physical function assessment begins with first seeing the elderly people and permeates the whole clinical visit. Careful observations of the elderly people will reveal important information about their function status. For example, observing gait when the person walks to the room. Self-care ability is observed when he/she unbuttons clothes for chest auscultation, removes clothes for blood pressure measurement, and takes off and puts on shoes for measuring height and weight. Transfer is observed when he/she gets on and off the examination bed. Table 4-5 provides a guide for assessing functional status.

二、功能状态的评估

为了保证老年人的安全，功能状态的评估必须在合适着装的条件下进行，比如穿合脚、硬底的鞋，这样也可避免误将外部影响因素当作功能改变。功能状态的评估从和老年人首次接触就已开始。仔细地观察老年人的动作、走路的姿势、步态和着装就可以获得很多初步信息。可在老年人解开衣物进行胸部检查，脱去衣袖进行血压测量，穿脱鞋子进行身高、体重测量时，评估老年人的自理能力。表4-5详细列举了功能状态的三个范畴、评估工具及评估工具所需要的时间。

Table 4-5　Assessment Tools for Functional Status

Domain	Assessment tools	Administration duration /minutes
Health-related physical fitness		
Cardiorespiratory fitness	Maximal exercise testing	30
	Submaximal exercise testing	20-30
	6-minute walk test	6
Body composition		
Weight	Calibrated scale with beam and moveable weights	2
Height	Stadio-meter	2
BMI	= (weight in kg)/ (height in meter)^2	1
Waist circumference	Tension-controlled tape	1
Waist-to-hip ratio	Tension-controlled tape	2
Skinfold Analysis	Caliper	5
Muscular fitness		
Muscular Strength	One repetition maximum Functional reach	Depends on muscle group tested
Flexibility	Range of motion	2
Physical function		
Transfer	Chair rise test	1
Lower extremity Strength	Timed chair rise test	1
Gait speed	Gait speed test	1
Balance	3-stand balance test	1.5
	Resistance to nudge	0.5
Mobility	Observation of ambulation and stair climbing	0.5
Overall physical function	SPPB	1
	PPF	5-10
	TUG test	1
Functional status		
AADLs	PASE	5-15
IADLs	The IADL Scale	2
BADLs	PSMS	2
	Katz Index of Independence in ADLs	2

Note. ADLs: Activities of Daily Living; AADLs: Advanced ADLs; BADLs: Basic ADLs; IADLs: Instrumental ADLs; PASE: The Physical Activity Scale for the Elderly; and PSMS: The Physical Self Maintenance Scale; TUG test: Timed Up and Go test.

表 4-5　功能状态的评估

项目	评估工具	测量时间 /min
健康相关体适能		
有氧适能	极量运动试验	30
	次极量运动试验	20～30
	6min 步行测试	6

项目	评估工具	测量时间/min
身体成分		
体重	体重计	2
身高	测距仪	2
BMI	= 体重（kg)/ 身高²（m²)	1
腰围	无张力软尺	1
腰臀比	无张力软尺	2
皮褶厚度	皮褶卡钳	5
肌肉适能		
肌肉力量	多次重复的最大值； 功能的实现	依据测量的肌肉群而定
关节灵活性	关节活动度	2
躯体功能		
移动	坐立试验	1
下肢力量	计时坐立试验	1
平衡力	3 种站姿的平衡测试 抗推试验	1.5 0.5
步速	步速测量试验	0.5
移动能力	观察移动和上下楼梯的能力	0.5
综合身体功能	SPPB PPF TUG test	1 5～10 1
日常生活活动能力		
AADLs	PASE	5～15
IADLs	IADL 量表	2
BADLs	PSMS Katz ADLs	2 2

注：ADLs；日常生活活动量表；AADLs；高级 ADL；BADLs；基本 ADL；IADLs；工具性 ADL；PASE；老年人身体活动量表；PSMS；自我维持身体活动量表；TUG 试验；定时起立行走试验。

i. Health-related Physical Fitness

Health-related physical fitness includes four components: cardiorespiratory fitness, body composition, muscular strength, and flexibility. There has been increasing interest in assessing health-related physical fitness in the elderly people for four reasons. First, a strong relationship between health-related physical fitness and good health has been repeatedly demonstrated. Second, health-related physical fitness is associated with the ability

（一）健康相关的体适能

健康相关的体适能有有氧适能、身体成分、肌肉适能及关节的灵活性四个部分。随着现代医疗的发展，健康相关的体适能在老年人中愈来愈受到重视，原因如下：体适能和健康密切相关；好的体适能有助于增强日常生活活动能力和质量；健康的体适能可以降低多种疾病的发病率（如冠心病、脑卒中、

to perform ADLs with vigor. Third, good health-related physical fitness reduces the risk for a variety of diseases (e. g., coronary artery disease, stroke, diabetes, cancers) and premature death. Last, health-related physical fitness can be enhanced through exercise.

This section provides an overview of how to assess health-related physical fitness. Readers interested in advanced study are referred to the American College of Sports Medicine's Guidelines for Exercise Testing and Prescription.

1. Cardiorespiratory Fitness　Cardiorespiratory fitness, or aerobic capacity, refers to the ability to use large muscles to perform dynamic, moderate to high intensity exercise for an extended period of time. It is traditionally measured using maximal oxygen consumption (VO_{2max}). Cardiorespiratory fitness is prone to aging effect, declining at about 10% per decade after 25 years of age and 15%-22% after 50 years of age in sedentary individuals [1% decline in $VO_{2max} = 5$ ml/ (kg · min)]. Low cardiovascular fitness increases the difficulty in carrying out ADLs. The good news is that aerobic exercise training can enhance cardiovascular fitness well into the 9th decade of life and reduce the extent of VO_{2max} decline (1%-7% decline/ decade in active the elderly people versus 15%-22% of their sedentary peers).

Maximal exercise test is often conducted for diagnosing cardiovascular disease, risk stratification in individuals with known cardiovascular disease, prescribing aerobic exercise, and evaluating treatment effects. Submaximal exercise testing is less physically demanding and predicts VO_{2max} from a submaximal work rate using standard formulas, but is criticized for the precision of their predictions. Both tests require special equipment (e. g., treadmill or cycle ergometer, electrocardiogram), and medical supervision by a physician is also needed for maximal exercise test, making them unsuitable for routine clinical use.

In contrast, field tests are relatively easy and safe to do, especially walking tests such as the Rockport one-mile fitness walking test and 6-minute walk test. The Rockport one-mile fitness walking test requires an elderly person to walk for a mile, while the 6-minute walk test asks the person to walk for six minutes. The time or distance walked or heart rate in the last minute of the test is used as indicators of cardiorespiratory fitness.

2. Body Composition　Body composition identifies the body make-up and includes the relative amount of body fat, muscle mass, and bone. Aging increases body fat and reduces muscle and bone mass. Muscle wasting (sarcopenia) is a strong predictor for

糖尿病和肿瘤）和过早死亡的风险；健康的体适能可通过运动提高。

本节将概述健康相关的体适能，感兴趣的读者可以进一步查阅美国运动医学院的运动测试和处方指南。

1. 有氧适能　有氧适能是指躯体的大肌群进行一定时间的中高强度有氧运动的能力。最大耗氧量（VO_2max）是测量有氧适能的指标。对于很少从事有氧运动的人更易衰老，最大耗氧量从 25 岁开始以每 10 年 10% 的速度降低，到 50 岁之后以每 10 年 15%～22% 的速度递减。但是，即便是 90 多岁的高龄老人，通过有氧运动仍可以有效保持和提高有氧适能。

极量运动试验通常用于诊断心血管疾病，对已知心血管疾病患者进行危险分层，制订有氧运动处方以及评价治疗效果。而次极量运动试验只需要运动到最大心率的 70%～85%，大多数老年人都可以承受。极量和次极量运动试验都可以用蹬车或跑步机进行测试，要求受试者运动到预定的心率水平，需要特殊仪器和人员配备。故而不适合普查。

相反，步行测试则相对简单、安全，特别是以一英里行走或 6 分钟行走测试为代表的步行测试，同时对场地、器材要求低，更为实用。一英里走所用的时间，6 分钟行走的距离及测试结束时的心率水平可以作为有氧适能的指标。

2. 身体成分　身体成分指身体中脂肪、肌肉和骨骼的相对重量。衰老会增加身体脂肪，减少肌肉和骨量。肌肉减少症是发病率和死亡率的强预测因子。骨量减少和骨质疏

mortality and morbidity. Reduced bone mass and density increases risk for osteoporosis and fractures.

Despite the lack of international standards, the current recommendations for normal percent body fat are 10%-25% for older men and 25%-37% for older women. The percent of body fat begins to increase after 45 years of age. Women tend to increase internal body fat, whereas men accumulate more subcutaneous fat. Excess body fat, especially excessive visceral fat, is linked to increased risk for many diseases (e. g. , diabetes, hypertension, metabolic syndrome, coronary artery disease, cancers).

Waist circumference, waist-to-hip ratio, and skinfold analysis can indirectly assess relative body fat quickly and economically without requiring substantial technical training. Waist circumference is measured around the narrowest part of the torso using a tension-controlled tape and can predict disease risk in each gender.

Woman: <70 cm indicating very low risk for diseases; 90 – 109 cm indicating high risk.

Man: <80 cm indicating very low risk; 100 – 120 cm indicating high risk.

Waist-to-hip ratio is the ratio of waist and hip circumferences. Health risk is very high for 60-69 years old men whose waist-to-hip ratiois > 1.03 and for 60-69 years old women whose waist-to-hip ratio is> 0.90.

Skinfold analysis assumes that subcutaneous fat is proportional to total body fat. The common skinfold site include abdominal, triceps, biceps, chest/pectoral, medial calf, midaxillary, subscapular, suprailiac, and thighs. All skinfold measures should be performed on the right side of the body in a standing position. Skin is pinched for 1-2 seconds, and caliper is placed directly on the skin surface perpendicularly and halfway between the crest and the base of the fold. Reading of the caliper should wait 1-2 seconds. Each site should be measured twice or more to ensure readings are within 1-2 mm. All sites should be measured before performing duplicate measures, so skin has time to regain normal texture and thickness for duplicative measures. The three-site or seven-site formulas are used to calculate body density for men and women respectively.

3. Muscular fitness Muscular fitness refers to the ability of groups of muscles to contract continuously without getting fatigue. Muscular strength is the aspect of muscular fitness that is particularly important to the elderly people and indicates the amount of force that can

松会增加骨折和骨质疏松的风险。

相对体脂比例是身体成分的主要指标，但国际上尚未有统一的相对体脂比例标准。目前普遍接受的老年人正常的相对体脂比是10%～25%（男性）和25%～37%（女性）。45岁后，人体脂肪含量逐渐增加。脂肪过多，尤其是腹部脂肪过多会增加老年人对糖尿病、高血压、代谢紊乱、冠状动脉粥样硬化、高血脂、癌症等疾病的易感性。

测量腰围、腰臀比和皮褶厚度可以简单、快速地筛查出相对体脂比例及对疾病的易感性。体重指数和腰围相结合对疾病的预测更准确。腰围是软尺测量躯干最窄的部分，可以预测不同性别的疾病风险。

女性腰围：<70cm提示疾病较低风险；90～109cm提示疾病高风险；

男性腰围：<80cm提示疾病较低风险；100～120cm提示疾病高风险。

腰臀比是指腰围和臀围的比值。对于60～69岁老年人而言，若男性的腰臀比＞1.03，女性的腰臀比＞0.90，则提示存在较高的健康风险。

皮褶厚度分析是指测量皮下脂肪占身体总脂肪比例。常见的部位包括腹部、肱三头肌、肱二头肌、胸部、小腿内侧、腋下、肩胛、腹部、大腿。所有的皮褶测量都应站立在受试者身体的右侧进行。测量时，将卡尺放置在皮肤表面垂直处，将皮肤捏1～2秒。每一个部位至少读数两次，以确保读数误差不超过1～2mm。为了使皮肤有足够时间恢复正常厚度，应将全部部位测量过后，再进行复测。

3. 肌肉适能 肌肉适能是指一组肌肉群能连续收缩而不感到疲惫的能力，它包括肌力和功能伸展。肌力通常指最大肌力，也就是肌肉在一次收缩后能产生的最大力度，而

be generated in a single muscle contraction. Muscular strength reaches its peak by 20-30 years of age and remains relatively stable until 45 years of age, but begins to decline subsequently and 1%-2% decline has been consistently reported after 60 years of age. Muscle strength is clinically measured using one repetition maximum test and functional reach. One repetition maximum test examines the heaviest weight that a person can successfully lift no more than one time without failing to complete a specified range of motion. Functional reach assesses muscular strength under conditions that match daily activities. Resistance training maintains and improves muscular strength in the elderly people.

4. Flexibility Flexibility or joint flexibility refers to the range of motion at a joint and includes static and dynamic flexibility. All joints should be evaluated including the neck, shoulders, trunk, lumbar, hips, knees, ankles, toes, elbows, and wrists. Static flexibility can be tested through passive range of motion, while dynamic flexibility requires older adult to actively move joints. If desired, goniometer can provide accurate measures of joint flexibility. Stretching exercise improves flexibility, although its effectiveness for reducing injuries and improving performance needs to be further evaluated in the elderly people.

ii. Physical Function

Physical function refers to the performance of specific physical tasks and includes five components: transfer, lower extremity strength, balance, gait speed, and mobility. Physical function is assessed using interview questions, questionnaires based on subjective reports, and performance-based tasks. Interview questions include whether an elderly person has experienced any changes in the ability to transfer, walk, maintain balance, and climb stairs, what the reasons are for such a change, and what type of assistance is needed, and who provides the assistance. Questionnaires are convenient and easy to do, but over-or under-reporting can be a problem. Performance-based tasks provide objective assessment, but only capture a snapshot of physical function at the time of assessment. Now, let's review the assessment of each component of physical function.

1. Transfer Transfer refers to the ability to transfer from one position to another and depends on lower extremity strength. A common way to evaluate transfer is to ask the elderly people to stand up from a seated position in a hard-back chair with arms folded across the chest. The inability to stand up indicates leg weakness and increased risk for disability.

功能伸展指在日常生活中的肌肉力度。两者都可以用测力计来测量。老年人由于老化导致肌肉力量下降，其降低的速度因人而异。肌肉强度在 20～30 岁前达到高峰，之后保持相对稳定，直到 45 岁开始下降。60 岁以后，肌肉力量以每年以 1%～2% 的速度下降，故对老年人而言，力量训练至关重要。

4. 关节的灵活性 关节的灵活性指一个关节的最大活动范围，可以通过被动活动范围（由评估者移动各个关节）和主动活动范围（由老年人自己主动移动各个关节）进行评估。应对所有的关节评估，即包括颈部、肩部、躯干、腰部、臀部、膝部、踝部、脚趾、肘部和腕部。必要时，可使用测角仪精确评估关节的灵活性。伸展运动可以促进关节的灵活性。

（二）躯体功能

躯体功能是指一个人能完成各种活动的能力，涉及转移、下肢力量、平衡力、步速和移动能力 5 个部分。躯体功能评估可使用问诊，基于主观报告的问卷调查和基于表现的任务来评估。问诊包括询问老年人是否经历了转移、走路、保持平衡、爬楼梯等能力的变化，原因是什么，需要什么样的帮助，以及谁提供帮助。问卷调查相对方便和易行，但易出现过度报告或是报告不足的问题。基于表现的任务可提供客观的评估，但只能在动作的瞬间观察到躯体功能。现在，让我们了解一下躯体功能各个组成部分的评估。

1. 移动 移动指老年人变换位置的平稳性和连贯性，主要取决于下肢力量。在和老年人接触时可以直接观察其移动能力，也可以让老年人做一些特定动作，如从椅子上站起，走到检查床边坐下。不能站立提示下肢无力，残疾的风险增加。

2. Lower extremity strength Lower extremity strength refers to the muscle strength of legs. It can be tested using the timed chair rise test which requires an elderly person to rise as quickly as possible from an armless chair five times in a row without using arms. Chairs should have no wheels and are placed against a wall for safety.

3. Balance Balance indicates the ability to maintain the center of gravity within the base of support and with minimal postural sway. Balance is tested using the 3-stand balance and resistance to nudge tests.

The 3-stand balance test measures the ability to maintain each stand for 10 seconds. Arms, bending knees, and moving body are allowed to help maintain balance without moving out of a stand:

Side-by-side stand: Standing with feet next to each other.

Semi-tandem stand: Standing with the front half of the inner side of one heel touching the back half of the inner side of the other heel.

Tandem stands: Standing with one foot in the front of the other with the heel of the front foot touching the toes of the other foot.

The resistance to nudge test assesses the ability to maintain balance when challenged. The clinician stands behind an elderly person, and gently and briskly pulls his/her shoulders back to observe if the older adult loses and regains balance. The clinician must be prepared to catch and ease the older adult to the floor should the older adult begins to fall.

4. Gait speed Gait speed refers to the speed that the elderly people walk at their usual pace. Gait speed predicts the risk for falls and future disability, and can be tested using gait speed test where a clinician records the time it takes the elderly people to walk 10 meters at usual speed. Assistive device like a cane or walker is allowed. Gait speed of > 13 seconds indicates fall risks.

5. Mobility Mobility refers to being in motion. Mobility is assessed by asking if the elderly people have any problems walking from room to room inside the house, climbing stairs, and walking around the community, or observing them walk and/or climb a flight of stairs.

6. Overall physical function While components of physical function allow assessing targeted area(s), tools evaluating overall physical function is more efficient and easier to administer, including the short physical performance battery (SPPB), performance-based physical function (PPF), and timed up and go test (TUG test).

2. 下肢力量 下肢力量指的是腿部肌肉的力量，可以通过记录老年人从椅子上连续起立五次所使用的时间来评估。为了保障老年人的安全，用来测试的椅子应该没有轮子，并靠墙而放，但要防止老年人头磕到墙上。

3. 平衡力 平衡力指身体通过最小晃动就能保持重心在支撑面内的能力。平衡测试使用三个站姿平衡和抗推试验来测试。

三种站姿的平衡测试是指每个姿势至少维持 10 秒的能力。只要不移动站立的位置即可，可通过手臂、弯曲的膝盖和移动的身体可以帮助保持平衡。

两只脚平行站立：双脚并拢。

半前后站立：双脚并拢后，一只脚向后移动半只脚的位置。

两脚前后站立：后脚的脚尖挨着前脚的脚跟。

还可采用抗推试验来评估平衡力。评估人站在老年人身后，轻轻地推老年人的肩膀，观察老年人是否失去平衡，但必须做好准备，及时抓住老年人，以防跌倒。

4. 步速 步速指日常生活中步行的速度，其可预测未来发生残疾的可能性。步速通过计时走 10m 所需的时间来测量。辅助设备，如手杖或助行器是可以使用的。10m 的用时 >13 秒提示老年人有跌倒的风险。

5. 移动能力 移动能力指走动的能力。询问老年人在社区和家里房间走动有无问题，并进一步通过观察老年人走动和上下楼梯来评估和判断其移动能力。

6. 综合身体功能 针对个人而言，评估具体的躯体功能是必须的，但在大规模筛查或首次临床体格检查等情况下，综合评估身体功能显得更为实用。可以同时评估多个身体功能的综合性量表便应运而生，包括简易躯体功能状况量表（SPPB）、基于性能的身体功能量表

The SPPB assesses balance, gait speed, and strength in about 10 minutes. The balance and strength subscales are administered the same as the 3-stand balance test and timed chair rise test described previously. The gait speed subscale uses a 4-meter course and is given twice with the faster speed used for scoring. Each subscale is scored from 0 to 4 with a total score of 0–12 (higher score indicating better function).

The PPF includes three previously described tasks (10-foot timed walk, timed chair rise test, and balance test) and grip strength (kilograms) of the dominant hand. Each test is scored from 0 to 4 points with a total score of 16 (higher scores indicating better physical performance). A score <10 has been linked to increased risk for incident Alzheimer's disease and other dementias.

The TUG test measures the time it takes the elderly people to rise from an arm chair, walk three meters, turn, walk back, and sit down. Inability to complete the task within 15 seconds indicates impaired lower extremity function. The TUG test has a positive predictive value of 0.91 and a negative predictive value of 0.92.

iii. ADLs

ADLs refer to routine activities that people tend to do in daily life and include three domains: AADLs, IADLs, and BADLs. AADLs are defined as activities undertaken to fulfill familial, community, and societal roles as well as participate in occupational and recreational activities. IADLs is defined as the ability to do household tasks such as doing laundry, preparing meals, doing housework, managing household finances, shopping, taking medications, driving or using public transportation, and using the telephone. BADLs outlines the ability to perform self-care activities such as eating, bathing, toileting, dressing, grooming, and transferring from bed to chair.

ADLs are assessed using interview questions, questionnaires based on subjective reports, and performance-based tasks. Similar to the assessment of physical function, the clinician can start by asking whether an elderly person has changed the way he/she does an ADL task, what the reasons are for such a change (e. g., due to a health-related problem), if and what type of assistance is needed, and who provides the assistance. It is particularly important to evaluate bathing because bathe difficulty is highly associated with disability and often the reason for requiring home services. Research has shown

（PPF）和起立 – 行走测试（TUGtest）。

SPPB 评估了平衡力、10m 步速和下肢力量。平衡力分量表同三种站姿的平衡测试，下肢力量分量表则是评估从椅子上连续起立。步速分量表要求老年人用最快的速度行走通过 4m 距离。各分量表的得分是 0～4 分，总分为 0～12 分（分数越高表示功能越好）。

PPF 包括了之前介绍的方法（计时行走、从椅子上连续起立和平衡测试）和用有利手进行握力测量。每部分测试的得分是 0～4 分，总分为 0～16 分（分数越高，表示躯体表现越好）。得分<10 分提示患阿尔茨海默病和其他类型痴呆的风险较高。

TUG 测试是记录老年人从椅子上站起、走 3m、转身、走回和坐下一系列动作所用的时间。若无法在 15 秒内完成这些任务，则提示老年人可能存在下肢功能障碍。

（三）日常生活活动能力

日常生活活动能力指每日生活中经常从事的活动，涵盖高级、工具性和躯体日常生活活动能力 3 个部分。高级日常生活活动能力（AADLs）指实现家庭、社区和社会角色需要及休闲、娱乐和工作所从事的活动；工具性日常生活活动能力（IADLs）指完成日常居家活动的能力，如洗衣服、做饭、理财、购物、服药、使用交通工具、打电话等；躯体性日常生活活动能力（BADLs）指自我照顾的能力，如吃饭、洗澡、上厕所、穿衣服等。自理能力通常是指工具性和躯体性日常生活活动能力，或者单指躯体性日常生活活动能力。

采集病史和使用量表是评估日常生活活动能力的主要办法。病史采集可以针对老年人及其家人，围绕日常生活活动能力的变化展开，集中于老年人完成各项日常活动时是否需要帮助。如果需要帮助，谁可以提供帮助等问题。如果有自理能力的变化，则需要进一步询问有关居家服务资源及使用情况。有研究表明，老年人往往会过高估计自己的能力，而照顾者倾向于低估老年人的能力。

that the elderly people tend to over-estimate their ADLs performance, while caregivers are inclined to under-estimate. Performance-based tasks provide objective assessment, but again only capture a snapshot of ADLs performance.

1. AADLs Usually, participation in social and occupational activities is assessed using interview questions described above due to a lack of clinical tools. Some tools do evaluate some AADLs in connection with other concepts, e. g. , the physical activity scale for the elderly (PASE) asks self-reported occupational, household, and leisure activities during a 1-week period to derive the amount and level of physical activity.

2. IADLs The IADL scale (IADLS) is one of the oldest scale for assessing IADLs. It contains eight items: using the telephone, shopping, food preparation, housekeeping, laundry, mode of transportation, responsibility for own medication, and ability to handle finances. Each item is scored as 0 or 1 with a total score of 0 (low function) to 8 (high function).

3. BADLs The physical self-maintenance scale (PSMS) and Katz index of independence in ADLs are frequently used to assess BADLs. The PSMS assigns a score of 1 (no impairment) to 5 (severe impairment) to each of six activities: toileting, feeding, dressing, grooming, ambulation, and bathing. Higher scores indicate greater dependence. The Katz ADLs rates the ability to perform bathing, dressing, toileting, transferring, continence, and feeding as 1 (no supervision, direction, or assistance) or 0 (with supervision, direction, older adult assistance, or total care). A total score of 6, 4, and ≤ 2 indicates full function, moderate impairment, and severe impairment, respectively.

The scales described above are based on the self-subjective assessment of the elderly, which may deviate from the actual activities of daily living of the elderly. In addition, there will be differences between the elderly their own estimation and the family's estimation of the ability of the elderly.

Box 4-3   Case Study

Let's review what we have learned about Mrs. Liu so far, she came to the clinic because her daughter is concerned about mom's functional decline. Mrs. Liu feels she is doing fine but did report some dizziness, balance, and memory issues, which made her drop some of her routine activities like knitting and some socialization. She still does square dance every evening.

1. **高级日常生活活动能力** AADLs 主要靠询问职业、社交、家庭和娱乐活动等的方面的日常生活活动和能力。目前并没有合适的临床量表，存在的量表大多专注于与这些活动相关的某方面，如老年体力活动量表（PASE）测量一周内与职业、家庭活动相关的运动量。

2. **工具性日常生活活动能力** 工具性日常生活活动量表（IADL 量表）是最常用的评估工具性日常生活活动能力的量表。该量表包括了八个条目，分别是打电话、购物、做饭、做家务、洗衣服、使用交通工具、用药和管理银行账号等活动。每个条目得分为 0 分或 1 分，总分为 0 ~ 8 分，分数越高，IADL 能力越好。

3. **躯体性日常生活活动能力** BADLs 包括洗漱、吃饭、穿衣和大小便等。可以用自我维持身体活动量表（PSMS）和 Katz 独立生活能力指标（Katz ADLs）进行评估。PSMS 包括了六种活动，即如厕、进食、穿衣、修饰、移动和洗澡。Katz ADLs 则评估老年人完成洗澡、穿衣、如厕、转移、控制大小便和进食的能力。

以上介绍的量表都是基于自我主观的评估，与老年人实际的日常生活活动能力可能存在偏差。此外，老年人自己的估计和家人对老年人能力的估计也会有区别。

Box 4-3   案例

现在我们来回顾刘女士的案例。大女儿很担心妈妈的身体状况，因而带她去诊所检查。刘女士自我感觉挺好的，就是有点头晕、腿脚不稳和记忆力下降，就她的年龄来说，她觉得自己是正常的。除了跳广场舞，她不进行别的活动。

Questions:

1. What domains of functional status will you specifically assess?

2. What interview questions and assessment tools will you use to assess Mrs. Liu's functional status?

3. What areas of functional status will you focus interventions on?

问题：

1. 功能状态评估的重点在哪里？

2. 如何选择评估功能状态的病史采集方法和评估量表？

3. 明确提高功能状态的干预重点是什么？

Section 5　Cognitive Function

I. Definition and Domains of Cognitive Function

Cognitive function is defined as cerebral activities that acquire, process, and output information and accumulate knowledge by which a person becomes aware of, perceives, or comprehends ideas. Cognition is typically categorized into four discrete domains as memory, executive functioning, visuospatial function, and language (Figure 4-3). More detailed classification further lists orientation, abstraction, judgment and problem solving, and attention domains. There are ongoing debates about whether orientation, abstraction, judgment and problem solving are indeed discrete cognitive domains. Is orientation a sub-domain of memory? Are abstraction, judgment, problem solving, and attention sub-domains of executive functioning? This section adopted the four domain categorizations used for dementia diagnosis, and introduces the components and normal-aging related changes of each domain.

i. Memory

Memory refers to the ability to store, retain, and recall information and includes explicit episodic memory and implicit procedural memory. Explicit episodic memory depends on the function of the hippocampus system and identifies a conscious process of recollecting previous events and experiences, which could be short-term (short-term memory) or long-term (long-term memory). Implicit procedural memory delineates the memory process that does not require conscious recollection to be activated and re-experienced, and can be established through brain mechanisms independent of hippocampus. Memory is formed via three steps: encoding which gets information into the memory system; storage where information are retained in the memory system; and retrieval which involves recalling information.

第五节　老年人认知功能的评估

一、认知功能的概念和范畴

认知功能指人脑通过收集、处理和传递信息而累积知识、灵活地观察、理解和推理事物间复杂关系的能力。最常用的临床分类方法将认知功能划分为记忆、执行功能、视空间功能和语言功能四大认知域（图4-3）。更细致的分类进一步区分定向力、注意力、抽象力、判断和解决问题能力为独立的认知域，但此分类颇有争议，比如注意力、抽象概括力、判断和解决问题能力是否隶属于执行功能的一个层面？本节沿袭临床，尤其是老年痴呆领域的传统，介绍四大认知域及总体认知功能。

（一）记忆

记忆是指对信息的编码、存储和提取能力，包括外显记忆和内隐记忆。外显记忆和内隐记忆的区别主要在于对以往事件和经验的储存是否需要经过海马和意识的参与，前者需要海马和意识的参与，而后者不需要。外显记忆可进一步分为近期记忆和远期记忆。

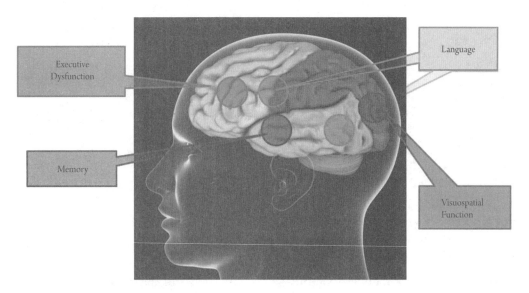

Figure 4-3　Cerebral substrates for cognitive domains

The elderly people perform less well than younger adults on encoding, storage, and recall of information with encoding particularly vulnerable to aging effect. It takes longer for the elderly people to process new information and retrieves well-learned information; however, slowed processing speed and motor function contributes significantly to performance on memory tasks. Slower encoding likely accounts for aging-related decline in short-term memory. Memory loss is the second most frequently reported problem by the elderly people after arthritis. Impaired short-term episodic memory is a telltale sign of Alzheimer's disease.

Long-term memory includes recognition and recall. Recognition does not decline with aging, but recall does. The extent of decline in recall depends on the extent of encoding difficulty. Long-term memory that spans months or years is usually well preserved into the seventh decade of life.

Orientation has a strong memory component and hence included here. Orientation refers to the mental process of being aware of time, place, and person. Disorientation often occurs in the sequence of time, place, and person. Orientation relies on learned knowledge, hence, remains stable in old age. It is unclear what the exact cerebral region is involved in orientation. Cerebral hemispheres and brain stem have been suggested to be the cerebral substrate for disorientation.

ii. Executive Functioning

Executive functioning is defined as a set of cognitive skills that organize, coordinate, and sequence goal-directed behaviors. Executive functioning consists of

增龄延长了信息的编码和提取过程，因此老年人经常出现短期外显记忆下降，但对内隐记忆影响很小。尽管如此，健忘仍是异常表现，短期外显记忆受损是阿尔茨海默病的典型症状。

长期记忆包括对信息的识别和提取能力。识别能力不受老化改变的影响，但与信息的提取能力和编码的难易程度相关。即便是70多岁的老人，他的跨时数月或数年的长期记忆都可以完好无损。

定向力是指对时间、地点和人物有意识的识别。它强烈地依赖于记忆，故而被划在记忆之下。老化改变不影响定向力。

（二）执行功能

执行功能通过其工作记忆、预备定势和抑制控制三个部分对有目标的行为进行组织、协调和排序。工作记忆是储存变化的口

three components: working memory, preparatory set, and inhibitory control. Working memory relates to the dorsolateral prefrontal cortical region and defines our ability to represent and integrate verbal and nonverbal changing information with past experience. Preparatory set is associated with the anterior cingulate prefrontal cortical region and determines our ability to organize and coordinate goal-directed behavior. Inhibitory control involves the orbital prefrontal cortical region and suppresses behaviors and information not pertinent to the task at hand.

Other aspects of executive functioning include attention, judgment and problem-solving, abstraction, and reaction time. Attention refers to the action of noticing someone or something, depends on the frontal cortical circuit, and includes both sustained and selective attention. Sustained attention refers to the ability to focus, while selective attention indicates the mental process of selectively concentrating on some aspects of the environment while ignoring others by allocating cognitive processing resources. Aging does not seem to affect either attention well into old age. Judgment and problem solving refers to the ability to evaluate evidence to make a decision or solve a problem, depends on orbitofrontal subcortical circuit, and tends to decline with aging. Abstraction is defined as the mental process of deriving higher concepts from classifying the general attributes of concrete concepts and involves frontal lobe. Reaction time refers to the time it takes to react and declines with aging with more complex tasks associated with longer reaction time. Executive function begins to show some decline at 60 years of age and substantial decline after 70 years of age.

Executive dysfunction is the predominant symptom of front-temporal dementia and other conditions that affect frontal lobe. Although impaired memory is the hallmark symptom for Alzheimer's disease, executive dysfunction can be the dominant or early symptom. However, subtle executive dysfunction is often neglected and not easily recognized by the elderly people, family members, or clinicians.

iii. Visuospatial Function

Visuospatial function outlines the cognitive process of perceiving, comprehending, and interpreting visual and spatial information. Intact visuospatial function allows efficient and accurate object and face recognition, safe environmental navigation, and skilled visuomotor movements like using a utensil. Visual object recognition primarily relies on the occipitotemporal visual pathways, while spatial perception involves predominantly the occipitoparietal regions.

头和行为信息，并将这些信息和过去经历整合到一起的能力；预备定势组织和协调有目的的行为；抑制控制则压制与手头任务无关的信息。

执行功能的其他方面包括注意力、判断和解决问题能力、抽象概括力和反应时间。注意力指意识到某人或某事，包括专心能力（持续的集中于某人或某事）和选择注意力（专注于整个环境中的一方面而忽略其他方面）。老化改变不影响注意力。判断和解决问题能力指通过评估证据来解决问题的能力。老化使老年人的判断和解决问题能力降低。抽象力指由具体形象到抽象概念的思维能力。抽象概括力随年龄增长而有所下降。反应时间指一个行为反应所需要的时间。反应时间随年龄增长而延长。执行功能在 60 岁以后开始下降，并在 70 岁以后加速下降。

执行功能障碍是前颞叶痴呆和其他影响额叶的疾病的主要症状。虽然记忆受损是阿尔茨海默病的标志性症状，但执行功能障碍可能是主要或早期症状。然而，微妙的执行功能障碍往往不容易识别，被老年人、家属或临床医生所忽视。

（三）视空间功能

视空间功能指对视空间信息的感觉、处理和解释能力。它使老年人能够认识事物和人物，并安全地在各种环境中活动和使用工具。视觉对象识别主要依靠枕颞视觉通路，而空间感知则主要涉及枕顶区。

The elderly people show some decline in visuospatial function, e. g. , decreased ability to perceive and reproduce figures in three dimensions, recognize embedded objects, and identify incomplete figures. Alzheimer's disease causes constructional apraxia, difficulty in assembling discrete components into multi-dimensional designs, which is related to greater difficulty in dressing, meal preparation, and hygiene.

iv. Language

Language refers to the ability to produce spontaneous speech, comprehend and repeat language, name objects, read, and write. Spontaneous speech is characterized by its rate, rhythm, volume, response latency, and inflection. Comprehension illustrates the ability to follow verbal and written instructions. Repetition defines the ability to repeat words, phrases, and sentences. Naming indicates the ability to name objects or part (s) of an object. Reading refers to the ability to read and comprehend what is read. Writing delineates an individual's ability to write complete sentences that are grammatically correct.

Some aging-related decline in semantic knowledge, the "tip-of-the-tongue" phenomenon, has been observed, however, significant declines are not found until 70 years old and older. Soft and monotone speech indicates Parkinson's disease. Word-finding difficulty is commonly seen in Alzheimer's disease.

v. Global Cognition

Similar to overall physical function, global cognition is widely used in cognitive research and clinical practice to capture multiple cognitive domains efficiently and holistically. Different cognitive domains could be included in various global cognition tools.

II. Assessment of Cognitive Function

Cognitive function is assessed using interviews and assessment tools. Cognitive interview begins when meeting the elderly people. Observation of their responses to interview questions provides initial insight into their cognitive function, and assessment tools provide quantifiable evidence.

Cognitive assessment requires special considerations. First, the environment is suitable for assessing cognition, e. g. , no distractions, right temperature, ample lighting. Second, the older adult can adequately see (e. g. , eyeglasses are worn) and hear (e. g. , hearing aid is on and in working condition), and is not distracted by discomfort. Third,

视空间功能随年龄增长而有所降低。如果出现不能把部分元件组成多维结构的结构性失用会使老年人在穿衣、做饭和洗漱方面遇到困难。

（四）语言功能

语言指一个人口头表达、理解、重复、命名、读和写的能力。口头表达指语速、语言运力、流量、反应潜伏期和语调；理解指明白和执行口头或书面指令的能力；重复是复述词、短语和句子的能力；命名是说出物品的名字；读是能读出并理解所读文字意义的能力；写指一个人写语法正确的句子的能力。语言还包括语义、词汇、句法和语音知识。除了语义学知识随老化有所下降外，语言的其他方面几乎没有明显的老化改变。

研究者已经发现了一些与年龄有关的语义知识的下降，即"舌尖"现象。然而，直到70岁及以上这一问题才会更加显著。柔和而单调的语言提示帕金森症。在阿尔茨海默病中，找词困难较为常见。

（五）总体认知功能

和总体功能状态类似，科研和临床经常使用总体认知功能来筛查认知障碍和监测医疗保健的有效性。不同的认知量表对所筛查的认知域有所不同。

二、认知功能的评估

使用访谈和评估工具评估认知功能。医护人员从和老年人接触开始，特别是在病史采集期间就要有意识地观察其认知功能。而评估工具则可以提供量化的证据。

但认知功能的具体评估需要特别注意以下四点：第一，要有合适的环境（如充足的照明、冷暖适宜、安静）；第二，确定老年人视力、听力和意识正常（如需要，老年人可戴眼镜和助听器）；第三，最佳实践是先分别

the best practice is to interview the elderly people and caregivers separately first and then together. For example, when interviewing the caregiver, the clinician asked about a recent memorable event that happened to the older adult (when, where, who, why, and how this event happened, etc.). When interviewing the older adult, he/she will be asked to give details about this event. Any discrepancies will aid the detection of memory problem. This practice will allow the clinicians to compare notes to understand the extent and awareness of cognitive impairment. If interviewed together only, the caregiver might dominate the conversations and/or the older adult might look for cues and validations from the caregiver.

A series of yes-no questions can be used initially to probe any perceived cognitive problems, starting with a global cognition question and moving through each cognitive domain (table 4-6). Any "yes" response should be followed with open-ended questions using OLDCART-I described in Section 2 Medical Conditions:

- Onset: When did this problem start?
- Location: Where has this problem been occurring? Home, community events, unfamiliar places, or others?
- Duration: How long has this problem been going on?
- Characteristics: How does this problem look like (e. g. , comes and goes, is always present, or gets worse over time)?
- Aggravating factors: What makes this problem worse?
- Relieving factors: What makes this problem better?
- Treatments: What have you done to relieve this problem? What's the effect?
- Impact: How does this problem affect your function?

III. Assessment Tools for Cognitive Function

Hearing impairment, visual impairment, and the level of consciousness must be screened first before administering assessment tools (table 4-6) to eliminate their impacts on cognitive performance and result interpretations. Corrective devices such as eyeglasses and hearing aids in good working conditions are to be applied as appropriate. Tools are only administered when the elderly people are fully alert.

面试老年人和其家人，然后再一起面试。这样可以先了解家人的看法和最近发生的老年人应该记得的事，然后咨询老年人的看法和对最近经历的描述，最后再一起会谈，观察老年人和家人之间的互动。用是与不是的问题可以快速地发现认知问题。一旦发现问题，则需更详细地询问问题的始发时间、地点、持续时间、特点、加重因素、减轻因素、采取的治疗措施及其效果。第四，一定要询问认知问题对功能状态的影响。

可以使用一系列"是－否"问题来评估认知功能（表 4-6）。回答应使用第 2 节"医疗条件"中所述的 OLDCART-I 进行开放式提问：

- 发作：症状何时开始？
- 位置：症状发生在哪里？家庭，社区活动，陌生的地方或其他地方？
- 持续时间：持续了多长时间？
- 特征：表现如何（例如，反反复复，持续存在或随着时间的推移而恶化）？
- 加剧因素：症状加剧的原因是什么？
- 缓解因素：好转的因素是什么？
- 治疗：您做了些什么来缓解症状？有什么作用？
- 影响：此症状带来哪些影响？

三、认知功能的评估量表

在使用评估工具（表 4-6）之前，必须首先筛选听力障碍、视力障碍和意识水平，以消除其对认知表现和结果解释的影响。在良好的工作条件下使用矫正装置，如眼镜和助听器。只有在老年人完全清醒的情况下才能使用工具。

Table 4-6　Interview Questions and Assessment Tools for Cognitive Function

Domain	Yes/No Interview Questions	Assessment Tools	Administration Time /min
Global cognition	Do you have any concerns about your cognition?	Mini-cog MoCA MMSE	5 5-10 5-10
Memory	Do you have difficulty remembering things that happened recently?	3-item recall HVLT-R	1.5 30
Executive function	Do you have trouble planning or solve problems?	CDT TMT	10 5
Visuospatial function	Do you have any problems with finding your ways around your community or unfamiliar places?	Copy designs of circle, square, cube, or intersecting pentagons	2
Language	Do you have trouble finding words, naming objects, reading, writing, or expressing yourself?	Objects naming, follow instructions, write a sentence	3

Note. CDT, The clock drawing test; HVLT-R, The Hopkins verbal learning test – revised; MMSE, The mini-mental state examination; MoCA, The Montreal cognitive assessment; and TMT, The trail making tests.

表 4-6　认知功能的评估

项目	是-否性访谈问题	评估工具	测试时间 /min
总体认知功能	您对自己的认知功能是否有顾虑？	Mini-cog MoCA MMSE	5 5~10 5~10
记忆	您记忆近期发生的事是否有困难？	三词语回忆测试 HVLT-R	1.5 30
执行功能	您在计划或解决问题方面是否感到困难？	CDT TMT	10 5
视空间功能	在您居住的社区或熟悉的地方您是否能找到回家的？	复制和画出不同图形如圆、方形、立方体或者五角星等	2
语言功能	您在组织语言、给物体命名、读书、写字、或表达自己的想法方面是否存在困难？	重复句子、命名物品、写句子等	3

注：CDT，时钟绘图测试；HVLT-R，霍普金斯语言学习测验 – 修订；MMSE，迷你精神状态考试；MoCA，蒙特利尔认知评估；TMT，开拓性测试。

i. Memory

Explicit episodic memory is tested with immediate and delayed wordlist recalls using the 3-word recall or and Hopkins verbal learning test -revised (HVLT-R). Delayed wordlist recall is especially effective at discerning memory impairment. The 3-word recall requires an elderly person to repeat three words that were said to ensure the words are registered in short-term memory, and then recall them

（一）记忆

短期外显记忆是用即时和延迟单词表回忆测试的，可使用三词回忆或霍普金斯言语学习测验（HVLT-R）。延迟单词表回忆在辨别记忆障碍方面尤其有效。三词回忆要求老年人重复所说的三个单词，以确保这些单词在短期记忆中被记住，几分钟后再回忆起来。

after a few minutes. Failing to recall all words indicates memory impairment.

The HVLT-R has six alternative forms. Each form has a 12-wordlist, three immediate recall trials, one delayed recall trial, and one recognition trial. In each immediate recall trial, an elderly person is instructed to listen carefully and memorize the same 12 words as they are read at one word every two seconds, and immediately recalls as many words as possible. Each correctly recalled word is awarded as 1 point. After 20-25 minutes, delayed recall is tested by asking the older adult to recall as many words as possible and each correct recall is counted as 1 point. In the recognition trial, 24 words are read and the older adult is asked to say "yes" to each word on the wordlist (12 targets) and "no" to each word not on the wordlist (12 distracters) to derive a discrimination index. A sum recall score < 20 and a discrimination index < 11 indicate impaired verbal memory and can correctly classify Alzheimer's disease with 94% sensitivity and 100% specificity. Although the HVLT-R spans 30 minutes, its actual administration is < 10 minutes because other assessments can be performed during the 20-25-minute delay. Its six different forms further allow repeated administrations over time without learning and practice effects.

Orientations to time, place, and person are usually assessed by asking a series of questions:

Time: What is today's date, day of the week, month, year, and time of the day? Answers to the first four questions must be exact, but time of the day can be within one hour of the actual time.

Place: Where are you now? What floor are we on? What city are we in? What province are we in? For the elderly people from out of the town, identified city landmarks are considered correct.

Person: What is your name? Who came with you today (if accompanied)?

ii. Executive Functioning

Executive functioning can be measured by the clock drawing test (CDT) and trail making tests (TMT), and the executive interview – 25 (EXIT-25). The CDT requires drawing a clock at a given time, and is considered normal if resembling a clock with the right time.

The TMT is a timed test with two parts. Practice on shorter sample tests is important to ensure that the elderly people understand the instructions of drawing the lines as fast as possible with lifting pencil from the paper. Part

不记得所有的单词表明记忆受损。

霍普金斯语言学习测试修订版（HVLT-R）有六种可选形式。每个形式有 12 个单词，三个即时回忆测试，一个延迟回忆测试和一个再认测试。在每一次即时回忆测试中，每隔 2 秒钟读一个词，要求老年人认真听并记忆，结束后立即让老年人回忆听到的词语。每正确回忆一个词语得 1 分。在 20~25 分钟后，进行延时回忆测试和再认测试，每正确回忆一个词语得 1 分。在再认测试中，阅读 24 个单词，要求老年人对单词表上的每个单词（12 个目标词）说"是"，对单词表上的每个单词（12 个干扰词）说"否"，从而得出一个辨别指数。回忆总分<20 和辨别指数<11 表示语言记忆障碍，能正确分类阿尔茨海默病，敏感性为 94%，特异性为 100%。尽管 HVLT-R 的时间跨度为 30 分钟，但其实际实施时间小于 10 分钟，因为在 20~25 分钟的延迟时间内可以进行其他评估。它的六种不同的形式进一步允许随着时间的推移，在没有学习和实践的情况下进行重复测试。

对时间、地点和人的定向通常通过问一系列问题来评估：

时间：今天的日期、星期、月份和年份和时间是什么？前四个问题的答案必须准确，但一天的时间可以在实际时间的一小时之内。

地点：你现在在哪里？我们在几楼？我们在哪个城市？我们在哪个省？对于来自外地的老年人，也可以回答的城市地标。

人：你叫什么名字？今天谁和你一起来的（如果有人陪同的话）？

（二）执行功能

执行功能可以通过画钟试验、连线试验以及执行功能测试 –25 来衡量。画钟试验要求绘制给定时间的时钟，如果类似于具有正确时间的时钟，也视为正常。

连线试验包含两部分，要求限时完成。缩短样本测试的练习对于确保老年人理解从纸上拿起铅笔尽快画线的说明非常重要。第

A requires an elderly person to connect numbered dots in the ascending order and. Part B asks the older adult to connect dots in the ascending order by alternating between numbers (1-13) and letters (A-M), e. g. , 1–A–2–B–3–C. Tests are terminated if the older adult makes ≥ 6 errors or does not complete within five minutes.

The EXIT-25 takes 15 minutes and consists of 25 performance-based items including number-letter task, word fluency, design fluency, anomalous sentence repetition, thematic perception, memory/distraction task, interference task, automatic behaviors, grasp reflex, social habits, motor impersistence, snout reflex, finger-nose-finger task, go/no-go task, echopraxia, Luria hand sequences, grip task, complex command task, serial order reversal task, counting task, utilization behavior, and imitation behavior. Each item is scored as 0 (no errors), 1 (complete task with prompting, repeat instruction, hesitant or other responses, or partial completion), or 2 (does not complete task) with a total score 0-50. Higher scores indicate greater executive dysfunction.

Attention can be assessed using the digit span tests and serial 7's test. The forward digit span test requires an elderly person to repeat a series of numbers with increasing length exactly the way they are said. Repeating <5 digits is abnormal. The backward digit span test asks the older adult to repeat a series of numbers with increasing complexity in reverse order of how they are said. Repeating <3 digits indicates abnormality. The serial 7's test requires the older adult to subtract seven from 100 and keep subtracting seven from each new number until five correct answers.

Judgment and problem solving can be assessed by asking an elderly person to solve a problem, e. g. , "If you are in a strange city, how would you locate a friend you want to see? " (call mutual friend or looking up in directory).

Abstraction is assessed by asking the older adult to tell the similarity and difference among objects, e. g. , how is an orange and an apple alike? (fruit). What is the difference between sugar and vinegar? (one sweet and one sour).

Response time is typically assessed as part of the TMT administration described previously.

iii. Visuospatial Function

Visuospatial function can be assessed by copying

一部分要求老年人按升序和顺序连接编号的点。第二部分要求老年人通过交替使用数字（1-13）和字母（A-M）按升序连接点，例如1-A-2-B-3-C。如果老年人出现≥6个错误或未在5分钟内完成测试，则终止测试。

执行功能测试-25需要15分钟，该测试由25个基于表现的项目组成，包括数字字母任务、单词流利性、设计流利性、异常句子重复、主题感知、记忆/分心任务、干扰任务、自动行为、抓握反射、社交习惯、运动不耐烦、口鼻反射、手指-鼻子-手指任务、进行/不进行任务、模仿动作、手序列、握力任务、复杂命令任务、序列顺序反转任务、计数任务、利用行为和模仿行为。每项得分为0分（无错误），1分（完成任务时有提示、重复指示、犹豫或其他反应，或部分完成），或2分（未完成任务），总分为0-50分。分数越高说明执行功能障碍越严重。

注意力可以通过数字广度测试和序列7测试来评估。前向数字广度测试要求老年人按照所说的方式重复一系列数字，长度不断增加。重复<5位是不正常的。向后数字广度测试要求老年人以与所说数字相反的顺序重复一系列越来越复杂的数字。重复<3位表示异常。序列7的测试要求老年人从100中减去7，并从每个新数字中减去7，直到5个正确答案。

判断和解决问题的能力可以通过让一位老年人解决一个问题来评估，例如，"如果你在一个陌生的城市，你将如何找到一个你想见的朋友？"（打电话给共同的朋友或在目录中查找）。

抽象性是通过让老年人说出物体之间的相似性和差异来评估的，例如，一个橘子和一个苹果有什么相似之处？（水果）。糖和醋有什么区别？（一甜一酸）。

响应时间通常作为前面描述的连线试验管理的一部分进行评估。

（三）视空间功能

视空间功能可以通过要求老年人复制和

design (s) such as a circle, diamond, cube, and/or intersecting pentagon. Inability to copy simple and complex designs signifies visuospatial impairment.

iv. Language

Comprehension is assessed by asking an elderly person to follow commands, e. g. , take this piece of paper, fold it in half, and put it inside the envelope. Repetition requires the older adult to repeat a sentence, e. g. , "no ifs, ands or buts." Naming asks the older adult to name objects such as a watch, pencil, and fingers. Reading requires the older adult to read a sentence in a newspaper and explain what he/she read. Writing is tested by asking the older adult to write a complete, grammatically correct sentence.

v. Global Cognition

The mini-cog, montreal cognitive assessment (MoCA), and mini-mental state examination (MMSE) are widely used for clinical assessment of global cognition. They are screening, not diagnostic, tools for dementia and cover different cognitive domains.

The mini-cog screens memory (3-word recall) and executive functioning (CDT) with 76%-99% sensitivity and 89%-93% specificity. An elderly person is asked to repeat the three words read to them, draw a clock of certain time, and then recall the three words. Failing to recall any words or to recall 1-2 words and have an abnormal clock indicates cognitive impairment.

The MoCA has gained popularity for detecting mild cognitive impairment and screen eight cognitive domains: executive function, visuo-constructional skills, naming, memory, attention and concentration, conceptual thinking, calculations, and orientation. The MoCA has a total score of 30 with a score of ≥ 26 considered normal and 92% sensitivity and 81% specificity.

The MMSE screens seven cognitive domains: orientation to time, orientation to place, registration, attention and calculation, recall, language, and visual construction. A score of ≤23 indicates cognitive impairment. The MMSE can be administered in 10 minutes and has 66%-87% sensitivity and 82%-99% specificity.

画出不同图形而测量评估。

（四）语言

让老年人根据指令做动作、重复句子、命名物品、读报纸、解释所读和写句子可以简单有效地筛查语言功能。

（五）总体认知功能

快速认知功能检测（mini-cog）、蒙特利尔认知评估（MoCA）和简易智能状态检测量表（MMSE）被广泛应用于全球认知的临床评估。它们是痴呆的筛查工具，而不是诊断工具，涵盖不同的认知领域。

快速认知功能检测包括筛选记忆（3字回忆）和执行功能（CDT），敏感性为76%～99%，特异性为89%～93%。要求老年人重复读给他们听的三个单词，并画一个特定时间的钟，然后回忆这三个单词。不记得任何单词或不记得1～2个单词，并且有一个画钟错误表明认知障碍。

蒙特利尔认知评估在检测轻度认知障碍和筛查八个认知领域方面已经获得了广泛的应用。这八个认知领域分别是执行功能、视觉构造技能、命名、记忆、注意力和集中力、概念思维、计算和定向。蒙特利尔认知评估总分为30分，≥26分视为正常，敏感性92%，特异性81%。

简易智能状态检测量表筛查了七个认知领域，分别是时间取向、地点取向、注册、注意力和计算、回忆、语言、视觉结构。得分≤23表示认知障碍。MMSE可在10分钟内给药，敏感性为66%～87%，特异性为82%～99%。

Box 4-4　Case Study

Assessment of functional status shows that Mrs. Liu does all her daily activities on her own. She hand washes clothes and has her own cell phone. Her daughter had hired house-keepers for her, but Mrs. Liu dislikes them and does not use them. Her daughter reported that mom's apartment is mess and smells urine. Mrs. Liu used to cook all meals, but nowadays she eats out some and skips some meals because "I don't feel hungry." and "Shopping is such a bother." She does not shop much because heavy grocery bag hurts her shoulders and hands. She rarely snacks. Mrs. Liu lives on the 3rd floor of a 20-story building. She used to walk upstairs, but begins to ride elevator 6 months ago. Her waist circumference is 95 cm and waist-to-hip ratio 1.6. She walked 425 meters in the 6-minute walk test, and scored 1 on balance, 3 on gait speed, and 3 on chair rise of the SPPB. Her IADLS is 6 and PSMS 4. Daughter added that mom's friends said that mom appears "aloof" in conversations and does not speak.

Questions:

1. What approach will you use to assess cognitive function?

2. How would you assess Mrs. Liu's cognitive function?

3. What areas of cognition will you focus on with interventions?

Box 4-4　案例

刘女士所有日常生活都自己做，不喜欢用保姆。她大女儿说妈妈家又脏又乱，还有一股尿味。刘女士现在很少买菜做饭，"买东西太麻烦，而且也不觉得饿"，所以就在外面吃。她住3楼，以前走楼梯，6个月前开始坐电梯。她的腰围是95cm，腰臀围比例1.6，6分钟走了425m，SPPB平衡分1，步速3，椅子起立3。IADL 6分，PSMS 4分。女儿说妈妈的朋友觉得妈妈很少谈话。

问题：

1. 认知功能的评估方法是什么？

2. 你如何选择认知功能的病史采集方法和评估量表？

3. 你怎样辨别提高认知功能的干预重点？

Section 6　Psychological Status

I. Definition and Domains of Psychological Status

Psychological status refers to one's mood states which are the display of emotions through body movements, facial expression, vocal tone, and self-description of own internal feeling. Disturbances in emotional state are not part of normal aging and occur in a wide variety of neuropsychiatric conditions such as dementia, schizophrenia, and Parkinson's disease. Although the entire spectrum of mood disorders can be presented in the elderly people, depression, anxiety, and grief are prevailing conditions. Anxiety and grief can often lead to depression. Table 4-6 outlines the interview questions and assessment tools for those conditions.

第六节　老年人心理状态的评估

一、心理状态评估的概念和范畴

心理状态指一个人通过肢体动作、面部表情、语调和自我描述等表现出来的情绪。老年人易发生多种情绪障碍，以抑郁、焦虑和悲痛最为普遍，其中，以抑郁症最为常见，焦虑和悲痛可以引发抑郁症。情绪障碍在阿尔茨海默病、精神分裂症、脑卒中等常见的精神、神经系统疾病中高发。总之，情绪障碍不是正常的老化改变，它对老年人的功能状态、身体健康和生活质量都有深远的影响。表4-6概述了针对这些条件的面试问题和评估工具。

i. Depression

The prevalence of depression is comparable between younger and the elderly people, but the elderly people often show atypical presentations. Instead of feeling depressed or sad, the elderly people more likely report lost pleasure in activities, memory loss, and/or difficulty concentrating. Feelings of worthlessness, inappropriate guilt, hypersomnia, weight gain, increased appetite, and suicidal ideation are less common. Major depression affects 1%-4% community-dwelling the elderly people, 10%-12% hospitalized the elderly people, and 10%-15% in nursing home residents. Depressive symptoms are more prevalent, affecting 6%-8% community-dwelling the elderly people, 20%-25% hospitalized the elderly people, and 20%-35% nursing home residents. Undiagnosed and untreated major depression is one of the most significant contributors to excess disability, morbidity, and mortality in the elderly people.

ii. Anxiety

Anxiety is a blanket term that covers several different forms of abnormal and pathological fear and anxiety, e. g., generalized anxiety disorder, panic disorder, panic disorder with agoraphobia, phobias, obsessive-compulsive disorder, and post-traumatic stress disorder. Anxiety is prevalent and creates significant burdens in the elderly people.

iii. Grief

Grief shows increasing prevalence in the elderly people because of increased chance of losing a loved one. Grief refers to the multi-faceted responses to loss, particularly the loss of someone or something with whom a bond was formed, and includes five stages: denial where a person is in a state of shock and a feeling of numbness is experienced; anger where the person feels angry that seems to have no limits; bargaining where the person is so overwhelmed with pain that he/she will reckon to do anything to avoid the loss; depression where the empty feeling occupies the person and grief enters on the deepest level; and acceptance where the reality of loss is accepted.

II. Assessment of Psychological Status

At this point, the following key pointers for assessing psychological status are probably old news to you as follows: assessment begins via observations of their verbal and nonverbal responses during the interview; a series of yes-no questions can be used initially to probe any perceived psychological problems (table 4-7); any "yes" response should be followed with open-ended

（一）抑郁症

抑郁症的患病率在年轻人和老年人之间存在差异，但老年人的抑郁症症状常不典型。老年人没有感到沮丧或悲伤，反而更有可能报告在活动中失去乐趣、记忆力丧失和／或注意力难以集中。毫无价值感、内疚感、嗜睡、体重增加、食欲增加和自杀意念不太常见。重度抑郁症见于 1%～4% 的社区老年人，10%～12% 的住院老年人和 10%～15% 的养老院居民。抑郁症状更为普遍，见于 6%～8% 的社区老年人、20%～25% 的住院老年人和 20%～35% 的养老院居民。未经诊断和治疗的抑郁症是导致老年人过度残疾、发病率和死亡率的最重要因素之一。

（二）焦虑

焦虑广义上指一系列异常和病态的焦急和恐惧。焦虑在老年人中非常普遍，是很严重的精神负担。

（三）悲痛

悲痛在老年人中越来越普遍，因为老年人失去亲人的机会越来越大。悲痛指的是对失去的多方面反应，特别是失去与之形成联系的人或物，它包括五个阶段：否认，当一个人处于震惊状态，并经历麻木的感觉；愤怒，当一个人感到愤怒，似乎没有限制；讨价还价，当一个人被痛苦压倒时，他／她会想尽一切办法避免损失；沮丧，当空虚的感觉占据这个人，悲伤进入最深的层次；接受，当损失的现实被接受时。

二、心理状态的评估

从本章第一节一路学下来，你应该可以猜到心理状态的评估沿袭其他维度的方法：在病史采集过程中观察老年人语言和非语言表现；用是否问题快速筛查；详细询问发现的问题；评估心理问题对功能状态的影响；进行量表测试。表 4-7 显示筛查心理状态的常

questions using a similar OLDCART described in Section 5 Cognitive Function; ask a question about the impact of the perceived psychological problem on physical function; and screen for psychological problem using a brief screening tool. Now, let's zero in on the three prevailing psychological problems in the elderly people: depression, anxiety disorder, and grief.

用量表及量表所需时间。

Table 4-7　Interview Questions and Assessment Tools for Psychological Status

Domain	Interview questions	Assessment tools	Test time /minutes
Depression	Do you feel depressed or sad? Do you feel you have lost pleasure in activities you used to enjoy?	GDS-15 GDS-4	5 1-2
Anxiety	Do you feel anxious or fearful?	GAI GAI-SF	5 1-2
Grief	Have you lost someone you love?	TRIG ICG-R	10 5-10

Note. GAI, The geriatric anxiety inventory; GAI-SF, The GAI short Form; ICG-R, The inventory of complicated grief-revised; and TRIG, The Texas revised inventory of grief.

表 4-7　心理状态的评估

项目	访谈问题	评估工具	测试时间 /min
抑郁	您感到悲伤或抑郁吗？ 您是否感觉对以往喜欢的事不再感兴趣？	GDS-15 GDS-4	5 1~2
焦虑	您感到焦虑或恐惧吗？	GAI GAI-SF	5 1~2
悲痛	您有没有亲人去世？	TRIG ICG-R	10 5~10

注：GAI，老年人焦虑量表；GAI-SF，GAI 简短格式；ICG-R，修订后的悲痛清单；和 TRIG，德州修订的悲痛清单。

i. Depression

Although the elderly people often do not report feeling depressed, a simple question, "Do you often feel sad or depressed?" still screens depression effectively with 0.71 and 0.77 positive and negative predictive values, respectively. The geriatric depression scale (GDS) with 15, 10, and 4 yes/no questions can be administered by the clinician or filled out by an elderly person. GDS-15 score ≥ 4 has 92.7% sensitivity and 65.2% specificity, GDS-10 score ≥ 4 has 80.5% sensitivity and 78.3% specificity, and GDS-4 score ≥ 2 shows 80.5% sensitivity and 78.3% specificity.

ii. Anxiety

Anxiety can be screened using "Do you feel anxious or fearful?" The geriatric anxiety inventory (GAI), or GAI short form (GAI-SF). The GAI consists of 20 agree/

（一）抑郁

询问是否感到抑郁仍是很有效的筛查抑郁症的方法。有 4、10 或 15 个条目的老年抑郁量表（GDS-4、GDS-10、GDS-15）也可以很敏感地筛查出抑郁症。

（二）焦虑

老年焦虑量表（GAI）及其简化版（GAI-SF）都可以有效地评估焦虑。GAI 包含 20 个问题，总分为 0～20。得分 <11 表示焦虑。GAI-

disagree questions based on self-report or interview with a total score 0-20. A score < 11 indicates anxiety with 84% sensitivity and 75% specificity. The GAI-SF includes only five items and a score ≥ 3 indicates anxiety with 75% sensitivity and 87% specificity.

iii. Grief

Grief is assessed by asking the elderly people if they have lost someone or something they love, the Texas revised inventory of grief (TRIG), and the inventory of complicated grief-revised (ICG-R). The TRIG has two sections: TRIG-past and TRIG-present. TRIG-Past includes eight items to assess the actions and feelings at the time of losing a loved one and the ability to maintain daily living tasks following the loss of a loved one. TRIG-present consists of 13 items to evaluate emotional feelings about the death of the loved one at present. Each item is rated as: 1 (completely true) to 5 (completely false). Higher sum scores for TRIG-present and TRIG-past indicate less grief. Low sum scores on both sections suggest prolonged grief. The ICG-R assesses a distinct cluster of grief symptoms that predicts long-term dysfunction and disabling health conditions if not treated appropriately. It includes 19 items (each rated on a 4-point Likert scale). A sum score > 25 indicates significant impairment in social, mental, physical, general health, and functioning.

Box 4-5　Case Study

Previously, we found Mrs. Liu having some memory issues that caused her to reduce social contacts and stop a longtime knitting hobby. Cognitive assessment further revealed that Mrs. Liu has trouble remembering recent events and keeping track of conversation threads. She is not worried: "It's all part of getting old. I'm 78 years old. What can you expect?!" The daughter relayed an argument with mom a few days ago because she donated some of dad's things. They had agreed to it, but mom got furious and denied agreeing to it. Mrs. Liu scored 22 on MMSE and drew wrong time on CDT.

Questions:

1. What mood disorder (s) is Mrs. Liu at risk for?

2. How would you assess Mrs. Liu's psychological status?

3. What interventions will be appropriate for Mrs. Liu?

SF 仅包含五个项目，得分 ≥ 3 表示焦虑，敏感性为 75%，特异性为 87%。

（三）悲痛

得克萨斯悲痛量表修订版（TRIG）和复杂悲痛量表修订版（ICG-R）均可以用来评估悲痛。得克萨斯悲痛量表修订版强调对过去和现在悲痛的检测，TRIG-past 包括八个项目，用于评估失去亲人时的行为和感受，以及失去亲人后维持日常生活的能力。目前，TRIG-present 包含 13 个项目，用于评估有关亲人死亡的情感感受。每个项目的等级为：1（完全正确）至 5（完全错误）。TRIG-present 和 TRIG-past 的总分越高，表示悲痛越少。而复杂悲痛量表则主要测量持续存在的病理性悲痛。它包括 19 个项目，总分 > 25 表示社交，精神，身体，总体健康和功能严重受损。

Box 4-5　案例

前面介绍过刘女士不记得花样也不再编织。她记不清近期事件，记不住聊天主题，但觉得这是老化的必然结果。女儿说几天前和妈妈因为捐爸爸遗物吵了一次，妈妈说她从来没同意捐。她的 MMSE 22 分，CDT 的时钟画错了。

问题：

1. 这个案例易感哪些情绪障碍？

2. 你如何选择评估心理状态的方法和量表？

3. 你该怎样根据评估结果来决定心理状态的干预重点？

Section 7　Social Status

I. Definition and Domains of Social Status

Social status refers to a person's standing and relationships within a society. It goes beyond social history on birthplace, residences, educational attainment, employment history, habits, hobbies, smoking, alcohol, and recreational drug use. Social status has six domains: social support, elder mistreatment, decisional capacity and competency, advance directives, financial situation, and spirituality (Figure 4-4).

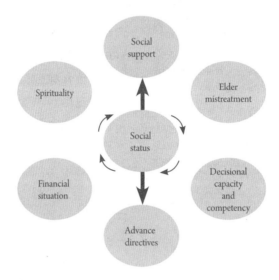

Figure 4-4　Domains of social status

i. Social Support

Social support describes the availability of family and friends who can provide personal support and assistance. The availability and quality of social support needs to be determined as it often determines if the elderly people will continue to live at home or be placed in nursing homes.

ii. Elder Mistreatment

Elder mistreatment is a broad term defining a variety of activities imposed on the elderly people by others, and includes elder abuse (physical, verbal, or both) and neglect (intentional or unintentional). The perpetrators are most often family members and caregivers. Elder mistreatment can occur in any settings, e. g. , home, nursing homes, hospitals, and adult day care services.

第七节　老年人社会状态的评估

一、社会状态的概念和范畴

社会状态指老年人在家庭、社区和社会中所处的位置和其社会关系。除了收集传统临床诊断包括的教育水平、工作经历、习惯、嗜好、烟、酒及娱乐和用药等信息外，老年人的社会状态评估强调6个范畴：社会支持、虐待、决策力和决策胜任力、委托、经济状况、精神信仰（图4-4）。

（一）社会支持

社会支持是指当老年人需要帮助时，是否有或有多少人可以提供帮助和护理服务。社会支持网络的质量往往决定一个老年人能不能继续安全地住在家里。

（二）虐待

广义上，老年人虐待指由他人强加于老年人的各种伤害性行为，如口头指责和身体惩罚等。家人和护理人员是虐待老年人的主要群体。虐待可以在任何场合发生。

iii. Decisional Capacity And Competency

Decisional capacity determines decisional competency. Decisional capacity refers to the ability to carry out a plan, whereas decisional competency is a legal term which portrays a judge's ruling about whether an individual is qualified and capable of making own decisions. Five elements are involved in decisional capacity: understanding, appreciation, reasoning, expressing a choice, and consistency of decisions.

(1) Understanding occurs when an elderly person demonstrates the ability to comprehend what is being communicated verbally or by writing, retain the communicated information long enough to recall it in discussions, and perceive the relationships between solutions and results.

(2) Appreciation is defined as the ability to recognize how the communicated information is related to one's own situations and to describe the advantages and disadvantages of a possible solution.

(3) Reasoning is demonstrated when an elderly person can manipulate information by comparing different alternatives and resultant outcomes, and provide rationales for making these comparisons.

(4) Expressing a choice describes the articulation of a clear choice to a decision.

(5) Consistency of the decision evaluates an elderly person's past decisions about similar issues.

Therefore, decisional capacity relies on language, short-term memory, and executive functioning, and is task specific, that is, incapacity to make decisions in one task does not mean incapacity to make decisions in another task. Clinically, decisional capacity is often triggered by three tasks: medical decisions, problems of self-care, and problems of finances. Medical decisions refer to the right to be informed before consenting to medical treatments, refuse medical treatment, and decide own health care.

iv. Advance Directives

Advance directives are legal documents which, when signed by the elderly people of sound mind, provide guidance about health care goals, preferences, and decisions in the event that they can no longer make such decisions. Advance directives include living will (describing overall health care goals and preferences) or durable power of attorney for health affairs (designated surrogate decision-maker for health care).

（三）决策力和决策胜任力

决策力决定决策胜任力。决策力指一个人是否有做决定的能力，而决策胜任力是法律术语，指法官决定的一个人是否有资格和能力自己做决定。决策力包括五个要素：理解、欣赏、推理、表达选择和决策的一致性。

（1）当老年人表现出理解口头或书面交流内容的能力，在讨论中保留足够长的时间来回忆交流信息，并感知解决方案和结果之间的关系时，理解就发生了。

（2）鉴赏力的定义是识别所传达的信息如何与自己的情况相关，并描述可能的解决方案的优缺点的能力。

（3）当老年人可以通过比较不同的选择和结果来操纵信息时，推理就得到了证明，并为进行这些比较提供了理论依据。

（4）表达一个选择，即描述一个明确的选择对一个决定的表达。

（5）决策的一致性，即评估老年人过去关于类似问题的决策。

因此，决策力依赖于语言、短时记忆和执行功能，并且是任务特定的，即不能在一项任务中做出决定并不意味着不能在另一项任务中做出决定。临床上，决策力通常由三项任务触发：医疗决策、自我照顾问题和财务问题。医疗决定是指在同意接受医疗、拒绝接受医疗、决定自己的医疗保健之前的知情权。

（四）委托

委托指由具有决策胜任力的老年人正式签署的、具有法律效力的生前预嘱和持久性的健康委托书。当老年人在失去决策胜任力时，它可以帮助医护人员决定如何提供其所需的医护服务。老年人也可以用持久性的健康委托书提前指定其医疗决策的代理人。

v. Financial Situation

The purpose of assessing the financial situation of the elderly people is to identify potential barriers to treatment compliance and possible governmental and nonprofit resources available to the elderly people. Understanding the elderly people's financial situation can help to initiate discussions and develop plans for meeting personal health care needs, especially for those with functional limitations.

vi. Spirituality

Spirituality identifies a person's belief system and is a process of making sense of self and the world from the social science perspectives. Spirituality is not synonymous with religion. It is more than religion and does not rely on a formal or informal religious affiliation. It is increasingly recognized that spirituality plays a role in disease risk, treatment responses, and mortality.

II. Assessment of Social Status

Social status can be assessed through interview questions or assessment tools. Table 4-8 describes the common interview questions, assessment tools, and their administration time.

（五）经济状况

经济状况指老年人的资产和各种医疗保险。询问经济状况的主要目的是帮助老年人申请使用社会资源，辅助决定诊断和治疗方案。

（六）精神信仰

精神信仰泛指一个人的信仰。精神信仰并不局限于宗教信仰，它对疾病的治疗和愈后有很大作用。

二、社会状态的评估

社会地位可以通过面试问题或评估工具进行评估。表 4-8 描述了常见的面试问题、评估工具及其评估时间。

Table 4-8　Interview Questions and Assessment Tools for Social Status

Domain	Interview questions	Assessment tools	Test time/min
Social support	"Do you live alone? " "Do you have a caregiver? " "Are you a caregiver? "		0. 5
Elder mistreatment	"Do you ever feel unsafe where you live? " "Has anyone ever threatened or hurt you? " "Has anyone been taking your money without your permission? "	H-S/EAST	3
Decisional capacity and competence	"Do you have trouble making decisions? " "Has anyone told you that you are not qualified to make your own decisions? "	EXIT-25 ≥ MMSE ≤ 10 MacCAT-T	15 5-10
Advanced directives	Explaining what advanced directives are before asking "Would you like more information about advanced directives? "	Living Will; Durable Power of Attorney for Health Affairs	Situation dependent
Financial situation	"Do you have health insurance or money to pay for your medical treatments, medications, or services? "		
Spirituality	"Is region or spirituality important to you and your health care? "	FICA Spiritual Assessment	15

Note. EXIT-25, the executive interview – 25; FICA, faith, belief, and meaning, importance and influence, community, and address/action in care; H-S/EAST, the Hwalek-Sengstock elder abuse screening test; MacCAT-T, the MacArthur competence assessment tool-treatment; and MMSE, the mini-mental state examination.

表 4-8　社会状态的评估

项目	访谈问题	评估工具	测试时间 /min
社会支持	"您是一个人居住吗？" "有没有人照顾您？" "家里有人需要您照顾吗？"		0.5
老年人虐待	"在您居住的地方，您有没有感觉到不安全？" "有没有人威胁或伤害过您？" "有没有人没有经过您的允许拿走您的钱？"	H-S/EAST	3
决策力和决策胜任力	"您在做决定上有困难吗？" "有没有觉得您不能够独自做决定？"	EXIT-25 ≥ MMSE ≤ 10 MacCAT-T	15 5~10
委托	提问前解释委托的含义 "关于委托，你希望得到更多信息吗？"	生前预嘱 持久性的健康委 托书	动态持续
经济状况	"您有医疗保险吗，是什么类型？"		
精神信仰	"您认为宗教或精神信仰对您的医疗保健重要吗？"	FICA 精神信仰评 估量表	15

注：EXIT-25，执行功能测试 -25；FICA，信仰、信念和意义、重要性和影响、社区和护理中的地址 / 行动；H-S/EAST，Hwalek Sengstock 老年虐待筛查测试；MacCAT-T，麦克阿瑟能力评估工具治疗；MMSE，简易智能状态检测量表。

i. Social Support

Emergency contact and social support network should be documented for the elderly people, even those who appear fully functional and independent. If assistance is needed, then the types of assistance needed and the quality of social support are to be evaluated. Gaps in care can be filled by home-care or community-based services. This is particularly important for frail the elderly people and those who lack social support.

ii. Elder Mistreatment

Cultural values might make the elderly people feel shameful or guilty to report abuse by their own children. A sensitive and non-judgmental approach is particularly important in screening elder mistreatment using the Hwalek-Sengstock elder abuse screening test (H-S/EAST) based on self-report. Although the original H-S/EAST has 15 items, studies have shown that a set of six questions is as effective as the 15-item test:

● Has anyone close to you tried to hurt or harm you recently?

● Do you feel uncomfortable with anyone in your family?

● Does anyone tell you that you give them too much trouble?

（一）社会支持

即便是完全可以独立自主的老年人，其紧急联系人及联系方式也必须记录在案。对需要帮助的老人，则需进一步评估具体需要哪方面的照顾，由谁提供照顾，有哪些社区服务资源。这点对独孤或空巢老人尤为重要。

（二）虐待

文化价值观可能会使老年人因举报受到自己的孩子虐待而感到羞耻或内疚。老人虐待筛查量表（H-S/EAST）可以筛查老年人虐待情况。老人虐待筛查量表包括 15 个条目和 6 个条目两个版本。适合文化、敏感和非批判的态度是让老年人承认被虐待的关键。尽管原始的 H-S / EAST 有 15 个项目，但研究表明，六个问题与 15 个项目的测试一样有效：

● 最近有没有人靠近你试图伤害过您?

● 您是否对家人感到不舒服?

● 有人告诉您，您给他们带来太多麻烦吗?

- Has anyone forced you to do things that you did not want to do?

- Do you feel that nobody wants you around?

- Who makes decisions about your life... like how you should live or where you should live?

iii. Decisional Capacity and Competency

Decisional capacity can be determined in three ways: formal neuropsychological testing of short-term memory, language, and executive function, observation of an elderly person's decision-making process, and the integration of the two:

(1) Assessment tools related to decisional capacity include the EXIT-25 and MMSE covered in Section 5 Cognitive Function based on the premise that diminished cognitive function likely diminishes decision-making capacity. To this end, EXIT-25 score $\geqslant 15$ and MMSE score $\leqslant 10$ suggest severe cognitive impairment and inability to make decisions.

(2) Observation of the decision-making process can be done using the MacArthur competence assessment tool -treatment (MacCAT-T) by evaluating the ability to make a specific medical decision using semi-structured interview in 10-15 minutes. After reviewing an elderly person's medical history, the clinician first discloses the nature of a condition, recommends treatment, explains the benefits and risks of the treatment, and describes alternative treatments and their associated benefits and risks. Afterward, the older adult is asked to make a treatment choice and explain how he/she made the choice. The clinician will ask questions to assess how well the older adult understand, appreciate, and reason about the disclosed information and to express a clear choice. The consistency of the choice is not assessed by the MacCAT. The MacCAT-T does not produce a sum score, but rates the older adult's responses as 2 (adequate), 1 (partial), or 1 (inadequate) to derive a summary score for understanding (0-6), appreciation (0-4), reasoning (0-8), and expressing a choice (0-2). The scores must be interpreted within clinical and other contexts.

(3) Combining (1) and (2) could be particularly useful for the elderly people with mild cognitive impairment (MMSE scores 11-23 and/or EXIT-25 score of < 15). The MacCAT-T will help assess decisional capacity in this population.

Temporary decisional incapacity can occur as a result of an acute medical condition such as stroke. Decisional capacity should be re-evaluated when the life-

- 是否有人强迫您去做不想做的事情？

- 您是否觉得没有人想要您在附近？

- 谁来决定您的生活……例如您应该如何生活或应该在哪里生活？

（三）决策力和决策胜任力

决策力可以通过三种方式来确定：对短期记忆、语言和执行功能进行正式的神经心理学测试，观察老年人的决策过程，以及两者的结合：

（1）与决策力相关的评估工具包括第5节认知功能中的执行功能测试–25（EXIT–25）和简易智能状态检测量表（MMSE）。前提是认知功能减弱可能会降低决策力。因此，EXIT–25得分≥15，MMSE得分≤10表明老年人没有决策力。

（2）决策过程的观察可以使用麦克阿瑟决策能力评估工具（治疗版）（MacCAT–T），通过在10～15分钟内使用半结构式访谈评估做出特定医疗决策的能力来完成。在回顾了一位老年人的病史之后，临床医生首先披露了病情的性质，推荐治疗，解释治疗的好处和风险，并描述替代治疗及其相关的好处和风险。之后，老年人被要求做出治疗选择，并解释他/她是如何做出选择的。临床医生将提出问题，以评估老年人对所披露信息的理解、欣赏和推理程度，并表达明确的选择。MacCAT不评估选择的一致性。MacCAT–T不产生总分，但将老年人的回答分为2（充分）、1（部分）或1（不充分），得出理解（0–6）、欣赏（0–4）、推理（0–8）和表达选择（0–2）的总分。分数必须在临床和其他情况下解释。

（3）结合（1）和（2）可能对轻度认知障碍的老年人特别有用（MMSE评分在11～23分和/或执行功能测试–25评分＜15分）。MacCAT–T将有助于评估这一人群的决策能力。

卒中等急性病可导致决策力暂时丧失。当危及生命的情况已经过去或损害范围已经

threatening circumstances have passed or the extenivt of damages becomes clear.

iv. Advance Directives

Advance directives rest upon intact decisional capacity to deal with hypothetical situations. Therefore, advance directives should be discussed as early as possible instead of at the time of need. The elderly people with even severe cognitive impairment could still make their medical preferences and wishes known. Living will document references for care such as medical resuscitation, mechanical ventilation, artificial nutrition, and end of life, and durable power of attorney for health affairs allows the elderly people to designate a surrogate decision-maker for health care if they can no longer do so. Both documents should be signed with copies included in medical records, and re-visited regularly and when better prognostic information becomes available. Signed documents should not be interpreted as "set in stone."

v. Financial Situation

The purpose of assessing financial situation is to ensure the feasibility of care plan and mobilize health resources. There is a fine line between clinical use and one's own curiosity about the elderly people's financial means. Only ask questions that will help optimize the care for the elderly people.

vi. Spirituality

The FICA spiritual assessment screens spirituality using a series of questions:

Faith, belief, and meaning: "Do you consider yourself spiritual or religious?" "Do you have spiritual beliefs that can help you cope with stress?" For the elderly people who answer "no", another question can be asked "What gives your life meaning?"

Importance and influence: "What importance does your faith and belief have in your life?" "Have your beliefs influenced you in how you handle stress?" "Do you have specific beliefs that might influence your health care decisions?"

Community: "Are you a part of a spiritual or religious community?" "Is this of support to you and how?" "Is there a group of people you really love or who are important to you?"

Address/Action in care: "How should the health care provider address these issues in your health care?"

明确时，应重新评估决策能力。

（四）委托

具有决策胜任力是签署委托的前提条件，所以必须尽早决定，而不是等出现需要时再做决定。通过生前预嘱，老年人可以表达对未来可能需要的治疗方法的意愿，如心肺复苏、呼吸机、人工营养、临终关怀。通过签订持久性的健康委托书，老年人可以指定其医护服务决策的代理人。需要强调的是生前预嘱和持久性的健康委托书并不是不可改变的，它们是一个动态变化的过程，需要定期回顾、探讨。

（五）经济状况

评估经济状况的目的是有效地利用社会资源来满足老年人的医疗保健需求，所问问题应该集中在这个方面。

（六）精神信仰

精神信仰对疾病的治疗和愈后有很大作用。FICA 精神信仰评估量表列举了一系列问题用以帮助医护人员对老年人的精神信仰进行评估：

信仰、信念和意义："你认为自己是个有精神或宗教信仰的人吗？""有什么精神信念可以帮你应对压力？"如果回答没有，"什么情况赋予你生活意义？"

重要性和影响力："信仰或信念对你来说有多重要？""信念怎样影响你应对压力？""有什么特别的信念会影响到你对医疗保健计划的决定？"

社区："你属于某个信仰或宗教团体吗？""这个团体对你提供什么样的支持？""你有没有特别爱的人或者说谁对你来说很重要？"

护理中的解决办法 / 行动："卫生保健提供者应如何在您的卫生保健中解决这些问题？"

Spiritual communities could serve as strong social support systems for some elderly people. Referral to or involvement of spiritual leaders could also provide valuable support to the elderly people and their families in making health care decisions conformant to their belief system.

Box 4-6　Case Study

Mrs. Liu denied depression, anxiety, and grief. She scored 24 on TRIG-past, 26 on TRIG-present, and 11 on GDS-15. She is a lifelong housewife and is financially supported by her children. There have never been any discussions about advance directives. The daughter once brought up Living Will, but mom got really mad feeling it was bad luck to talk about death. Mrs. Liu has 3 children who all live remotely with her oldest daughter closest (8-hour train ride away). All children are involved in mom's life and decision-making, and they try to visit her regularly in different times of the year.

Questions:

1. What components of social status will you assess?

2. How would you assess Mrs. Liu's social status?

3. What interventions are appropriate to improve Mrs. Liu's social status?

Section 8　Health Care Goals, Values, and Preferences

I. Definitions of Health Care Goals, Values, and Preferences

Health care goals are defined as the perception of the aims or desired outcomes of health care. Values are the judgment of what is important is health care and life. Preferences refer to the expression of desirability or selection of one course of health care actions and outcomes in contrast to other courses. Preferences are built on a person's health care goals and values. Eliciting preferences is foundational to evidence-based practice and patient-centered care (figure 4-5).

某些信仰社区可能是某些老年人的重要社会支持。及时让信仰团体参与医疗保健计划的制订和实施可以为老年人及其家人提供有价值的服务和帮助临床决策。

Box 4-6　案例

刘女士否认有任何情绪障碍。她的 TRIG-past 24 分，TRIG-present 26 分，GDS-15 11 分。她是家庭主妇，有三个孝顺孩子，孩子们给妈妈提供经济帮助并探讨解决妈妈的各种需要。妈妈拒绝谈论遗嘱。她女儿有一次提到生前预嘱话题，刘女士非常生气，她认为谈论死亡是非常不吉利的事。刘女士的三个孩子都住的很远，离她最近的大女儿也有 8 小时的火车车程。所有孩子都参与妈妈的生活问题决策，她们每年都有规律地在不同时间探望妈妈。

问题：

1. 这个案例社会状态的评估重点是什么？

2. 你如何评价刘太太的社会地位？

3. 你如何根据评估结果来决定社会状态的干预重点？

第八节　老年人医疗保健目标、价值观和意愿的评估

一、医疗保健目标、价值观和意愿的概念

医疗保健目标指老年人对医疗保健服务渴望达到的结果。价值观是指老年人对医疗保健各类服务的评价和看法，由老年人决定哪些医疗保健和生命的方面更为重要。意愿指在有多个选择时，老年人自己所偏向的选择。医疗保健目标和价值观直接影响意愿。医疗保健目标、价值观和意愿是循证实践的基石（图 4-5）。

II. Steps for Eliciting Health Care Goals, Values, and Preferences

Eliciting health care goals, values, and preferences is required of all health care decisions, and are typically obtained through interviews during initial clinical encounter and periodically over time. The extent and depth of assessment will depend on each person's unique context, and follows three steps in sequence (figure 4-5).

二、医疗保健目标、价值观和意愿的评估

了解老年人的医疗保健目标、价值观和意愿需要 3 个步骤：识别意愿敏感情况、充分剖析不同治疗保健方案的利弊、咨询老年人意愿（图 4-5）。

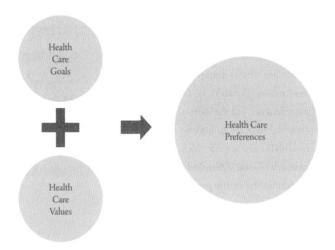

Figure 4-5. Foundations of patient-centered care

i. Recognize a Preference-sensitive Situation

Clinicians need to recognize a preference-sensitive situation that refers to the situation when multiple options are available or a difficult decision-making event occurs. Examples of preference-sensitive situations include, but are not limited to:

1. More than one reasonable treatment options, e. g., drug therapy plus lifestyle modification versus surgery.

2. Different treatment outcomes, e. g., treatment A (aggressive chemotherapy) prolongs life, but has unpleasant side effects, while treatment B (palliative care) enhances quality of life, but doesn't prolong life.

3. Treatments with uncertain benefits, e. g., experimental drugs / devices / procedures.

4. Significant change in an elderly person's condition, e. g., relocation to a nursing home, death of a family member, exacerbation of a chronic condition, or decline in physical function.

（一）识别意愿敏感情况

临床医生需要认识到一个偏好敏感的情况，指的是当多种选择可用或困难的决策事件发生的情况。偏好敏感情况的示例包括但不限于：

1. 不止一种合理的治疗方案，例如药物治疗加上生活方式改变与手术。

2. 不同的治疗结果，如一种治疗方案（积极化疗）延长生命，但有不愉快的副作用，而另一种治疗方案（姑息治疗）提高生活质量，但不能延长生命。

3. 疗效不确定的治疗，例如实验药物 / 设备 / 程序。

4. 老年人的状况发生重大变化，如迁往养老院、家人去世、慢性病恶化或身体功能下降。

ii. . Adequately Inform the Elderly People and Their Families

Once recognizing a preference-sensitive situation, clinicians must adequately inform the elderly people and their families of expected benefits and risks of different care options. The keyword here is "adequately inform", which means that clinicians need to present all care options, their respective benefits (e. g. , prevent, slow, or cure a condition), risks (e. g. , side effects and their likelihood of occurrence), feasibility (e. g. , time commitment and costs), and health care outcomes (e. g. , extended survival or function improvement). For example, donepezil is the first-line treatment for Alzheimer's disease. Clinicians consider the benefits of donepezil (reducing cognitive decline) outweighs risks (side effects of nausea and dizziness tolerable), but the elderly people might consider nausea and dizziness significantly interfere with their function and ability to enjoy life since donepezil will not cure Alzheimer's disease. Adequately informing is particularly important for the elderly people with multimorbidity because treatments for one disease could worsen other disease(s) and/or predispose them to geriatric syndromes. A decision-tree approach could be used to outline the details of each treatment option (time and effort, benefits, risks, outcomes) for easy comparison. While adequately informing might appear arduous, its significance cannot be over-emphasized.

iii. Elicit Preference after Adequate Informing

After adequately informing, clinicians can elicit the elderly people's health care goals, values, and preferences to guide care decisions. Table 4-9 illustrates steps for eliciting health care goals, values, and preferences. Nonetheless, clinicians need to be aware of three pitfalls. First, the health care goals, values, and preferences are not equivalent to health care decisions. Clinicians honor and support the elderly people's health care goals, values, and preferences to the extent possible, but need to make clinical decisions based on their own expertise and sound rationales. Second, health care goals, values, and preferences change over time and are fluid. For instance, preferences might change from "doing everything you can to keep me alive" at initial cancer diagnosis to "just making me comfortable and pain-free" after a couple bouts of chemotherapy. Hence, health care goals, values, and preferences need to be re-evaluated when the elderly people's conditions change. Last, respecting and considering health care goals, values, and preferences do not mean that the elderly people can demand any treatments without a reasonable expectation of benefits.

（二）充分剖析不同治疗保健方案的利弊

在这一步，医护人员要为老年人及其家属充分剖析不同治疗保健方案的利弊，包括用法（剂量、使用频率、途径、使用方法等）、好处（预防、减缓，还是治愈疾病）、副作用（出现副作用的可能性、对老年人的影响）、可行性（疗程、费用）和期待的结果（延长寿命、提高功能）。比如多奈哌齐不能延缓、治愈阿尔茨海默病，但可以短期缓解认知障碍，50% 以上的老年人会有恶心、头晕等副作用。医护人员认为此药利大于弊，但老年人认为头晕会严重影响他／她的生活质量，且多奈哌齐不能治愈阿尔茨海默病，弊大于利。充分剖析不同治疗保健方案的利弊对有共患疾病的老年人尤为重要。

（三）咨询老年人意愿

确认老年人已充分了解各种治疗方案的利弊之后，才能让其表达意愿。医疗保健决定都应该以意愿为准，但是意愿并不代表医疗决策。表 4-9 说明了医疗保健目标、价值观和意愿的评估步骤。此外，医疗保健的目标、价值观和意愿是随环境而变化的，尤其是当患者对疾病、治疗的认识逐步加深之后。最后，最大限度地满足患者的意愿不等于患者可以无理地要求尝试任何治疗措施。

Table 4-9　Steps for Eliciting Health Care Goals, Values, and Preferences

Step	Focus
1	Recognize a preference-sensitive situation
2	Adequately inform the elderly people and families
3	Elicit preference after adequate informing

Note. The duration of time needed to complete each step is highly variable depending on the complexity and extent of the situation.

表 4-9　医疗保健目标、价值观和意愿的评估步骤

步骤	侧重点
1	识别意愿敏感情况
2	充分剖析不同治疗保健方案的利弊
3	咨询老年人意愿

注：完成每个步骤所需的时间长短取决于情况的复杂性和程度。

III. Importance of Health Care Goals, Values, and Preferences

Thanks to an exponentially growing body of research, evidence-based practice is increasingly adopted in health care practice worldwide. An important cornerstone for evidence-based practice is patients' health care goals, values, and preferences. It is not uncommon that even the strongest evidence such as systematic reviews and meta-analyses do not yet incorporate health care goals, values, and preferences of the elderly people into their recommendations. Hence, it is vitally important for clinicians to intentionally integrate health care goals, values, and preferences into care plans in the context of the elderly people's unique contexts (medical conditions, geriatric syndromes, functional status, cognitive function, psychological status, social status, genetic disposition, environment, and lifestyle).

Except for those with a cognition-altering condition such as advanced Alzheimer's disease and dementia, the elderly people are fully able to evaluate the feasibility and impact of different health care choices. They are capable of taking into consideration of their pertinent clinical, personal, and cultural contexts about health and health care, and articulate their goals, values, and preferences for care. The best practice, thus, considers the elderly people's health care goals, values, and preferences in all clinical decisions.

三、医疗保健目标、价值观和意愿的评估

老年人越来越多地参与到临床科研中，指数递增的科研成果使循证实践在老年医疗保健领域得到日益广泛地应用。尽管医疗保健目标、价值观和意愿是循证实践的重要基础，系统分析、综述和临床指南这些最有力的科研证据很少考虑到老年人的医疗保健目标、价值观和意愿。这个问题在有共患疾病的老年人中尤为突出。

除有认知功能障碍的老年人外，老年人享有充分的临床决策力。他们可以综合、全面、深入地比较权衡各种诊断治疗方案的利弊，表达自己的医疗保健目标、价值观和意愿，做出适合自己身体、家庭等各方面情况的决定。因而，所有医疗保健决策都应老年人以意愿为准。

Box 4-7　Case Study

Mrs. Liu completed schooling and was married at 18 years old. She has lived in her neighborhood for >20 years and knows her neighbors. Her husband died 1.5 years ago. She lost her sister-in-law, a close friend who lived in the same city, 2 months ago due to brain infarct, which is a main reason for her daughter's visit. Mrs. Liu cared for her sister-in-law in the last 6 months of her life, but her sister-in-law did not recognize her and was in a lot of pain.

Questions:

1. What are some potentially preference-sensitive situations?

2. How do you explain to Mrs. Liu and her daughter the importance for Mrs. Liu to articulate her health care goals, values, and preferences?

3. How will you assess Mrs. Liu's health care goals, values, and preferences?

Section 9　Genes, Environment, and Lifestyle

I. Definitions of Genes, Environment, and Lifestyle

Genes refer to loci or regions of DNA and are the molecular units of heredity. Environment is the physical and cultural settings that an individual lives in. Lifestyle is defined as the way an individual life. Genes, by themselves and via interactions with environment and lifestyle, influence most biological traits, disease susceptibility, and treatment responses. Figure 4-6 depicts the interaction of genes, environment, and lifestyle.

II. Assessment of Genes, Environment, and Lifestyle

Genes are analyzed in laboratories using genetic, molecular, and cellular techniques. Genetic analyses are beyond the scope of this chapter.

Environmental assessment includes two components: safety of home environment and accessibility

---

Box 4-7　案例

刘女士完成义务教育，18 岁结婚，在现在的社区生活了 20 多年。丈夫 1 年半前去世。她的小姑子兼好朋友 2 个月前因脑梗过世，她一直照顾小姑子，但后来她小姑子每天都和疼痛做斗争，而且后来几个月都不认识刘女士。

问题：

1. 你可以举出几个潜在的意愿敏感的情况吗？

2. 你如何解释医疗保健意愿、价值观和偏好在医疗保健中的重要性？

3. 你怎样来评估刘女士的医疗保健意愿、价值观和喜好？

第九节　老年人基因、环境和生活方式的评估

一、基因、环境和生活方式的概念

基因是指 DNA（脱氧核糖核酸）分子上具有遗传信息的特定核苷酸序列；环境指老年人生活中自然、人为和文化因素的总称；生活方式指衣、食、住、行、休息、娱乐等物质生活和精神生活的价值观、道德观和取向。基因本身及其与环境、生活方式的协同作用决定一个人对疾病的易感性和治疗效果。图 4-6 描述了基因、环境和生活方式的相互作用。

二、基因、环境和生活方式的评估

基因是在实验室里利用遗传、分子和细胞技术进行分析的。遗传分析超出了本章的范围。

环境评估包括两个组成部分：家庭环境安全和所需服务的可及性。理想情况下，跨

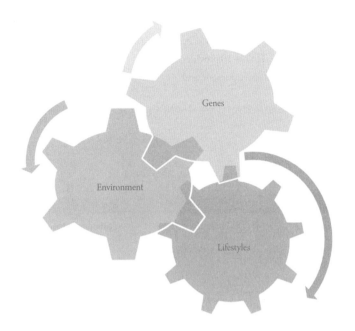

Figure 4-6　Foundations of precision medicine

to needed services. Ideally, at least one member of the interdisciplinary team should visit the elderly people's residence to perform a home-safety inspection. Even a single visit could yield invaluable health information. If home visit is not feasible, the elderly people can be asked to complete a home-safety checklist:

(1) Are there handrails on both sides of the stairs and steps?

(2) Are there a lot of lights at the top and bottom of the stairs?

(3) Are there small rugs scattered around the house that can easily trip a person?

(4) Are the stairs clean all the time?

(5) Are there nightlights in the bedroom, hall, and bathroom?

(6) Is there a non-slip mat in the tub or shower?

(7) Does the tub or shower have a non-skid bottom?

(8) Are there grab bars in the tub or shower?

(9) Are any spills wiped up as soon as they happen?

Accessibility to needed services evaluates the adequacy of access to personal and health care services by assessing the needs, readiness for outside assistance or services, and availability of services.

Lifestyle has seven components: nutrition, exercise, sleep, stress management, sun exposure, social contact, and enjoyment. For each component, ask detailed questions using the 5 Ws: what, when, where, why and

学科团队中至少有一名成员应该访问老年人的住所，进行家庭安全检查。哪怕是一次访问也能产生宝贵的健康信息。如果进行家访不可行，可以要求老年人填写一份家庭安全检查表：

（1）楼梯和台阶两边都有扶手吗？

（2）楼梯的顶部和底部有很多灯吗？

（3）房子周围是否有容易绊倒人的小地毯？

（4）楼梯一直干净吗？

（5）卧室、大厅和浴室里有夜灯吗？

（6）浴缸或淋浴间有防滑垫吗？

（7）浴缸或淋浴有防滑的底部吗？

（8）浴缸或淋浴间里有扶手吗？

（9）一旦发生泄漏，是否立即清除？

所需服务的可及性通过评估需求、外部援助或服务的准备情况以及服务的可用性来评估获得个人和保健服务的充分性。

生活方式有七个组成部分：营养、锻炼、睡眠、压力管理、阳光照射、社交和享受。对于每个部分，使用5个W问详细的问题：

how to identify any problems. For example, what exercise do you do? When do you do it? Where do you do it? Why do you do it? And how do you do it? Table 4-10 provides a summary of the assessment of genes, environment, and lifestyle.

什么、何时、何地、为什么以及如何识别任何问题。例如，你做什么运动？你什么时候做？你在哪里做的？你为什么这么做？你是怎么做到的？表 4-10 总结了对基因、环境和生活方式的评估方法。基因的分析主要由实验室完成。

Table 4-10　Assessment of Genes, Environment, and Lifestyle

Domain	Assessment Method
Genes	Laboratory-based tests
Environment	
Safety of home environment	Home visit
Accessibility to needed services	Questionnaire or interview
Lifestyle	
Nutrition, exercise, sleep, stress management, sun exposure, social contact, and enjoyment	5 W questionnaire or interview

Note. 5 Ws include what, when, where, why, and how.

表 4-10　基因，环境和生活方式的评估

项目	评估方法
基因	实验室检测
环境	
家居环境安全	家庭访视
服务需求的可获得性	问卷调查或访谈
生活方式	
营养、运动、睡眠、压力管理、晒太阳、社交、娱乐活动	5 W 问卷或访谈

注：5W 是指 what, when, where, why and how。

III. Importance of Genes Environment, and Lifestyle

Genes, environment, and lifestyle play important roles in the development and evolvement of precision medicine. Precision medicine is a medical model that proposes to customize medical care by tailoring health care decisions, practices, and/or products to each individual patient. Precision medicine came into existence because of the lack of effective means to prevent or treat many diseases and the tremendous variability among individual genetic makeup, environment, and lifestyle. Under this model, diagnostic testing of a patient's genetic and other molecular and cellular contents is analyzed to aid the selection of appropriate and optimal therapies. Precision medicine does not mean that drugs or medical devices that are unique to a patient will be created. Instead, it classifies individuals into groups that differ in disease susceptibility,

三、基因、环境和生活方式的重要性

基因、环境和生活方式对精确医学的发展和演变起着重要作用。精准医疗是一种医疗模式，它通过为每位患者量身定制医疗决策、实践和／或产品来定制医疗服务。精确医学的出现是由于缺乏有效的手段来预防或治疗许多疾病，以及个体基因组成、环境和生活方式之间的巨大差异。在这个模式下，诊断测试病人的遗传和其他分子和细胞内容进行分析，以帮助选择适当和最佳的治疗方法。精确医疗并不意味着将创造出患者独有的药物或医疗设备。相反，它将个体分为不同的组，这些组在疾病易感性、对特定治疗的反

responses to a specific treatment, and/or prognosis and concentrate treatments to those groups who will benefit based on genes, environment, and lifestyle.

Precision medicine has demonstrated great success in cancer treatment, namely precision oncology. However, it is not currently in use for most diseases. Tremendous financial resources have been devoted to extend the success of precision oncology to other diseases such as diabetes, heart disease, obesity, Alzheimer's disease, and mental illness in the U.S.A.

应和/或预后方面不同，并将治疗集中在那些基于基因、环境和生活方式受益的组。

精确医学在癌症治疗方面取得了巨大的成功，即精确肿瘤学。然而，它目前并没有用于大多数疾病。在美国，大量的财政资源被用于将精确肿瘤学的成功推广到其他疾病，如糖尿病、心脏病、肥胖症、阿尔茨海默病和精神疾病。

Box 4-8   Case Study

Mrs. Liu stated that her goal is to continue to do what she is doing now and dies at home with families around. She does not want extraordinary measures to save her life because "I'm ready to go and join my husband and sister-in-law." She does not want to spend all her savings and children's money just to live longer, which is why she does not like hospitals, "too expensive". Since her sister-in-law passed, she does not have a local emergency contact. She does know her neighbors well. Here children feel very guilty leaving mom alone and agree to do everything for mom. They all offered to have mom move in, but mom does not want to because she wants to be where her husband and sister-in-law was.

Questions:

1. What environmental and lifestyle factors can promote Mrs. Liu's health care?

2. How would you personalize the care plan based on all the descriptions of the case study so far?

(YU Fang)

Box 4-8   案例

刘女士的目标是继续她现在的生活，将来在家里，在亲人的氛围中去世。她不想去医院花掉孩子们的大笔钱，用复杂的治疗来延长寿命。她说我已经准备好了去见我的丈夫和小姑子。自从她小姑子去世以后，她在当地就没有了紧急联系人。她和周围的邻居很熟悉。孩子们因为妈妈一个人留在这里感觉到非常的惭愧。他们都愿意为妈妈做些事情，都提出让妈妈搬去和他们一起住，但是妈妈不愿意离开这个她和丈夫及嫂子一起建设起来的家。

问题：

1. 你如何利用环境和生活方式来帮助刘女士满足她的医疗保健需求？

2. 根据这个案例所提供的全部数据，你如何制订一套综合的以人为本的医疗保健方案？

（于　放）

Key Points

1. Geriatric assessment describes a comprehensive and multi-dimensional diagnostic and management process for evaluating and managing health in the elderly people. It's typically conducted by an interdisciplinary team over multiple clinical visits at a variety of settings.

2. The goals of geriatric assessment are to generate comprehensive assessment data to support diagnoses, inform a patient-centered care plan, evaluate health care outcomes, and realize high care safety, quality, and coordination.

本章要点

1. 老年人健康评估是一门深入、多维度的综合学科。它适用于老年人复杂的诊疗过程。老年人健康评估的运作方法灵活多样，强调跨学科合作，通过多次随访完成。

2. 老年人健康评估深入、全面地诊疗老年人的健康问题，通过对医疗保健目标、价值观、意愿及基因、环境和生活方式的考虑充分制订以人为本的医疗保健计划，达到促进医疗保健的安全性、持续性和协调性。

3. Geriatric assessment has eight dimensions, including medical conditions; geriatric syndromes; cognitive function; functional status; psychological status; social status; health care goals, values, and preferences; and genes, environment, and lifestyle.

4. Health care goals, values, and preferences as well as genes, environment, and lifestyle provide the overall, intersecting context for the other six dimensions, and all eight dimensions interact with each other reciprocally.

5. Functional status occupies the central role in geriatric assessment, and the elderly people's ability to function at a level consistent with their lifestyles should be an important consideration in all health care planning.

6. Medical conditions are assessed using the conventional health assessment through health history and physical examination. The emphasis is on distinguishing abnormal signs and symptoms from normal aging-related changes, which is not always possible.

7. Geriatric syndromes disproportionately affect the elderly people and share common risk factors and physiopathological pathways. They are not normal aging. Many geriatric syndromes are under-reported, recognized, or treated.

8. Cognitive function is defined as cerebral activities that acquire, process, and output information and accumulate knowledge by which a person becomes aware of, perceives, or comprehends ideas. It includes four discrete domains: memory, executive functioning, visuospatial function, and language.

9. Psychological status refers to one's mood states which are the display of emotions through body movements, facial expression, vocal tone, and self-description of own internal feeling. Depression, anxiety, and grief are prevailing conditions in the elderly people, although the entire spectrum of mood disorders can occur.

10. Social status refers to a person's standing and relationships within a society, and includes social support, elder mistreatment, decisional capacity and competence, advanced directives, financial situations, and spirituality.

11. Preferences are built on a person's health care goals and values. Eliciting preferences is foundational to evidence-based practice and patient-centered care.

12. Precision medicine takes into account individual differences in genes, environment, and lifestyle to prevent and treat diseases. Genes, by themselves and via

3. 老年人健康评估包括疾病，老年综合征，功能状态，认知功能，心理状态，社会状态，医疗保健目标、价值观和意愿，基因、环境和生活方式8个维度。

4. 医疗保健目标、价值观和意愿以及基因、环境和生活方式为疾病、老年综合征、功能状态、认知功能、心理状态、社会状态提供整体背景。这8个维度协同作用。

5. 功能状态是老年人健康评估的核心。一切医疗护理干预都应以其对功能状态的影响为准则。

6. 老年人疾病评估的重点在于辨别正常老化与异常病理性变化，其步骤和传统临床诊断类似。

7. 由多种因素引起的多器官系统损伤导致老年人应激能力下降，出现老年综合征。老年综合征属异常变化，常常没有被医护人员及时发现和治疗。

8. 认知功能指人脑通过收集、处理和传递信息而累积知识、灵活地观察、理解和推理事物间复杂关系的能力。认知功能包括记忆、执行功能、视空间功能和语言功能四大认知域。

9. 心理状态指一个人通过肢体动作、面部表情、语调和自我描述等表现出来的情绪。老年人易发生多种情绪障碍，以抑郁、焦虑和悲痛最为普遍。

10. 社会状态指老年人在家庭、社区和社会中所处的位置和其社会关系。老年人的社会状态评估强调6个范畴：社会支持、虐待、决策力和决策胜任力、委托、经济状况和精神信仰。

11. 医疗保健目标和价值观直接影响意愿。医疗保健目标、价值观和意愿是循证实践及以人为本的医疗保健模式的基石。

12. 精准医疗模式是指进一步根据患者的基因、环境和生活方式的差异给予有针对性地预防和治疗。

interactions with environment and lifestyle, influence most biological traits, disease susceptibility, and treatment responses.

Critical Thinking Exercise

1. What are the dimensions of geriatric assessment and their relationships?

2. What domains does each dimension of geriatric assessment include?

3. Why is geriatric assessment important?

4. What are normal aging-related changes and abnormal findings in the elderly people?

5. How do you assess each domain of the eight dimensions of geriatric assessment?

6. How do you interpret the findings from geriatric assessment?

7. How do you synthesize data from geriatric assessment to design interventions?

批判性思维练习

1. 老年人健康评估包括哪些维度？它们的关系是什么？

2. 老年人健康评估的各个维度涵盖什么范畴？

3. 老年人健康评估为什么重要？

4. 怎样区分老龄过程中的正常老化和异常变化？

5. 怎样评估老年人健康评估的维度及其范畴？

6. 怎样解释老年人健康评估的结果？

7. 如何用老年人健康评估的结果来指导医疗护理干预？

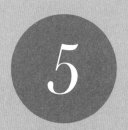

Chapter 5　Medication Management
第五章　老年人安全用药的护理

Learning Objectives

On completion of this chapter, the reader will be able to:

- Describe the characteristics of medication use in elder adults;

- List medications that are best avoided in elder adults;

- Identify potential risk factors for adverse drug reactions;

- Describe the pharmacokinetic and pharmacodynamic changes associated with aging and the implications for drug therapy;

- State the impact that drugs may have on an elder adults quality of life;

- Describe issues related to the optimal use of psychotropic, cardiovascular agents, and antimicrobials;

- Anticipate the effects of increased availability of nonprescription and herbal remedies on patient self-management;

- Identify risk factors for non-adherence and suggest strategies to improve adherence.

学习目标

学完本章节，应完成以下目标：

- 描述老年人的用药特点；

- 列举老年人应避免使用的药物；

- 辨别老年人药物不良反应的潜在危险因素；

- 描述与老龄相关的药代动力学和药效动力学的改变及药物治疗的副作用；

- 叙述药物可能对老年人生活质量产生的影响；

- 描述精神科药物、心血管药物及抗生素的最佳用药方法；

- 预见非处方药和草药使用的增加对老年患者自我管理的影响；

- 辨别老年人服药不依从的危险因素并提出促进依从性的策略。

Medications have important and often essential roles in the management of acute or chronic health conditions and maintenance of well-being in elder adults. At least 94% of adults aged 65 to 74 take medications of some type. Of these, more than 84% regularly take prescription medications, 46% for over the counter medications and 53% dietary supplements. The prevalence of medication use increases even more for those 75 years old or older. Medication can be vital contributors to health and well-being, but more or less, all medications carry certain degree of risks. For elder adults, these risks may be dangerous and even life-threatening. This chapter explains aging-related changes in pharmacodynamics and pharmacokinetics, and provides guidelines for promoting safer and more effective drug therapy. An emphasis is placed on the role of nurse in ensuring improved outcomes for elder adults.

Box 5-1　Case Study

An 82-year-old man with a history of congestive heart failure is taking a number of prescriptions, including psyllium (Metamucil), digoxin (lanoxin), phenytoin (Dilantin), and cimetidine (Tagamet).　He is 175 cm tall and weighs 63 kg.

Questions:

1. On the basis of potential drug interactions, identify the relevant assessment priorities.

2. What factors place this patient at risk for drug toxicity?

Section 1　Introduction

When caring for elder adults, it is important for nurses to understand special considerations for medication use in the elder population. Medications act differently in elder adults than in younger adults and require careful dosage adjustment and monitoring. Elder adults are also more likely than other populations to take more than one medication regularly, increasing the risk of interactions and adverse reactions. To ensure optimal health outcomes, it is important to understand how the pharmacokinetic and pharmacodynamic processes change with aging.

用药在维持老年人健康中起着重要的作用。65～74 岁的老年人中，至少有 94% 服用某种药物。其中，84% 以上的老年人规律服用处方药，46% 的老年人服用非处方药，53% 的老年人服用保健药物。75 岁及以上服用药物的老年人所占的比例更多。药物对人体的健康产生巨大作用，但所有药物都有一定程度的危害性，尤其是对于老年人，这些危害甚至是危及生命的。对护理人员来说，为了确保最佳的健康状况，理解衰老及衰老对药物在体内的作用过程是十分重要的。本章将解释衰老和药物的作用关系，并对老年人安全有效地用药提供指导。

Box 5-1　案例

一位 82 岁患有充血性心力衰竭的男性患者，正在服用几种处方药，包括洋车前子、地高辛、苯妥英钠和西咪替丁。他身高 175cm，体重 63kg。

问题：

1. 请根据潜在的药物相互作用，明确相关的评估重点。

2. 哪些因素使这位老人有药物中毒的危险？

第一节　概述

在照顾老年人时，仔细考虑老年人药物的使用对护士来说是非常重要的。药物在老年人体内的代谢与年轻人不同，用药时需要认真调整剂量并监测。与其他人群相比，老年人更有可能定期服用一种以上的药物，从而增加了药物间的相互作用和不良反应的风险。为了确保最佳的健康结果，了解药物代谢动力学和药效学过程如何随年龄变化是很有意义的。

I. Pharmacokinetic Change

When a medication is taken orally, it begins a journey of four phases that are absorption, distribution, metabolism, and excretion. What the body does to the drug during the four phases of this journey is known as pharmacokinetics. The normal physiologic changes that occur with aging can alter pharmacokinetics.

i. Absorption

Absorption refers to the movement of a drug from the site of administration to the systemic circulation. The primary alteration of absorption occurs with medications taken orally or via feeding tubes. To be absorbed, orally administered medications need first to enter the stomach and intestines. With aging there is decreased secretion of gastric acid, slowed gastric emptying and decreased gastrointestinal motility, decreased absorptive capacity, and decreased blood flow to the stomach and intestines. Although these effects may slow absorption of oral medications, they do not substantial affect the amount of medication absorption that ultimately occurs; therefore age-related changes in absorption of most drug are usually insignificant; however, the first dose of a new medication may take longer to take effect. Topical medications also face barriers to absorption. Aged skin has decreased water, relative decrease in lipid, and decrease in tissue perfusion. These changes may result in impaired absorption of some medications that are administered via lotions, creams, ointments, and patches.

ii. Distribution

Distribution refers to movement of the drug from the systemic circulation to the site of action. Distribution is affected by the relative amounts of total body water, fat, and protein binding. Elder adults have alterations in each of these three areas and have affect distribution. Total body water gradually decreases with aging. Because there is less water for dilution, this may result in a higher concentration of highly water-soluble drugs. Because hydrophilic drugs have a tendency to stay within circulation longer, this will be reflected by a higher serum drug level on laboratory studies. If the risk of toxicity is to be decreased, smaller doses of hydrophilic medications such as digoxin, lithium, atenolol, and amino-glycosides may be needed for elder adults. Conversely, elder adults have a decrease in lean body mass, so the percentage of fat is increased in comparison with younger adults of similar weight. As a consequence of this higher proportion of fat, there will be an increase in the distribution of highly fat-

一、老年人药物代谢动力学特点

药物经口服入时，一般经历四个阶段的过程：吸收，分布，代谢和排泄。人体在这一过程的四个阶段中对药物做出的反应被称为药物代谢动力学。随着年龄的增长，药物代谢动力学会随着正常的生理变化而发生改变。

（一）药物的吸收

药物的吸收是指药物从给药部位进入体循环的过程。最初期药物的吸收变化发生在口服给药或通过鼻饲管给药。口服药物首先要进入胃和肠道被吸收。随着年龄的增长，胃酸分泌减少，胃排空减慢，肠蠕动减弱，吸收能力下降，胃和肠道的血液流动减少。虽然这些影响可能会减缓口服药物的吸收，但它们不会对最终发生的药物吸收量产生实质性的影响，因此，与年龄相关的药物吸收变化通常是微不足道的；然而，新药物的第一剂可能需要更长的时间才能起作用。局部用药也面临吸收障碍。老化的皮肤水分减少，脂质相对减少，组织灌注减少。这些变化可能会导致洗液、霜剂、软膏和贴片给药的吸收障碍。

（二）药物的分布

药物的分布是指药物从体循环后向各组织器官及体液转运的过程。药物分布受到体液量、脂肪量和与血浆蛋白结合量的影响。老年人在这三个方面都有变化，并且影响分布。随着年龄的增长，体液总量逐渐减少。因为用于稀释的水分较少，这可能导致高水溶性药物的浓度更高。由于亲水药物有停留在循环中更长时间的趋势，这点在实验室研究中反映出较高的血清药物水平。如果要降低毒性的风险，在亲水药物的用量上老年人可能需要小剂量用药，如地高辛、锂、阿替洛尔和氨基糖苷。相反，老年人的身体肌肉量会减少，所以与体重相似的年轻人相比，脂肪的比例会增加。由于脂肪比例的增加，高脂溶性（亲脂性）药物的分布也会增加。

soluble (lipophilic) drugs. As a result, lipophilic drugs such as benzodiazepines and some anesthetics may exhibit extended effects.

iii. Metabolism

Metabolism refers to the reactions that transform drugs into metabolites that can be more easily excreted. There is a generalized decrease in all metabolic processes with aging. In addition to metabolic processes, adequacy of hepatic circulation to direct drugs to the liver for metabolism must be considered. There is a 40%-65% decrease in hepatic blood flow in older age. This is particularly relevant in regard to the role of first-pass metabolism. First-pass metabolism is a process in which a large percentage of drugs absorbed from stomach or intestines first enters the portal circulation of liver and is metabolized (inactivated) before reaching the systemic circulation. A decrease in hepatic blood flow can result in a decrease in the amount of a drug diverted to live for transformation before it enters the systemic circulation. With decreased first-pass metabolism, a greater amount of active drug enters the systemic circulation; consequently, there is an additional risk that standard doses of drugs will more likely result in toxic effects. The implications of these alterations are that metabolism of some drugs may be slowed, thus leading to a prolonged drug half-life and all increased risk of drug accumulation and toxic effects; however, this cannot be generalized to all elder adults. Individualization of medication regimens and careful assessments for signs or symptoms of toxic effects or complications are necessary while dosing schedules are being optimized.

iv. Excretion

Excretion refers to the elimination of drugs from the body which occurs primarily via the kidneys. When renal function is decreased, half-life increases and drugs can accumulate to toxic levels. This has important implications for elder adults because, for most, renal function decreases with aging, especially for those who have conditions such as hypertension or heart disease. The kidney blood flow of the elderly decreased with aging, kidney weight decreased, kidney units decreased, glomerulus effective filter surface reduced, so that the glomerular filtration rate is reduced, it is easy to cause cumulative intoxication. At the same time, kidney tubules secretion and re-absorption function are significantly reduced in the elderly so the kidney function is reduced; the ability to excrete drugs by the kidneys is reduced. These changes cause the drug in the elderly can not be quickly excreted, it is easy to accumulate in the body,

因此，亲脂性药物，如苯二氮䓬类药物和一些麻醉剂可能会表现出延伸效应。

（三）药物的代谢

药物的代谢是指将药物转化为更容易排泄的代谢物的反应。随着衰老，所有代谢过程都有普遍的降低。除了代谢过程外，还必须考虑到肝循环是否足以将药物引导到肝脏进行代谢。老年人肝血流量和细胞量比成年人降低40%～65%。这在首过效应方面尤其重要。首过效应是大部分从胃肠道吸收的药物，经门静脉系统进入肝脏，在肝脏进行首次代谢，使进入体循环的药量减少的过程。肝血流量的减少会导致药物在进入体循环之前被转送到靶器官的药量的减少。随着首过效应的减少，更多的活性药物进入体循环。因此，就会出现标准剂量的药物将有可能导致毒性风险。这些改变的影响是，某些药物的新陈代谢可能减慢，从而导致药物半衰期延长，并增加药物积累和毒性反应的风险。在优化用药方案时，必须进行个性化设计，并仔细评估药物毒性作用和药物副作用引起的症状和体征。

（四）药物排泄

药物排泄是指药物从体内被清除，大多数药物经过肾脏排泄。当肾功能下降时，药物半衰期延长，药物可能在体内积累到毒性水平。这对老年人有重要影响，因为对大多数人来说，肾功能会随着年龄的增长而降低，尤其是对那些患有高血压或心脏病等病症的老年人。随着老化的作用，老年人肾血流量减少，肾重量减轻，肾单位减少，肾小球有效过滤表面减少，使得肾小球过滤率降低，易引起蓄积中毒；同时，老年人肾小管分泌和重吸收功能均明显降低，故肾功能减退，经肾脏排泄药物的能力减少。这些变化造成药物在老年人身上无法迅速排出，

and cause cumulative intoxication. Therefore, medication should be taken with caution, so as not to endanger kidney function, such as some antibiotics including streptomycin, cantimycin, neomycin, and carnamycin.

In summary, the change of drug metabolism in the elderly is particularly, so nurses should pay attention to monitor the dynamic change. Most drugs' effect and blood drug concentration is consistent, and changes in blood drug concentration can reflect the change law about drug's absorption, distribution, metabolism, excretion processes. At the same time, it is necessary to adjust medication for the elderly with combining clinical indications.

II. Pharmacodynamic Change

Physiological alterations which associated with aging can also alter the elder adult's response to drugs. Pharmacodynamics refers to what the drug does to the body, is the term used to explain the body's response to a drug. As people age, pharmacodynamics is altered by the number of receptors and their affinity for drugs, as well as by alterations in response to receptor stimulation. As a result, drug sensitivity may be either increased (e. g. , increased sedative effects of benzodiazepines) or decreased (e. g. , decreased bronchodilator response to beta agonists such as albuterol). In both respects, the altered sensitivity is unrelated to the drug level. Furthermore, the bodily processes that maintain homeostasis become less effective; consequently, the elder adult may be less able to tolerate the effects and side effects of certain drugs.

容易蓄积于体内，引起积蓄中毒。因此，用药时须谨慎，以免危及肾脏功能，如某些抗生素，包括链霉素、庆大霉素、新霉素及卡那霉素等。

综上所述，老年人药物代谢的变化有其特殊性，在护理工作中要注意监测血药浓度的动态变化，大多数药物的药效强度与血药浓度是一致的，血药浓度的变化可反应药物吸收、分布、代谢、排泄等过程的变化规律，同时要结合临床指征，随时调整老年人的用药。

二、老年人药效动力学特点

药物效应动力学（pharmacodynamics in the elderly）简称药效学，是研究药物对机体的作用及作用机制的科学。老年药效学改变是指机体效应器官对药物的反应随年龄增长而发生的改变。老年药效学改变的特点：对大多数药物的敏感性增高、作用增强，对少数药物的敏感性降低，药物耐受性下降，在多种药物联合应用时，如不减少剂量，常不能耐受，使药物不良反应发生率增加。例如，由于老年人大脑耐受低血糖的能力较差，易发生低血糖昏迷。因此，要教会老年糖尿病患者和家属识别低血糖的症状，随身携带糖果、饼干和糖尿病卡，便于发生意外时的救治。另外，老年人个体差异较大，多种药物联合应用时常发生药物的相互作用，使协同作用或拮抗作用增强，故药物的相互作用在老年人中可引起严重的不良反应。如利尿药、镇静药、安定药各一种并分别服用，耐受性较好，能各自发挥预期疗效；但若同时合用，则患者不能耐受，易出现直立性低血压。因此，要根据个体差异调整药物的用量。

Section 2　Principles of Medication Management in the Elderly

Rational drug use is defined by the World Health Organization (WHO) as: "The drugs that patients accepted are appropriate to their clinical needs, drug dosages should be consistent with the patients individually, course appropriate, the drugs are most inexpensive on patients and their communities." Therefore, the rational drug use contains essential elements for safety, availability and affordability. Safety is the basic premise of rational drug use; it involves risks and benefits of the medication. Because organ functional reserves decline with aging, as well as the stability of the body, the degree of drug tolerance and safety margins in the elderly have decreased markedly. According to statistics, the rates of adverse drug reactions (ADR) of the elderly are higher than those of young people, and increases with aging: ADR rate among people 51-60 years old is 14.4%; it rises to 15.7% in people aged 61-70; 18.3% in 71-80 years old, and 25% in 81 years old or over. Therefore, in order to improve medication safety, certain principles of drug use for the elderly should be followed.

I. Principle of Benefit

The principle of benefit means medicine used for the elderly must be weight to ensure the benefit. First of all, a clear indication of the drug use is needed. Secondly, the drug benefit/risk ratio should be greater than 1. Even if there are indications, but drug benefit/risk ratio is less than 1, the drug should not be given. Meanwhile, the drug with good efficacy and small side effects should be selected. For example: for the elderly with arrhythmia, sudden cardiac arrest is rare when structural heart disease or blood flow dynamic disorder are absent. However, arrhythmia can be induced by long term use of antiarrhythmic drug, which increases mortality. Therefore, such patients should take antiarrhythmic drugs as little as possible.

II. Principle of Five Drugs

Principle of five drugs refers to the use of drugs in the elderly cannot exceed 5 kinds. This principle is based on the relationship between number of drug use and ADR

第二节　老年人用药原则

世界卫生组织（WHO）将合理用药（rational drug use）定义："合理用药要求患者接受的药物适合其临床的需要，药物剂量应符合患者的个体化要求，疗程适当，药物对患者及其社区最为低廉。"因此，合理用药包含的基本要素为安全性、有效性及经济性。安全性是合理用药的基本前提，它涉及用药的危险和效益。老年人由于各器官贮备功能及身体内环境稳定性随年龄而衰退，因此，对药物的耐受程度及安全幅度均明显下降。据有关资料统计，老年人的药物不良反应（ADR）发生率较年轻人高，且随年龄增加而增加：51～60 岁 ADR 发生率为 14.4%，61～70 岁为 15.7%，71～80 岁为 18.3%，81 岁及以上为25%。因此，老年人用药要遵循一定的用药原则，以提高用药安全性。

一、受益原则

受益原则是指老年人用药必须权衡利弊，以确保用药物对患者有益。首先，老年人用药要有明确的用药适应证，另外还要保证用药的受益／危险比大于 1。即便有适应证但用药的受益／危险比小于 1 时，就不应给予药物治疗。同时选择疗效确切而毒副作用小的药物。例如：患有心律失常的老年人，如果无器质性心脏病又无血流动力学障碍，则发生心源性猝死的可能性很小，但在长期使用抗心律失常药时可能发生药源性心律失常，增加死亡率，故此类患者应尽可能不用或少用抗心律失常药。

二、五种药物原则

五种药物原则是指老年人同时用药不能超过 5 种，这一原则是根据用药数目与 ADR发生率的关系提出的。据统计，同时使用 5

rate. Polypharmacy refers to describe the use of multiple medications by a patient, especially when too many forms of medication are used by a patient. It has been an issue of great concerns in gerontological nursing. According to statistics, ADR rate increases with the number of medications used by the elderly. ADR rate is 4% when using 5 kinds of drugs; it rises to 10% for 6-10 type of drugs, 25% for 11-15 types, and 54% for 16-20 types. It is common to see the elderly with more than 2 kinds of chronic diseases, so they often use a variety of drugs for treatment, which not only increase the financial burden in patients but also increase ADR. In the implementation of principle of five drugs, following should be kept in mind:

(1) Understand the limitations of drugs, many diseases have no effective drugs for treatment. If too much drugs are used, the harm of ADR may be greater than the disease itself.

(2) Select major drug according to health condition. If the effect is not obvious, and the patient has poor tolerance, or not taking drugs according to doctor's advice, the drug should be stopped.

(3) Use the drugs with therapeutic effects for both diseases: such as to choose Beta receptor blockers or calcium antagonist for the treatment of hypertension and angina pectoris.

(4) Pay more attention to non-drug treatment, such as for the early diabetic, diet therapy can be used firstly.

III. Principle of Low Doses

Principle of low doses refers to controlling the drug dosage for elderly people at the lowest effective dose to ensure drug safety and efficacy. For most drugs, the principle of low dose mainly applies at the beginning stages of drug use. In order to get satisfactory effects and minimal side-effects, the initial dose normally starting from 1/5-1/4 of adult dose with slow increments to adjust the dose as clinical response. For drugs require initial loading dose for rapid effects in the first time, such as lidocaine, lower bound of doses are available for the first time, principle of low dose mainly reflects in the maintenance dose. In addition, the drug dosage of the elderly should be individualized. To analyze specifically base on the age, health status, body weight, liver and kidney function, protein binding rate, clinical situation, treatment index of

种药物以下的 ADR 发生率为 4%，6～10 种为 10%，11～15 种为 25%，16～20 种为 54%。老年人因多病共存，常采用多种药物治疗，这不仅加重患者经济负担，降低依从性，而且导致 ADR 的发生率增高。同时，使用 2 种药物的潜在药物相互作用发生率为 6%，5 种药物为 50%，8 种药物增至 100%，虽然并非所有药物相互作用都能导致 ADR，但这种潜在的危险性无疑是增加的。当用药超过 5 种时，就应考虑是否都是必要用药，以及依从性和 ADR 等问题。在执行 5 种药物原则时要注意：

（1）了解药物的局限性，许多老年性疾病（如钙化性心脏瓣膜病）无相应有效的药物治疗，若用药过多，ADR 的危害反而大于疾病本身。

（2）根据病情需要，选主要药物治疗。凡疗效不明显、耐受差、未按医嘱服用药物的应考虑终止。

（3）选用具有兼顾治疗作用的药物：如高血压合并心绞痛者，可选用 β 受体阻滞剂及钙通道阻滞剂。

（4）重视非药物治疗，如早期糖尿病可采用饮食疗法。

三、小剂量原则

小剂量原则是指将老年人用药剂量控制在最低有效剂量，以保证用药的有效性和安全性。对于大多数药物来说，小剂量原则主要体现在开始用药阶段，一般开始用成年人剂量的 1/5～1/4，缓慢增量，然后根据临床反应调整剂量，以获得满意疗效和最小副作用为准则。对于需要使用首次负荷量的药物，如利多卡因、胺碘酮等，为了确保迅速起效，老年人首次可用成年人剂量的下限，小剂量原则主要体现在维持量上。另外，老年人用药剂量的确定，要遵循剂量个体化原则。应根据老年人的年龄、健康状态、体重、肝肾

the elderly . If the purpose of treatment can be achieved with a smaller dose, it is not necessary to use a large dose.

功能、蛋白结合率、临床情况、治疗指数等情况具体分析，能用较小剂量达到治疗目的的，就没有必要使用大剂量。

IV. Principle of Timing

The principle of timing refers to select the most appropriate time for drug use based on the principles of biology time and pharmacology time, to maximize drug action and minimizing side effects. The onset, aggravating and mitigation of many diseases have circadian rhythm, such as variant angina pectoris, cerebral thrombosis, asthma often attack during the night. In addition, pharmacokinetics and pharmacodynamics also have rhythm. For example, the hypoglycemic effect of insulin in the morning is greater than in the afternoon. Therefore, determination of the best time of drug use should be based on disease outbreaks, pharmacokinetics and pharmacodynamics of circadian rhythm changes. Timing should also refer to the adverse events. For example, diuretics should be given in the morning, so the patient would not run to the bathroom all night.

四、择时原则

择时原则是指根据时间生物学和时间药理学的原理，选择最合适的用药时间进行治疗，最大限度地发挥药物作用，尽可能降低毒副作用。由于许多疾病的发作、加重与缓解具有昼夜节律的变化，如变异型心绞痛、脑血栓、哮喘常在夜间发作，急性心肌梗死和脑出血的发病高峰在上午等；另外，药代动力学、药效学也有昼夜节律变化。例如，白天肠道功能相对亢进，因此白天用药比夜间吸收快、血液浓度高；药效学也有昼夜节律变化；胰岛素的降糖作用上午大于下午。因此，应根据疾病的发作、药代动力学、药效学的昼夜节律的变化来确定最佳用药时间。

V. Principle of Suspending Medication

Principle of suspending medication refers to the evaluation of drugs used by elderly, when the ADR is suspected; the drug use should be monitored carefully. Any new symptoms, including body, cognition, or emotional symptoms, should be observed closely. They may be signs of ADR, or indicators of disease deterioration. These two conditions need to be distinguished. For ADR, the drug needs to be stopped, but for disease deterioration dosing need to be adjusted. For the new symptoms occur with drug use in the elderly, withdrawal medication can be more beneficial than increasing, so suspending medication principle is one of the easiest and most effective interventions.

五、暂停用药原则

暂停用药原则是指对老年人所用药物予以评价。当怀疑 ADR 时，要在监护下停药一段时间。在老年人用药期间应注意密切观察，一旦发生任何新的症状，包括躯体、认知或情感方面的症状，都应考虑 ADR 或病情进展，因为这两种情况处理截然不同，前者需停药、后者则应调整药量。对于服药的老年人出现新症状，停药受益可能多于加药受益，所以暂停用药原则作为现代老年病学中最简单、最有效的干预措施之一。

Box 5-2 Risk Factors for Medication Errors

- Use of multiple medications.
- Cognitive impairment.
- Hearing deficits.
- Arthritic or weak hands.
- History of noncompliance with medical care.

Box 5-2 用药失误的危险因素

- 服用多种药物。
- 认知障碍。
- 听力缺陷。
- 患关节炎或手部力量弱。
- 有服药不易从医嘱经历。

- Lack of knowledge regarding medications.
- Limited finances.
- Illiteracy.
- Lack of support system.
- History of inappropriate self-medication.
- Presence of expired or borrowed medications in home.

- 缺乏相关服药知识。
- 经济能力有限。
- 文盲。
- 缺乏支持系统。
- 有不适当的自己服药经历。
- 在家里有过期药物和借用的药物。

Section 3　Commonly Used Medications and Adverse Drug Reactions

This section reviews major drug groups and the main concerns related to their use in the elder population. This section is not intended to be an all-inclusive drug review; readers are advised to consult with current drug references and pharmacists for comprehensive information.

I. Psychotropics

Psychotropic medications, which include antipsychotics, anti-depressants, sedative-hypnotics, and anxiolytics, are often prescribed for the elder adults, because financial worries, deaths, illness, and many other problems commonly faced by elder adults give legitimate cause for the problems as anxiety, depression, etc.

i. Anxiolytics and Hypnotics

Insomnia and anxiety are problems that commonly plague elder adults. Many drugs are used to treat these problems that have the potential for bothersome and dangerous adverse effects in elder adults. Because insomnia and anxiety often occur as secondary to medication side effects or secondary to medical conditions

第三节　老年人常用药物及不良反应

本节回顾主要的药物组和老年人使用这些药物相关的主要问题。本节并非是涵盖一个全面的药物回顾；建议读者查阅现有的药物参考资料和药剂师以获得更全面的信息。（老年人的药物不良反应随着年龄的增长而增加。另外，老年人感官功能及认知功能的衰退，也对老年人的安全用药造成了隐患。例如，听力、视力及注意力减退，都能使老年人对药物的治疗目的、服药方法和服药时间、剂量不能正确理解和执行，影响用药的安全性和疗效。因此，了解老年人常用药物的不良反应，指导老年人安全用药是护理人员的重要职责。）

一、精神科药物

精神科药物常应用于老年人，包括抗精神病药、抗抑郁药、镇静催眠药和抗焦虑药。老年人通常面临的经济问题、死亡、疾病和许多其他问题都是引起老年人焦虑、抑郁等问题的原因。

（一）抗焦虑药和催眠药

失眠和焦虑是困扰老年人的常见问题。许多用于治疗这些疾病的药物在老年人群中使用时可能产生危险的副作用。由于失眠和焦虑往往也继发于药物副作用、痴呆、甲状腺功能异常或抑郁等，因此，对失眠或焦虑

such as dementia, thyroid abnormalities, or depression, proper diagnosis and treatment of any underlying causes of insomnia or anxiety can decrease the appropriate use of these medications. Nonpharmacologic interventions are often effective but tend to be underused; therefore, a trial of nonpharmacologic treatment is initially preferred whenever possible, before initiation of pharmacologic therapy in elder adults.

Benzodiazepines, which are commonly prescribed for both problems, are also concerns for elder adults. Benzodiazepines with long half-lives such as diazepam (valium) should be avoided because of the increased toxicity; in addition all benzodiazepines, including shorter-acting ones such as lorazepam can cause excessive sedation, impaired memory, decreased psychomotor performance, and balance disturbances, and may lead to drug dependence. If a benzodiazepine is required, it is best to give the smallest dose possible and monitor closely for side effects. Benzodiazepines should not be used for extended periods. It is important to assess for an effects and continued need of these medications so that they can be discontinued in a timely manner.

ii. Antidepressants

All antidepressants are generally effective for managing depression in elder adults; however, some are better tolerated than others. Older tricyclic antidepressants have been used to treat depression, as well as insomnia and neuropathic pain; however, significant side effects occur even in low doses and before therapeutic levels are reached. As a treatment for insomnia, tricyclic antidepressants are generally too sedating and can cause daytime somnolence. Additionally tricyclic antidepressants possess anticholinergic side effects that can create problems for many elder adults.

Selective serotonin reuptake inhibitors (SSRIs) are generally the antidepressant of first choice for elder adults because they are better tolerated. However, they may cause dose-related gastrointestinal disturbances, including gastrointestinal bleeding, and central nervous system arousal effects. Fortunately, most side effects of the SSRIs last only a few days.

Selection of an antidepressant is often based on side effect profiles, which differ among available agents. For instance, mirtazapine (Remeron) has more potential for sedation than some SSRI antidepressants. It can also reduce anxiety and increase appetite; therefore, if the patient suffers depressive symptoms of anxiety,

的任何潜在原因进行正确的诊断和治疗会减少这些药物的使用。非药物干预通常有效，但往往未得到充分利用；因此，在开始对老年人进行药物治疗之前，应尽可能先进行非药物治疗。

苯二氮䓬类药物是治疗失眠和焦虑这两种老年人关注问题的常用药物。应避免使用半衰期较长的苯二氮䓬类药物，如安定，因为其毒性会增加；此外，所有的苯二氮䓬类药物，包括短效的药物，如劳拉西泮，均会引起过度镇静、记忆受损、精神运动能力下降和平衡失调，并可能导致药物依赖。如果需要使用苯二氮䓬类药物，最好给予尽可能小的剂量，并密切监测副作用。苯二氮䓬类药物不能长期使用，评估这些药物的效果和继续使用的必要性是很重要的，以便及时停药。

（二）抗抑郁药

所有的抗抑郁药一般都对控制老年人的抑郁有效；然而，有些人比其他人更能耐受药物。较经典的三环类抗抑郁药已被用于治疗抑郁症、失眠和神经性疼痛；然而，即使在低剂量和在达到治疗水平之前的剂量也会出现明显的副作用。作为一种治疗失眠的药物，三环类抗抑郁药镇静作用过大，会导致白天嗜睡。此外，三环类抗抑郁药具有抗胆碱能副作用，会给许多老年人带来一些问题。

选择性5-羟色胺再摄取抑制剂（SSRIs）通常是老年人的首选抗抑郁药物，因为它们的耐受性更好。然而，它们可能引起剂量相关的胃肠紊乱，包括胃肠出血和中枢神经系统的觉醒效应。幸运的是，SSRIs的大多数副作用只持续几天。

抗抑郁药物的选择通常是基于其副作用的范围，这和其他药物的选择有所不同。例如，米氮平（Remeron）比一些SSRIs抗抑郁药有更强的镇静作用，它还可以减少焦虑，增加食欲；因此，如果患者出现焦虑、失眠、

insomnia, and lack of appetite, then mirtazapine may be an appropriate choice to help the patient with sleep, increase appetite and reduce anxiety. On the other hand, a patient exhibiting depressive symptoms such as increased sleepiness, decreased affect, and decreased socialization may benefit from a more stimulating antidepressant like sertraline (Zoloft) or venlafaxine (Effexor). Thus, the side effect profile of an antidepressant may be used to identify the most appropriate medication for depressive symptom pattern.

iii. Antipsychotics

Antipsychotics can control the symptoms of excitement, restlessness, hallucinations and delusions without affecting conscious consciousness. Therefore, such drugs are mainly used in schizophrenia, so also known as schizophrenia drugs. Chlorpromazine is the representative of this kind of drugs, there are more than 10 kinds of antipsychotics, including perphenazine, haloperidol and clozapine, there is no significant difference in the efficacy of each drug. The main side effects of antipsychotic drugs are: a. sleepy, dry mouth, blurred vision, these problems don't need special treatment ; b. constipation, the use of laxatives can solve this problem ; c. external cone reaction; d. some drugs such as chlorpromazine, clozapine are easy to cause postural hypotension reaction, the patient should be slowly to prevent from fainting, if change posture from sitting or lying position to standing position; e. anxiety, depression side effects should be treated with anti-anxiety and antidepressant treatments; f. rare and serious side effects are malignant symptoms (high fever, silence and stiffness), severe rash, drug fever and granulocyte deficiency, the drug should be stopped immediately and give the patient internal medicine treatment.

II. Cardiovascular Medications

Cardiovascular medications are taken by large numbers of elder adults because of the high prevalence of cardiovascular disorders in this population. The majority of people older than 65 has hypertension. In the United States, the Joint National Committee on Prevention, Detection, Evaluation, and Treatment of High Blood Pressure (JNC) is the foremost provider of evidence-based clinical guidelines to grade hypertension management. The drugs recommended for management of hypertension are also used in the management of a number of other cardiovascular conditions.

1. Beta-blockers Beta-blockers (BBs) have been demonstrated to improve mortality rates for patients

食欲缺乏等抑郁症状，那么米氮平是帮助患者改善睡眠、增加食欲、减少焦虑的合适选择。另外，表现出如嗜睡、情绪低落和社交活动减少等症状的抑郁症患者，可能会受益于刺激性更强的抗抑郁药，如舍曲林（Zoloft）或文拉法辛（Effexor）。因此，抗抑郁药的副作用范围可以被用来确定选择治疗抑郁症最合适的药物模式。

（三）抗精神病药

抗精神病药可在不影响意识清醒的条件下，控制兴奋、躁动、幻觉及妄想等症状。因此类药主要用于精神分裂症，故也称精神分裂症药。氯丙嗪是这类药物的代表，较为常用的还有奋乃静、氟哌啶醇和氯氮平等10多种，各药疗效无明显差异。抗精神病药物的副作用主要有：①困倦、口干、视物模糊，此类情况不需特殊处理；②便秘，可应用通便药缓解便秘；③锥体外系反应；④有些药如氯丙嗪、氯氮平等容易引起直立性低血压反应，改变体位时如由坐位或卧位起立要缓慢，以防晕倒；⑤出现焦虑、抑郁副作用时，应辅以抗焦虑及抗抑郁药治疗；⑥少见而严重的副作用是恶性症状群（高热、缄默和木僵）、严重皮疹、黄疸、药物热及粒细胞缺乏，应立即停药并进行内科处理。

二、心血管药物

由于心血管疾病在老年人群中患病率较高，许多老年人服用心血管药物。例如，多数65岁以上的人都患有高血压病。在美国，全国高血压预防、检测、评估和治疗联合委员会（JNC）是高血压管理分级的首要循证临床指南提供者。推荐用于治疗高血压的药物也用于治疗其他心血管疾病。

1. β-受体阻滞剂 β-受体阻滞剂（BBs）已被证明可改善有心血管病史患者的死亡率。

with a history of cardiovascular disease. They decrease angina symptoms, cardiac workload, and oxygen demand through reduction of heart rate, cardiac output, and atrioventricular conduction. This provides a cardio-protective effect for patients with a history of ischemia or myocardial infarction.

2. Calcium channel blockers Calcium channel blockers (CCBs) have a beneficial effect in decreasing cardiac workload through decreasing peripheral resistance. For this reason, they are an alternative choice for patients with severe reactive airway disease or with a high degree of heart blockage where a BBs might be contraindicated.

3. Angiotensin-converting enzyme inhibitors and angiotensin receptor blockers The angiotensin-converting enzyme inhibitors (ACEIs) and angiotensin receptor blockers (ARBs) also have demonstrated value in decreasing the chance of cardiac mortality in patients with heart failure. They also confer renal protection, which is particularly beneficial for patients with diabetes.

Because elder adults are likely to have more comorbidities (eg., diabetes, reduced kidney function, and heart disease), JNC recommends selecting hypertensive treatment based on comorbid conditions or compelling indication. For example, a 70-year-old patient with hypertension and diabetes would benefit from thiazide-type diuretics and an ACEI or ARB. On the other hand, if the patient had hypertension with ischemic heart disease, the optimal management may be a thiazide diuretic with a BBs.

The main concerns with the use of antihypertensive medications in elder adults are an increased risk of orthostatic hypotension and dehydration, especially with volume-depleting agents and vasodilators. The aging person has reduced kidney function and decreased ability to maintain fluid and electrolyte balance. In addition, some elder adults may have decreased appetite and sense of thirst and subsequent decreased oral intake of food and fluid and increased risk of dehydration. Subsequently, it is not surprising that dehydration is common among elder people and is a frequent reason for admission to the hospital. Assessing for the adverse effects of antihypertensive treatment is essential in maintaining the health of elder patients and reducing complications and hospitalizations.

4. Diuretics The elderly with heart failure has poor appetite, and it will affect the normal intake of electrolytes, coupled with liver and kidney function reduction, poor regulatory ability. It is easily to occur the

它们通过降低心率、心排血量和房室传导来减少心绞痛症状、心脏负荷和氧需求量。这为有缺血或心肌梗死病史的患者提供了心脏保护作用。

2. 钙通道阻滞剂 钙通道阻滞剂（CCBs）可通过降低外周阻力而有效降低心脏负荷。因此，当 BBs 被禁用时，对于严重的反应性气道疾病或严重的心脏阻滞患者，CCBs 是另一种选择。

3. 血管紧张素转换酶抑制剂和血管紧张素受体阻滞剂 血管紧张素转换酶抑制剂（ACEIs）和血管紧张素受体阻滞剂（ARBs）在降低心力衰竭患者的死亡率方面也有价值。它们还能保护肾脏，这对糖尿病患者尤其有益。

由于老年人可能有更多的共病（如糖尿病、肾功能减退和心脏病），JNC 建议根据共病情况或强制性的指征选择高血压治疗。例如，70 岁的高血压和糖尿病患者可以从噻嗪类利尿剂和 ACEI 或 ARB 中获益。另一方面，如果患者患有高血压并伴有缺血性心脏病，最理想的治疗方法是服用噻嗪类利尿剂和 BBs。

老年人使用抗高血压药物的主要问题是增加直立性低血压和脱水的风险，特别是使用能量消耗的药物和血管扩张剂。老年人肾功能下降，维持体液和电解质平衡的能力下降。此外，一些老年人的食欲和口渴感可能会降低，因而食物和液体的摄入量会减少，脱水的风险也会增加。所以脱水在老年人中很常见，并且是住院的常见原因。评估抗高血压治疗的不良反应对于维持老年患者的健康、减少并发症和住院治疗至关重要。

4. 利尿剂 老年人在心力衰竭时食欲较差，会影响正常的水电解质的摄入，加上肝肾功能减退，调节能力差，易发生水电解质紊乱及酸碱失衡，故在应用排钾利尿剂时，

electrolyte disorder and acid-base imbalance, so when the potassium excretion diuretics is applied, nurses should pay more attention to monitor blood gas and blood electrolytes, in order to detect imbalances early and adjust timely.

5. Digoxin　In addition to medications used in management of hypertension and related disorders, many elder adults are prescribed Digoxin. Digoxin is sometimes used to treat heart failure because it increases the force of cardiac contraction; however, although this will increase cardiac output, research has shown that it does not necessarily reduce morbidity and mortality. For this reason, its use in management of heart failure has become controversial, and it is no longer considered as first line therapy. Digoxin remains a beneficial agent for the management of atrial tachyarrhythmia, because it slows the heart rate, allowing for adequate ventricular filling.

Because the renal function of the elderly is decreased, the drug excretion rate is slowed down and the half-life is prolonged, the blood concentration of drug should be monitored regularly to avoid poisoning. For the chronic heart failure patient with sever gastrointestinal congestion, the drug effect will be affected by poor absorption. Deslanoside (cedilanid) can be injected intravenously, but the injection should be slowly, and the nurse should pay more attention to monitor patient's heart rate and heart rhythm.

6. Anti-arrhythmic agent　The treatment of arrhythmia in the elderly should be preferred for drugs with less side effects, and the dose should be determined mainly on the basis of clinical results, rather than simply considering the plasma concentration, otherwise other types of arrhythmia may occur due to the high dose of the drug. When anti-arrhythmia drug is applied by intravenous, in particular, should be careful, and should monitor the patient's electrocardiogram and blood pressure.

III. Antimicrobial

An antimicrobial is an agent that kills microorganisms or inhibits their growth. Antimicrobial medicines can be grouped according to the microorganisms they act primarily against. Infections in elder adults can result in devastating health events because of generally decreased physiologic reserves. Urinary tract infections (UTIs) and respiratory infections (especially pneumonia and exacerbations of chronic lung diseases) are common and

应注意监测血气及血电解质情况，以便早期发现失衡现象，及时补充调整。

5. 地高辛　除了用于治疗高血压和相关疾病的药物外，许多老年人还服用地高辛。地高辛因能够增加心肌收缩力而用于治疗心力衰竭；虽然地高辛能增加心排血量，但是研究表明，它不一定减少发病率和死亡率。因此，它在心衰治疗中的应用备受争议，也不再被认为是一线治疗方法。但地高辛仍然是一种有益的药物，因为它能够减慢心率，使心室能够充分充盈，故可用于控制房性心动过速。

由于老年人肾功能减退，药物排泄速度减慢，半衰期延长，故应定期监测血药浓度，以免发生中毒。对慢性心力衰竭胃肠道淤血较重者，会因吸收不良而影响药效，可用去乙酰毛花苷（西地兰）静脉注射，但注入要缓慢，并须注意监测心率及心律。

6. 抗心律失常药物　老年人心律失常的治疗应首选副作用小的药物，并主要依据临床效果确定剂量，而不能单纯地考虑血药浓度，否则可能会因用药剂量大而发生其他类型的心律失常。在经静脉应用抗心律失常药物时，尤其应谨慎，须有心电图、血压的监测。

三、抗生素

抗生素是一种杀死微生物或抑制其生长的物质。抗生素可根据其主要作用的微生物分类。老年人感染通常由于减少了生理储备可导致严重的健康事件。尿路感染和呼吸道感染（尤其是肺炎和慢性肺部疾病的恶化）是常见的，往往会导致住院。

often lead to hospital admissions.

Pharmacologic treatment of infections has the potential to achieve cures, but problems related to their use persist. Because many elder adults have reduced renal function, dosage adjustments may be needed for certain antibiotics such as aminoglycosides. Antibiotic resistance, an increasing problem, may hinder the efforts for finding the right treatment mix for complicated infections. Even for less serious infections in elder adults, common antibiotic side effects such as diarrhea can create significant and even dangerous shifts in fluids and electrolytes. Nausea can result in decreased intake, further contributing to this problem.

The use of antibiotics in the elderly must be very carefully, due to the decline of body organ function with the aging process. If we use antibiotics carelessly, there will be serious results. There are some points should be noted as following:

1. When antibiotic is used to patient at the first time, nurse should pay more attention to observe the presence of allergic reaction, it can be avoided by skin allergy test or used small dosage.

2. When using antibiotics for the elderly with poor liver and kidney function, nurse should pay attention to the signs of liver toxicity and renal toxicity. For example, kidney function should be monitored because cephalosporin and aminoglycosides may cause renal toxicity.

3. Pay attention to the presence of repeated infections, especially in elderly patients who have been treated with antibiotics for a long time. Curative effects should be assessed, and try not to use the same type of antibiotics for a long time.

4. More than two antibiotics in the human body will produce synergy or antagonizing effects. For example, beta-lactam (penicillin, cephalosporin) and aminogins, quinolones are applied at the same time, will produce synergies, that is, enhanced effects, while the simultaneous application of chloramphenicol, macrolides (red mycomycin), will produce antagonist, that is, the effect is weakened.

药物治疗感染有可能获得治愈，但与它们的使用有关的问题仍然存在。由于许多老年人肾功能减退，某些抗生素如氨基糖苷类可能需要调整剂量。抗生素耐药性是一个日益严重的问题，它可能会阻碍寻找多重感染的治疗组合。即使对老年人感染不那么严重的情况，常见的抗生素副作用，如腹泻，也会在体液和电解质方面造成重大甚至危险的变化。恶心会导致摄取量减少，进一步导致这个问题。

抗生素的使用在老年人的身上必须十分谨慎，因在人体老化过程中全身器官功能衰退，抗生素使用不慎，会造成严重后果。以下是使用抗生素的几点注意事项：

1. 第一次使用抗生素时应特别注意观察有无过敏反应的出现，可通过皮肤过敏试验或先予以小剂量等方法避免。

2. 肝肾功能不佳的老人使用某些抗生素时，要注意肝毒性或肾毒性现象。如头孢菌素及氨基糖苷可能引起肾毒性，应监测肾脏功能。

3. 注意观察有无重复感染的现象，尤其是长期接受抗生素治疗的老年患者，应评估抗生素的药效，尽量不要长期使用相同种类的抗生素。

4. 两种以上的抗生素在人体内会产生协同作用或拮抗作用。如 β- 内酰胺类（青霉素类，头孢菌素类）与氨基糖苷类、喹诺酮类药物同时应用，会产生协同作用，即作用加强；而同氯霉素类、大环内酯类（红霉素）同时应用，则产生拮抗作用，即作用减弱。

IV. Nonprescription Agents

Elder adults are the largest consumers of nonprescription drugs. They believe that drugs that are available over-the-counter (OTC) are always safe; however, many of the prescription drugs that have been reclassified to over the counter medications [eg., nonsteroidal anti-inflammatory drugs (NSAIDs) and sedating antihistamines] have a potential for significant harm in elder populations.

Elder adults usually do not voluntarily report information about the use of over-the-counter medications. Missing out on the chance of health education related to drug application and the checking of interaction of the drugs may worsen patients' current health status. The need for education is complicated by the reality that many elder adults have decreased visual acuity, cataracts, macular degeneration, and other visual problems that limit the ability to read finely-printed labels and instructions. Further, a recent nationwide study in China found that 46% of patients taking prescription medications also taking nonprescription drugs, thus increasing the potential for drug-drug interactions.

The first challenge for nurses regarding nonprescription drugs is to remain informed regarding all medications that patients are currently taking. It is necessary to verify that there are no contraindications or significant interactions with prescribed medications. It is also important to be aware that patients may against certain products that may interact negatively with other medications or with their particular medical condition(s).

V. Dietary Supplements

Dietary supplements are an overarching category of drugs that include vitamins, minerals, herbal remedies, and alternative medicines. The use of dietary supplements is an established practice among many elder adults. According to a recent study, almost half of elder adults living in the United States take some sort of dietary supplement on a regular basis. The same study identified that more than half of elder adults who take prescription medications also take supplements, which increases the potential for drug-drug interactions. The most common dietary supplements identified in this study were vitamins or minerals and system-specific remedies such as omega-3 fatty acids, garlic, and coenzyme Q for the cardiovascular problems;

四、非处方药物

老年人是非处方药的最大消费者。他们相信非处方药总是安全的；然而，许多处方药已被重新分类为非处方药。非甾体抗炎药和镇静类抗组胺药对老年人有潜在的严重危害。

老年人通常不会主动报告非处方药的使用情况。因此，错过了与药物有关的健康教育机会和检查处方药的相互作用可能使患者目前健康状况恶化。由于许多老年人视力下降、白内障、黄斑变性和其他视觉问题限制了他们阅读标签和说明书的能力，这一现实使教育的需求变得复杂。此外，中国最近的一项全国性研究发现，46% 服用处方药的患者也服用非处方药，从而增加了药物相互作用的可能性。

对于护士来说，非处方药的第一个挑战是了解患者目前服用的所有药物。有必要确认与处方药物没有禁忌证或明显的相互作用。同样重要的是要意识到，患者可能会反对某些产品，这些产品可能与其他药物或他们的特定医疗条件产生负面影响。

五、保健药物

保健药物包括种类繁多，常见的有维生素、钙剂、铁剂、中草药和替代类药物。据统计，大约 50% 的老年人规律地服用保健药物，而且同样大约 50% 多的老年人在服用保健品的同时服用处方药。许多保健品的疗效和安全性都没有经过系统的研究，因此，虽然一些保健品能够对老年人健康有益处，但也有潜在不良反应。如可能影响正常的生理过程而引起对健康的损害。因此，老年人对保健品的选择要慎重。

glucosamine-chondroitin for joint problems; and saw palmetto for prostate problems.

There are a number of additional concerns regarding the use of dietary supplements. They are not regulated for safety and efficacy by the Food and Drug Administration (FDA) in the same manner as prescription drugs, which undergo a rigorous drug approval process. As a result, there is a lack of predictable product quality and potency. The fact is that many herbs are available in their natural unprocessed state which can further complicate predictability. Beyond these concerns, the use and safety of these products in elder adults, especially in elder adults with comorbidities, have not been adequately studied.

As with any drug, dietary supplements have inherent adverse effects, particularly when taken in large doses. Although some dietary supplements may be beneficial, or at least not harmful, they may also interact with certain diseases and normal physiologic processes, which may lead to delayed improvement.

Section 4 Nursing Interventions for ADR Prevention in Elderly

According to statistics, among 50 million hospitalized patients each year in China, at least 2.5 million patients' admissions to hospital are ADR related. The incidence among the elderly is three times higher than in other groups and accounted for half of all ADR related deaths. So, nursing care of adverse drug reactions in the elderly is important.

Box 5-3 Introduction of *the 2015 America Geriatrics Society Beers Criteria*

The 2015 American Geriatrics Society (AGS) Beers Criteria are presented; it was updated from the 2012 version. It includes the lists of potentially inappropriate medications to be avoided in older adults. New to the criteria are the lists of select drugs that should be avoided or have their dose adjusted based on the individual's kidney function and select drug-drug interactions documented to be associated with harms in older adults. *The 2015 AGS Beers Criteria* are applicable to all older adults with the exclusion of those in palliative and hospice care. Careful application of the criteria by health professionals, consumers, payors,

人们对于使用营养补充剂存在许多额外顾虑。处方药需要通过食品和药品监督管理局的一系列严格药物审批流程，而营养补充剂却不同于处方药，并未经过同样的流程，无法监控其安全性和有效性。因此，无法预测营养补充剂的产品质量和功效。事实上，很多草药是在自然未加工状态下获得的，这增加了预测其功效的复杂性。除了这些顾虑外，老年人，尤其是多病共存的老年人，其使用这些产品的安全性尚未得到充分的研究。

正如任何药物一样，营养补充剂也有副作用，特别是在大剂量使用时。尽管一些营养补充剂可能有效，或是至少无害，但这些营养补充剂也会与特定疾病和正常生理过程发生相互作用，从而可能延缓其改善作用。

第四节　预防老年人用药不良反应的护理措施

据统计，我国每年5 000万住院患者中，至少有250万人的入院与ADR有关，其中重症ADR 50万人，死亡19万人，其中老年人数量比成年人高3倍以上，在所有ADR致死病例中占一半。因此老年人用药不良反应的护理是护理工作中重要的内容。

Box 5-3 《2015年美国老年医学会啤酒标准》介绍

介绍了《2015年美国老年病学会（AGS）啤酒标准》，从2012版更新。它包括老年人要避免的潜在不适当的药物清单。标准的新内容是应该避免的选择药物的列表，或者根据个体的肾功能调整其剂量，并选择记录为与老年人危害相关的药物－药物相互作用。《2015年AGS啤酒标准》适用于所有老年人，不包括姑息治疗和临终关怀护理。卫生专业人士，消费者，付款人和卫生系统认真适用

and health systems should lead to closer monitoring of drug use in older adults.

标准应对老年人使用药物进行监测。

I. Assessment of Drug Use

Nursing staffs should conduct a comprehensive assessment of drug use in the elderly for the purposes of preventing or eliminating adverse drug reactions. It includes the following aspects:

1. History of medication　Nurses should assess the indications for medications, and conduct detailed assessment of patient medication history including past and present records of drug use, drug allergies, causes of ADR, as well as elderly adult's perception for the drug use.

2. Ability of medication administration　Nurses need to assess elder people's intellectual status, such as reading, comprehension, memory, sight, and hearing. Meanwhile, nurses need to assess the ability of drug preparation, taking drug on time, detecting ADR in time, and ability of swallowing. Furthermore, nurses need to assess if the elder adults know why they are taking it, how they should be taking it, and what they actually take, and reasons for not taking the way as prescribed as well. Ability to pay for drugs should be assessed.

3. The function of body systems　Nurses need to carefully assess the function of body systems, such as biochemical markers of liver and renal function to facilitate judgment of rationality of drug use. Meanwhile, nurses should know clearly the therapeutic window of the drugs which the elderly taken.

4. Psychosocial conditions　Nurses should assess elder people's education level, dietary habits, and family financial status and family support. It is important to assess their understanding of drug use, and psychological reactions to drug use, such as dependence on the drug, expectations, and fears to drugs.

II. Health Education on Medication Management for the Elderly and Their Families

i. Explanation of Drug Use

Nurses should explain to the elderly and families about: type of drug, drug name, dosage, and duration of effects, adverse drug reactions correct ways of administration, and significance of adherence.

一、老年人用药评估

护理人员应全面评估老年人的用药情况，预防或消除药物不良反应。主要包括以下几个方面：

1. 老年人的用药史　详细评估老年人的用药史，建立完整的用药记录，包括既往和现在的用药记录、药物的过敏史、引起不良反应的药物，以及老年人对药物的认知情况。

2. 老年人服药的能力　评估老年人的智力状态如理解力、阅读能力、记忆力等，视力、听力、准备药物的能力、准时准量服药的能力及时发现不良反应的能力、吞咽能力等。此外，评估老年人是否知道为什么服用，应该如何服用，服用什么药，以及不按规定服用的理由。支付药费的能力也应该进行评估。

3. 老年人各系统的老化程度　仔细评估老年各脏器的功能情况，如肝、肾功能的生化指标。以判断药物使用的合理性。同时，护士应明确了解老年人用药的治疗窗口。

4. 老年人的心理–社会状况　评估老年人的文化程度、饮食习惯、家庭经济状况，对当前用药方案的了解、认识程度和满意度，家庭的支持情况，对药物有无依赖、期望、恐惧等心理。

二、家庭和老年人的用药健康教育

（一）加强老年人用药的解释工作

护理人员要以老年人能够接受的方式，向其解释药物的种类、名称、用药方式、药物剂量、药物作用、不良反应和药效时长等，同时，要反复强调正确服药的方法和重要性。

ii. Encouraging Non-drug Therapy as First Choice

Sometimes lifestyle changes can improve conditions and eliminate the need for medications. These can include diet modifications; regular exercise, effective stress management techniques, and regular schedules for sleep, rest, and elimination. Non-drug therapies have grown in acceptance and popularity among consumers and can offer effective and safe approaches to managing health conditions. It is crucial for nurses to be aware of the uses, limitations, precautions, and possible adverse reactions associated with alternative therapies, so that they can help elder adults be informed consumers.

iii. Discourage for Non-prescription Medication

Nurses should guide the elderly to take medication strictly follow the physician's orders. All adjustments of type or dosage of medication require physician's instruction, no matter the conditions are improving or deteriorating.

iv. Strengthening Drug Safety Education for Family Members

Family members have important roles of assisting and supervising the elderly administering medication. Nurses should pay more attention to drug safety education for family members, as well as the elderly to prevent accidents caused by improper use, especially for families with demented elderly.

III. Strategies for Improving Adherence

Drug compliance refers to the patient's obedience to or compliance with the doctor's order, refers to the patient's behavior and the degree of compliance with the clinical doctor's order, it is a kind of behavior that compliance with doctor's order. The elderly patients, especially those suffering from chronic diseases, their treatment effect is often not satisfactory, in addition to the etiology, pathogenesis is not clear, and lack of effective drugs, the important problem is the poor compliance with the doctor's order. The reasons for poor drug compliance in the elderly are due to memory decreased, it is easy for the elderly to miss or mistake drugs; because of reduced economic income, the life of the elderly is relatively tight, so they reduce or stop taking drugs by themselves; the elderly are worry about the side effect of the drugs, so they stop taking them; lack of the support from the family

（二）鼓励老年人首选非药物性治疗

有时生活方式的改变可以改善病情，减少药物治疗。这些包括饮食调整；有规律的锻炼；有效的压力管理技巧；有规律的睡眠，休息和排便。非药物治疗在消费者中越来越受到认可和欢迎，提供有效和安全的方法来管理健康状况。对护士来说，了解替代疗法的用途、局限性、预防措施和可能的不良反应是至关重要的，这样他们才能帮助老年人成为知情的消费者。

（三）指导老年人不擅自购买及服用非处方药物

护士应严格按照医嘱指导老年人服药。无论情况改善或恶化，所有药物的类型或剂量的调整都需要医生的指导。

（四）加强家属的安全用药知识教育

家庭成员在协助和监督老年人用药方面起着重要的作用。护士应重视对家庭成员和老年人的药物安全教育，防止因使用不当而造成的事故，特别是对有痴呆老人的家庭。

三、提高老年人服药依从性

服药依从性是指患者对医嘱的服从或遵从，是指患者求医后其行为与临床医嘱的符合程度，为遵循医嘱的行为活动。老年患者，尤其是患有慢性疾病的老年人治疗效果不满意，除与病因、发病机制不明，缺乏有效的治疗药物外，还有一个重要的问题，就是老年患者服药的依从性差。老年人服药依从性较差的原因有：①由于记忆力减退，容易漏服或错服药；②经济收入减少，生活相对拮据，导致擅自减药或停药；③担心药物副作用，自行停药；④家庭社会的支持不够，如长期服药治疗的慢性患者，没有家人的协助就医、服药，造成不能持续用药。提高老年

and community, such as chronic patients with long-term medication treatment. They have no family members to help them to see doctor and take medicine, resulting in the inability to continue measures to improve drug compliance in the elderly are as follows:

i. Promote Health Education

The patient's good treatment compliance is closely related to the patient's health concept and knowledge level. Therefore, whether in outpatient clinics, wards, or in the community, nursing staff can use special lectures, group discussions, developing materials, individual guidance and other comprehensive education methods, to carry out health education actively with the medical activities. Health education for elderly patients can improve their awareness of diseases and related knowledge, promote their adoption of a beneficial lifestyle, and consciously improve their drug compliance.

ii. Set up Collaborative Nurse-patient Relationship

The health belief model based on patient's feelings holds that if the patient subjectively feels that taking the drug according to the doctor's advice will benefit, the more likely it is to adopt compliance with the behavior. Nursing staff should encourage the elderly and their family members to participate in the formulation of treatment program and nursing plan, guide family members to observe changes of the patient's condition, supervise and guide patient to take medication, improve drug compliance. Additionally, and issue family drug records card to remind patient to take medication according to the record everyday, to avoid missing and taking more, and clearly record the number and time of the patient's medication, it is also an effective way to improve drug compliance.

iii. Interventions of Behavioral Therapy

Behavioral therapy measures include behavioral monitoring which maintain requiring elderly patients to keep a diary of their medication, self-observation records of their condition, etc. ; stimulation and control include linking the drug behavior of elderly patients to daily habits, such as setting an alarm to remind the time of taking medication; strengthening behavior involves giving recognition when the patient has good compliance, otherwise giving a reminder.

For different elderly people, different methods can be used to improve drug compliance:

1. For the elderly who is hospitalized, nursing

人服药依从性的护理措施如下：

（一）开展健康教育

患者良好的治疗依从性与患者的健康观念、知识层次密切相关。因此，无论是在门诊、病房、还是在社区，护理人员可采用专题讲座、小组讨论、发宣传材料、个别指导等综合性教育方法，在医疗活动中积极开展健康教育。对老年患者进行健康教育，提高对疾病以及相关知识的认识水平，促使其采取有益的生活方式，自觉地提高其服药依从性。

（二）建立合作性护患关系

以患者感受为核心基础的健康信念模式认为：患者若主观感受到采取遵医嘱服药行为将受益，则采取依从性行为的可能性越大。护理人员要鼓励老年人及其家属参与治疗方案与护理计划的制订，指导家属学会观察病情变化，监督指导患者服药，提高服药依从性；另外，发放家庭用药记录卡，提醒患者每日根据记录服药，避免漏服、多服的情况，并清楚记录患者的服药次数和时间，也是提高服药依从性的有效方法。

（三）行为治疗措施

行为治疗措施包括：①行为监测：要求老年患者记录服药日记、病情自我观察记录等。②刺激与控制：将老年患者的服药行为与日常生活习惯联系起来，如设置闹钟提醒服药的时间。③强化行为：当患者依从性好时给予肯定，反之给予提醒和指正。

针对不同的老年人，可以采取不同的方法提高服药依从性：

1. 对住院的老年人，护理人员应严格执

staff should strictly implement the procedures for administering medication, medication is delivered to the patient on time, and ensure that they take it.

2. For the elderly who still need to continue taking their medication after discharge from the hospital, the nursing staff should explain the name, dosage, effect, side effect and time of the drug to the elderly by oral or written ways. For example, the dose and time of the drug are indicated with a larger label in order to be recognized and remembered by the elderly. In addition, it is helpful to improve the drug compliance that community nurses visit to the home of the elderly regularly, and to count the remained number of pills based on prescription.

3. For the elderly with poor memory, the daily drug can be put in a special medicine box, this box includes a number of small boxes, each small grid indicates the time of the drug, and put the drug in a prominent position, to promote elderly patients to develop the habit of taking the drug on time.

4. For the elderly with dysphagia and confusion, medicine is generally administered through the nasal feeding tube. For the elderly who are conscious but have dysphagia, the drug can be processed into a paste and then given.

5. For external application, the nurses should elaborate and put a prominent label on the outside of the box, stating that it is not oral and inform the family members.

IV. Monitoring Adverse Drug Reactions in Elderly

i. Observation of Adverse Drug Reactions

Nurses should observe the adverse drug reactions which may occur after the administration to the elderly, and treat it in time. For example, when Digoxin is prescribed for the elderly, nurse should measure heart rate of old people before administering the medication, and ask whether there are Digoxin poisoning symptoms, such as yellow-green sight.

ii. Observation of Contradiction Reactions of Drugs

Contradiction refers to a special adverse drug reaction which is the opposite effect of the medication. Elder people are prone to drug contradiction. For example, Nifedipine is used to treat angina pectoris, but angina may get aggravated after use, or it may induce arrhythmia. Hence, nurses should observe carefully after

行给药操作规程，将药物按时送到患者床前，并确保其服下。

2. 对出院后仍需继续服药的老年人，护理人员要通过口头或书面的方式，向老年人解释药物名称、用量、作用、副作用和用药时间。如用字体较大的标签注明用药的剂量和时间，便以老年人识别和记忆。此外，社区护理人员定期到老年人家中根据处方清点其剩余药片的数目，也有助于提高老年人的服药依从性。

3. 对记忆力较差的老年人，可将每天需要服用的药物放置在专用的服药盒内，盒子若干小格，每个小格标明服药的时间，并将药品放置在醒目的位置，促使老年患者养成按时服药的习惯。

4. 对吞咽障碍及神志不清的老年人，一般通过鼻饲管给药。对神志清楚但有吞咽障碍的老年人，可将药物加工制作成糊状物后再给予。

5. 对于外用药物，护理人员应详细说明，并在盒子上外贴醒目标签，注明不可口服，并告知家属。

四、监测老年人用药不良反应

（一）密切观察药物不良反应

要注意观察老年人用药后可能出现的不良反应，及时处理。如对服用洋地黄类药物的老年人，服药前要测心率，经常询问老年人是否有黄绿视等洋地黄中毒症状。

（二）注意观察药物矛盾反应

老年人在用药后容易出现药物矛盾反应，即用药后出现与用药治疗效果相反的特殊不良反应。如用硝苯地平治疗心绞痛反而加重心绞痛，甚至诱发心律失常。所以用药后要细心观察，一旦出现不良反应时宜及时停药、

administrating medication which may have contradiction effects.

iii. Selects Dosage Form Easily Taken by Elderly

For old people with dysphasia, tablet and capsule are difficult to take, liquid dosage form, such as granules, oral liquid are better choice. If it is necessary, injection may be chosen for the elderly with dysphasia. The elderly with unstable gastrointestinal function should not take release inhibitor, because gastrointestinal function changes affect absorption of the drug.

iv. Ensure Appropriate Medication Time and Medication Interval

According to the ability of taking drugs and living habits of the elderly, drug administration should be as simple as possible. When therapeutic effect is similar between oral and injection drugs, oral drugs should be chosen first. Some drugs have interactions with food, so those drugs should be avoid taking at meal time. In addition, if the interval of administration is too long to achieve the therapeutic effect, and frequent administration is easy to cause drug poisoning. Therefore, when nurses plan medication schedule and interval, it is necessary to consider the schedule of the elderly and ensure effective blood concentration.

v. Other Measures to Prevent Adverse Drug Reactions

For old people with poor outcomes of medical treatments, nurses need to assess patients' adherence to treatment. For the old people with long-term drug use, blood concentration of the medication need to be monitored.

(GUO Hong)

Key Points

1. Achieving positive therapeutic outcomes and reducing ADRs requires knowledge of age related alterations that determine how elder adults react to drugs. Understanding of the unique problems attributable to aging, and awareness of resources to address problems and concerns related to medication use will facilitate nurses practice responsibility in improving patient medication management.

就诊，根据医嘱改服其他药物，保留剩药。

（三）选用便于老年人服用的药物剂型

对吞咽困难的老年人不宜选用片剂、胶囊制剂，宜选用液体剂型，如冲剂、口服液等，必要时也可选用注射给药。胃肠功能不稳定的老年人不宜服用缓释剂，因为胃肠功能的改变影响缓释药物的吸收。

（四）规定适当的服药时间和服药间隔

根据老年人的服药能力、生活习惯，给药方式尽可能简单，当口服药物与注射药物疗效相似时，则采用口服给药。由于许多食物和药物同时服用会导致彼此的相互作用而干扰药物的吸收。如含钠基或碳酸钙的制酸剂不可与牛奶或其他富含维生素D的食物一起服用，以免刺激胃液过度分泌或造成血钙或血磷过高。此外，如果给药间隔过长达不到治疗效果，而频繁地给药又容易引起药物中毒。因此，在安排服药时间和服药间隔时，既要考虑老人的作息时间又应保证有效的血浓度。

（五）其他预防药物不良反应的措施

由于老年人用药依从性较差，当药物未能取得预期疗效时，更要仔细询问患者是否按医嘱服药。对长期服用某一种药物的老年人，要特别注意监测血药浓度。

（郭　宏）

本章要点

1. 若要达到有效的治疗结果及减少药物不良反应，护理人员应该掌握增龄相关的药代动力学及药效动力学改变；理解与增龄相关的用药特殊问题；注意解决用药问题的方法，这样能够有助于护理人员在促进老年患者用药管理中实践其职责。

2. Elder adults consume a large proportion of pharmaceutical products. The use of inappropriate medications results in significant morbidity and mortality and adds economic burden to patients and health care systems.

3. Elder adults may be at risk for adverse drug reactions because of age related changes, multiple chronic illnesses, polypharmacy, non-adherence, and lack of knowledge.

4. A reduction in drug dosage is often required for elder adults with decreased renal or hepatic function and ability to excrete medications.

5. Knowledge of clinically important drug interactions is essential in planning alternative medication regimens and preventing potential serious ADRs.

6. Medication problems should always be suspected in patients experiencing overt or subtle changes in cognitive or physical function.

7. Nurse can play a key role not only in assessing patients for risk factors that may reduce compliance but also in developing strategies to reduce or to eliminate these risks.

8. For most medications prescribed for elder adults, it is necessary to start low, go slow, and periodically review medication regimens.

Critical Thinking Exercise

1. List age-related changes that affect the way in which drugs behave in elder persons.

2. What key points would you include in a program to educate senior citizens about safe drug use?

3. What interventions could you employ to aid an elder adult who has poor memory to safely administer medications?

4. Review major drug groups and identify problems that could potentially be managed with non-pharmacologic means.

5. A home care nurse is seeing an 81-year-old man who is taking a complex medication regimen. He cannot remember when he last took several of his medications, and his wife states she is confused by the recent switch of several drugs to other generic brands. What questions should nurse ask to establish list of risk of patient noncompliance?

2. 老年人消费是药物产品的很大一部分。不适当用药可造成患病率和病死率的增高，同时增加了患者及医疗系统的经济负担。

3. 增龄、患有多种慢性病、多重用药，用药不依从以及缺乏用药知识等因素均是老年人发生药物不良反应的危险因素。

4. 肾功能和肝功能减退的老年人排泄药物的能力减退，用药时需考虑减少剂量。

5. 临床中重要的药物之间相互作用的知识是计划替代性治疗和预防潜在的严重药物不良反应的基础。

6. 当患者经历明显或细微的认知或生理功能变化时，药物问题也应该被考虑到。

7. 护理人员不但在评估患者用药不依从的危险因素中承担重要角色，而且有责任发展减少不依从因素的策略。

8. 对于大多数服用处方药的老年人，从低剂量开始逐渐加量直至到最有效剂量，并且定期复查疗效是必要的。

批判性思维练习

1. 列举因增龄引起的老年人用药行为的变化。

2. 在对老年人做安全用药的健康教育计划中，你会给出哪些主要建议？

3. 你将运用哪些措施去帮助一个记忆力不好的老年人安全用药？

4. 回顾老年人常用药物种类，辨别可以用非药物疗法管理的健康问题。

5. 一位家庭护士看护一位81岁的老人，他进行着复杂的药物治疗方案。他记不住最近什么时候服用了几种药物，他的妻子述说她将最近更换的几种药和其他普通品牌的药混淆了。护士在建立患者服药不依从的计划单时应提出哪些问题？

Chapter 6 Home and Institutional Care

第六章 养老与照护

Learning Objectives

On completion of this chapter, the reader will be able to:

- Describe the impacts of social changes on long-term care of elder adults;

- Distinguish the categories and types of long-term care models;

- Describe the characteristics of different kinds of institutional care and the corresponding requirements;

- Describe a good living environment for improving the health of the elderly;

- List common issues related to home care;

- Discuss strategies to improve home care quality;

- Explain the meaning of quality of care for institutional care;

- List the strategies to improve the quality of institutional care.

学习目标

学完本章节，应完成以下目标：

- 描述社会变化对老年人长期照护的影响；

- 区分不同类型与形式的长期照护模式的特点；

- 描述不同类型的机构照护的特点及相应要求；

- 描述促进老年人健康的良好居住环境的特点；

- 列举居家照护中的常见问题；

- 讨论促进居家照护质量的策略；

- 解释机构照护质量的含义；

- 列举促进机构照护质量的策略。

Traditionally, elders are usually cared by their family members at home in China. As increased prevalence of long-term disability among older adults and decreased ability of informal support system to take care of frail elders, institutional care for the elderly is needed to supply long-term care in China. Institutional care will serve individuals who need the most care which are not available in the community. In this chapter, home and community-based care and institutional care are described in detail, and quality issues on institutional care and corresponding strategies to improve the quality are discussed.

中国的传统是老年人在家庭中养老，由家人提供养老照护。但在当今社会，随着老年人口寿命的增长，疾病所导致的失能老人人数逐渐增多，而家庭照护系统的功能却逐渐减弱。机构养老照护逐渐成为家庭照护的一个必要的补充。机构养老照护可以为那些无法获得家庭和社区照护系统的，但是又需要大量照护的老年人提供最终的照护场所。本章将详细阐述家庭与社区照护以及机构照护的特点及相应的问题，同时对于某些可促进照护质量的策略进行了相应的讨论。

Section 1　Social Impact on Elder Care

As the high prevalence of co-morbidity and disability among the elder population, many elders need assistance with care either related to daily living or disease management. This section will introduce different models of long-term care of the older adults.

I. Long-term Care Models for Elderly

The term of "long-term care" is most accurately used to describe a collection of health, personal, and social services provided over a prolonged period to people who have lost or never acquired functional capacity. Majority of the recipients of long-term care are older adults. Long-term care services range from supportive care to very complex care. According to the complexity of care provided and amount of skilled care and services required by the residents, long-term care settings can go from more structured to less structured as one moves from institutional setting to community-based programs to home setting. Table 6-1 illustrates this continuum of long-term care settings.

According to the settings of long-term care, there are two major kinds of long-term care models for elderly. They are community-based elderly care as well as institution-based elderly care.

第一节　社会变化对养老照护的影响

随着老年人多病共患与失能人数的增长，越来越多的老年人或者需要日常生活照料的辅助，或者需要疾病的管理。本节将对不同形式的长期照护模式及其特点进行介绍。

一、常见的养老照护模式

长期照护这个词汇常用于描述那些为失去功能的人群所提供的一系列与健康相关的、个体的，以及社会化的服务。长期照护服务的接受者大部分为老年人。长期照护提供的服务包含内容较广，可以由支持性的服务到比较复杂的服务。根据所提供的照护服务的特点，如所需的专业性照护的量和照护持续时间的长短，提供长期照护的场所可以从非机构性场所过渡到机构性的场所照护。表 6-1 中介绍了不同长期照护场所下可提供的养老照护模式。

根据提供的长期照护的场所的不同，可将长期照护模式分为两类，即以社区为基础的养老照护和以机构为基础的养老照护。

Table 6-1　Continuum of Long-term Care Settings

Home	Community	Institutional
Home health nursing	Adult day care center	Nursing facility
Home health rehabilitative services	Senior center	Assisted living
Homemaker	Congregate meal programs	Special care units
Home-delivered meals	Hospice	Continuing care retirement communities
Adaptive devices to home environment		Hospice
Hospice		

表 6-1　不同长期照护场所的照护服务

居家	社区	机构
居家健康照护	成人日间照护中心	养老院
居家健康康复服务	老人活动中心	有助聚居
家务服务	集体就餐服务	特殊照护单元
送餐服务	临终关怀	连续照护型退休社区
居家宜居辅助设备		临终关怀
临终关怀		

i. Community-based Elderly Care

Community-based elderly care services usually include home health care, community-based alternative programs, respite care, adult day care programs, senior citizen centers, and other access services.

1. Home health care　The purpose of the home health care is to help the elderly who has a physical or cognitive impairment at home. An older adult with a specific diagnosis may receive home health care for a limited time and be provided with assessment, observation, teaching, certain technical skills and personal care. In addition, after a concrete assessment, homemaker services could be provided either in short-term or long-term period.

2. Adult day care services　It provides a variety of health and social services to the elderly who live alone or with their families in the community. The role of adult day care programs is to help delay institutionalization for older adults who need some supervision but without need continuous care. Thus, older adults, who are physically frail and/or cognitive impaired and need ADLs assistance and monitoring, are eligible for this service. Most of adult day care services operate 5 days a week during typical business hours. Key services may include assistance with personal

（一）以社区为基础的养老照护

以社区为基础的养老照护模式包括居家健康照护、社区选择性服务、喘息照护、成人日间照料服务、老年人社区活动中心及其他一些可及的服务。

1. 居家健康照护　此服务的目的是帮助那些具有生理或者认知功能受损的老年人尽可能在家中生活。有特殊疾病诊断的老年人，他们所需的居家健康照护可以是短期的，主要是对患者提供评估、观察、指导或提供某些特别的技术或者个人照护服务。另外，经过具体的评估之后，也要短期或者长期地给予日常家务服务。

2. 成人日间照护服务　它可以为独自在社区生活的或者与家人共同生活的老年人提供多种服务。这种服务的目的是延迟那些需要某些部分而非持久性照护的老年人入住养老机构的时间。因此，对于那些有生理功能受损、认知功能受损、需要部分日常生活照料和监护的老年人可以使用这种服务形式。大部分日间照护中心每周开放 5 天，每天开

care, nursing and therapeutic services, meals, recreational activities, and transportation to and from the facility. Some programs only accept elderly with dementia. The services allow family members to provide home care for their older relatives and maintain their employment at the same time.

3. Respite care Respite care provides short-term relief or time off for family members providing home care for ill, disabled, or frail older relatives. The difference between respite care and adult day care program is respite care is usually provided at home or in institutional settings (e. g. , specially designated hospital or nursing facility units). In-home and institutional respite care can be provided on a regular schedule (e. g. , 6 hours a week) or for longer time intervals (e. g. , 1 week, a weekend). Respite staff usually includes healthcare personnel, trained volunteers, and personal care attendants.

4. Homemaker services These services include something as housekeeping, laundry, food shopping, meal preparation, and running errands. Individuals who provide the care usually do not need to be licensed or certificated. However, background checks and letters of recommendations are often requested as the qualifications for the positions.

5. Nutrition services These services provide the elderly with inexpensive, nutritious meals at home or in group settings. Home-delivery programs (e. g. , Meals-on-Wheels) deliver hot meals to home once or twice a day, 5 days a week, even with some special diets. The frequencies are based on clients' needs. Home-delivery nutrition services can also give a chance to the volunteer delivering the meal to check on the older adult daily and report any problems to the supervisor. Congregate meal sites provide meals in group settings such as churches, senior centers, and senior housing. The congregate meal services provide social opportunities for older adults who are otherwise socially isolated.

6. Transportation services Some communities provide transportation services for disabled elderly through public or private agencies. The transportation usually accommodates wheelchairs. The fee for such transportation services is usually minimal. Many care facilities for elderly also freely provide their own transportation services.

放时间与社会工作时间相一致。日间照护中心会提供个人照护、治疗性护理服务、饮食服务、娱乐活动，以及相应的交通服务。某些日间照护中心则只对痴呆患者开放。总之，日间照护中心这种服务形式使得家庭成员能正常上班，保留工作；同时家人又能将老年人留在家中在下班时间或者周末给予照顾。

3. 喘息照护 喘息照护是给家中的患者、失能者或者衰弱的老年人提供照护并给家庭照顾者提供短期的休息机会。此服务形式与日间照护中心的区别是喘息照护通常在患者的家中或者机构中提供服务。这种服务可以是定期提供的（如每周6小时的服务）或者更长一些间隔时间（如持续一周，或者一个周末等）。喘息照护的服务提供者应该包括健康专业人员、受过训练的志愿者、个人卫生服务人员等。

4. 家务服务 这种养老服务形式提供多项服务内容，包括清扫房间、洗衣服、做饭、帮助购物及随时供差遣等服务。服务提供者不需要证书或者专业培训，但是他们的背景资料往往在雇佣前需要被审查，以保护被照顾者的安全。

5. 营养配餐服务 此种服务为老年人提供便宜的、营养的居家食物。上门送饭服务可以每天1~2次，每周5天，甚至可以为老年人提供某些特别的饮食。这种上门服务也可以使得送饭上门的志愿服务者能每天观察老年人的状况，如有异常可以马上报告给相关人员。营养服务也可以为一组老年人提供服务，可以将老年人聚集在某些场所，然后集中提供营养服务，同时也使得就餐老年人间彼此有一定的社交机会。

6. 交通运送服务 一些社区也为老年人和有残障的老年人提供交通运送服务。这种运送往往可以将轮椅搬上搬下，服务费用也很便宜。很多老年人服务项目都为老年人免费提供相应的交通运送服务。

7. Hospice services　These services are provided by an interdisciplinary team consisting of the client's own physician, hospice physicians, nurses, medical social workers, bereavement coordinators, and volunteers. Team members use their expertise and skills to meet the needs of dying persons and their families. These needs include but not limited to teaching family and friends how to administer medications, helping dying persons maintain as much mobility and activity as possible, and listening and responding to a dying person's needs. Help from the hospice team is available 24 hours a day. One member of the team is always on call and will make home visits as needed any time. However, the dying person and his or her family direct the care and are directly involved in the decision-making process. Historically, most hospice programs are provided at the dying person's own home. Now it is not necessary for a terminally ill person to be homebound or to have a skilled nursing aid. Hospice team consults and supports the family in their commitment to care for the hospice client. If the person does not have any family caregivers, the hospice program can still maintain the dying individuals in their homes. Hospice services can across different settings in which care provided, such as in nursing homes or hospitals.

ii. Institution-based Elderly Care

As mentioned in table 6-1, long-term care for elderly can be provided in institutions. Persons living in these institutional facilities are called residents. The facility is their permanent or temporary home. Some residents stay for a short time to recover from an acute illness, surgery, or injury. After the recovery, they return home. Other residents require nursing care in nursing facilities until death. There are several kinds of institution-based elderly care which are illustrated as the follows:

1. Skilled nursing facilities　Skilled care is delivered by nurses and others to residents. Care may be sub-acute (short stay) or chronic for frail elderly residents requiring help with activities of daily living.

2. Assisted living programs　Assisted living facilities have been considered as a place between home care and the nursing facility in the continuum of long-term care. Assisted living settings are homelike and offer a variety of services, including assistance with dressing and bathing, preparing meals, personal laundry and house-keeping services, social and recreational programs, transportation, 24-hour security, and emergency call

7. 临终关怀服务　这种服务往往由一组专业人士组成，包括医生、护士、社会工作者、葬礼安排人员和志愿者等。这组人员用他们的专业知识和技能满足临终患者和其家人的需求，如指导家人如何给临终患者服用药物，如何尽可能地帮助患者进行力所能及的活动，如何满足临终患者的需要等。来自这支专业队伍的帮助可以是24小时的。小组成员中每天都有1个人通过电话进行24小时的值班，以保证需要时的家庭出诊。临终患者和家人均参与照护活动和照护决策。既往的临终关怀服务是在临终患者家中提供的，但是现在这种服务还可以扩展到护理院等机构内。

（二）以机构为基础的养老照护

如表6-1所示，老年人的长期照护也可以通过机构照护的形式加以实现。某些老年人只是短暂停留在养老机构，如养老院里。他们入住的原因可能是由于术后的恢复需要，或者处于某些疾病或者伤害的康复期。当他们身体健康恢复到一定程度后，就可以回到自己的家中。还有一些老年人会在养老机构中一直居住到死亡。机构照护的形式有多种：

1. 护理院　护理院的专业性照护和技能性照护需要护士和其他相关专业人士给予提供。照护可以针对老年人的亚急性（短期停留）或者慢性病老年人的需要而提供日常功能照护。

2. 有助聚居　有助聚居被认为是介于居家和护理院之间的一种形式。有助聚居机构的环境很类似于居家的环境，同时提供各式服务，如帮助穿衣和洗澡、帮助准备饭菜、帮助洗衣服和做家务，以及安排一些社交和娱乐活动等。有助聚居还可以提供24小时保安和急救运送、给药、少量的医疗处置以及

system, health checks, medication administration, and minor medical treatments. Residents purchase the services based on their needs. There are more opportunities for health care personnel to incorporate both health promotion and illness care into the model.

3. Special care units Started from 1980 in the US, special care unit (SCU) is designed to meet the caring needs of people with Alzheimer's disease and other types of dementia-related illness. In the SCUs, behavioral manifestations of dementia are managed in the environment without use of chemical or physical restraints whenever possible.

4. Continuing care retirement communities Continuing care retirement communities (CCRC) is a type of retirement community where a number of aging care needs, from assisted living, independent living and nursing home care, may all be met in a single residence. These various levels of shelter and care are housed on different floors or wings of a single high-rise building or in physically adjacent buildings. Typically, elderly candidates move into CCRC while still living independently, with few health risks or healthcare needs, and will remain reside there until end of life. As patrons progress in age, and medical needs change, the level of nursing care service increases proportionally in response. If greater illness or injury warrants hospitalization, the patron may return to his or her residence after recovery, and should receive appropriate treatment and care. CCRC are ideal for seniors that may be living in isolation, and would like to be immersed in a hospitable environment with other people of the same age. Typically, a range of activities and amenities are provided for both recreation and resource. However, CCRCs are costly, and vary widely in entrance and recurring fees.

5. Hospice services Except the difference on the setting of providing care, the content of services is as same as the one provided at the dying person's own home. Hospice services in the institutions still emphasize the multidisciplinary work. Hospice professionals need to prepare a family for the loss of a dying person. Various types of bereavement services are also available after the patient' death, such as family counseling, bereavement volunteer visits, and grief classes.

健康查体等服务。

3. **特殊照护单元** 开始于 1980 年的美国，主要用于照护阿尔茨海默病的患者或者其他类型的痴呆患者。在特殊照护单元，对于痴呆患者的行为问题的管理不主张使用物理或者化学性的约束方法，而应该尽可能地改善环境，使其符合痴呆老年人的现存能力，进而减少痴呆行为的发生。

4. **连续照护型退休社区** 连续照护型退休社区是由一系列的养老服务形式所组成的，从独立居住、有助聚居到护理院照护，全部都可以在一个居住社区得以实现。不同类型的照护服务被安排在这个大社区的不同的区域或者楼层中。一般情况下，最开始进入这个社区的老年人是能相对独立生活的，相对较健康。他们在这个社区里一直生活到去世。随着机体健康的变化，照护需求的增长，老年人对护理照护的需要也逐渐增加。老年人可以因为某些急性病或者严重的健康问题入住医院进行治疗，出院后即回到这个社区，根据患者的不同健康需要被安排在不同的照护区域，最终至能最大限度地相对独立生活。退休社区适合于资源不足的老人，在退休社区中他们可以得到与同年龄段老人一样的医疗照护和其他服务。但此种照护形式花费较高。

5. **临终关怀服务** 除了所提供临终关怀服务的场所不同之外，服务的内容与居家临终服务是基本一致的。在机构内的临终服务仍然强调由不同专业人士组成的服务小组为临终患者和其家庭提供服务，如为临终患者提供直接照护，为家庭成员进行指导、咨询，提供葬礼服务等。

II. Impact of Social Changes on Long-term Care for Elderly

By the end of 2018, there were 2.49 million people 60 years of age or over, accounting for 17.9% of total population in China. It is estimated that China could have about 487 million people 60 years of age or over by 2050. Traditionally, family-based care is the predominant model for the older adults. However, as life expectancy and the size of the older adult population increase, the possibility of a person entering a nursing facility at some point also grows.

China has changed dramatically in recent years, including the changing of family structure. In traditional Chinese society, the elderly used to live with one of their children. But nowadays, more and more young adults are moving out, leaving their elderly parents alone. A nationwide survey found that about 23 percent of China's seniors over the age of 65 live by themselves. Family-based care is now impractical because most middle-aged children have little time to take care of their parents. So one of the things the elderly have to face nowadays is how to arrange their late years when their families cannot take care of them.

The demographic trends suggest that the demand for the kinds of long-term care services now being provided mainly by nursing homes is certain to increase. In addition to the effects of health status on survival, changes in health status may directly affect the chance of institutionalization for the elderly. For instance, with increasing numbers of person over 85 years old, there may be an increase in survival and increased number of people with chronically morbid, and physically and mentally impairment. This would increase the demand for intensive nursing home care.

Despite the increasing challenge of caring for current and future elders, family support for frail elders will continue to be the key care pattern in China which is consistent with Chinese culture. It is still critical to develop community-based long-term care services and programs to help informal caregivers support their elders.

In addition, improved longevity over the past two decades is causing an increase in the prevalence of chronic disease and disability in the population. China is currently working to develop policies and initiatives around elderly care, especially innovative approaches to providing support via health care and social care, and challenges that

二、社会变化对老年人长期照护的影响

在中国，截止到 2018 年年底，60 岁及以上老年人口已经达到 2.49 亿，占全国总人口的 17.9%。预计到 2050 年，中国 60 岁及以上的老年人口将达到 4.87 亿。传统上，家庭照护模式是中国老年人养老的最主要的模式。但是，随着人口寿命的增长和老年人数目的增加，老年人进入机构进行养老的可能性也在增长。

中国社会近年来发生了较大的变化，包括家庭结构的改变。既往老年人常和自己的子女生活在一起，但是现在越来越多的年轻子女离开老年人而独自生活。一项全国范围的调查发现，中国 65 岁以上的老年人中约有 23% 独自生活。家庭式的照护模式在目前的中国受到冲击，这是因为大部分的子女因为工作的原因很少有时间照护他们的老年人。因此，老年人们在晚年时将要面临的一个问题就是谁来照护他们。

中国人口学数字的变化也提示对于护理院等长期照护的需求在增长。除了生存年限增长这个原因外，健康状况的变化也是导致老年人入住养老机构的一个原因。如随着 85 岁以上的老年人越来越多，他们可能伴有的慢性疾病就越多、功能受限的可能性就越大，需要大量护理的可能性就越高。

虽然中国社会面临老年人养老的挑战，但是依据中国的传统，家庭式的照护目前还将是中国社会的主要养老模式。同时，发展相应的以社区为基础的养老照护模式也是迫切需要的，这样就可以帮助家庭照顾者将老年人尽可能留在家中接受照护。

此外，随着人口寿命的增长，老年群体中慢性疾病的发生率和失能率也在逐渐增加。中国政府正在制订相关的政策和方法来面对这一严峻挑战，特别提出通过医养结合的方式来照护老年人，使他们在得到照顾的同时

elderly patients face in access to medications. The long-term care system should reflect the characteristics of the combination of medical care and living support.

还得到良好的医疗和护理。中国的长期照护体系也要将医养结合的理念融入到其工作实践中，以更好地解决老年人的养老问题。

Section 2　Home Care

第二节　居家养老照护

Home care refers to any type of care given to the elderly in their own homes. Home care is an old-age insurance socialized service supported by community and society, aiming to offer services to the aged people in their own homes. It includes professional health care services, life assistance services and psychological comforts. Care received in the home provides the elderly with the opportunity to maintain control over significant aspects of their lives. Being cared at home, the aged can gain a steady sense of belonging, which is of great significance for fostering self-respect and a complete self-image of the elderly.

居家养老照护是由社区和社会帮助家庭为居家老年人提供生活照料、医疗护理和精神慰藉等方面服务的一种社会化的养老服务形式。居家养老对老年人获得自尊和保持完整的自我有着重要的意义。

I. Environmental Arrangements for Home Care

The environment within which older persons live can profoundly affect their health, well-being, independence and quality of life, particularly when they are vulnerable, and the influence of care environments on patients has long been a fundamental concern to nurses. The worse an individual adapts to the environment, the greater the risk to their security and well-being is. Creating a good living environment is very significant for promoting the health of the elderly and improving the quality of life of older persons.

i. Home Physical Environment

There is a direct relationship between health and housing. When an individual is in poor health, impaired, or having functional declines due to aging, health concerns are virtually indistinguishable from housing concerns, particularly in an aging housing condition. To compensate for and help manage health conditions, the physical environment of homes can be both prosthetic and therapeutic. As a prosthetic environment, the home can compensate for limitations in functional abilities to enable individuals to carry out basic activities associated with daily living safely and independently, participate in social roles, and receive personal assistance from caregivers as

一、居家养老的环境安排

营造良好的生活环境，对促进老年人的健康，提高老年人的生活质量有着重要的意义。

（一）家庭内的物理环境

为了适应老年人的健康状况，应重视居室环境的改善。居室环境的改善要遵循的原则是自理、安全、方便和舒适。

needed. Therapeutically, the environment can facilitate health maintenance and management by supporting health-promoting behaviors and provision of health care services. Home adaptation or modification can provide elder friendly living so older occupants may continue to live in comfort home. The focus of making a home elder-friendly should always be on increasing and improving the following four elements: self-sufficiency/self-reliance, safety/security, comfort and convenience.

1. Lighting　Light affects older people's ability to see, function and move around, and consequently his or her orientation. Good lighting improves safety and reduces some types of fatigue. Light can come from natural or artificial sources. Older adults require higher light levels and may have a greater sensitivity to glare. Lighting must be adequate, particularly in potentially hazardous areas such as on the staircase. Glare should be avoided and diffuse lighting is more desirable than that of very high levels. Use blinds, shades, or curtains to minimize glare from windows. Provide general or ambient light throughout the room to eliminate dark areas and allow for good visibility for people to move around. Keep brightness levels within a room and the adjacent spaces about the same. Identify where visual tasks will be performed, and put extra light at those places. Install switches near room entrances and near the bed for easy access.

2. Color contrast　Different colour schemes can influence mood or activity, for example pale, clear blue and green provide a relaxing environment, yellows are cheerful, and touches of bright red encourage activity. Color contrast is important for people to be able to see stairs or food. A coloured object on a white surface is preferable to the other way around because bright surfaces reflect up to 80 per cent of the light falling on it; a dark surface reflects no more than 20 percent. Identify steps, stairs, drop-offs, and edges by using a bright color paint and texture provided by sand additives. Paint the edge of each step, the top and bottom of ramps, and the edges of walkways. The edges of doorways and windows can be identified by having the molding done in a dark color if the walls are light, or in white if the walls are bright colors.

3. Temperature, humidity and ventilation　Adequate thermal comfort, both in summer and winter, boosts the mood, increases performance and in some cases prevents and alleviates diseases. The ability to adapt to changes in humidity or temperature is directly related to comfort. Most older adults feel comfortable at a room temperature of 22-24℃ with the humidity at 50%±10%. An individual who has difficulty adapting

1. **光线**　房间里光线应充足，避免强光照射。安装夜灯，每个房间的入口处和床旁应安装电灯开关，方便老年人使用。

2. **颜色**　色彩对人的情绪和行为有一定的影响。使用不同的颜色可以产生不同的情绪反应。台阶、楼梯踏步、扶手采用鲜艳的颜色，便于老年人行走。

3. **温湿度和通风**　老年人体温调节能力差，室温应以 22～24℃较为适宜，合适的湿度则为（50%±10%）。开窗通风可以调节室内湿度，保持空气新鲜，减少室内污染。

to high temperature may experience a rapid rate, cramps, nausea, and vomiting. Severe inability to adapt to heat can result in heat stroke and death. An individual who has difficulty adapting to lower temperature may experience a change in behavior, depressed vital signs and eventual unconsciousness. Extremes of heat or cold increase the incidence of infection and add to discomfort. Temperatures can be regulated with air conditioners and dehumidifiers. An adequately ventilated room should contain a comfortable amount of moisture and is free of (if there are) irritating pollutants, odors, or noxious fumes. Proper ventilation can reduce airborne contaminants.

4. Living room The doorways should be wide enough to allow a person to pass a wheel chair. The threshold should be flush with the floor and there should be no barrier on the way from room to room. Scatter rugs and loose throw rugs should be removed. Textured strips or nonskid wax on hardwood and tile floors should be used to prevent slipping. Do not have electrical cords trailing across the floor.

Stairways can present problems, particularly for falls. Railings should be installed on both sides of the stairs, and must be securely attached to provide adequate support. Stairs are free of clutter and debris. Stair treads are dry, not wet or icy. Treads should preferably have slip resistant surface or at least non slip stripes at the edge to avoid slipping. The treads and risers may have contrasting colors to make them clearly defined for elderly with poor vision.

The location of furniture should be arranged to make the elderly parent can hold on to something as they move around the house and avoid clutter. All remaining furniture should be stable and without sharp corners, to minimize the effects of a fall.

5. Bathroom The bathroom is one of the most dangerous places in the home for the elderly. It is preferable if the bathroom door can be unlocked from the outside. Bathroom lighting should be adequate so that puddles of water or other potential hazards will be easily visible. Floors in bathroom should have non-slip tiles. Use of rubberized mats in shower area will minimize falls caused slipping. Grab bars (preferably steel) should be strategically placed along water closets, urinals, wash basins and shower areas which aim to assist the elderly persons to perform their daily actives with ease. All the accessories in the bathroom should be accessible to the person in a wheel chair. There should be clear and safe access to windows or an extractor fan to allow adequate ventilation. Water temperature controls are properly installed and clearly

4. 起居室 门口足够宽，方便轮椅通过，避免设置门槛。室内地板选用防滑材料，去除松散的地毯，地板上不能有电线。

楼梯装设扶手，避免堆放杂物，阶梯边缘有醒目标志，阶梯边缘最好加上防滑贴条，避免跌倒。

调整家具的位置，以便于老年人在室内行走时扶握，家具牢固固定，避免杂乱摆放。家具的转角应尽量用弧形，以免碰伤老年人。

5. 浴室 浴室是老年人家中最危险的地方之一。浴室的门应从外面可以打开，光线应充足。地面铺防滑砖，在沐浴区放置橡胶垫以防跌倒。确保轮椅上的老年人可以使用浴室中的所有设施。浴室内安装扶手和通风装置，同时应安装水温控制装置以防烫伤。

labeled. All hot water in the older person's home should be controlled thermostatically to a maximum temperature of 120 degrees Fahrenheit to avoid burns.

6. Kitchen areas Flooring should not be slippery and should be having a non-glare surface. Kitchen ventilation system or range exhausts should be in proper working order and utilized when cooking. Place towels, curtains, and other things that might catch fire away from the kitchenware. Avoid wearing clothes with long loose-fitting sleeves while cooking. Do not use the gas range or the oven to heat the home. Kitchen wall cabinets cannot be too high to be easily reached.

ii. Family Social Environment

The family social environment mainly refers to the inter-personal relationships in the family, including relationships between spouses, parents and kids, siblings, mothers-in-law and daughters-in-law, and grandparents and the kids. These relationships form an interrelated and interactive family relationship network. Tension of any of these relationships can bring harms to the steady and harmony of the family. Among these relationships, spousal relationship is the core, and relationship between parents and kids is also attached with great importance.

1. Relationship between spouses Relationship between spouses is seen as the core. Among family members, the spouse has the biggest possibility of talking to the aged partner from the heart and offering tender help. A spouse provides financial support, daily caring as well as psychological comforts, irreplaceable by the children. Whether male or female, the spouse is always seen as the first to look after the partner besides him/herself. In psychological comforting, spouse is the first choice for the aged to communicate, children coming next. Due to the great importance of spouse, once the spouse is lost, great hurt will be caused to the aged. For the elders, losing spouses equals to psychological loneliness and the loss of daily caring.

With the prolonging of life expectancy, the increasing elder couples depend on each other for late years. According to some researches, under normal conditions, the aged with spouses enjoy better life quality than those who lost spouses or were divorced. However, the role of the caring played by the spouse declines with age.

2. Relationship between generations It is very clear that a large majority of the Chinese elderly live with their children, and the higher the age, the higher the proportion living with their children. Elderly females of

6. **厨房** 厨房地面应防滑，安装通风装置。毛巾、窗帘和其他易燃物品应远离灶台。不要使用煤气灶或烤箱加热室内。厨房吊柜不宜太高，以方便老年人取物。

（二）家庭内的社会环境

家庭内的社会环境主要指的是家庭内的人际关系，包括夫妻关系、亲子关系、兄弟姐妹关系、婆媳关系、祖孙关系等。这些关系共同构成了一个互相联系、互相影响的家庭关系的网络。其中任何一种家庭关系的紧张，都有可能影响到整个家庭的稳定与和谐。在这些家庭关系中，夫妻关系是核心，父母子女关系是重点。

1. **夫妻关系** 夫妻关系是家庭关系的核心。在所有的家庭成员中，配偶最可能成为老年人的知心人和提供救助。配偶在经济支持、日常生活照护和精神慰藉方面都发挥着儿女们无法代替的作用。由于配偶角色的重要性，一旦失去配偶就会对老年人的身心造成很大损伤。对于老年人来说，丧偶意味着精神上孤独和生活上无人照料。

随着预期寿命的延长，更多的老年夫妻依靠彼此支持和照护来度过晚年。研究显示，有配偶的老年人比丧偶者或离婚的老年人享有更好的生活质量。但是，随着年龄的增长，配偶所扮演的关怀角色将逐渐减少。

2. **代际关系** 在老年人的非正式照护网络中，子女是老年人照护的重要基础。照护内容包括了对老年人的经济支持、日常生活照料、精神疏导和患病情况下的护理等。

all age groups are more likely to live with their children, because elderly women are more likely to be economically dependent and widowed. Chinese elderly more rarely live with other people than with offspring and spouses. In the informal support network of older people, children are the foundation. Caring includes financial support, daily caring, psychological comfort and caring during sickness.

Adult children are often involved in direct caregiving activities for their older parents. The legal responsibility of adult children to support their older parents has been a Chinese tradition for thousands of years. It is children's responsibility to show their filial piety when their parents become elderly. When the People's Republic of China was established in 1949, this tradition was written into the Constitution. Filial piety includes both feeding and respecting. "Feeding" mainly refers to providing financial support and caregiving to the aged. "Respecting" is related to the spiritual respect, emotional and social support for older family members. The sense of filial responsibility revives and social pressure remains strong when one parent falls ill or dies. Adult children often take over functions that older parents can still fulfill-even with difficulty. Actually, too much loving protection can be destructive to aging parents. The wish to protect an older person who is becoming increasingly frail is natural; however, this is usually the last thing an older person wants or needs.

Due to declining fertility, urban drift, increasing divorce rate, extremely rapid population aging, and the increased participation of women in the workforce, the traditional family structure of the country has greatly changed. The "4-2-1" family structure and the "empty nest" have occurred. The "4-2-1" family structure refers to the pyramid of four grandparents, two parents, and one single child in a family. It is extremely difficult for an adult couple to provide support for their combined four aging parents and/or grandparents while taking care of their own child and maintaining successful careers in an increasingly fast-paced Chinese society. The modernization of China has created enormous opportunities for young adults determined to improve their living standards. Many young adults have left their parents to pursue freedom and economic prosperity, which leads to the increasing prevalence of "empty nests", where older adults live alone. Older adults living alone, particularly those residing in the countryside, are the most vulnerable population. Empty nests threaten the viability of the traditional way of caring for older Chinese. The collapse of big families and the fading of family affections both have enlarged the

中华民族有敬老、爱老的美德。儒家文化也素来强调孝敬父母。中国宪法规定"父母有抚养教育未成年子女的义务，成年子女有赡养扶助父母的义务。"赡养老年人是家庭传统的功能。由于我国传统家庭结构和规模发生了变化，代际关系出现"重心下移"，尊老孝道观念需要继续保持和加强。

随着出生率下降、城市化进程加快、农村人口外出打工率上升，离婚率增加、人口老龄化、女性就业者增加等原因，我国的传统家庭结构发生了巨大变化，"4-2-1"家庭和空巢老人带来的社会问题越来越多。"4-2-1"家庭是指由四位祖父母，一对夫妇，以及这对夫妇的一个孩子所组成的家庭结构。对一对成人夫妇而言，他们同时要照顾四位父母甚至他们的祖父母，还要照顾孩子和工作，面临非常大的困难。随着中国社会的发展，越来越多的年轻人都离开家乡到其他城市中寻求更好的发展，导致中国出现很多的空巢家庭，老年人单独生活，特别是生活在农村的空巢老人，是非常脆弱的人群，需要特别的关注。传统大家庭的分散和家庭感情的淡漠影响了代系间的亲情关系，使得传统的家庭养老方式逐渐减弱，并且无法满足未来老年人口增长的需求。

gaps between generations, which impacts the mood and life quality of the aged. Today, generation relationship has shifted its focus. As a result, the traditional pattern of family support as a way of caring for the older Chinese is weakening and will not meet the needs of the booming older population in the upcoming decades.

iii. Social Environment

As the older population increases and family structure changes, the domestic function of providing for the aged has been weakening gradually. Naturally, the family's obligation to provide for the aged has been shared by the society. Social environment can play an important role in caring the elderly.

1. Government China has not been well-prepared for meeting the health needs of its growing elderly population. The Chinese government has only recently acknowledged the consequences of the rapid population aging and has started to address them in various policies and programs. Though public funding for the long-term care of the elderly in China is still limited, the Chinese government has started to allocate more funding in this area. The Chinese government has gradually established a uniform basic old-age insurance system in urban areas that covers all the employees of different types of enterprises, persons engaged in individual businesses of industry or commerce, and people who are employed in a flexible manner. It has begun to study the establishment of an old-age social security system in rural areas in order to guarantee the basic livelihood of the elderly people there. China will establish a subsidy system for elder care services, which will enable low-income senior citizens who are physically challenged or lived alone, to move to nursing homes or enjoy home care services on government subsidies. In addition, part of residents over 80 years old will be entitled to a unified monthly allowance across China.

At present, the country has developed a full set of law system, covering retirement, health care, life care service, maintenance of rights, spiritual life and so on, and the career of caring the aged is institutionally secured.

2. Community With the acceleration of population aging, community is playing a more and more important role in social development. Therefore, community's involvement in the aged care becomes an inevitable tendency. The community-based system for providing care to the elderly is a model which allows the elderly to continue living at home by providing

（三）社会环境

随着老年人口的增加和家庭结构的变化，家庭养老的功能逐渐减弱。社会承担的养老责任越来越重要。

1. **政府** 中国政府已经意识到人口老龄化带来的问题，并已开始制订各种政策和方案解决这些问题。目前，中国已经逐步在城市和农村地区建立了相应的基本养老保险制度和社会保障制度。此外，身体残障或独居的低收入老年人能够入住养老机构并享受政府补贴的养老金。部分 80 岁以上的中国居民可根据户籍地政策按月领取津贴。

目前我国已经基本形成了一套涵盖养老、医疗、生活照料服务、权益维护、精神文化生活等多方面内容的老龄政策法规体系，老龄事业的发展有了较好的制度保障。

2. **社区** 随着人口老龄化速度加快，社区参与养老是必然的趋势。目前，我国已经初步形成了一套较为完备的社区居家养老服务运作体系，各地努力探索社区居家养老模式，已经积累了一些经验。在部分大中城市已初步形成了设施服务、定点服务和上门服

additional support through community centers and institutions. At present, a relatively complete set of home care operating system has been formed, and various places are trying to explore community home care mode, and a lot of experience has been captured. In most big cities, a community care service mode has been formed, with facility service, service at regular time and home service as the main forms. There are a variety of community-based programs and services that can help senior citizens live safely and comfortably at home. The traditional domestic service primarily focused on providing services such as laundry, cooking, shopping and cleaning. The community-based service is an upgrade of the domestic service and also includes education in medical knowledge and health preserving, medical rehabilitation, psychological care and safeguard of the elderly legal rights. In order to improve mental alertness, staff will also read letters, newspapers or books to the elderly.

Although community-based care has been improved in recent years, there are still some inevitable difficulties. These facilities are still small in number, of varying standards, and are often too expensive for many elderly and their families. The low qualities of care providers result in a lack of professional abilities. Care providers are mostly the laid-off workers and people having difficulties in seeking employment. Influenced by traditional values, many of them think that serving the old is dirty, tired, and inferior to others. Another problem worth considering is that the real wage of these care providers is at the lowest or even less than the minimum wage of the temporary workers, which is unfavorable to stabilize the team of care providers.

3. Civil society organizations Civil society organizations, bridges gaps between government and the public, are playing a very important role in home care. Civil society organizations, under the guidance and support of government, could largely motivate social forces and sufficiently make the best of sources of different sections to provide socialized service for the aged. Civil society organizations include non-government organizations (e. g. Community Alliance), civil rights associations, charity organizations and public interest organizations (Red Cross, Senior Citizens Foundation, etc.). Volunteer's groups are highly welcomed to join the home care service. In some cities, aged people are recruited in the community, and "Time Deposit Service", a mutual-help project, is performed. The Time Deposit Service uses an interest-based system to take care of the old today for the benefit of the service providers in the future. Every minute a service provider spends caring for the elderly today will be

务为主要服务形式，以生活照料、医疗保健、心理保健、文化娱乐、参与社会以及权益保护为主要服务内容的社区养老服务格局。

尽管近年来基于社区的养老护理有所改善，但仍然存在一些不可避免的困难。一方面，社区养老机构数量不足，服务标准不一，多数费用昂贵。另一方面，养老机构人员专业护理能力不足、工资待遇低，造成护理人员团队不稳定。

3. **民间组织** 民间组织作为政府和社会公众联系的桥梁和枢纽，在居家养老服务中发挥重要作用。民间组织在政府的主导和推动下，可以广泛动员社会力量，充分利用多方资源为老年人提供社会化服务。大力倡导志愿者队伍参与居家养老服务。一些城市在社区内招募老年群体，开展"时间储蓄"式的老年人互助活动。服务者提供的每一分钟的为老服务都会被详细记录，等到未来提供服务者成为需要照护的老人时，他人也会为其提供同样时间的照护服务。一些退休的具有医学背景的社区志愿者还组建了相应的志愿者团队，为那些独居的老年人提供每月一次的上门诊断服务，或者为低收入的老年人

recorded and when the service provider is old, someone will look after him/her for the same amount of minutes. Some retired medical professionals establish volunteer teams and provide door-to-door diagnosis once a month for those who live alone or are very old for a low fee.

II. Common Issues during Home Care

Home care advocates that the aged receiving life care in their homes or communities, which fits their living habits and meets their psychological needs, beneficial for their late years. However, there are still some common issues during home care, such as the caregivers facing stress and challenges, abuse and neglect of the aged and delayed first aid for empty-nest elderly.

i. Stress and Challenges of Family Caregivers

The older population is growing in number, and life expectancy is increasing. In general, good health becomes less probable with increasing age, especially after age 75. For those impaired elderly, activities of daily living become increasingly difficult, which makes them more independent. In recent years, family caregivers have emerged as important members of the patient's healthcare team. The caregiver may be a spouse, a daughter, a son, a daughter-in-law, a sibling, a friend or any other family member. Caregivers help with many things such as grocery shopping, house cleaning, cooking, shopping, paying bills, giving medicine, bathing, using the toilet, dressing and Eating. While daughters were the primary caregivers of older parents in the past, more men are becoming involved in caregiving roles.

There are some personal rewards associated with caregiving for an older family member. Caregivers have a feeling of giving back to a loved one. It can also make caregivers feel needed and can lead to a stronger relationship with the person receiving care. Although family caregivers perform an important service for society and their relatives, they do so at considerable cost to themselves. Caregiver stress is a daily fact of life for many caregivers. Caregiving often takes a great deal of time, effort, and work. Many caregivers struggle to balance caregiving with other responsibilities including full-time jobs and caring for children. Constant stress can lead the caregiver into "burnout" and health problems.

1. Stress of caregivers Providing care to someone-whether full-time, part time, or long distance-takes a huge toll. Family caregivers are experiencing multidimensional stress, including physical, emotional, financial and social problems.

提供相应的医疗服务。

二、居家养老过程中的常见问题

居家养老虽然可以为老年人提供熟悉的生活环境，满足他们的心理需求，但是同时也面临着下列众多的挑战。

（一）家庭照顾者的压力与挑战

老年人的生活自理能力逐渐下降，其照料工作由家庭照顾者来完成。家庭照顾者主要包括老年人的子女和配偶。照顾者为老年人提供穿衣、吃饭、沐浴、如厕、做饭、喂药、打扫卫生、购物及支付账单等活动。

尽管照顾老年人是亲情的体现和家庭、社会责任感的要求，但是照顾老年人也付出了巨大的代价。照顾者不仅需要付出大量的时间和精力照护老年人，而且还要完成自己的事务，因此照顾者面临着很大的压力，会产生疲惫感和健康问题。

1. 照顾者的压力 无论是提供何种类型的照护，家庭照顾者承受的压力都会来自多个方面：

(1) Physical stress: Research suggests that caregivers may also be more likely to have health problems than non-caregivers. Obvious physical signs of stress include, but certainly are not limited to, fatigue, high blood pressure, irregular heartbeat or palpitations, chest pain, back, shoulder or neck pain, frequent headaches, digestive problems, and hair loss. Long-term caregiving appears to exact a toll on the immune system of caregiver. They experience more infections and more stress-related illness such as hypertension and heart disease than non-caregivers. Very often, caregivers neglect his or her own health issues, which are usually compounded by stress, because he or she has other responsibilities outside of caregiving. Additionally, the caregiver may be missing meals or eating an unhealthy diet for a period of time, so that their weight either increases or decreases dramatically.

(2) Psychological stress: Studies have shown that caregiving can adversely influence the caregivers' psychological health by added strain, stress and depression. The emotional experiences involved with providing care can strain even the most capable person. Emotional signs of stress are usually not easily observed. These signs include a gamut of feelings, including but not limited to anxiety, depression, irritability, frustration, lack of control, and isolation. A stressed caregiver may also report or exhibit mood swings, memory problems, and/or general unhappiness with their position as a caregiver, including resentment toward the care recipient and family members who do not contribute in any meaningful way. Individuals suffering from caregiver stress are also prone to depression. Feelings of depression can become a serious problem for some caregivers. Ironically, many of those caregivers with the most severe depression do not know or recognize that they are depressed. Consequently, they often do not seek medical help for their condition. Caregivers tend to drink alcohol more often than non-caregivers. They also tend to use more psychotropic drugs such as those that induce sleep or relaxation. A note of caution: problem will arise when those stressed caregivers accidentally combine alcohol with a relaxant drug. Combining drugs with alcohol is dangerous and should be avoided.

(3) Financial stress: The cost of caregiving can place a burden on the finances of many families. Unless the care recipient can finance all or most of the goods and services required for care, the family caregiving network will need to subsidize the cost of the long-term care. Medication purchases often prove to be the first of the financial shocks as chronically ill adults usually take several prescription medications. The responsibility of an in-home caregiver

（1）生理压力：研究表明，照顾者比非照顾者更易于出现健康问题。躯体方面常表现为疲劳、高血压、心律不规则、胸痛、肩背或颈部疼痛、头痛、消化不良及脱发等。经历持续压力的照顾者可以出现免疫功能下降。

（2）心理压力：照顾者的心理健康问题常常被忽视，心理方面常表现为焦虑、抑郁、烦躁、沮丧、缺乏控制感和孤独；还可以表现为情绪波动、记忆力下降及对处于照顾者角色的不满意，严重时会产生抑郁。

（3）经济压力：照顾者必须放弃或减少工作时间来照护老年人，使收入减少。日常支出的医疗费用也会增加照顾者的经济压力。

is usually of full-time or overtime, meaning that the majority of caregivers are not able to keep their jobs outside of the home, even if the job is only a part-time one. Caregivers must sacrifice gainful employment to care for a family member, and the income lost may place the family unit in a crisis of survival. As doctor bills and other treatment fees accrue, and as less energy is left for work, caregivers often find themselves facing financial pressures as well.

(4) Social stress: Caregiving also places limits on the caregiver's social life. An overwhelmed caregiver will often miss or delay their appointments, as they often give up their 'me' time. They will stop engaging in their usual activities and often lose connections with friends and family. Further, they may stifle feelings of anger and frustration, which then surface as angry outbursts directed at family, friends, co-workers, or even strangers.

2. Factors affecting caregiver stress　Caregiver burdens are influenced by several factors. Those factors are grouped into three categories: caregiver factors, patient factors and environmental factors.

(1) Caregiver factors: The factors of caregivers can influence the stress perceived by caregiver, including gender, educational level, income status, kinship ties, time spent per day and coping strategies. Gender is an influence on the perception of caregiver stress. Women are likely to be regarded as the most appropriate caregivers for family members.

The education level has a negative correlation with caregiver's burden. It was assumed that the higher the level of education one gets, the higher the salary he/she will earn. High salary would decrease financial problems related to providing care for an ill family member. The caregiver with higher level of education also tends to have more knowledge to deal with the stressful events. Therefore caregiver's education level influences the burden of the caregiver.

Income may have influence on the burden of the caregiver. Low income is associated with a higher degree of burden on the caregivers. Lower income is a stressor that can heighten the feeling of stress during providing care for an ill family member. Besides providing care for ill members, caregivers also have to solve financial problems and find out source of money.

Kinship ties (spouse, child, and siblings) are other factors that can influence caregiver stress. In general, closer kinship ties are associated with increased caregiver burden. Adult children experience more caregiver burden than more distant relatives.

（4）社会压力：照顾者参加社会活动的机会减少，牺牲亲情和友情。照顾者出现的愤怒、沮丧等情绪，影响照顾者与他人的和睦相处。

2. 照顾者压力的影响因素　照顾者压力的影响因素分为三类：照顾者因素，被照顾者因素和环境因素。

（1）照顾者因素：照顾者的性别、教育程度、经济收入、与老年人的关系、照护时间以及应对方式等影响照料者所承受的压力。

受教育程度与压力成负相关。通常受教育水平越高薪水就越高，照护所带来的财务问题会越少。教育水平越高的护理人员往往具备更多的知识来应对压力事件，因此照顾者的教育水平会对照顾者负担有影响。

同样，低收入增加了照顾者的负担。特别是照顾生病的老年人带来的经济压力更大。低收入导致照顾者感知到的照顾压力增加，除了要提供照护之外，照顾者还要寻找解决经济困难的方法。

亲属关系（配偶，孩子和兄弟姐妹）的紧密程度也可影响照顾人员的压力。一般而言，紧密程度越高，照顾者的照顾压力越大。成年子女比远方亲戚承受更多的照料者负担。

Time spent for caregiving per day is related to burden. There was a significant positive correlation between hours of care per day and caregiver burden. The higher the number of hours a caregiver spends on providing cares per day, the greater the burdens he/she will bear. The more the time a caregiver spends with an ill family member, the more the objective burdens he/she will get. When caregivers spend more time with their ill family members, they will have less time for themselves. Finally, it will increase the burdens of the caregivers and affect his/her daily activities.

Caregivers' coping strategies influence their perceptions of caregiver stress. There are two types of coping strategies. One is emotion-focused coping dealing with the feelings associated with major strain, and the other one is problem-focused coping aiming to confront the reality of major strains by dealing with the tangible consequences. Female caregivers tend to apply more emotion-focused coping, while males use problem-focused coping strategies a lot, and problem-focused or mixed coping strategies are found to be the most effective.

(2) Patient factors: Variables pertaining to the illness that affect family caregivers are the stage of illness (i. e., onset, long haul, end stage, etc.) and the duration of illness (i. e., lifetime vs. old age). There is also a strong relationship between care-recipient behaviors and caregiver burden. Care-recipient behaviors that are known to be especially burdensome include incontinence, severe functional impairments, hallucinations, suspiciousness, agitation, wandering, catastrophic emotional reactions, disruptiveness at night, behaviors dangerous to the patient, and the need for constant supervision. Because many of these characteristics are common among dementia patients, it is believed that caregiving for an elderly person with dementia is more difficult than providing care to an elderly person with physical rather than mental limitations.

(3) Environmental factors: The environment surrounding caregivers can influence the perceived stress, including culture and social support. Culture shapes one's perceptions of familial responsibilities and thus also influences caregiver stress. Caucasian caregivers tend to report greater depression and appraised caregiving as more stressful than African American (AA) caregivers. In fact, AA caregivers experience similar amounts of caregiver stress but express it differently from Caucasian caregivers.

照顾者每天花费在护理上的时间越长，他/她承受的负担也越大。照顾者每天花费在照护方面的时间越长，越没有给予自己的时间。久而久之，会逐渐增加其照顾压力，影响其日常活动。

面对压力，照顾者的应对策略各有不同。应对策略可分为情感型应对和解决问题型应对。情感型应对是处理与压力相关的情绪反应，而问题型应对则是面对现实解决压力所带来的结局。女性照顾者倾向于采用情感型应对方式，而男性多从解决问题的角度来应对压力，解决问题型应对或者两者混合式的应对方式被认为是比较有效的应对方法。

（2）被照顾者因素：老年患者的病情、患病持续时间会影响照顾者的压力。此外，被照护者的行为症状与照顾者的压力之间有非常大的相关性。特别是老年患者存在大小便失禁，严重功能障碍，幻觉，躁动，昼夜作息颠倒、有激越行为、徘徊行为的老年人更难护理并且需要持续的监护。由于这些问题在痴呆症患者中是常见的，因此患有痴呆症的老年人更难护理。

（3）环境因素：文化背景和社会支持等环境因素可以影响照顾者的压力感知。不同的文化背景可以塑造不同的家庭责任观，因此也影响了照顾者的压力。在亚洲文化中，家庭承担的照顾责任较重，但成员间沟通合作不足，导致对照顾者的社会支持和情感支持减少。

Among Asian cultures, a greater sense of responsibility to care for elderly family members and the reluctance to discuss family problems lead to less social and emotional supports for caregivers.

The perceived social support and family function have negative correlations with caregiver burden. Better family function has an impact on better adaptation that is associated with effective coping. Utilization of formal support received has a positive correlation with burden. Caregiver's burden increases when informal support could not meet caregiver's need. Supporters could reduce the burden if they fulfill the unmet needs of the caregivers.

3. Potential for harm In general, family members may be challenged to find the capacity or ability to provide care. Caregivers can place their family members at risk in two ways, and both situations are preventable. Firstly, despite their good intentions and hard work, if caregivers do not have the knowledge and skills to perform their work, they may unintentionally harm their loved ones. This risk of injury is directly associated with the lack of knowledge and competence, which can be improved through caregiver education and support. For example, a recent study confirmed that care recipients had many negative outcomes when untrained informal caregivers managed their home enteral nutrition or tube feeding. Problems include tube displacement, tube clogging, infection, and dehydration—all of which can lead to a stressful caregiving situation and hospital readmission.

A second concern is that the demanding work of caregiving can put caregivers at risk of engaging in harmful behaviors toward their care recipients, particularly among caregivers of persons with cognitive impairments. Depressed caregivers are more likely to harm their elderly family members. Caregivers who are at risk of depression while caring for elderly family members with significant cognitive or physical impairments are more likely to engage in neglect or abusive behaviors, such as screaming and yelling, threatening to abandon or use physical force, withholding food, hitting, or handling roughly. More detailed explanation on elderly abuse is described in Chapter 7.

4. Interventions to decrease the burden of family caregivers Caregiving brings many negative consequences to caregivers, so it's very important to take measures to support family caregivers.

(1) Education and training: Lack of education and training can contribute to caregiver stress, so it is important for health care professionals to provide information and training for caregivers. Health care professionals should

感知社会支持和家庭功能与照顾者压力成负相关。良好的家庭功能会使照顾者更加有效应对压力，从而减轻负担。当非正式的支持不能满足照顾者需求时，照顾者的压力增加。当支持者可以满足照顾者的需要时，照顾者的压力就会相应降低。

3. 照顾者压力的潜在危害 照顾者压力可以给被照顾者带来两方面的危害，一方面是由于缺乏知识和技能使被照顾者有受伤害的风险。例如，未经培训的非专业人员实施肠内营养或管饲护理时，可能会有很多不良后果。问题包括饲管移位，饲管堵塞，感染和脱水等。这些情况会导致更大的护理压力和再住院风险。

另一方面有认知障碍（如抑郁）的照顾者可能对老年人产生一些虐待的行为。具体有关虐待的相关内容介绍请见第七章。

4. 减轻照顾者压力的策略 采取措施缓解家庭照顾者的压力非常重要。

（1）教育培训：缺乏照护知识和技能会影响照顾者压力，因此要向照顾者提供知识和技能培训。医务工作者应该先了解家庭需要

ask the family what they want to know, as well as provide them with information they need to know. An individual or group-based intervention for families should focus on the provision of information. One of the goals of education should be to help caregivers build the confidence that they can do a task or take an action. It is crucial to give caregivers an opportunity to practice skills in a learning environment that is non-threatening and psychologically safe. It is vital to discuss the barriers caregivers may face in the real world and ways to overcome these barriers. Sharing printed information is another important way to provide education. Educational materials should be easy to read, with bullet points, definitions of difficult terms and illustrations. Materials should be written in plain language and avoid medical terms. Another resource for families is the Internet. Many health and caregiving organizations offer a variety of helpful information through their websites.

(2) Supporting group: Support groups may be professionally led (usually time-limited) or peer led (usually open-ended and ongoing). The former are often conducted in certain facilities such as hospitals or clinics, whereas the latter are typically held in communities. Some support groups are oriented to specific diseases such as cancer group, and others are for family caregivers in general. A support group can be a place where caregivers get advice, gain information about their older relatives' medical conditions and problems, share experiences and feelings, develop new coping strategies, and learn about community resources and care alternatives. A support group also may provide an acceptable outlet for socializing.

(3) Respite program: Respite programs are services that are designed for the family members, and are offered in part to give the family caregiver a break from caregiver responsibilities. Services offered are both in-home and in-agency institutional settings for short periods of time ranging from a few hours per day to a week or two while the caregiver may be out of town. Studies show that respite care can potentially improve the well-being of the caregiver as well as possibly delaying the institutionalization of the older person in their care. The primary intended beneficiaries of respite services are caregivers, care receivers can also benefit from the services. In many cases, respite care providers may be the only source of out-side-the-family socialization for care receivers. Care receivers will also benefit from caregivers being more "refreshed" after a break in caregiving.

哪些知识和技能的培训，这样才能提供给他们所真正需要的。无论是做家庭的个体干预还是群体干预，都一定要先满足其需要。对照顾者进行教育的一个目的就是要增强他们照护老年人的自信心。要为照顾者提供一个安全的、无威胁的学习环境。与照顾者讨论他们在照顾过程中遇到哪些困难、使用了哪些方法去解决。为照顾者提供打印出来的教育资料，便于阅读的，有详细解释的。教育资料一定是用易懂的语言、避免医学术语。同时也可以为照顾者提供一定的网络学习资源。

（2）支持性团体的帮助：支持性团体可以为照顾者提供有关特定疾病的咨询、教育培训，以及社区资源和照护服务；也可以为照顾者之间分享经验和感受提供机会；同时也为照顾者参加社会活动提供机会。

（3）喘息服务项目："喘息服务"是指提供临时性照护服务，让照顾者在短时间得到休息，也能使身心得到放松。同时也可以使接受照护的老年人受益。

ii. Delayed First Aid for Empty-nest Elderly

The Chinese have traditionally been happy with big-sized families, which often place several generations under one roof, but now great changes have taken place. The number of empty-nest families, in which there is only an elderly couple or one aged person, is on the rise, particularly in some inland mountainous rural areas. This occurrence is closely related to China's overall economic environment, due to the accelerated process of urbanization, the imbalance of economic development between the inland and coastal regions, and the flow of rural surplus labor to big cities on the eastern coast. Some farmers have established their careers in those cities and become urban dwellers, while their parents are left behind in rural homes. It is obvious that the social and medical problems of the empty-nest elderly will become a critical issue in the near future. One widespread social concern among empty nesters is delayed first aid.

1. Causes　According to the statistics from an emergency center in Tianjin city, 20% of elder patients had died when doctors rushed to the scene, of which 80% was due to delayed first aid. There are some factors related to these phenomena, including mental health factors, physical care and access to the health-care delivery system.

(1) Psychological factors: The empty nest syndrome is a maladaptive response to the post-parental transition. Parents, especially mothers, may suffer from all kinds of symptoms when their children leave home, like a sense of loss, grief and depression. Depression damages the health of the elderly, decreases their social and physical activities, generate unsociability and reduce the quality of life.

(2) Factors related to daily care: Adult children have traditionally been expected to provide care for their parents. In fact, older adults have to increasingly rely on themselves. Empty nest is a time when older individual's health and energy levels may decline. Some people are diagnosed with chronic illnesses. Symptoms of these diseases can limit normal activities and even long-enjoyed pastimes. Health issues related to midlife may begin to occur and can include: hypertension, weight problems, arthritis, menopause, osteoporosis, heart disease, depression or stress-related illnesses. Physical health problems and irreversible decrease in function capacity may inhibit people from interacting with friends or family members in leisure or work, and decrease social integration. If older individual's health is good, he or she can still take care of himself. Once health status declines, due to the lack of life care from child adults, older adults will suffer from inconvenience. Seriously, their lives

（二）空巢老年人居家急救不及时

随着城市化进程的加快，空巢老年人面临着社会和医疗问题，其中引起社会广泛关注的一个问题是居家急救不及时。

1. **原因**　据天津急救中心统计，医生赶到居家意外现场时，20% 的老年患者已经死亡，其中 80% 是因为急救不及时。造成老年人急救不及时的原因主要包括心理因素、生活照料因素和医疗护理因素。

（1）心理因素：空巢综合征是老年人在子女成家立业独立生活之后，由于适应不良出现的一种综合征，表现为失落、悲伤和抑郁。抑郁可损害老年人的健康，减少老年人的社交活动和体力活动，从而导致老年人的生活质量下降。

（2）生活照料因素：空巢期老年人的身体健康水平和活动能力下降，大多患有慢性疾病。这些疾病损害了老年人的躯体健康，影响了老年人的活动能力，阻碍老年人的社会生活。一旦身体状况发生改变，再加上缺乏子女的照护，老年人就会遭遇不便，甚至生命受到威胁。

are often threatened.

(3) Factros related to healthcare: Elderly people have low income, especially empty-nest elderly. It is even worse in the inland mountainous rural areas in China, where the elderly depend on their children to take care of them, and their income comes mainly from their children. They also pay most of their medical costs out of pocket because they are not insured. The financial situation of empty-nest dwellers is worse in rural areas than in cities. Rural areas are frequently characterized by poorly developed, fragile economic infrastructures, resulting in fewer available per capital hospital beds, doctors, nurses, and other health-care services. In addition to socioeconomic hardships, rural residents face substantial physical barriers, including the lack of public transportation, difficult terrain, and long distances to services. The condition restricts empty-nest elderly to accessing to health care.

2. Interventions　The empty nest problem is related to family, community, government and the society as a whole and requires joint efforts from all parties concerned. In our country, respect and caring for the elderly has long been considered the traditional Chinese virtues. Adult children should often visit and care elderly parents, and should be familiar with the conditions of elderly related to physical and mental aspects. The traditional vertical support of elderly people, which places the responsibility on the children and the work units, is supposed to switch to modern horizontal style, which consists of mutual care within the couple and care from the local community.

Additionally, the set of emergency call can be used for elder empty nester. Seniors living by themselves are especially vulnerable to potentially dangerous situations. Empty-nest elderly can get a personal home medical alarm for protection. Older individuals probably have phone numbers of family and friends and that can provide some assurance for them, but it really isn't enough. If they have a sudden medical emergency, they might find themselves unable to reach the phone to summon help. The alarm itself is set within a wrist band or pedant which an older adult wears around his neck. It contains a large button which he can press in case of an emergency. The patient's condition will be immediately sent to an emergency command center. The set also shows the patient home address and telephone information. A good medical alarm can help older individual contact with a professionally-trained staff within seconds. The alarm does not only make elderly access assistance quickly, but also reduces their anxiety about accidents and increases their confidence in performing everyday activities.

（3）医疗护理因素：空巢老年人收入低，尤其是内陆农村地区的老年人，他们的收入主要依靠子女提供。他们没有保险，无力支付医疗费用。农村地区经济不发达，基础设施少，医疗服务缺乏。此外，交通不便、地势险要、距离医疗机构远等障碍，限制了老年人获得及时的医疗保健。

2. **对策**　要解决空巢家庭面临的问题，需要国家、社会和家庭的共同努力。尊重和照护老年人是我国的传统美德，子女应该经常回家看望年老的父母，并了解老年人身体和精神方面的状况。同时，传统的家庭代际支持应该转变成夫妇之间的相互照料和社会支持。

此外，在空巢老年人家中安装紧急呼叫系统。独居的老年人发生意外事故时，该系统可帮助老年人获得医疗救助。在紧急情况下，只需要按一键，指挥中心将显示老年人的住址和其他信息。紧急呼叫系统不仅使老年人在短时间内联系到专业人员，迅速获得帮助，而且可以减少老年人担心意外事故发生的焦虑，增加执行日常活动的信心。

III. Strategies to Improve Home Care Quality

Based on the current condition in our country, home care service in the community is feasible. Targeting at issues related to home care presently, improvements should be performed through reasonable design.

1. Completing law and policy system   Home care service should be led and administrated by the government, which coordinates different sections macroscopically, as planned and following certain steps, thus completing the social welfare system. Meanwhile, the government has to perfect relative law for home care, making sure there are laws to abide by, and should increase financial investment to community health services. The government should strengthen the supervision system, qualify the service standard and improve the service quality.

2. Building service network for home care   Building service network of home care service includes quickening the constructions of community service centers and facilities in city and countryside communities. Integrated home care service center and basic service facilities will be built in cities and countryside, providing life care, health care, entertainment and psychological comforting to the aged, laying a solid material foundation for home care service.

3. Fostering staff providing home care service   Sparing no effort to build a huge service staff with both professionals and volunteers as members is of vital importance for the overall development of home care service. Staff must receive related training and be examined strictly, and cannot work officially only without being given the certificate. Meanwhile, moral education and skill training of staff must be strengthened, continuously enhancing their political capabilities and services. In additional, more volunteers' organization and members should be recruited, encouraging volunteers to provide more services for the aged through their professional knowledge, skills and physical strength. For example, there is a time deposit system, which encourages the younger elder to look after aged people, and in turn, receive help when they are aged.

4. Support from the family   For home care, family should also play its own role to support home care. It is every citizen's responsibility and obligation to strengthen the work of media and publicity on elderly care, to promote China's virtues on elderly care, and to

三、提高居家养老质量的策略

根据我国目前的情况，在社区开展居家养老服务是切实可行的途径。针对目前居家养老服务中所存在的一系列问题，需要通过合理设计予以改善。

1. 完善法律和政策体系   居家养老服务应该由政府牵头管理，有计划、有步骤地从整体上协调，健全社会保障体系。同时，政府要完善居家养老相应的法律法规，使居家养老事业的发展有法可依。

2. 构建居家养老服务网络   加快城乡社区服务机构、设施的建设，在城市和农村建立综合性居家养老服务中心和基础性的服务设施，真正在社区构建起为老年人提供生活照料、医疗康复、文化娱乐、精神慰藉等多项服务，为居家养老服务奠定坚持的物质基础。

3. 加强居家养老服务队伍建设   从事养老护理等相关服务的人员必须经过相关职业培训，严格考核，取得从业资格证书才能正式上岗。同时，要加强服务人员的职业道德教育和岗位技能培训。此外，还要大力发展居家养老服务的志愿者组织和人员，鼓励志愿者为老年人提供多种形式的养老服务。如推行时间储蓄制度。

4. 家庭全力支持   加强舆论宣传，弘扬中华民族的传统美德，广泛开展敬老、养老、助老的道德教育，强化赡养老年人是每个公民的责任和义务的意识，使全社会形成家庭

widely carry out moral education with respecting the elderly and caring the elderly. Doing so can foster the atmosphere of home care in the society. Adult children should consciously build up the awareness of caring the elderly, respecting the old and loving the elderly, actively performing the duties to take care of the elderly. We should not only provide materials to the elderly, but also provide the spiritual comfort and enhance their sense of happiness and the quality of life.

养老的良好氛围。成年子女自觉树立养老、敬老、爱老的责任意识，主动履行对老年人的"反哺"义务。

Section 3   Institutional Care

With the increasing challenge of caring for current and future elders, the development of institutional care for elderly calls attention due to its vital supplemental role to the long-term care system. Institutional care provides the last caring setting for elders who need the most care but who do not have appropriate care available in the community.

I. Characteristics of Institutional Care and Requirements

Currently, China has two systems that provide institutional care for elders: the first one is the social welfare system. This is run by Departments of Civil Affairs at various levels and operates welfare institutes, homes for the aged, and veteran care facilities; and the second one is the medical care system which is operated by the National Health and Family Planning Commission of the People's Republic of China. This system usually manages geriatric hospitals, nursing facilities, rehabilitation wards, and mental health hospitals for elders with mental health problem such as dementia. These two systems have separate funding mechanisms and policies that create different segments for long-term care. Geriatric hospitals and rehabilitation wards in general hospitals are usually operated and managed by the local department of health. Many medical expenses are covered by medical insurance. Veteran care facilities provide LTC services to veteran soldiers who are functionally disabled and are elders. Welfare institutes and homes for the aged have played the most important role in providing institutionalized long-term care services. Other private, nonprofit Long-term care facilities have been set up to compensate public

第三节   机构养老照护

随着老龄化社会的发展，机构照护成为长期照护体系中一个非常重要的补充部分。机构照护可以为那些在社区中没有相应照护资源的老人提供最终的照护。

一、机构养老照护的特点

目前，中国有两个体系可以为老年人提供机构照护。一个是社会福利体系，由民政部门管理，开设有相应的福利院、养老院、老年公寓、军人福利院等类型的机构照护；另外一个则为中华人民共和国国家卫生健康委员会负责，常设有老年病医院、护理院、康复病房、老年精神病房等各种形式的养老机构。这两个体系的基金来源和政府管理方式不同。在当今中国，民政部门开设的社会福利机构在机构照护中起到主要的作用。在中国，为老年人所提供的机构照护尚在发展过程中。因此，本节所介绍的有关机构照护的一些内容主要来自国外的经验，希望对中国机构照护的发展有所启示。

facilities during the recent years. Institutional care for older adults in China is still in the developing process. Thus, in this section, more information on institutional care from foreign countries is introduced.

i. Characteristics and Requirements for Nursing Acilities

1. In the United States, all nursing facilities must function under the federal regulations.

2. Medical, nursing, dietary, recreational, rehabilitative, social, and spiritual care is usually provided.

3. An ideal long-term care facility is a combination of both medical and social models without exclusive one or the other. The medical model places residents in a sick role and in need of direct help from health care personnel. Compliance with the medical regimen is emphasized and residents are expected to comply with staff and medical decisions. In addition to the traditional medical concerns, social model emphasizes that residents' social and psychological health need to be considered. Thus, subjective evaluations of their quality of life need to be valued. Residents should have their rights to make decision and choose exercise they want to participate.

4. A nursing facility must provide or arrange for the provision of nursing and related services, and specialized rehabilitative services to attain or maintain the highest practicable physical, mental, and psychosocial well-being of each resident. These services must be provided in accordance with the comprehensive assessment and plan of care. Pharmacy, dental, dietary, and related social services, as well as an ongoing program of activities must be available and must meet professional standards of quality.

5. Nurse aide training and competency evaluations are required for nurse aides employed in long-term care.

ii. Characteristics and Requirements for Assisted Living

1. Assisted living is a philosophy of care and services promoting independence and dignity.

2. Assisted living is an elder care alternative on the continuum of care for older adults, for whom independent living is no longer appropriate but who do not need the 24-hour medical care provided by a nursing home.

（一）护理院的特点

1. 在美国，所有护理院的开设都必须遵守国家的相关政策。

2. 在护理院，应该提供涵盖医疗、护理、康复、饮食、娱乐、社交及精神照护等各种服务。

3. 理想的护理院的管理模式应该是医疗模式和社会模式的相结合。医疗模式强调要给老年人提供符合其生理需求的疾病照护和治疗；而社会模式则关注老年人的心理和社会健康。在全部照护过程中，老年人有权利参与自己的各种照护方案。

4. 应该对护理院中的老年人进行详尽的评估，在评估基础上为老年人提供相应的生理、心理和社会的治疗与护理。药物指导、口腔卫生指导、饮食调节及相关的社会活动安排也应该在护理院中有所体现。

5. 护理院中的护工一定要经过培训，具备相关的照护能力。

（二）有助聚居机构的特点

1. 有助聚居机构的开设目的是促进老年人自理和维护其尊严。

2. 有助聚居机构为那些需要一定帮助的老年人提供服务，但是这些老年人又不需要24小时的类似于护理院所提供的医疗照护。

3. People who live in assisted living facilities usually have their own private apartment. It may resemble a dormitory or hotel room consisting of a private or semi-private sleeping area and a shared bathroom. There are usually common areas for socializing, as well as a central kitchen and dining room for preparing and eating meals.

4. Household chores are performed that sheets are changed, such as laundry is done, and food is cooked and served. Grocery service is often available too. Some homes even have a beauty parlor on site.

5. There is usually no special medical monitoring equipment that one would find in a nursing home, and their nursing staff may not be available at all hours. But they are available by phone or e-mail 24 hours out of the day, to ensure proper teaching and/or education of staff available. Trained staff is usually on-site around the clock to provide other needed services.

iii. Characteristics and Requirements for Special Care Units

Special care units (SCUs) for dementia mainly differ from "traditional" integrated units in their philosophies and goals, physical design and other environmental features, staff composition and training, and family involvement. The characteristics and requirements for special care units are:

1. Patient care philosophies and goals Six concepts are often used to explain and justify the particular physical design features and patient care practices used in a given special care unit or recommended for special care units generally. The concepts also have important implications for staff composition and training and the individualization of care. These six concepts are something can be done for individuals with dementia; many factors cause excess disability in individuals with dementia. Identifying and changing these factors will reduce excess disability and improve the individuals' functioning and quality of life; individuals with dementia have residual strengths. Building on these strengths will improve their functioning and quality of life; the behavior of individuals with dementia represents understandable feelings and needs, even if the individuals are unable to express the feelings or needs. Identifying and responding to those feelings and needs will reduce the incidence of behavioral symptoms; many aspects of the physical and social environment affect the functioning of individuals with dementia. Providing appropriate environments will

3. 在有助聚居机构生活的老年人通常有他们自己的房间。同时也有共享的社交区域、餐厅、中央厨房等。

4. 有助聚居机构内提供家务服务，如更换床单、清扫房间、帮助烹调食物、帮助购买物品等。部分有助聚居机构还会有相应的美容美发店。

5. 有助聚居机构看不到在护理院中所见的医疗设备，护士也不需要24小时在机构内工作。但是一定有异常情况，护士是24小时都可以通过电话获取到的。受过培训的护工可在一定的时间段为居住的老年人提供相应的服务。

（三）特殊照护单元的特点

特殊照护单元（SCU）与既往传统的照护病房不同，主要体现在照护理念、照护目标、环境设置、人员组成、家庭参与度等几个主要方面。它的特点是：

1. **患者照护的理念和照护目标** 有6个理念常用于体现SCU的特点，它们是与普通老年人的照料相比，为痴呆患者同样可以做很多事情；很多因素可以导致痴呆患者的功能过度丧失。通过确认和改变这些因素可以减少痴呆患者的功能过度丧失，促进和维持个体的功能，提高其生活质量；痴呆患者仍有其残留的能力。在其残留能力的基础上提供适宜的照护可以促进痴呆患者的功能，提高痴呆患者的生活质量；痴呆患者所产生的行为问题意味着患者有某些特殊的需求或者情感需要，确认这些需求和情感需要并对其做出适当的反应将会减少行为问题的发生；很多物理的和社会的环境因素可以影响痴呆患者的功能；提供合适的物理和社会环境可以促进患者的功能，提高其生活质量；痴呆患者和其家庭成员是一个整体。了解家庭成

improve their functioning and quality of life; individuals with dementia and their families constitute an integral unit. Addressing the needs of the families and involving them in the individuals' care will benefit both the individuals and the families.

2. Physical design and other environmental features   A variety of physical design and other environmental features have been proposed for SCUs. Most of these features are intended to compensate directly for residents' cognitive impairments, but some are intended to compensate for physical impairments that may exacerbate an individual's fictional deficits. Several environmental features considered to be important for SCUs are as follows:

(1) Arrangement of residents' bedrooms: It will be better that the bedrooms are arranged around a common, central area and location of the nurses' station to facilitate resident supervision and staff/resident interaction, locked units and freedom of movement. When the dementia unit is locked, staff does not have to worry about residents leaving the facility. Residents can wander freely within the unit. This freedom enhances their autonomy and avoids power struggles with staff. Encouraging this activity is helpful, because it gives patients something to do and also tires them out, reducing behavior problems during the day and sleep problems at night.

(2) Other environment cues: SCUs typically use environmental cues to help residents identify their own rooms. For example, rooms or doors to rooms are painted different colors; patient picture is placed outside the room especially a picture taken several years earlier, because patients may not recognize their current appearance, but they remember how they looked in the past. Objects should be well-defined, for example, black on white or navy blue with yellow; patterned and floral designs may not be best.

员的需求并将家属纳入痴呆患者的个体照护活动中将是患者和其家庭的双重受益。

2. 环境设计和其他环境特点   SCU 有多种多样的物理环境设计特点，但主要出发点还是为了适应痴呆患者的认知功能损害，同时还有一部分设计要满足由于疾病进展而导致的患者失能的问题。一些重要的环境因素列举如下：

（1）照护单元中痴呆患者的房间安置：照护单元中痴呆患者的房间安置最好以护士站或者某一公共活动区域为中心呈环形设计，以方便工作人员对痴呆患者的观察和监管，同时促进工作人员和痴呆患者之间的互动；照护单元针对痴呆患者而言是相对封闭的，患者是不能随便外出的。但是在照护单元内，痴呆患者可以毫无限制地活动。照护单元相对封闭的特点，可以减少工作人员担心患者走失的负担。同时，由于痴呆患者可以自由地在照护单元内徘徊，这种自由使得患者感知到的自主性和控制感增强，减少了与工作人员之间的冲突。同时，单元内环境的设计也很重要。环形的设计可以让痴呆患者没有障碍地进退自如。

（2）其他环境特征：SCU 特别使用环境的特征来帮助痴呆患者确认他们自己的房间。如房间和门可以漆成不同的颜色方便患者进行区分；患者自己的照片可以放在房门外，这个照片尽可能是患者多年前拍摄的而不要用近期拍摄的照片，因为痴呆患者近期记忆的受损程度更重于远期记忆，患者不能辨认出照片中最近时期的自我影像，但是却相对容易地辨认出远些时候的自我图像。物品一定是被痴呆老人容易辨识的，如白配黑或者黄配海军蓝的颜色都容易被痴呆老人所辨认，但是图案或者花卉的设计形式一般要避免。

(3) Sensory stimulation: One of the most important but often neglected design issues is the amount of sensory stimulation that exists in patients' environments—in particular, light and noise. Appropriate light (e. g., no bright lights in the middle of the night) and lower level of noise can be helpful to decrease the incidence of behavioral problems.

(4) Structured activities: A well-designed dementia special care program can engage patients in activities that appropriate to their cognitive and functional abilities and allow them to use their remaining capabilities. These activities can include singing, dancing, exercises, painting, crafts, games, parties, pet therapy, field trips, reality orientation, sensory and cognitive stimulation, reminiscence therapy, religious services, housekeeping, cooking, gardening, and sheltered workshop activities.

3. Staff composition and training   The literature on SCUs emphasize the need for staff members who are knowledgeable about dementia and skilled in caring for individuals with dementia. Therefore, formal and informal training can be especially focused on dementia patients' needs. In the US, some state regulations have prescribed that all staff require several hours (i. e., 40 hours) of training before they "assigned" to the SCUs and several hours (i. e., 2 hours) of in-service training intermittently. Several state regulations for SCUs require that an interdisciplinary team develop an individualized plan of care for each new resident and review the plan on a quarterly basis.

4. Family involvement   Many SCUs have special programs to involve, inform, and support residents' families, such as inviting a family member to attend care plan meetings and establishing a family support group.

（3）适宜的感知觉刺激：即灯光和噪声的问题。白天的时候应保持足够的照明，夜晚时暴露于过强的光照下，也能改变痴呆患者的睡眠－觉醒周期，使得患者非常不容易入睡。因此，当工作人员在半夜里需要帮助患者时，一定要尽可能地将光线调到最弱，使得患者明显地感知到所处的时刻是夜晚，这样才能更容易让患者再次入睡。噪声往往导致激越行为的出现，因此，SCU 中要尽量控制噪声，尽可能减到最小。

（4）精心设计的符合痴呆患者认知功能和自理能力的活动：可以让痴呆患者继续使用他们尚存的能力。这些活动应该每天都开展，而且最好白天和晚上都有。如唱歌、跳舞、健身、画画、手工、游戏、联欢会、宠物治疗、现实定位活动、感知和认知功能刺激活动、回想治疗、园艺活动等。这些活动一定要建立在患者既往的经历和所具备的能力上，安排患者参加他们各自适合的活动，而不要再让痴呆患者重新去学习一个新的技能。

3. **人员构成和培训**   在 SCU 工作的人员一定要经过相关的培训，使得他们掌握照护痴呆老年人的知识和技巧。在美国，一些州已经明确规定工作人员在进入 SCU 工作前一定要完成相应学时的培训（如 40 个小时的培训），工作后还应该间断性地接受在职教育。美国一些州还明确规定在 SCU 中的工作人员应该是多专业协作的团队，而且应针对每一个痴呆患者共同制订符合其自身特点的治疗与照护计划。这些计划需要每个季度进行再一次评估和更新。

4. **家庭参与**   与养老机构普通单元的患者的家庭成员相比，SCU 的患者的家庭参与痴呆患者照护的程度更高。让家庭参与痴呆患者照护计划的制订对于提供痴呆患者个体化的照护是非常重要的。同时，很多 SCU 都建立有家庭成员支持小组，帮助照顾者调整他们的积极情绪，更好地参与 SCU 内痴呆患者的照护活动。

II. Issues on Quality of Institutional Care

The quality of long-term care has raised concerns over many years among national policy makers, the public, and the users of services and their families. The long-term care quality is usually multidimensional, comprising clinical, functional, psychosocial, and other facets of residents' health and well-being. There are several issues on quality of institutional care which need to be considered.

i. Lacking Measurements to Evaluate the Care Quality

There is a lacking of a stable and reliable measurement model for evaluating deficiencies on institutional care quality. Historically, many studies have used only one or a few indicators of the quality of nursing home care (e. g., resident satisfaction, pressure ulcers, and mortality rate). Those limited measures could not adequately reflect the total configuration of the quality of care.

ii. Work Force

Institutional care requires an adequate, skilled, and diverse work force. Registered nurses and nursing assistants or aides represent the largest component of personnel in institutional care. Other professionals are also needed, including physicians, social workers, therapists (physical, occupational, and speech), mental health providers, dietitians, pharmacists, podiatrists, and dentists. They provide different kinds of essential services to consumers who use the institutional care. Non-professionals, who provide the majority of personal care services, such as assistance with eating or bathing, have a major impact on both the health status and the quality of life of long-term care users.

Institutional care services are labor intensive so the quality of care depends largely on the performance of the caregiving personnel. The numbers, training, and competence of staff are widely viewed as critical to the quality of services. In foreign countries, many researchers report the relationship between quality of institutional care and the number and type of staff and their expertise and skills related to nursing homes. In addition to staffing levels, a key issue is whether the work force in long-term care has adequate education and training to provide high quality of care to individuals. In foreign countries, there are many regulations to set for some personnel in nursing homes and home health agencies. However, in China, it is stilled lacked.

二、机构照护中的常见问题

长期照护机构中的照护常见问题是多年来国家政策制订者、老年人及其家庭特别关注的问题。长期照护质量通常是多维度的，由临床指标、功能状态、心理社会及其他方面的健康指标所构成。影响机构照护质量的几个因素：

（一）缺少稳定可信的测量工具测量机构照护的质量

既往研究所关注的质量评价指标往往过于单一化，如老年人满意度、压疮发生率及病死率等。这些有限的测量工具不能很全面地反映养老机构的照护质量。

（二）人员的问题

机构照护需要一批质量合格的、有相应技能的、多种背景的工作人员。注册护士和护工在养老机构的人员构成中占有主要比例。其他专业人士则包括医生、社会工作者、治疗师、精神健康治疗师、牙医、药剂师、饮食治疗师等。这个队伍的人员在一起密切工作以为老年人提供良好的机构照护。非专业人士，如提供饮食照护、协助洗澡和个人卫生的工作人员，同样也对老年人的照护质量起到重要的影响作用。

机构护理服务是劳动密集型的，因此护理质量在很大程度上取决于护理人员的素质。这些人员的数目、是否经过培训、各自的能力等因素都被认为是影响机构照护质量的重要因素。在国外，很多研究已经发现工作人员的类型组成、专业能力等与机构照护的质量相关。在国外，对于机构照护中的人员组成有相应的规定，但是我国目前尚缺乏此方面的信息。

iii. Reimbursement Methods

Many researchers have argued about the effects of reimbursement methods and rates on institutional quality of care. In China, the reimbursement regulation is not very clear for institutional care. Foreign researchers have reported that higher reimbursement rates have a positive relationship with staffing levels, but no consistent results showed higher reimbursement rates are positively associated with higher quality of institutional care. More studies are needed. In addition, the effects of payment systems and reimbursement methods on the accessibility of institutional care and quality of services need to be explored in future.

III. Strategies to Promote Quality of Institutional Care

The followings are some strategies that have been proposed to improve quality of care and life in nursing facilities. There are three categories to group these strategies: increasing mandatory external pressure on nursing facilities to improve quality of care; increasing voluntary external incentives to improve quality of care; and changing nursing facilities' internal operations.

i. Increasing Mandatory External Pressure

1. Direct regulation　The most important part to improve quality of care and life in nursing facilities is direct regulation. Facilities cannot operate unless they are licensed by the province in which they are located, and they cannot receive government funding unless they are certified as meeting the national quality standards. Most of the recent studies reveal that the inadequate regulation involves allegations of weak enforcement rather than inadequate nursing home quality standards.

2. Improving information systems for quality monitoring　Valid, reliable, and timely data about nursing facility residents and the care they receive are essential both to outside regulators and to individual providers. In the US, key data about all nursing home residents are collected as part of the federal-mandated minimum data set (MDS). The MDS has been originally designed for needs assessment and care planning, but later it has been used to periodically collect information on resident functional and medical status. Since June 1998, all nursing homes have been required to submit the MDS information electronically to the government on a quarterly basis.

（三）养老花费支付办法

很多研究发现不同的养老花费支付办法与机构照护质量相关。在中国，养老花费支付体系尚不完善，缺少相应的研究。国外研究发现较好的养老花费支付办法和较高的支付率与机构内的人员组成结构成正相关，但是否与照护的高质量相关尚未定论。我国机构照护的养老花费支付体系与机构照护质量间的关系尚需要进一步的探讨。

三、促进机构照护质量的策略

以下列举出有助于促进机构照护质量的三大类促进策略：增加外界的强制性策略；增加外界公众的呼吁；改变养老机构的内部运转特点。

（一）增加外界强制性策略

1. 直接管理　养老机构必须经过政府审批同意后才可以开设。他们必须符合一定的政策要求和质量标准后才可以得到国家的相应补贴。

2. 促进质量监管的信息系统的建设　关于养老机构照护质量的有效的、可信的数据对于保证照护质量是非常重要的。在美国，所有养老机构的老年人需要被评估，并将评估数据填入最小评估数据集（minimum data set，MDS）。MDS 不仅被用于患者的评估和制订计划，目前也被用于周期性地评价老年人的信息和其功能状态。在美国，从 1998 年开始，护理院被要求每个季度提供一次该院老年人的基本信息，即使用 MDS 去统一评定。

Box 6-1 The Long-term Care Minimum Data Set (MDS)

The long-term care minimum data set (MDS) is a standardized, primary screening and assessment tool of health status that forms the foundation of the comprehensive assessment for all residents in a Medicare and/or Medicaid-certified long-term care facility. The MDS contains items that measure physical, psychological and psychosocial functioning. The items in the MDS give a multidimensional view of the patient's functional capacities and helps staff to identify health problems.

3. Strengthening the caregiving workforce

The first strategy is to increase the amount of personnel in nursing homes by mandating higher minimum staffing ratios; the second strategy is to increase the required minimum training of people who work in nursing facilities, especially certified nurse assistants. The final approach is to improve wages, benefits, and working conditions in nursing homes to attract and retain "better", more qualified staff. In the United States, the number of personnel per resident varies widely across facilities. Non-sufficient staff cannot provide nursing and related services to attain or maintain the "highest practical level" of physical, mental, and psychosocial well-being of every resident. But the national regulation does not provide specific standards or guidance as to what constitutes "sufficient" staffing. A number of studies have found that a positive association between nurse staffing levels and the processes and outcomes of care. Higher nurse staffing hours were associated with fewer nursing home deficiencies.

4. Staff training　Without adequately training, staff cannot provide good quality of care. Especially with the increased acuity of nursing home residents and the greater complexity of care needed today, one strategy to improve quality of care is to significantly increase training requirements for all types of nursing home staff. Currently, certified nurse assistants make up the largest proportion of caregiving personnel in nursing homes and provide most of the direct care, but they receive little formal training. In the US, the government requires nursing assistants to receive a minimum of 75 hours of entry-level training, to participate in 12 hours of in-service training per year, and to pass a competency examination within 4 months of employment.

Box 6-1　长期照护机构中的最小数据集（MDS）

长期照护机构中的最小数据集是一个标准化的测评工具，用于基本筛查和随后评估在长期照护机构中入住人群的健康状况，它是对这些居住在由美国医疗照护保险认可的长期照护机构中的人群进行综合评估的基础。MDS测评生理、心理和社会等各方面的功能。这个测评工具对入住人群的多维度功能进行了描述，以帮助机构中的照护者确认这些入住人群的健康问题。

3. **加强养老机构中的人力资源配置**　可以通过规定养老机构中最低人力配置标准来保证养老机构中有最低限度的人力资源。另外，还可以对养老机构中人员的培训活动提出政策性要求，特别是那些获得证书的护工。最后，通过增加工资待遇、福利，改善工作环境等方法吸引那些更好的员工加盟。

4. **员工培训**　养老机构中的员工一定要经过合适的培训，否则不能提供符合要求的高质量的服务。政府要制订相应的最低培训要求和培训标准。如在美国，政府规定护工要接受75小时的上岗前培训，工作后要每年接受12小时的继续教育，员工在接受雇佣后4个月内要通过相应的能力考核。

ii. Increasing Voluntary External Incentives

1. Providing consumers with more information Providing consumers and their families with more information about quality of care in individual nursing homes can help them choose facilities which provide better care to use. The market competition will force improvements in quality of care of nursing homes. In the US, there are some "Nursing Home Compare" websites to provide information about individual nursing homes. The information include the general characteristics of the facility (e. g. , for-profit or nonprofit) and residents (e. g. , percentage of residents who are very dependent in eating), citations for deficiencies in meeting the federal certification standards, and staffing ratios.

2. Strengthening consumer advocacy Consumer advocacy programs can play a range of functions, assisting with individual complaints and mediating conflicts, advocating public policies to improve quality of care, educating public policies to improve quality of care and consumer protection, and raising the salience of quality-of-care issues.

3. Increasing medical insurance reimbursement Currently, most nursing home residents pay the service fees by themselves. The reimbursement policy for nursing home residents is still in the developing process. Studies from foreign countries show that there is a relationship between lower reimbursement rates and poor quality of care in nursing homes. In addition, the reimbursement policy is very critical to the level of resources available to nursing homes.

iii. Changing Nursing Facilities' Internal operations

1. Developing and implementing practice guidelines It is no doubt that nursing homes must take responsibility for changes at the micro level, where individual caregivers interact with individual nursing home residents. In order to help care providers to provide better direct care, practice protocols should be developed for a number of conditions, including incontinence, restraints, pressure ulcers, pain and depression.

2. Changing the culture of nursing facilities With the new goal of making nursing homes more homelike, less institutional, and less medical, the innovations on the social, cultural, and physical environments in nursing facilities have developed. These innovations are appealing and appear to address many of the quality-of-life problems in traditional nursing homes. For instance, it emphasizes community by linking the

（二）增加外界公众的呼吁

1. **为消费者提供更多的信息** 国家要为老年人及其照顾者提供更多的关于每个机构照护质量的相关信息，这样个体可以选择到照护质量更好的机构接受照护。这种良性的市场竞争会使得各个照护机构要立足于提高自己的照护质量。如在美国，就有比较各个照护机构质量的网站，使得公众能够了解这些照护机构的基本特点和基本质量状况，以及入住人员的基本功能状况。

2. **加强养老机构使用者的呼吁** 养老机构的使用者呼吁项目可以帮助养老机构中的个体报告不良的照护经历、药物错用情况，呼吁相关政策的改变等。

3. **增加医疗保险赔付比例** 目前，很多养老机构的老年人是自己付养老机构的费用。对于养老机构医疗保险赔付的政策制订尚在发展中。发展完善的医疗保险赔付制度有可能促进机构照护的质量，同时也可能会扩展养老机构可以获取到的资源。

（三）改变养老机构中的内部运转机制

1. **发展和实施相应的实践指南** 为了使得机构内的照顾者能为老年人提供较好的照护质量，应该制订可以参照实施的各种实践指南，如失禁老年人的照护指南、约束的使用条件、压疮、疼痛和抑郁患者的照护指南等。

2. **改变照护机构内的环境氛围** 提倡养老照护机构内的氛围应更接近于家庭的环境，而不要像医疗机构那样。在养老照护机构内发展较好的人文社会环境非常重要，如养老照护机构应有较宽敞的外界庭院，可以养花草树木和宠物，也可以有儿童和老年人互动的场所。这种新的环境文化理念会相应提高

facility to the outside world in which plants and animals abound and children interact with residents. Encouraging these new care models might improve quality of care and life.

Quality of care in nursing facilities remains a major problem for which there are no simple solutions. All of the possible strategies for reform face some political and financial barriers. More studies need to be done to address the efficacy of the strategies.

(LIU Yu)

Key Points

1. According to the complexity of care provided and the amount of skilled care and services required by the residents served, Long-term care settings can go from more structured to less structured as one moves from the institutional setting to community-based programs to the home setting.

2. Community-based elderly care services usually include home health care, community-based alternative programs, respite care, adult day care programs, senior citizen centers, and other access services.

3. Institutional-based elderly care facility is elder's permanent or temporary home. There are different kinds of institutional-based care program which are skilled nursing facilities, assisted living programs, special care units, continuing care retirement community, and hospice care.

4. Home care is an old-age insurance socialized service supported by community and society, aiming to offer services to the aged people in their own homes.

5. Home adaptation or modification can provide friendlier elder living so older occupants may continue to live in the comfort of home. The focus of making a home elder-friendly should always be on increasing and improving the following four elements: self-sufficiency/self-reliance, safety/security, comfort and convenience.

6. The family social environment mainly refers to the inter-personal relationships in the family, including relationships between spouses, parents and kids, siblings, mothers-in-law and daughters-in-law, and grandparents and the kids. These relationships form an interrelated and interactive family relationship network. Tension of any of these relationships can bring harms to the steady and harmony of the family.

养老机构的照护质量。

要促进养老机构的照护质量，没有单一的方法可以促成。而且这些促进策略可能还会受到国家政策和经济因素的制约，同时也需要更多的研究去探讨可行的质量促进策略。

（刘　宇）

本章要点

1. 根据所提供照护的复杂性、所需要的照护技能的数量以及所需要的服务特点，长期照护的场所可以由居家、社区照护机构或者机构照护等不同的场所来提供。

2. 以社区为基础的养老照护服务通常包括家庭健康服务、社区替代性服务、喘息服务、成人日间照料、社区老人中心，以及其他可利用的服务等。

3. 以机构为基础的养老照护是老年人临时的或者永久居住的场所。有各种不同类型的居家照护服务方式，包括护理院、有助聚居、特殊照护单元、连续照护型退休社区以及临终关怀服务等。

4. 居家照护是由社区和社会所支持的一种养老方式，目的是为居家老人提供相应的养老照护服务。

5. 家庭环境改造和调整可以为老年人提供一个更加友好和舒适的可以持续居住的环境。适老化居家环境调整的重点在于以下四个方面：自主、安全、舒适以及方便。

6. 家庭中的社会环境是指家庭成员间的交往，包括配偶间的关系、父母与孩子之间的关系、兄弟姐妹间的关系，婆媳间关系、祖孙辈之间的关系等。这些关系形成了一个相关联系和相互影响的关系网。任何关系中的紧张都会影响整个家庭关系的稳定与和谐。

7. There are some common issues during home care including the caregivers facing stress and challenges, abuse and neglect of the aged and delayed first aid for empty-nest elderly. All these issues need to be paid more attention by health care personnel.

8. The physical and social environment in which care occurs must be modified to facilitate maintenance of function and reduce the possibilities of harms to elderly.

9. There are corresponding characteristics and requirements for different kinds of institutional care facilities.

10. There are three categories to group these strategies: increasing mandatory external pressure on nursing facilities to improve quality of care; increasing voluntary external incentives to improve quality of care; and changing nursing facilities' internal operations.

Critical Thinking Exercise

1. An 87-year-old woman is being treated for a cardiac disorder. She is interested in her care and she is alert too. However, she has a hearing deficit and does not have a hearing aid. On teaching her about her cardiac medication, you notice that she often gets confused about the names, dosing schedules, and side effects of each medication. You know she has a daughter living with her.

Questions:

(1) How will you do to offer several strategies to help her remain independent and maintain accurate medication schedules and monitoring?

(2) What will you do to strengthen the family caregiver's roles?

2. A 92-year-old man has been living with his 65-year-old son for many years. The son is suffering from complications of long-term diabetes and feels that he is no longer capable to take care for his dad. No other family members are available to take care of the old man or take him into their home.

Question: How would you go about determining the options available to the dad?

7. 在居家照护中要关注一些问题，包括照顾者面临的照护压力与挑战，老年人虐待，空巢老人居家急救不及时。这些问题需要健康保健人员加以关注。

8. 物理环境和社会环境调整的目的是可以促进和维持老年人的功能、减少老年人受到伤害。

9. 不同的机构照护场所具有不同的特点和要求。

10. 有助于促进机构照护质量的三大类促进策略是增加外界的强制性策略，增加外界公众的呼吁，改变养老机构的内部运转特点。

批判性思维练习

1. 一位87岁高龄的女士正在接受有关心脏系统疾病的治疗。她意识敏捷，对自己的疾病照护也很感兴趣。但是听力不佳，也没有相应的助听设备。在护士进行有关心血管药物服用的知识宣教时，发现她经常对每种药物的名字、剂量、副作用等感到困惑。她的女儿现在和她一起居住。

思考：

（1）你怎么做可以帮助她维持生活的独立以及按照医嘱正确服用药物和监测药物的作用？

（2）你将如何帮助家庭照顾者更加胜任她的照顾者角色？

2. 一位92岁的男士和他65岁的儿子已经一起生活了很多年。儿子多年来一直受糖尿病并发症的影响，越来越感觉到自己没有能力照护好自己的父亲了。其他家庭成员也没有能力来照护这位92岁的老人。

思考：你如何为家庭成员提供可执行的老年人照护方式？

Chapter 7 Protection of Rights and Interests of Elderly

第七章 老年人权益与保护

On completion of this chapter, the reader will be able to:

- Describe the significance of the national strategy to actively respond to population aging;

- Describe the purpose of the *Law on the Protection of the Rights and Interests of the Elderly*;

- List the changes in the new version of the *Law on the Protection of the Rights and Interests of the Elderly*.

学完本章节，应完成以下目标：

- 描述积极应对人口老龄化国家战略的意义；

- 描述老年人权益保障法的目的；

- 列举新版《老年人权益保障法》的变化。

The elderly is a vulnerable group. Due to the natural physical aging and the readjustment of interest and distribution, the needs of some elderly people are easy to be ignored, which limits their ability to meet their own needs. *The Law of the People's Republic of China on the Protection of the Rights and Interests of the Elderly*, promulgated and implemented in 1996, is the first law in Chinese history that specifically protects the elderly, which provides a legal basis in China. This chapter will introduce the national strategy to actively respond to aging and the relevant contents of China's *Law on the Protection of the Rights and Interests of the Elderly*.

老年人属于社会人口中的弱势群体。生理的自然衰老及社会变迁过程中利益关系和分配关系的重新调整等原因，部分老人的需求容易被忽视，使老年人满足自身需求的能力也受到限制。1996年颁布实施的《中华人民共和国老年人权益保障法》是我国历史上第一部专门保护老年人权益的法律，使得我国老年人权益保障有了法律依据。本章将介绍积极应对老龄化的国家战略以及我国老年人权益保障法的相关内容。

Section 1 National Strategy for Actively Responding to Population Aging

China actively responds to the aging population, constantly introduces new policies, improves the social security system, and actively responds to the challenges brought by aging. The *"suggestions of the CPC Central Committee on formulating the 14th five year plan for national economic and social development and the long-term goals for 2035"* adopted at the Fifth Plenary Session of the 19th CPC Central Committee proposed to "implement the national strategy to actively respond to population aging". The implementation of the national strategy to actively respond to population aging is related to the overall development of the country and the well-being of the people.

I. Great Significance of Implementing the National Strategy to Actively Respond to Population Aging

The implementation of the national strategy to actively respond to population aging is an important embodiment of fulfilling the original mission of the party and adhering to the people-centered development thought. The implementation of the national strategy to actively respond to the aging of the population, so that every elderly person can live at ease, calm and comfortable, realize the aspirations of the majority of the elderly and their families for an increasingly happy life, and give full play to the positive role of the elderly in economic and social construction, will further highlight the original mission of the party and the superiority of our socialist system.

第一节　积极应对人口老龄化国家战略

我国积极应对人口老龄化，不断出台新政策，完善社会保障制度，积极应对老龄化带来的挑战。党的十九届五中全会通过的《中共中央关于制定国民经济和社会发展第十四个五年规划和2035年远景目标的建议》提出"实施积极应对人口老龄化国家战略"。实施积极应对人口老龄化国家战略，事关国家发展全局，事关百姓福祉。

一、实施积极应对人口老龄化国家战略的重大意义

实施积极应对人口老龄化国家战略，是践行党的初心使命、坚持以人民为中心的发展思想的重要体现。实施积极应对人口老龄化国家战略，让每位老年人都能生活得安心、静心、舒心，实现广大老年人及其家庭对日益增长的美好生活向往，发挥老年人在经济社会建设中的积极作用，必将进一步彰显党的初心使命和我国社会主义制度的优越性。

The implementation of the national strategy to actively respond to population aging is an important consideration in maintaining national population security, social harmony and stability, and achieving the second Centennial goal. Promoting the active response to population aging as a national strategy is conducive to the further consensus of the whole Party and society, enhancing the sense of risk, responsibility, mission and urgency, coordinating the resources and forces of all parties, and responding in a timely, scientific and comprehensive manner.

Implementing the national strategy to actively respond to population aging is an important measure to promote high-quality development and accelerate the construction of a new development pattern. The rolling "silver wave" not only brings great challenges and impacts to China's economic and social development, but also contains valuable development opportunities and hopes.

The implementation of the national strategy to actively respond to population aging is conducive to turning danger into opportunity, seeking opportunities in danger, hedging adverse effects, and actively transforming aging risks into social benefits; It is conducive to further promoting the supply side structural reform, comprehensively liberalizing the elderly care service market, giving birth to new industries, new formats and new models of the silver economy, and cultivating new drivers of economic growth; It is conducive to expanding elderly consumption, continuously expanding domestic demand, enriching the domestic cycle, and promoting the benign interaction between domestic and international cycles.

The pension policy is the concrete embodiment of the concept and attitude of coping with population aging, and the sum of public policies adopted to adjust the contradiction between aging and social, political, economic and cultural development. With the deepening of China's aging, in recent years, China has made great efforts to cope with the aging of the population by issuing pension policies in the form of notices and laws through the State Council, the national office for aging, the Ministry of human resources and social security and other departments, focusing on national education, pension services, social security, talent training and other aspects. The quantitative change trend of pension policies generally reflects the positive correlation between pension demand and policy supply.

实施积极应对人口老龄化国家战略，是维护国家人口安全和社会和谐稳定、实现第二个百年奋斗目标的重要考量。把积极应对人口老龄化提升为国家战略，有利于全党全社会进一步凝聚共识，增强风险意识和责任感、使命感、紧迫感，统筹各方资源力量，及时应对、科学应对、综合应对。

实施积极应对人口老龄化国家战略，是推动高质量发展、加快构建新发展格局的重要举措。滚滚而来的"银发浪潮"，既给我国经济社会发展带来巨大挑战和冲击，也蕴藏着宝贵的发展机遇和希望。

实施积极应对人口老龄化国家战略，有利于化危为机、危中寻机，对冲不利影响，积极转化老龄风险为社会收益；有利于深入推进供给侧结构性改革，全面放开养老服务市场，催生"银发经济"新产业、新业态、新模式，培育形成经济增长新动能；有利于拓展银发消费，持续扩大内需，充实国内大循环，促进国内国际双循环良性互动。

养老政策是应对人口老龄化在理念与态度上的具体体现，是调整老龄化问题与社会政治经济文化发展矛盾所采取的公共政策的总和。随着中国老龄化的不断加深，近年来，我国通过国务院、国家老龄办、人力资源和社会保障部等部门发布通知、法律等形式的养老政策，围绕国情教育、养老服务、社会保障、人才培养等方面积极应对人口老龄化，养老政策数量变迁趋势总体上体现出养老需求与政策供给的正相关性。

II. Attach Importance to Education of Aging National Conditions

The national education on population aging is to make the whole society realize that population aging brings about economic and social problems under the background of social age structure changes, development problems and major social transformation problems. Enhance the awareness of the whole society to actively respond to aging, condense social consensus and form a joint force.

In 2018, the national office on aging issued the notice on carrying out national education on population aging, which aims to improve the aging awareness of Party and government cadres, teenagers and the elderly through national strength education, and create a good atmosphere to actively respond to population aging, which is of strategic significance for building the general pattern of aging work. Article 8 of Chapter 1 of the law of the people's Republic of China on the protection of the rights and interests of the elderly stipulates that the state should carry out education on the national conditions of population aging and enhance the awareness of the whole society to actively respond to aging. The whole society should carry out extensive publicity and education activities to respect, provide for and help the elderly, and establish a social custom of respecting, caring for and helping the elderly.

III. Layered Security to Meet the Needs of Elderly Care in Multiple Directions

With the development of population aging in China, the scale of elderly groups such as the elderly, disabled and semi-disabled, empty nest elderly and lost independence is becoming larger and larger. In view of the insufficient allocation of formal and informal resources, and the problems still existing in low-income elderly groups, the Chinese government formulates different elderly care services and social security policies according to the location, income, physical condition, etc. of different elderly groups to meet the growing variety of elderly care services Social security and other needs to promote healthy aging. In 2019, *the Guiding Opinions on Establishing and Improving the Elderly Health Service System* was put forward, which requires to meet the multi-level and diversified health service needs of the elderly, provide comprehensive and continuous whole process services. By 2022, a comprehensive and continuous elderly health

二、重视老龄化国情教育

人口老龄化国情教育，就是要让全社会都能认识到，人口老龄化带来的是社会年龄结构变化背景下的经济社会问题，是发展的问题，是重大社会转型问题。增强全社会积极应对老龄化的意识，凝聚社会共识，形成合力。

2018 年全国老龄办发布《关于开展人口老龄化国情教育的通知》旨在通过国强教育重点提高是党政干部、青少年和老年人的老龄意识，营造积极应对人口老龄化的良好氛围，对于构建老龄工作大格局具有战略意义。《中华人民共和国老年人权益保障法》中第一章第八条规定国家要进行人口老龄化国情教育，增强全社会积极应对老龄化意识。全社会应当广泛开展敬老、养老、助老宣传教育活动，树立尊重、关心、帮助老年人的社会风尚。

三、分层保障，多方位满足养老需求

随着我国人口老龄化的发展，高龄、失能半失能、空巢、失独等老人群体规模日益庞大，针对正式资源、非正式资源配置不足，低收入老年群体仍然存在的问题，我国政府根据不同老年群体的地区、收入、身体状况等，制定不同养老服务以及社会保障政策，满足不同老年群体日益增长的各种养老服务、社会保障等需求，促进健康老龄化。2019 年提出了《关于建立完善老年健康服务体系的指导意见》（国卫老龄发〔2019〕61 号）要求以满足多层次、多样化的老年人健康服务需求为导向，兜底保障，提供综合连续的全程服务。到 2022 年，综合连续、覆盖城乡的老年健康服务体系基本建立，老年人的健康服

service system covering urban and rural areas will be basically established, and the health service needs of the elderly will be basically met.

IV. Optimize Resource Allocation and Explore a New Mode of Providing for the Aged

The new elderly care model refers to a model based on the "combination of medical care and elderly care" and "smart elderly care", in which governments, institutions, individuals, etc. use the Internet, big data, etc. to provide health care, life care, spiritual comfort, etc. for elderly groups with different physical conditions.

The combination of medical care and elderly care refers to the integration of medical care, elderly care and rehabilitation to promote the construction of a social service system "based on home-based elderly care, supported by community services and supplemented by institutional elderly care". The smart elderly care service policy refers to the policies issued by the state, including the development goals, service contents and service methods of smart elderly care services, to regulate the healthy development of smart elderly care. The development of smart elderly care industry is to meet the practical needs of the development of the elderly care market, solve the disadvantages of traditional elderly care, adapt to the "Internet +" era, and actively respond to the national population aging policy. From 2017 to 2020, the state successively issued policies to promote the integration of medical care and elderly care and smart elderly care. In 2019, the "several opinions on further promoting the development of the integration of medical care and elderly care" (Guo Wei Lao Sheng Fa [2019] No. 60) put forward opinions on promoting the reform of "decentralized management and service" of medical care and elderly care institutions and increasing government support and security in view of the current problems that still exist, such as the need for further connection between medical care and elderly care services, At the same time, the national medium and long term plan for actively responding to population aging requires the in-depth implementation of the innovation driven development strategy, taking technological innovation as the first driving force and strategic support for actively responding to population aging, further promoting the development of smart elderly care, promoting the combination of online and offline, realizing the optimal allocation of resources, and meeting the medical and elderly care needs of the elderly.

务需求得到基本满足。

四、优化资源配置，探索养老新模式

新型养老模式是指基于"医养结合"与"智慧养老"，由政府、机构、个人等利用互联网、大数据等为不同身体状况的老年群体提供健康医疗、生活照料、精神慰藉等的模式。

医养结合是指医疗、养老、康复为一体，促进"以居家养老为基础、社区服务为依托、机构养老为补充"的社会服务体系的建设。智慧养老服务政策是指国家出台的包含智慧养老服务发展目标、服务内容服务方式等来规范智慧养老事业健康发展。发展智慧养老产业是满足养老市场发展、破解传统养老弊端、适合"互联网+"时代、积极响应国家人口老龄化政策等方面的现实需要。2017年到2020年国家陆续出台促进医养结合与智慧养老的政策，其中2019年《关于深入推进医养结合发展的若干意见》（国卫老龄发〔2019〕60号）针对当前仍存在医疗卫生与养老服务需进一步衔接等问题，提出了推进医养结合机构"放管服"改革、加大政府支持力度与保障的意见，同时《国家积极应对人口老龄化中长期规划》要求深入实施创新驱动发展战略，把技术创新作为积极应对人口老龄化的第一动力和战略支撑，进一步推进智慧养老的发展，促进线上与线下结合，实现资源的优化配置，满足老年人的医疗、养老等需求。

Section 2 *Law on the Protection of the Rights and Interests of the Elderly*

I. Overview of *Law on the Protection of the Rights and Interests of Elderly*

The *Law of the People's Republic of China on the Protection of the Rights and Interests of the Elderly* (hereinafter referred to as *Law on the Protection of the Rights and Interests of the Elderly*) was adopted at the 21st Meeting of the Standing Committee of the Eighth National People's Congress on August 29, 1996. It is the first law in China's history that specifically protects the rights and interests of the elderly and another important law in China to protect the rights and interests of special groups of citizens. It marks the legalization of the protection of the rights and interests of the elderly in China. The promulgation and implementation of *Law on the Protection of the Rights and Interests of the Elderly* met the objective requirements of the development of China's aging population and the protection of the rights and interests of the elderly at that time, reflected China's national conditions, maintained Chinese tradition, and reflected the wishes of the elderly. It is a law with Chinese characteristics to protect the legitimate rights and interests of the elderly. After three amendments in 2009, 2012 and 2018, the full text of the latest version of *Law on the Protection of the Rights and Interests of the Elderly* includes general provisions, family support and support, social security, social services, social preferential treatment, livable environment, participation in social development, legal liability and supplementary provisions, with a total of 85 articles in nine chapters.

II. Purpose of *Law on the Protection of the Rights and Interests of the Elderly*

From family pension, home-based pension to institutional pension, every revision and improvement of *Law on the Protection of the Rights and Interests of the Elderly* is to protect the legitimate rights and interests of the elderly, develop the cause of the elderly, carry forward the virtues of respecting, providing for and helping the elderly of the Chinese nation, enhance the sense of responsibility of the whole society, improve the conditions for safeguarding the rights and interests of the elderly, and achieve a sense of security, a sense of medical care, a sense of action, a sense of learning, and a sense of happiness for the elderly.

第二节 《老年人权益保障法》

一、《老年人权益保障法》概述

《中华人民共和国老年人权益保障法》（以下简称《老年人权益保障法》）是 1996 年 8 月 29 日第八届全国人民代表大会常务委员会第二十一次会议通过，是我国历史上第一部专门保护老年人权益的法律，是我国保护公民特殊群体权益的又一部重要法律，标志着我国老年人权益保障工作从此走上法制化的轨道。《老年人权益保障法》的颁布实施适应了当时中国人口老龄化发展和老年人权益保障的客观要求，体现了中国国情，保持了中国传统，反映了老年人的心愿，是一部有中国特色的保护老年人合法权益的法律。经2009 年、2012 年和 2018 年三次修正，最新版的《老年人权益保障法》全文包括总则、家庭赡养与扶养、社会保障、社会服务、社会优待、宜居环境、参与社会发展、法律责任、附则，共九章八十五条。

二、《老年人权益保障法》的目的

从家庭养老、居家养老到机构养老，每一次《老年人权益保障法》的修改与完善，都是为保障老年人合法权益，发展老年事业弘扬中华民族敬老、养老、助老的美德，增强全社会的责任意识，改善维护老年人权益的各种条件，实现老有所养、老有所医、老有所为、老有所学、老有所乐。

III. Changes in the New Version of *Law on the Protection of the Rights and Interests of the Elderly*

1. Take active response to population aging as a long-term strategic task of the country. The general provisions stipulate that the state should carry out national education on population aging to enhance the awareness of active aging in the whole society; Attach importance to and support scientific research on aging, and establish a statistical investigation and release system for the cause of aging, aging work and the situation of the elderly. This regulation clarifies the strategic positioning of dealing with aging.

2. The family pension has been repositioned. Change "the elderly care mainly depends on family" to "the elderly care is based on home". At present, the average number of people in each family in China is only 3.1. The miniaturization of the family has significantly weakened the function of family pension. It is stipulated that the elderly pension is based on home, which emphasizes the role of the state and society in the elderly pension.

3. Emphasize the daily services and spiritual needs of the elderly. The current *Law on the Protection of the Rights and Interests of the Elderly* stipulates that "local people's governments at all levels, relevant departments and grass-roots mass autonomous organizations should incorporate elderly care service facilities into the construction planning of supporting facilities in urban and rural communities, establish service facilities and outlets to meet the needs of the elderly, such as life services, cultural and sports activities, daily care, disease care and rehabilitation, and provide services to the elderly nearby." In addition, the new law adds the construction of an elderly friendly environment and stipulates the principles for the state to promote the construction of a livable environment for the elderly.

In terms of meeting the spiritual needs of the elderly, the current *Law on the Protection of the Rights and Interests of the Elderly* stipulates that family members should care about the spiritual needs of the elderly and should not ignore or neglect the elderly. Dependents who live separately from the elderly should often visit or greet the elderly. At the same time, it stipulates that employers should guarantee the right of dependents to visit elder parents and take leave in accordance with relevant regulations, which solves the practical problems of many job seekers.

4. Gradually improve the level of preferential treatment for the elderly. People's governments at all levels

三、新版《老年人权益保障法》的变化

1. 将积极应对人口老龄化作为国家的一项长期战略任务。总则中规定国家进行人口老龄化国情教育，增强全社会积极老龄化意识；重视和支持老龄科学研究，建立老龄事业、老龄工作和老年人状况统计调查和发布制度。这一规定明确了应对老龄化的战略定位。

2. 对家庭养老做了重新定位。将"老年人养老主要依靠家庭"改为"老年人养老以居家为基础"。我国目前平均每个家庭只有 3.1人，家庭的小型化使得家庭养老的功能明显弱化，规定老年人养老以居家为基础，就更强调了国家和社会在老年人养老上的作用。

3. 注重老年人的日常服务和精神需求。现《老年人权益保障法》规定"地方各级人民政府和有关部门、基层群众性自治组织，应当将养老服务设施纳入城乡社区配套设施建设规划，建立适应老年人需要的生活服务、文化体育活动、日间照料、疾病护理与康复等服务设施和网点，就近为老年人提供服务。"另外，新法增加了宜居环境建设，对国家推进老年宜居环境建设做了原则规定。

在满足老年人精神需求方面，现《老年人权益保障法》规定家庭成员应当关心老年人的精神需求，不得忽视、冷落老年人。与老年人分开居住的赡养人，应当经常看望或者问候老年人。同时规定用人单位应该按照有关规定保障赡养人探亲休假的权利，解决了很多在外求职者的实际问题。

4. 逐步提高对老年人的优待水平。各级人民政府和有关部门应当为老年人及时、便利

and relevant departments shall provide conditions for the elderly to receive pensions, settle medical expenses and enjoy other material assistance in a timely and convenient manner. At the same time, it is stipulated that art galleries, museums, libraries, memorial halls and other places should be free or preferential to the elderly.

5. Protect the rights of the elderly to participate in public affairs. The current *Law on the Protection of the Rights and Interests of the Elderly* stipulates that "the formulation of laws, regulations, rules and public policies involving major issues of the rights and interests of the elderly should listen to the opinions of the elderly and their organizations. The elderly and their organizations have the right to put forward opinions and suggestions on the protection of the rights and interests of the elderly and the development of the cause of aging to state departments."

IV. Abuse of Elderly

The abuse of the elderly is a social problem worldwide. The physical and mental health of the elderly has been damaged due to abuse, the mortality rate has increased, and the medical cost has increased significantly, which has seriously affected their later life. The problem of elder abuse occurs in both developing and developed countries, but its existence is generally underestimated in the world. Nurses play a very important role in identifying and preventing elder abuse.

WHO's definition of abuse of the elderly: "in any relationship that should be trusted, single or repeated behaviors that cause injury or pain to the elderly, or lack of appropriate actions to take care of the elderly." In the WHO/ International Study on the Prevention of Abuse, the abuse of the elderly could be divided into three categories: neglect, including isolation, abandonment and social exclusion, violation of personal, legal and medical rights, deprive of choice, decision, status, finance and respect. The severity of the consequences of maltreatment of the elderly depends on the type of injury or damage suffered, the intention of maltreatment, severity, frequency and duration. Timely access to health care and social assistance will affect the final outcome. The key to dealing with the abuse of the elderly lies in prevention and intervention.

The elderly are the contributors, who have made or still make contributions to national construction, social development, national progress and family life, and laying the foundation for today and future development. In the construction of a socialist harmonious society, we should strengthen the protection of the rights and interests of

地领取养老金、结算医疗费和享受其他物质帮助提供条件。同时规定，美术馆、博物馆、图书馆、纪念馆等场所，应当对老年人免费或者优惠开放。

5. 保障老年人参与公共事务的权利。现《老年人权益保障法》规定："制定法律、法规、规章和公共政策，涉及老年人权益重大问题的，应当听取老年人和老年人组织的意见。老年人和老年人组织有权向国家机关提出老年人权益保障、老龄事业发展等方面的意见和建议。"

四、老年人虐待的问题

老年人虐待的现象是一个世界性的社会问题和健康问题，老年人因被虐待导致身心健康受到伤害，死亡率升高，医疗费用大幅上升，严重影响了老年人的晚年生活。虐待老人的问题在发展中国家和发达国家都有发生，但全球却普遍低估它的存在。护士在识别和预防虐待老人方面起着非常重要的作用。

WHO 对虐待老年人的定义："在任何理应相互信任的关系中，单次或重复性导致老人受到伤害或痛苦的行为，或缺乏照顾老年人的适当行动。"在世界卫生组织 / 国际防止老年人虐待的研究中，老年人将虐待分为三大类：忽视，包括孤立、遗弃和社会排斥；侵犯人身、法律和医疗权利；剥夺选择、决定、地位、财政和尊重。虐待老年人造成的后果的轻重程度，取决于所受的伤害或损害的类型、虐待的意图、严重程度、频率和延续时间。能否及时得到保健及社会帮助将影响到最终结果，应对虐待老年人问题的关键在于预防和干预。

老年人是劳动者，曾经或依旧为国家建设和社会发展、民族进步以及家庭生活做出贡献，为今天和未来的发展奠定了基础。在建设社会主义和谐社会建设中，要加大保护老年人权益的力度，不断完善《老年人权益

the elderly, constantly improve *Law on the Protection of the Rights and Interests of the Elderly*, and maximize the protection of the rights and interests of the elderly.

保障法》，最大限度地保护老年人的权益。

Key Points

1. The implementation of the national strategy to actively respond to population aging is an important embodiment of fulfilling the original mission of the party and adhering to the people-centered development thought; It is an important consideration to maintain national population security, social harmony and stability, and achieve the second Centennial goal. It is an important measure to promote high-quality development and accelerate the construction of a new development pattern, which is conducive to turning crisis into opportunity and promoting economic growth.

2. We should strengthen the national education on the conditions of population aging and establish a social custom of respecting, caring for and helping the elderly.

3. We should actively explore a new pension model based on "combination of medical care and elderly care" and "smart pension".

4. *Law on the Protection of the Rights and Interests of the Elderly* is the first law in China's history that specifically protects the rights and interests of the elderly, marking that the protection of the rights and interests of the elderly in China has since embarked on the track of legalization.

5. *Law on the Protection of the Rights and Interests of the Elderly* aims to improve the conditions for safeguarding the rights and interests of the elderly, so as to achieve a sense of security, a sense of medicine, a sense of action, a sense of learning and a sense of happiness for the elderly.

6. The abuse of the elderly is a worldwide social and health problem, which seriously affects the old life of the elderly. The world health organization divides abuse into three categories: neglect, aggression and deprivation.

Critical Thinking Exercises

"The elderly have a sense of security, a sense of medical care, a sense of action, a sense of learning, and a sense of happiness for the elderly" is the legislative goal of China's *Law on the Protection of the Rights and Interests of the Elderly*. Please discuss its specific content with examples.

本章要点

1. 实施积极应对人口老龄化国家战略，是践行党的初心使命、坚持以人民为中心的发展思想的重要体现；是维护国家人口安全和社会和谐稳定、实现第二个百年奋斗目标的重要考量；是推动高质量发展、加快构建新发展格局的重要举措，有利于化危为机，促进经济增长。

2. 要加强人口老龄化国情教育，树立尊重、关心、帮助老年人的社会风尚。

3. 要积极探索基于"医养结合"与"智慧养老"的新型养老模式。

4.《老年人权益保障法》是我国历史上第一部专门保护老年人权益的法律，标志着我国老年人权益保障工作从此走上法制化的轨道。

5.《老年人权益保障法》旨在改善维护老年人权益的各种条件，实现老有所养、老有所医、老有所为、老有所学、老有所乐。

6. 老年人虐待现象是一个世界性的社会问题和健康问题，严重影响老年人的晚年生活。世界卫生组织将虐待分为忽视、侵犯和剥夺三类。

批判性思维练习

"老有所养、老有所医、老有所为、老有所学、老有所乐"是我国《老年人权益保障法》立法目标，请结合实例讨论其具体内容。

Chapter 8 Care for Elderly with Common Chronic Disease

第八章　老年人常见慢性病的护理

Learning Objectives

On completion of this chapter, the reader will be able to:

- Discuss factors affecting the incidence of chronic diseases for the elderly;

- Differentiate between healing and curing;

- List care goals for chronic diseases;

- Discuss methods to maximize the benefits of traditional treatments for the elderly with chronic disease;

- List alternative therapies that could benefit the elderly with chronic diseases;

- Discuss strategies for the elderly health promotion.

学习目标

学完本章节，应完成以下目标：

- 探讨老年人发生慢性病的相关因素；

- 区分治疗和治愈；

- 列举慢性病的照护目标；

- 探讨使老年慢性病患者治疗效果最大化的方法；

- 列举有益于老年慢性病患者的替代疗法；

- 探讨老年人健康促进的策略。

Modern medical technology has helped many people survive illnesses that once would have killed them; greater numbers of people are reaching old age, in which the incidence of chronic disease is higher. Common chronic diseases among the elderly, including hypertension, diabetes mellitus, arthritis, heart disease and osteoporosis, are fully introduced in the book of *Medical-Surgical Nursing* instead of this book. Other chronic conditions such as dementia, skin problems, hearing and visual impairment, and so on will be discussed in the following chapters. Since chronic diseases are highly prevalent in the elderly population, gerontological nurses often are involved in assisting patients with the demands caused by chronic conditions. The manner in which a chronic disease is managed can make a huge difference between a high-quality life and an unsatisfying suffering. In this chapter, basic knowledge about chronic diseases and goals for chronic care will be discussed, as well as the principles to manage chronic conditions.

Box 8-1　Case Study

Eighty-three-year-old Mr. Li has been diagnosed with diabetes mellitus for years. According to physical examination, his excess weight is contributing to his problem. He and his wife, who is also obese, have been counseled and educated on the need to reduce weight and to follow good dietary practices.

At his first follow-up visit Mr. Li is found to have gained 4 kg. When questioned, he admits to not following his dietary plan and instead eating the fat meat, fried foods, and cakes that his wife continues to prepare. The record indicates that Mr. Li has been advised that he has circulatory and visual problems that are most likely related to his diabetes, so he has been informed of the risks associated with noncompliance.

Questions:

1. What is primary health problem for Mr. Li?

2. How to balance Mr. Li's eating habits and his health condition?

3. What action should Mr. Li take?

现代医疗技术的进步帮助了越来越多的人免于因疾病而死亡，人类的预期寿命因此不断延长，与此同时，慢性病的发生率也在不断增高。老年人常见的慢性病包括高血压、糖尿病、关节炎、心脏病和骨质疏松等。老年人慢性病的发生率较高，不同的慢性病管理方法对于患者的生活质量会产生巨大影响。因此对于老年专科护士来说，准确认识老年人慢性病管理中的挑战和目标是非常重要的。本章节将介绍老年慢性病的相关基本知识，探讨老年慢性病的照护目标以及慢性病管理策略。

Box 8-1　案例

李先生今年83岁，他患有糖尿病多年。体检结果显示，体重超标是导致李先生健康问题的主要原因。李先生和他的夫人都存在肥胖问题，近期他们针对降低体重和合理饮食进行了咨询，并接受了健康教育。

在第一次家庭随访时，医护人员发现李先生的体重增加了4kg。当问及此事，李先生承认其并未遵从饮食计划，反而吃了他妻子准备的肥肉、油炸食品和甜食。健康档案显示，医护人员已告知李先生，他的糖尿病极易引起循环系统和视力问题，李先生也知道不遵医嘱行为将导致的风险。

问题：

1. 李先生最主要的健康问题是什么？

2. 如何帮助李先生平衡他的饮食习惯和健康状况？

3. 针对李先生的问题，该采取哪些措施？

Section 1　Basic Information about Chronic Disease

Chronic disease, short for non-communicable chronic disease (NCD), is a disease of long duration and generally slow progression. A chronic disease is one lasting 3 months or more, by the definition of the U. S. National Center for Health Statistics.

I. Characteristics of Chronic Disease

Chronic diseases are complex and vary in terms of their natures, etiology, and the extent of their impacts on the community. They include four major types listed by the WHO (box 8-2). Chronic diseases do not often recover spontaneously, and are rarely cured completely. Comorbidity and multi-morbidity are common features of chronic diseases and are associated with worse health outcomes, complex clinical interventions and management, and increased care burden.

Box 8-2　Four Major Types of Chronic Disease

● Cardiovascular diseases (including cerebrovascular disease, heart failure, ischemic cardiopathy) .

● Cancers.

● Chronic respiratory diseases [such as chronic obstructive pulmonary disease (COPD) and asthma].

● Diabetes mellitus.

II. Epidemiology of Chronic Disease

For a variety of reasons, including the fact that more people live longer and the medical technology is improved, the incidence of chronic diseases have increased over the years. Chronic diseases represent the major global health problem of the 21st century. Data from the WHO show that chronic disease is the major cause of premature death, even in places where infectious diseases are rampant.

All age groups and all regions are affected by chronic diseases. And the ageing of the population is the major force driving the epidemic of chronic diseases. Eighty-eight percent of people over the age of 65 or over suffer from two or more diseases.

第一节　慢性病概述

慢性病是慢性非传染性疾病（NCD）的简称，是指病程长，进展缓慢的一类疾病。根据美国国家健康统计中心的定义，一般持续时间超过 3 个月。

一、慢性病的特点

慢性病较为复杂，不同的慢性病在性质、病以及其对社会的影响程度等方面都存在差异。常见的慢性病包括四类（box 8-2）。慢性病患者一般无法自行痊愈，且很少被治愈。慢性病可导致残疾，甚至死亡。

Box 8-2　慢性病的四大类型

● 心血管疾病（包括脑血管疾病、心力衰竭、缺血性心脏病）。

● 肿瘤。

● 慢性呼吸系统疾病（如慢性阻塞性肺病、哮喘）。

● 糖尿病。

二、慢性病的流行病学

在多种原因的影响下，慢性病的发生率逐年增高，已成为 21 世纪全球主要的健康问题。世界卫生组织的数据显示，慢性疾病是导致过早死亡的主要原因，即使在传染病猖獗的地区也是如此。

不同年龄、不同地区都会受到慢性病的侵袭，老年人是慢性病的主要发患者群。65 岁及以上的老年人群中 88% 存在多病共存的问题。

III. Risk Factors of Chronic Diseases

Chronic diseases are driven by complex gene-environment interactions acting across the lifespan and being modulated by socio-economic determinants, psychological factors, gender and age (figure 8-1). Ageing, rapid unplanned urbanization, and the globalization of unhealthy lifestyles are the major risk factors associated with chronic diseases.

三、慢性病的危险因素

慢性疾病是在复杂的基因 – 环境相互作用下产生的，受到社会经济因素、心理因素、性别和年龄影响（图 8–1）。老龄化、过快的城市化发展、不健康生活方式的全球化是慢性病的主要危险因素。

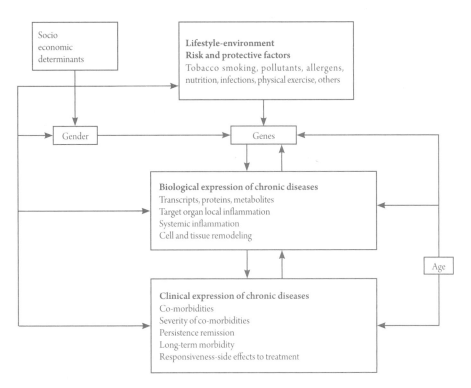

Figure 8-1　Risk factors related with chronic diseases

i. Modifiable Behavioral Risk Factors

Tobacco use, physical inactivity, unhealthy diet and the harmful use of alcohol are modifiable behavioral risk factors of chronic diseases.

ii. Metabolic/Physiological Risk Factors

The behaviors mentioned before lead to four key metabolic/physiological changes that increase the risk of chronic diseases: raised blood pressure, overweight/obesity, hyperglycemia (high blood glucose levels) and hyperlipidemia (high levels of fat in the blood). In terms of attributable deaths, the leading metabolic risk factor

（一）可纠正的行为风险因素

吸烟、缺乏运动、不健康的饮食和有害的饮酒会增加慢性疾病的风险。

（二）代谢和生理相关危险因素

上述的行为可导致血压升高、超重或肥胖、高血糖和高血脂。就死亡原因而言，全球主要的代谢危险因素是血压升高（占全球死亡人数的 18%），其次是超重、肥胖和血糖升高。

globally is elevated blood pressure (to which 18% of global deaths are attributed) followed by overweight and obesity and raised blood glucose.

IV. Socioeconomic Impacts of Chronic Disease

The rapid rise in chronic diseases is predicted to impede poverty reduction initiatives in low-income countries, particularly by increasing household costs associated with health care. Vulnerable and socially disadvantaged people get sicker and die sooner than people with better social-economic status, especially because they are at greater risk of being exposed to harmful products, such as tobacco or unhealthy food, and have limited access to health services.

Section 2　Assessment of Chronic Disease

As for different kinds of chronic diseases, the assessment tools vary a lot, from symptoms experience to quality of life with specific chronic disease. As far as the detail content about the assessment introduction for specific chronic disease, readers could find more information in *Medical-Surgical Nursing* books. In this section, it will give some knowledge about the assessment of chronic care needs, which is also important to direct the care goals and plans.

I. Assessment of Self-care Capacities of the Elderly

Self-care capacities can vary considerably among persons who have chronic conditions. The self-care capacity of the same individual will also vary at different times throughout the course of the illness. The nurse should review the elderly individual's capacity to fulfill each of the health-related requirements.

II. Assessment of Care Capacity of the Family

A majority of elderly people with chronic conditions manage their conditions in the community, with family support or involvement; therefore, assessment must consider the capacity of the family to assist and cope with caregiving as well.

The nurse cannot assume that the presence of family

四、慢性病对于社会经济的影响

慢性病发病率升高带来医疗费用增加对发展中国家的影响更大。相比具有较高社会地位的人群，社会中的弱势人群病情加重和死亡的风险更高。因为弱势人群暴露于有害环境（例如烟草或不健康食品）的风险更大，而医疗资源的可及性不足。

第二节　慢性病的评估

不同慢性病的评估工具非常多，读者可参考内科护理学或外科护理学。本节将介绍关于慢性病照护需求评估的相关内容。

一、针对老年人自我照护能力的评估

慢性病患者的自我照护能力差异很大。同一个体的自我照护能力在病程的不同阶段也会有所不同。护士应评估老年人的能力，判断其能力是否能够满足每个健康相关需求及疾病的影响。

二、针对家庭照护能力的评估

大多数老年慢性病患者居住在社区环境，因此评估不仅要考虑个体自我照护能力，还包括家庭协助和照护的能力。

护士不能假定家庭照护者都能够补偿患

members guarantees compensation for the patient's care deficits. Sometimes the caregivers may not have the physical, mental, or emotional abilities to meet the elderly patient's care needs. For instance, the family may not want to provide care because of the imposition on their lifestyle or their feelings toward the patient. These factors must be considered before care is delegated to family members.

Identified care needs direct goals and plans for care. Setting goals is important in helping patients and their families understand the realistic outcome of the condition. And the patient and family caregivers should accept care plan priorities and goals.

Section 3　Management of Chronic Disease

People living with chronic illnesses often must manage daily symptoms that affect their quality of life, and experience acute health problems and complications that can shorten their life expectancy. This section provides information about chronic disease management and health promotion.

I. Goals of Chronic Care

Since elderly patients with chronic disease cannot eliminate their disease, care measures focus on helping patients effectively live in harmony with the condition, which means healing is of utmost importance. Healing indicates the mobilization of the body, mind, and spirit to control symptoms, promote a sense of well-being, and improve the quality of life. Healthcare professionals should differentiate acute care and chronic care clearly and orient appropriate care goals for the elderly with chronic diseases. The following goals are realistic to chronic care:

i. Maintain or Improve Self-care Capacity

Chronic diseases often place extra needs on the elderly people. They may be required to obtain special diets, modify their regular activities, administer medications, perform treatments, or learn to use assistive devices or equipment. Nurses may need to assist patients in improving their abilities to meet these needs.

ii. Manage the Condition Effectively

Elderly with chronic disease need to be knowledgeable about their health conditions and related care. However,

者的自理能力缺失。有时照顾者在身体、心理或情绪方面的能力不足，难以满足老年慢性病患者的护理需求。此外，有的家庭可能由于生活方式或情感方面的原因，不愿意提供照护。

因此明确护理需要，对指导护理目标和护理计划的制订非常重要。而后者有助于帮助患者及其家庭对患者当前的健康状况进行合理预期。

第三节　慢性病的管理

慢性病并发症发病率高，影响寿命和生活质量，患者日常生活中要控制症状。本节将介绍有关慢性病管理和健康促进的相关知识。

一、慢性病照护的目标

老年慢性病患者的护理重点是帮助患者和疾病和谐共处，控制症状，促进幸福感，提高生活质量。应区分急性期疾病和慢性病的护理，针对老年慢性疾病确定一个适当的护理目标。下述内容是慢性病照护的常见合理目标：

（一）保持或提高自我照护能力

老年慢性病患者有更高的照护需求。例如需准备特殊饮食，调整日常活动，服用药物，接受治疗或是学习使用辅助器具。护士需要帮助老年人保持或提高自我照护能力，以满足需求。

（二）有效管理症状

患有慢性病的老年人需要了解自己的健康状况和护理方法。自我激励是调动自我照

self-motivation is necessary to mobilize knowledge and skills in self-care, so assessing motivational factors and planning and strategies to enhance motivation are necessary aspects for gerontological nursing.

iii. Prevent Complications

Complications must be prevented because they could weaken self-care capacity, increase disability, and hasten decline. Whether a patient with diabetes lives an active life or becomes a blind amputee is largely determined by the extent to which treatment plans are followed and complications are actively prevented.

iv. Achieve the Highest Possible Quality of Life

Consideration should be given to helping elderly patients participate in activities that bring pleasure, stimulation, and reward. The nurse should assess the extent to which recreational, social, spiritual, emotional, and family needs are met and provide assistance to fulfill those needs. It is crucial for health professionals to regularly evaluate the extent to which treatment of the condition promotes or prohibits a satisfying lifestyle.

II. Maximizing the Benefits of Chronic Care

The main challenge regarding chronic diseases is to understand their complexity. With similar diagnoses and care requirements, the final treatment outcome of individuals may vary a lot. Hence, patients should be placed at the center of the care system and management of multiple chronic diseases requires a transformation in health care.

i. Establish Chronic Care Model

The chronic care model (CCM) identifies the essential elements of a health care system that encourage high-quality chronic disease care. These elements are the community, the health system, self-management support, delivery system design, decision support and clinical information systems. CCM overcomes the deficiencies of traditional management of chronic disease, like lack of care coordination and planned care, lack of active follow-up to ensure the best outcomes and patients inadequately trained to manage their illnesses.

ii. Using a Chronic Care Coach

The chronic care coach can be a family number, friend, or someone with a similar chronic condition. The coach may accompany the patient to have office visits and check on the patient's status routinely. Also, the coach can encourage patient to comply with care demands and

护知识和技能的必要条件。因此评估激励因素，制订提高老年人自我激励的计划和策略是老年护理的重要方面。

（三）预防并发症

并发症会弱化个体自我照护的能力，增加残疾，并加速功能下降，因此必须积极预防并发症。

（四）尽可能获得较高的生活质量

医护人员应定期评价不同治疗方式对于老年慢性病患者生活质量的影响。护士应评估老年患者在娱乐、社交、精神、情感和家庭等方面需求得到满足的程度，并提供帮助以满足这些需求。

二、慢性病照护效果的最大化

慢性病的最大挑战在于了解其复杂性。尽管诊断和护理要求类似，不同个体最终的临床结局可能会相差很大。因此，患者是照护系统的中心，针对多种慢性病的管理模式应有所转变。

（一）建立慢性病照护模式

慢性病护理模式（CCM）涵盖了一个卫生保健系统的基本要素。这些要素包括社区、卫生系统、自我管理支持、转运系统设计、决策支持和临床信息系统。该模式有助于克服传统慢性病管理模式中的不足之处，取得更好的照护效果。

（二）使用慢性病照护教练

慢性病照护教练可以是一个家庭成员、朋友或病友。老年专科护士可以列出日常训练的基本步骤，为慢性病照护教练提供专业的建议和支持（box 8-3）。

provide inspiration and hope. Gerontological nurses can advise and support persons who function as chronic care coaches by outlining some of the basic steps of this process (box 8-3).

Box 8-3　Steps in Chronic Care Coaching

- Contact: Schedule regular telephone or face-to-face contact to check on the patient's status.

- Observe: Be attentive to comments, mood, body language, energy, general status, presence of symptoms, compliance.

- Affirm: Reinforce care plan and actions, and recognize patient's efforts and accomplishments.

- Clarify: Ask questions, validate observations, correct misconceptions, and reinforce information.

- Help: Offer assistance when self-care capacity is diminished; locate and negotiate resources.

- Inspire: Encourage patient to comply with care plan, build on positive experiences and accomplishments; offer hope.

- Nurture: Provide education, information, support.

- Guide: Assist in setting realistic goals, developing plans, prioritizing, seeking resources.

iii. Locating a Support Group

Support groups can be important for the elderly people with chronic diseases; they provide the opportunity not only for valuable information but also for perspectives from those living with similar situations. Patients may be more willing to ask questions and express concerns with their peers than with health care professionals.

iv. Making Smart Lifestyle Choices

Patients with lifelong health conditions need to choose smart lifestyle which could maximize their health and quality of life, such as compliance with the prescribed treatment plan, healthy and balanced dietary, regular exercise, stress management, and development of a healing attitude.

v. Using Complementary and Alternative Therapies

More and more elderly people use complementary and alternative therapies for health promotion and illness management. Common complementary and alternative therapies for people with chronic conditions include acupuncture, guided imagery, herbal medicine, massage

Box 8-3　慢性病照护教练的基本工作步骤

- 联系：定期电话或面对面联系，以检查患者的情况。

- 观察：关注言谈、情绪、肢体语言、整体状况等。

- 核实：强化照护计划和行动，识别患者的努力和成果。

- 明确：询问、证实观察结果、纠正误解、强化信息。

- 帮助：当患者自我照护能力下降时，提供帮助；提供资源。

- 启发：鼓励患者依从护理计划，加强积极的体验，提供希望。

- 培育：提供教育、信息和支持。

- 指导：协助慢性病患者制订合理目标，建立计划，寻求资源。

（三）确定支持团体

支持团体对于老年慢性病患者非常重要，通过支持团体不仅可以获得宝贵信息，并且可以从病友身上获得经验。相比医护人员，患者可能更愿意向病友提问并提出疑虑。

（四）明智地选择生活方式

对于慢性病患者来说，明智地选择健康的生活方式，可以最大限度地提高他们的健康水平和生活质量，如遵守治疗方案、养成良好的饮食习惯、定期运动、进行压力管理等。

（五）使用补充和替代疗法

常见的补充和替代疗法包括针灸、指导意象、中草药、按摩、冥想、气功、太极和瑜伽。护士可以帮助患者评估补充和替代疗法的有效性。患者应与医生讨论这些疗法。

therapy, meditation, Qigong, Tai chi and Yoga. The nurse plays a significant role in helping the patient evaluate the effectiveness of complementary and alternative therapies and use only safe practices. Patients should be encouraged to discuss these therapies with their healthcare providers.

III. Health Promotion for Elderly with Chronic Diseases

According to the Center For Disease Control And Prevention (CDC), a lot of the sickness, disability, and even death associated with chronic disease can be avoided through preventive measures. The CDC suggests that the elderly can lessen the possibility of the onset of chronic disease in later years by:

i. Practicing a Healthy Lifestyle

Adoption of healthy lifestyles is the most effective way of staying healthy. WHO suggested that the risks of developing chronic diseases at an older age can be significantly reduced by adopting healthy behaviors, such as being physically active, eating a healthy diet, avoiding the harmful use of alcohol and tobacco products.

ii. Taking Regular Health Examination and Screens

It is helpful to take regular use of early detection and testing such as breast, prostate and cervical cancer screenings, diabetes and cholesterol screenings, and bone density scans, etc. The main purpose of health examination is to detect diseases at an earlier stage, for the better control of diseases and hence decrease risk of complications and reduce disability and mortality in some cases.

iii. Providing Health Education

Health education increases individuals' knowledge of health and health care, and makes them informed about their health care choices. Providing health education for old people is an important way of health promotion. The main objective of health education is to provide individuals and society with assistance so that they can lead a healthy life through their own efforts and actions. Similarly, it makes changes in the beliefs and value systems of individuals, their attitudes and skill levels, in other words, it changes their lifestyles.

(XI Xing)

三、老年慢性病患者的健康促进

与慢性病相关的许多不适、残疾，甚至死亡，都是可以通过预防措施避免的。老年人可以通过以下方法，减少在未来几年发生慢性病的可能性：

（一）践行健康的生活方式

采用健康的生活方式是保持健康最有效的方法。WHO 建议，采取健康的行为，如适当活动、健康饮食、避免酗酒和吸烟，可以显著降低老年人发生慢性病的风险。

（二）定期体检

定期检查的项目包括乳腺癌、前列腺癌和宫颈癌筛查，糖尿病和胆固醇检查，骨密度扫描等。健康检查的主要目的在于早期发现疾病，从而更有效地控制疾病，降低并发症和残疾的风险。

（三）提供健康教育

健康教育可以增加个人的健康知识，使他们了解自己的医疗选择。为老年人提供健康教育是健康促进的重要途径。健康教育可以改变个人的信仰和价值体系，态度和技能水平，换句话说，它改变了老年人的生活方式。

（奚 兴）

Key Points

1. Gerontological nurse should assess the self-care capacities of the elderly and the care capacity of the family, so that identified care needs could direct goals and plans for care.

2. Healthcare professionals should differentiate acute care and chronic care clearly and orient an appropriate care goals for the elderly with chronic diseases, including maintain or improve self-care capacity, manage the condition effectively, prevent complications and achieve the highest possible quality of life.

3. Many elderly people can benefit from taking a combination of conventional and complementary and alternative health practices for the care of their chronic diseases.

4. Elderly can lessen the possibility of the onset of chronic disease in later years by practicing a healthy lifestyle, taking regular health examination and screens and providing health education.

Critical Thinking Exercise

1. If you developed a chronic disease, how your life would be changed? What additional problems would be for the elderly if they faced this same situation?

2. Review the common chronic diseases affecting the elderly population and identify the threats to the quality of life which are associated with the chronic diseases.

3. Discuss the approaches that could help to empower an elderly adult who has a chronic disease to realize self-management.

本章小结

1. 老年专科护士应评估老年人的自我照护能力和家庭的照护能力，以便明确护理需求，从而有助于制订护理目标和计划。

2. 针对老年慢性疾病需确定一个适当的护理目标，包括保持或提高自我照护能力、有效地管理状况、预防并发症的发生和尽可能获得较高的生活质量。

3. 许多老年慢性病患者可以通过使用传统疗法、补充疗法、替代疗法相结合的方式而获益。

4. 老年人可以通过践行健康的生活方式、定期体检和接受健康教育等方式，降低发生慢性病的风险。

批判性思维练习

1. 若你患了慢性病，你的生活会如何改变？如果是老年人面对同样的情况，他（她）又会遇到哪些新的问题？

2. 总结老年人群的常见慢性疾病，找出与慢性病相关的可能影响老年人生活质量的因素。

3. 探讨如何通过向老年慢性病患者授权，从而实现患者自我管理的方法。

Chapter 9 Care of Elderly with Geriatric Syndrome and Frailty

第九章 老年综合征与衰弱老年人的护理

Learning Objectives

On completion of this chapter, the reader will be able to:

- Distinguish concept of geriatric syndromes and frailty;
- Identity risk factors contribute to geriatric syndromes and frailty;
- Explain the importance of identifying and assessing frailty among elder people;
- Apply the principles and intervention strategies to care geriatric disorders.

学习目标

学完本章节，应完成以下目标：

- 区分老年综合征和衰弱的概念；
- 识别引起老年综合征和衰弱的危险因素；
- 解释在老年人中识别和评估衰弱的重要意义；
- 应用照护原则和干预策略为存在老年综合征的患者提供照护。

Aging is sometimes described as a progressive deterioration of physiological function, an intrinsic age-related process of loss of viability and increase in vulnerability. Normal aging is accompanied by a number of physiologic changes both in appearance and functions, such as gradual reduction in height, weight loss, lower metabolic rate, longer reaction times, and declines in memory functions, decreased sexual activities, and menopause in women. The elderly people often experience functional declines in kidney, pulmonary, endocrine and immune systems, and lowered or lost function in audition, olfaction, and vision. Along with aging, the incidence of a number of pathologies increases such as type 2 diabetes, heart disease, cancer, arthritis, and lung disease. Aging is a complex process composed of several features, for example, physiological changes that lead to functional degeneration; increased susceptibility to co-morbidity and an exponential increase in mortality. With the elder population expanding all the time, it will take lots of health care resources for frail elderly and increase the burden to the whole society. Under this situation, it is critical to advance the knowledge of geriatric syndrome and frailty and to improve the nursing quality in order to prepare to the coming challenge. This chapter will cover two sections, geriatric syndromes and frailty.

正常的老化常伴有一系列躯体和功能的生理改变，如身高逐渐降低，体重下降，代谢率降低，反应时间延长，记忆力下降，性行为减少，女性绝经等。衰老是一种进行性的功能衰退，身体各部分器官系统（如泌尿、呼吸、内分泌和免疫系统等）的功能逐渐衰退的过程，是一种内在的、必然的、与年龄有关的不可逆过程，可伴有脆弱性的增加。此外，慢性病在老年人中的发生率增加，常见的慢性病有 2 型糖尿病、心脏病、肿瘤、关节炎、呼吸系统疾病等。或者说，衰老即伴随着广泛的生理变化，限制人们正常的生理活动，使人们更容易发生疾病和死亡。随着人口老龄化的日益严峻，衰弱的老年人将需要更多的医疗卫生资源，并会给整个社会造成巨大的负担。如何促进老年人维持自身功能的独立性，提高老年人的生活质量，减低老年人不良健康结局的发生，是全世界所面临的难题，而加强对老年综合征和衰弱的认识，提高老年护理质量至关重要。本章包括老年综合征和衰弱两部分。

Box 9-1 Case Study

Mr. Lin is a 72-year-old male who has lived alone since his wife died approximately 1 year ago. He is brought to the hospital by his son who is concerned that his father became unsteady on his feet and he has recently falls for three times without serious injury at home. Mr. Lin has been in good health with the exception of hypertension, which is well controlled. Mr. Lin spends most of his time watching news on television and he refused to go out door for social activity. His physical examination is normal. According to Mr. Lin's health condition record, he has lost more than 5 kg over the past year.

Questions:

1. What is most possible health problem for Mr. Lin? And why?

2. What do you need to screen in a suspected frail patient?

3. What is your health suggestion for Mr. Lin?

Box 9-1 案例

林先生，男，72 岁，自去年老伴去世后，独居生活。林先生近年来腿脚不便，近期在家中已发生 3 次跌倒，所幸并无大碍，但林先生的儿子非常担心，将父亲送入医院检查。林先生患有高血压，但控制较好，他的总体健康状况良好。平时林先生不爱出门参加社交活动，大部分时间是在家看电视新闻。经检查，林先生身体无异常。其健康档案提示，在近一年里，林先生的体重下降超过 5kg。

问题：

1. 目前林先生最有可能存在的健康问题是什么？为什么？

2. 对于怀疑存在衰弱问题的老年人，如何进一步确诊？

3. 你对于林先生的健康方面有何建议？

Section 1　Care of the Elderly with Geriatric Syndrome

Decline of homeostatic reserve capacity of all organ systems with increasing age is the primary principle of geriatrics. Exposure to multiple individual risk factors causes individual decline in organ function and the organ function is further affected by chronic health conditions. Usually atypical disease presentations are typical for geriatric medicine and currently referred to as "geriatric syndrome". Geriatric syndromes are defined as "The multi-factorial health conditions that occur when the accumulated effects of impairments in multiple systems render an older adult vulnerable to situational challenges." They include hearing loss, visual impairment, falls, polypharmacy, pain, sleep disorders, urinary incontinence, delirium, cognitive impairment, and substance abuse as described in Chapter 4 Section 3 *Geriatric Syndromes*. General information with respect to the definition, assessment, prevention and treatment principle of geriatric syndromes is provided in this section. More detailed information with specific geriatric syndrome will be introduced in the following chapters.

I. Basic Information on Geriatric Syndrome

i. Concept of Geriatric Syndrome

The term syndrome "is not specific disease factors, but a chain of physiologic processes, the interruption of which at any point produces the same ultimate impairment of body function". Cushing's syndrome is a good example of a traditional medical syndrome wherein disruption of a single physiological process (excessive cortisol secretion) results in multiple common clinical manifestations. These clinical manifestations may include general signs (hypertension, moon facies, truncal obesity), endocrine problems (impaired glucose tolerance, hyperlipidemia), skin problems (plethora, hirsutism, acne), skeletal manifestations (osteopenia, myopathy) and psychiatric disturbances (depression, psychosis).

The term "syndrome" applied to geriatric conditions has been at odds with the traditional use of "syndrome" from earlier times. The outcome of geriatric syndrome is a single phenomenology rather than a spectrum of symptoms and signs, and results from numerous rather than a single disruption. Geriatric syndromes are groups of specific signs and symptoms that share many common

第一节　老年综合征

随着年龄的增长，老年人各器官系统的稳态储备能力下降，这也是老年医学面临的重要问题。多种危险因素可导致个体器官功能下降，另外还受慢性疾病的影响。老年综合征指老年人由多种疾病或非疾病原因造成的同一种临床表现或健康问题的老年病症。常见的老年综合征有听力障碍、视力受损、跌倒、多重用药、疼痛、睡眠障碍、尿失禁、谵妄、认知受损和物质滥用等。本节将介绍老年综合征的定义、评估、预防和治疗原则。后续章节中将分别介绍常见的老年综合征。

一、老年综合征的概述

（一）老年综合征的概念

综合征是指一系列病理过程中，当出现一个症候时，同时会伴有另外几个症候。一个综合征的各种症状可看作是由一个基本原因所引起的表现，例如典型的库欣综合征主要是由于皮质醇的长期过多分泌而引起了一系列的临床表现。这些临床表现包括了一般症状（高血压、满月脸、向心性肥胖）、内分泌问题（糖耐量受损、高脂血症）、皮肤问题（多毛、痤疮）、骨骼表现（骨质疏松、肌肉无力）和精神障碍（抑郁、精神病）。

与传统的医学模式中单一疾病或原因导致的综合征不同，老年综合征强调多种疾病或原因导致同一症状。也就是说，老年综合征是一组特殊的症状和体征，它们具有许多共同特征，在老年人中非常普遍，尤其是衰弱的老人。老年综合征强调导致同一临床表

features and highly prevalent in older adults, especially the frail elderly. It emphasizes multiple causation of a unified manifestation. In geriatric syndromes, it is multiple abnormalities that "run together" to cause a single phenomenology. For example, in delirium, the cumulative effects of multiple contributors (impaired cognition, severe illness, dehydration, etc.) result in the delirium phenomenology (figure 9-1). Delirium can be seen in elders with dehydration, it can also be seen in patients with urinary track infection.

Geriatric syndromes have a devastating effect on the individual's quality of life as they progress, may lead to significant disability, and are part of the "cascade to dependency" that can often result in institutionalization. An elderly patient whose chief complaint is a result of a geriatric syndrome will often present with symptoms that are difficult to attribute to the organ system causing the initial pathology.

现的多重因果关系，如老年人的谵妄，可能是多种因素（认知障碍、严重疾病、脱水等）的累积效应所导致（图9-1），既可以出现在认知功能受损的老年人中，也见于病重或脱水的老年人。

老年综合征可因多种因素相互作用，最终造成多种器官系统受损。老年综合征可引起老年人自理能力受限，甚至影响其日常生活活动，生活质量下降，最终不得不入住养老机构。当老年人的主诉提示某种老年综合征时，往往会伴有一系列相关的症状，难以推断是某一个器官或系统的问题。

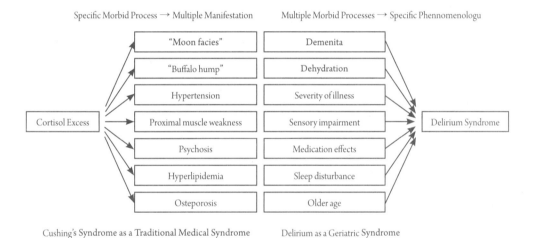

Figure 9-1　Traditional medical syndrome vs. geriatric syndrome

ii. Risk Factors Contributing to Geriatric Syndromes

Known risk factors reported by literature include normal changes of aging, multiple diagnoses (comorbidity), multiple medications (polypharmacy), multiple care providers, adverse effects of therapeutic interventions, as well as impaired cognitive function and decreased mobility. Geriatric syndromes share many common aging-related risk factors, indicating that they usually have more than one cause, and involve several different organ systems. Geriatric syndromes acknowledge the complex interplay between age-related physiologic changes, chronic disease, and functional stressors in older adults. Multiple underlying factors, involving

（二）老年综合征的影响因素

导致老年综合征的危险因素有很多，可能是多个常见的衰老相关的危险因素重合的结果，涉及多个不同的器官系统。虽然老年综合征的概念仍然没有明确的界定，文献中报告的确定的风险因素包括正常老化、多种疾病共病、多重用药、多人轮替照料、治疗干预的副作用、认知功能受损以及功能下降和活动减少。一项基于社区老年人的队列研究调查了存在跌倒、失禁和功能障碍的老年人，结果提示四肢肌肉无力、视力听力下降、

multiple organ systems, tend to contribute to geriatric syndromes. In a population-based cohort of community-dwelling elderly patients with falls, incontinence, and functional dependence, researchers found 3 independent predisposing factors: upper and lower extremity weakness, decreased vision and hearing, and anxiety or depression. Similarly, in a systematic review of studies about risk factors for pressure ulcers, incontinence, falls, functional decline, and delirium and researchers found that older age, functional impairment, cognitive impairment, and impaired mobility were shared risk factors.

II. Assessment for Geriatric Syndrome

Clinicians should attempt to treat or manage a geriatric syndrome even though a single cause may not be able to be identified. Whereas in a younger person a workup may look primarily for single diseases, the interaction of multiple physiologic changes and comorbidities in an older adult warrant a broader perspective. Diagnostic testing that would be relevant in a younger person may not be as beneficial in an older person, and may lead to unnecessary treatment or harm for the patient. Currently, there is lack of consensus on how to assess geriatric syndromes at the same time and quickly. Recent literature has described some tools for the identification of geriatric syndromes, but few were specifically designed for general practice, and even those that exist suffer important limitations.

The Fulmer SPICES (box 9-2), an acronym for the geriatric syndromes, has been widely used as an efficient and effective way to conduct assessment. The SPICES acronym is easily remembered and may be used to recall the common problems of the elderly population in all clinical settings. Although psychometric testing of SPICES validity and reliability has not been conducted, widespread utilization provides indication of its significant usefulness.

Box 9-2 Fulmer SPICES

- S: Sleep Disorders.
- P: Problems with Eating or Feeding.
- P: Pain.
- I: Incontinence.
- C: Confusion.
- E: Evidence of Falls.
- S: Skin Breakdown.

焦虑或抑郁为独立危险因素。此外，一项针对压疮、失禁、跌倒、功能障碍和谵妄的系统评价结果显示，高龄、功能受损、认知受损和行动能力受损是这些老年综合征的共同危险因素。

二、老年综合征的评估

尽管难以明确病因，老年综合征仍需引起医护人员重视。老年综合征涉及多个生理功能改变和共病的相互作用，治疗时应综合考虑。有些适用于年轻患者的诊断性测试往往不适合老年人。目前，对如何定义和评估老年综合征还缺乏共识。文献报告了多种用于识别老年综合征的工具，但都存在局限性，不利于临床实践。

Fulmer 的 SPICES 指标（box 9–2），已广泛用于老年人评估。SPICES 是由评估项目的首字母组成，用于评估老年人常见问题。目前尚未有研究对 SPICES 的信度和效度进行测试。

Box 9-2 Fulmer SPICES

- 睡眠障碍。
- 进食或喂食障碍。
- 疼痛。
- 尿失禁。
- 意识障碍。
- 跌倒。
- 皮肤完整性受损。

III. Management of Geriatric Syndrome

Switching from a single disease framework to a broader holistic approach helps tailor care planning to the individual patient and maximizes the overall treatment benefit. In other words, interventions may be effective in preventing some of these shared risk factors for geriatric syndromes and therefore managing more than one issue. For example, strategies for management of delirium also may reduce falls, and Tai Chi may be helpful in preventing both falls and cognitive decline.

Geriatric syndromes have high impacts on patient morbidity and mortality. They can limit older adults' abilities to carry out basic daily activities, threaten their independence and lower their quality of life. However, providing care for elder people with geriatric syndromes is complicated because geriatric syndromes normally have problems in more than one system, and one geriatric syndrome often contributes to another syndrome.

Patients with complex geriatric syndromes have more care needs than most primary care patients. Unlike patients with intermittent, acute problems, patients with complex geriatric syndromes have multiple chronic diseases and daily symptoms, and frequently require services from different practitioners in the hospital, home, community, and outpatient settings. Clinically, we manage each geriatric syndrome the same way we manage disease. Since geriatric syndromes do not belong to an organ system, a separate assessment of them must be done. Because of frequent care needs, geriatric patients have high utilization of healthcare services and are among the most costly patients in the health care system.

Nurses and family caregivers need to be informed about the geriatric syndromes so that they can provide efficient care to patients. Assessing relative risk is the first step in a patient's plan of prevention. Failing to identify, diagnose, or treat geriatric syndromes can adversely affect an older adult's health and longevity. Use best-practice exemplars of effective prevention programs to care for older adults with geriatric syndromes. These exemplars in corporate an interdisciplinary team approach as well as a strong geriatric nurse-centered approach. Proper managing these conditions leads to better outcomes, including lower disability and mortality, less nursing home placement, shorter length of stay, and less hospital readmission.

三、老年综合征的管理

老年医学的重点在于评价功能状况、衰弱和其他老年综合征的同时，治疗疾病。因此应综合考虑治疗方案，考虑患者整体健康状况，实现个体化的整体护理。例如，治疗谵妄的同时也可预防跌倒，太极锻炼在预防跌倒的同时缓解认知能力下降。

老年综合征对患者疾病发病率和死亡率有很大影响。老年综合征会限制老年人的基本日常活动能力，使其自理能力下降，生活质量降低。然而，老年综合征的护理较为复杂，因为老年综合征通常存在不止一个系统的问题，而且一个老年综合征常常导致另一个综合征。

伴有复杂老年综合征的老年人，对于照护的需求不同于其他患者，他们对于医院、家庭、社区、门诊的照护需求更大，因而针对老年综合征患者的照护更加复杂。在临床上，我们对每一种老年综合征的治疗方法与对疾病的治疗方法相似。由于老年综合征不属于某一个器官系统的问题，必须对它们进行单独的评估。另外，老年患者护理需求繁杂，医疗服务的占用率高，是医疗系统中花费最高的患者之一。

护士和家庭照顾者需要掌握老年综合征的知识，以便提供高效的护理服务。在临床实践中识别和评估老年综合征是进行老年综合征管理的第一步，若不能识别、针对和处理潜在的老年综合征病因（如感知觉障碍、衰弱、皮肤问题），会进一步影响老年人的健康。推荐医护人员使用最佳实践方案预防老年综合征。这些方案大多整合多学科团队资源，以护士为主导进行干预。适当的护理措施可以使老年综合征得到预防或延迟，降低残疾和死亡率，减少入住养老院的概率，缩短住院日，减少再入院。

Detailed information of nursing care of geriatric syndromes will be introduced in the subsequent chapters.

后续的章节中将具体介绍不同老年综合征的护理。

Section 2　Frailty

第二节　衰弱

The concept of frailty came across from last century in 1970s. Although there has no consensus of the definition and measurement of these concepts, more and more research has shown their clinical applications and importance to gerontological care. The aim of this section is to widen the knowledge of gerontology nurses and researchers about theory and clinical application of frailty.

衰弱这一概念是在 20 世纪 70 年代最先被提出的。虽然对衰弱的概念和评估方法尚无共识，但越来越多的研究表明其临床应用的有效性和在老年护理中的重要性。本节介绍衰弱的理论和临床研究进展。

I. Basic Information on Frailty

i. Concept of Frailty

The definition of frailty in dictionary is the state of being weak in health or body (especially from old age). Frailty is an important concept in geriatrics and has been described as "the overarching geriatric syndrome" due to its importance in predicting treatment benefit and prognosis (figure 9-2). During the three decades of frailty study, there were plenty of models, criteria and measurements to identify frailty, but still no consensus yet and the concept is evolving all along.

一、衰弱的概述

（一）衰弱的基本概念

衰弱是指身体处于缺乏力量和健康而容易受到伤害的状态或特质；也有学者定义衰弱为自我平衡失调而致的不稳定状态；有学者定义为功能受损合并自评健康状况低下，还有学者定义为多领域（包括心理、认知、社会、环境等）的功能失调而导致的脆弱状态（图 9-2）。在三十年的衰弱研究中，有大量的模型、标准和测量方法被用来识别衰弱，但至今仍没有达成共识，而且衰弱概念一直在演变。

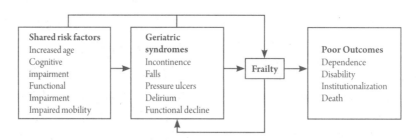

Figure 9-2　The relationship among risk factors, geriatric syndromes and poor outcomes

Different operational definitions of frailty exist in the literature and make the dimensions of instruments with multiple aspects of physiology, psychology, social and function. Each dimension has several factors. Physical dimension includes nutritional status, physical activity, mobility, strength and energy; psychological dimension

文献中对衰弱的操作性定义不同，使得衰弱评估工具的维度具有生理、心理、社会、功能等多方面的特征，每个维度都包含诸多方面。身体维度包括营养状况、身体活动、活动能力、体力和能量；心理维度包括认知

includes cognition and mood; social dimension includes social contacts and social support. The concept of frailty is discussed for quite a long time. The debate has centered on whether frailty should be defined purely in terms of biomedical factors or whether psychosocial factors should be included. Although different perspectives of frailty exist, there is a consensus that frailty is a dynamic state and increases the risks for adverse health outcomes like fall, hospitalization, impaired physical functions, and death in the future.

The most widely used definition is what Fried published that frailty is a biologic syndrome of decreased reserve and resistance to stressors, resulting from cumulative declines across multiple physiologic systems, and causing vulnerability to adverse outcome. A key component in the frailty syndrome is sarcopenia, the loss of muscle mass and strength with ageing. Markers of frailty include age-related weakness, weight loss, declines in strength and endurance, progressive functional worsening as well as psychological, emotional and social problems, resulting in adverse health outcomes.

In the *Chinese Expert Consensus on Assessment and Prediction of Elderly Patients' Weakness* in 2017, frailty is defined as a non-specific state in which the decline of elderly patients' physical reserve leads to increased vulnerability and decreased anti-stress ability. A series of clinical negative outcomes can be caused by frail people experiencing small external stimulation. frailty involves multiple system pathological and physiological changes, including neuromuscular, metabolic and immune systems.

ii. Related Theories and Pathogenesis of Frailty

Frailty is a state in which the physical reserve energy of an individual is reduced to a certain level (close to the threshold), its internal dynamic balance is out of balance, its health, function and integrity are damaged, its susceptibility to stressors is increased, and it is easy to cause clinical outcomes. Once the body's reserve energy decreases, its ability to restore its own balance weakens. The more serious the individual is damaged, the less likely it will be to recover its basic health and function after the disease. On the contrary, the reserve energy can also be enhanced through pre intervention or care compensation.

At present, the mechanism of frailty is not clear. According to the detection of blood biomarkers in the frail people, it is generally believed that frailty is related

维度和情绪维度；社会维度包括社会交往和社会支持。长期以来，人们一直在讨论衰弱的概念。争论的焦点在于，衰弱是应该仅仅根据生物医学因素来定义，还是应该包括心理社会因素。尽管不同学者对衰弱的概念有不同的解释，但都包括一些共同的要素，即衰弱是一个进展性的动态过程与状态，该类人群处于易受伤害及易发生不良健康结局的危险中，如跌倒、住院、功能障碍、若干年后的死亡等。

目前各个领域最常用概念是 Fried 等提出的：衰弱是身体各系统机能进行性下降而表现出的躯体症状，具体表现为身体储备能力和防御能力下降，更易出现不良结局。衰弱的一个关键因素是肌少症，即随着年龄的增长，肌肉的质量和力量的损失。衰弱的标志包括与年龄有关的无力、体重减轻、耐力和力量下降、渐进性功能恶化以及心理、情感和社会问题，最终导致不良的健康结果。

在 2017 年的《老年患者衰弱评估与干预中国专家共识》中，衰弱被定义为老年人生理储备下降导致机体易损性增加、抗应激能力减退的非特异性状态。衰弱老年人经历外界较小刺激即可导致一系列临床负性事件的发生。衰弱涉及多系统病理、生理变化，包括神经肌肉、代谢及免疫系统等。

（二）衰弱的相关理论和发病机制

衰弱是个体生理储备能力降低到一定程度（接近阈值），其内部动态平衡失调，健康、功能和完好性受损，对于压力源的易感性增加，易引发临床事件的一种状态。一旦机体的储备能力下降，其恢复自身平衡的能力就削弱了。个体受损越严重，则其在疾病之后，生理功能下降，机体系统失调，恢复基本健康和功能的可能性就越小。相反，储备能力也可通过干预手段或照护补偿来增强。

目前衰弱的发生机制尚不明确，根据对衰弱人群的血液标记物进行检测，一般认为衰弱与慢性炎性反应有关。而肌肉减少症是

to chronic inflammatory reaction. And sarcopenia is the nuclear pathological basis of frailty. Sarcopenia is a kind of syndrome characterized by progressive systemic and generalized decrease of skeletal muscle mass and muscle strength. It is the result of imbalance of muscle synthesis and catabolism caused by many factors.

iii. Prevalence and Consequences of Frailty

The prevalence of frailty varies according to different regions and diagnosis criteria. Generally, it is estimated that the prevalence of frailty is 4%-59.1% based on the existing studies. In a cross-sectional study, it is reported that the prevalence of frailty among community-dwelling elders is 11.1% in China. It predicts that in 2020 to 2050, the population of elders in China will reach more than 300 million. According to the national statistics, among the elders over 60, 53.9% of them have chronic disease; each person has 2 to 3 diseases in average. Under this situation, it is critically important for the health system to screen for frailty and provide intervention to elders in case of irreversible adverse outcomes.

Frailty has a transitional progression. Prefrailty is defined as the transitional stage between the non-frail and frail state. Pre-frail individuals have a significantly higher risk of developing adverse outcomes than non-frail people, and frail individuals have a still higher risk. Without any appropriate intervention, the state will get worse and the next stage is frailty. Frail older people are at an increased risk for developing other geriatric syndromes, morbidity, institutionalization and death, resulting in burden to individuals, their families, health care services and society. Frailty can result in physical disability, affecting the ability of managing activities of daily life. Frail elders need care from family numbers and community. Research indicated that it disturbs normal life plan of family caregivers and raises self-report health problems. Long time caregiving leaves heavy burden to the caregivers not only physiologically but also emotionally, and socially. Under the traditional family view, it will influence vastly with the modern family structure changing.

Frail elderly people are more vulnerable to environmental stressors and damages leading to more serious consequences. Among the elders with heart failure, more than 50% were frail. During the hospitalization, new environment, using new medication, activities restriction and acute disease affect the elders who are already in the unstable state. After discharge, physical function and the ability of self-care will decline, resulting in worse quality of life.

衰弱的核心病理基础。肌肉减少症是指进行性的全身广泛性的骨骼肌质量（含量）下降和力量（强度）降低为特征的一类综合征，是多种因素引起的肌肉合成和分解代谢失衡的结果。

（三）衰弱的流行病学

因不同地区衰弱的诊断标准不一，各地衰弱发生率约在 4%～59.1%。我国一项横断面调查显示，社区老年人中衰弱的发生率约为 11.1%。据预测，2020 年至 2050 年，中国老年人口将超过 3 亿。据国家统计，60 岁以上老年人中，慢性病占 53.9%；每个人平均有 2 到 3 种疾病。

衰弱是渐进发展的。衰弱前期被定义为非衰弱和衰弱状态之间的过渡阶段。处于衰弱前期的个体发生不良后果的风险明显高于非衰弱者，而衰弱个体的风险更高。如果没有任何适当的干预，衰弱前期的状态将恶化，下一个阶段就是衰弱。衰弱导致躯体功能障碍，影响了个人的自理能力。衰弱的老年人需要配偶、子女或其他家庭成员的照护，同时需要社区的协助。研究显示，因为照护衰弱老年人，家属的正常生活计划被打乱，且自评存在健康问题。长期照护衰弱老年人，可对照护者造成了情感、身体、社会等方面的负担。在传统家庭观念的影响下，随着我国家庭结构的改变，照护衰弱老年人将给家庭带来巨大的影响。

衰弱老年人易受创伤和环境的压力的影响，产生的结果更为严重。在心力衰竭的老年人中，超过 50% 的老年人属于衰弱。住院期间，陌生的环境、使用新的药物、限制活动及急性病都会对自身平衡系统紊乱的老年人产生影响。出院后，衰弱老年人的躯体功能和自我照护能力下降显著，进而导致生活质量下降。

Study shows after exposure to stressors, frail elderly encounter more functional deficits and are at higher risk of comorbid disorders and even death than robust elders. Different levels of frailty also indicate different prognoses.

iv. Factors Contributing to Frailty

Frailty is the result of a series of factors. Brown put the factors into 2 major categories: individual and environmental. Individual factors are gender, health status, nutrition and cognition. Environmental factors mean economic condition, living environment and law. These factors are also major parts of holistic nursing. A theoretical framework that includes bio–psycho–social–spiritual factors as contributors to frailty is recommended as the most useful framework for gerontological nursing.

1. Advanced age Because physiologic decline is an inherent feature of aging, the occurrence of frailty inevitably rises with age. It is believed that frailty is more prevalent in 80 years old than 65 years old. However, frailty is not synonymous with aging, as individual differences in organ reserves may protect against or mitigate the consequences of the decline. The size of the reserves determines the degree of frailty, with elderly people with low reserves being more vulnerable and prone to functional deficits and comorbid disorders.

2. Physical factors According to a systematic review, physical factors are referred most times. Physical factors relate to musculoskeletal system and function. Theoretical model and studies have already demonstrated that low activity led to sarcopenia which was the main reason for frailty. Deterioration of the musculoskeletal system is a key component of the frailty syndrome. Function disability includes impairment of sensory, difficulty in ADL and IADL, decline in mobility and sensitivity.

3. Disease Disease contributes to frailty, like various individual diseases, a summation of the number of diseases or chronic low-grade inflammation resulting from a normal aging-related change. Theoretical studies not only focus on a specific disease, but also on the whole framework that discuss the role of morbidity. Further clarification is needed about which diseases are contributing to frailty and how they are doing this.

4. Cognitive/psychological factors The contribution of cognitive/psychological factors to frailty is identified in most of the studies according to a systematic review. Fried and Nourhashemi et al identified cognition as a factor contributing to frailty, while Strawbridge et al.

研究显示，衰弱老年人预后不良，发生日常活动功能障碍、跌倒、髋部骨折、入住医院、死亡的危险高于健壮的老年人，不同衰弱程度的老年人，在发生不良事件后的预后也不相同。

（四）衰弱的影响因素

衰弱是由一系列影响因素造成的，即个人和环境因素：个人因素指性别、身体状况、营养状况、认知状况等；而环境因素包括了经济、居住条件、法律因素等。这些都是整体护理关注的重点，反映了人的生物、心理、精神、社会等方面的整体性。

1. 高龄 随着年龄的增长，与年龄相关的生理功能受损将不可避免，个体健康储备不断被透支，导致累计健康缺失随之增长，衰弱程度加重。衰弱在老年人中的发生率较高，年龄越大，衰弱发生率越高。然而，衰弱并不是老化的同义词，因为器官储备存在个体差异，而这种差异影响衰弱的结局。

2. 身体因素 身体因素是最主要的影响因素。身体因素可分为两大类：肌肉骨骼和身体功能。理论模型和研究证实活动减少导致肌肉骨骼无力，是衰弱发生的主要原因。功能障碍包括感知觉的缺失、日常生活活动或工具性生活活动出现困难、行动力和灵敏度的下降。

3. 疾病因素 疾病因素包括不同的个体疾病，慢性轻度炎症等。理论性的研究并不在意某一具体疾病，而是在整体框架中讨论疾病的角色。今后需要进一步澄清究竟是哪些疾病导致了衰弱，以及二者之间的作用机制。

4. 认知和心理因素 根据一项系统评价报告，多个研究显示认知和心理因素会影响衰弱的发生。有学者将自评健康状况纳入衰弱的定义中。精神是影响老年人健康的重要

included cognition as part of their operational definition. Dayhoff et al used the psychological measure of self-rated health as part of their operational definition. Spirituality also has been identified as a contributing factor to elders' health and wellbeing. It may be useful for future researchers to examine the relationship between frailty and spirituality more closely.

5. Nutritional factors　Malnutrition can lead to frailty. The assessment includes body weight and body mass index (BMI). It is of vital importance to have gold standards to reflect malnutrition and figure out the relationship between sarcopenia, malnutrition, low activity and frailty.

6. Social factors　More and more attention is paid to the social factors of frailty. Nouhashemi found that social activity like taking holidays, joining elders' activities are negatively related to frailty; meanwhile family and friends' visits are positive related. Brown found that social disengagement is also part of frailty, so lack of social support and activity are the potential factors of frailty.

II. Assessment for frailty

Identifying frailty in an elder often can change the trajectory of care, because frailty is a dynamic state and can be reverted back to less or no frailty. Existing instruments are divided into two kinds; one is based on frailty phenotype which was developed by Fried and her colleagues, another one is based on clinical diagnoses and number of impaired functions, including indexes of cognition, signs, symptoms and diseases. There is no gold standard to measure frailty. However, several studies have compared and contrasted some of the frailty scales and they found all of them to be effective in predicting mortality among community-dwelling older adults. Researches can choose the following instruments according to their perspective of frailty.

i. Frailty Phenotype

It is suggested by Fried that frailty phenotype consists of 5 aspects: shrinking (unintentional weight loss), weakness, exhaustion, slowness, and low activity. Frailty is determined by the presence of three or more components, prefrail stage means 1 or 2 criteria are met, and if someone meets no criteria, then he or she is robust. Most researchers use this phenotype as a framework and modify the instrument based on the purpose of their studies.

因素，在今后的研究中，学者也可进一步探讨衰弱和精神的关系。

5. **营养状况因素**　营养不良会导致衰弱，评估指标包括体重和身体质量指数（BMI）。寻找反映营养不良的金标准，同时阐明肌少症、营养不良、身体活动与衰弱之间的关系至关重要。

6. **社会因素**　社会因素对于衰弱的影响越来越得到关注。Nouhashem 发现社会活动如休假、参加老年活动与衰弱成负相关，而家人朋友的慰问则与衰弱成正相关。Brown 发现社会参与度也是衰弱的一部分，社会支持和社会活动的不可及是造成衰弱的潜在因素。

二、衰弱的评估

识别老年人衰弱往往可以改变护理的方向，因为衰弱是一种动态状态，是可能逆转的。目前不同学者对衰弱的操作性定义不能统一。然而，多项研究对不同衰弱量表进行了比较，结果发现所有量表都能有效预测社区老年人的死亡率。研究人员可以根据自身对于衰弱的认识选择以下工具。

（一）衰弱表型
衰弱表型是 Fried 等提出的 5 个躯体功能指标，即非故意的体重下降、握力下降、自诉疲惫、走路速度缓慢、身体活动量低，占有其中至少 3 项指标，则为衰弱，只有 1~2 项定义为衰弱前期，没有任何 1 项为强健。很多研究者基于衰弱表型的条目，在修改和补充具体的测量方式后，进行了更多的研究。

ii. Frailty Index

Based on the concept of cumulative health impairment of individual, Rockwood and Mitnitski invented frailty index (FI) to measure frailty (box 9-3). This index includes 70 items like the degree of disease, ADL and IADL, physical symptom, clinical examination results. If one item is met, then one score is got. The advantage of the index is easy to understand and have a better prediction, but also time consuming.

（二）衰弱指数

衰弱指数是 Rockwood 和 Mitnitski 在个体健康累积损失的概念上开发的衰弱测量工具（box 9-3）。该量表涵盖了70个可能的缺陷，例如现存疾病的严重程度、日常生活能力、躯体症状、临床检查结果等，每项1分，最后根据评分判断该老年人在群体中的水平。该法优点在于易理解，预测能力强，但过于烦琐耗时。

Box 9-3　List of variables used by the Canadian Study of Health and Aging to construct the 70-item CSHA frailty index

- Changes in everyday activities
- Head and neck problems
- Poor muscle tone in neck
- Bradykinesia, facial
- Problems getting dressed
- Problems with bathing
- Problems carrying out personal grooming
- Urinary incontinence
- Toileting problems
- Bulk difficulties
- Rectal problems
- Gastrointestinal problems
- Problems cooking
- Sucking problems
- Problems going out alone
- Impaired mobility
- Musculoskeletal problems
- Bradykinesia of the limbs
- Poor muscle tone in limbs
- Poor limb coordination
- Poor coordination, trunk
- Poor standing posture
- Irregular gait pattern

- Falls

- Mood problems
- Feeling sad, blue, depressed
- History of depressed mood
- Tiredness all the time
- Depression
- Sleep changes
- Restlessness
- Memory changes
- Short-term memory impairment
- Long-term memory impairment
- Changes in general mental functioning
- Onset of cognitive symptoms
- Clouding or delirium
- Paranoid features
- History relevant to cognitive impairment or loss
- Family history relevant to cognitive impairment or loss
- Impaired vibration
- Tremor at rest
- Postural tremor
- Intention tremor
- History of Parkinson's disease

- Family history of degenerative disease

- Seizures, partial complex
- Seizures, generalized
- Syncope or blackouts
- Headache
- Cerebrovascular problems
- History of stroke
- History of diabetes mellitus
- Arterial hypertension
- Peripheral pulses
- Cardiac problems
- Myocardial infarction
- Arrhythmia
- Congestive heart failure
- Lung problems
- Respiratory problems
- History of thyroid disease
- Thyroid problems
- Skin problems
- Malignant disease
- Breast problems
- Abdominal problems
- Presence of snout reflex
- Presence of the palmomental reflex

- Other medical history

Box 9-3　加拿大健康和老年研究所用的70条目衰弱指数变量列表

- 每日活动量的变化
- 头颈部疾病
- 颈部肌肉紧张
- 面部肌肉紧张
- 穿衣服受限
- 沐浴受限
- 个人修饰受限
- 尿失禁
- 如厕受限
- 日常生活受限
- 直肠疾病
- 胃肠道疾病
- 做饭受限
- 吸吮受限
- 独自外出受限
- 行动受限
- 骨骼肌疾病
- 四肢运动迟缓
- 四肢肌张力差
- 肢体协调性差
- 躯体协调性差
- 站姿不良
- 不规则步态
- 跌倒

- 情绪问题
- 情绪低落
- 抑郁病史
- 疲劳
- 抑郁
- 睡眠改变
- 不安
- 记忆下降
- 短期记忆力下降
- 长期记忆力下降
- 一般心理功能变化
- 出现认知症状
- 谵妄
- 偏执特征
- 认知受损病史
- 认知受损的家族史
- 震颤受损
- 静止性震颤
- 姿势性震颤
- 意向性震颤
- 帕金森病史
- 退行性疾病家族史

- 复杂部分性癫痫发作
- 全身癫痫发作
- 晕厥或黑矇
- 头痛
- 脑血管疾病
- 脑卒中病史
- 糖尿病病史
- 高血压
- 脉搏
- 心脏病
- 心肌梗死
- 心律失常
- 充血性心力衰竭
- 肺部疾病
- 呼吸受限
- 甲状腺疾病病史
- 甲状腺疾病
- 皮肤问题
- 恶性肿瘤
- 乳房疾病
- 腹部疾病
- 出现口噘嘴反射
- 出现掌颏反射
- 其他病史

iii. Clinical Frailty Scale

After Canadian aging and health survey in 2005, Rockwood and his colleague developed clinical frailty scale (CFS), which has high area under the receiver operating characteristic curve for predicting adverse outcomes within 70 months. The instrument is based on the comprehensive geriatric assessment by physician. According to the ability of ADL, elders are categorized into 7 scales; the higher scale is, the more seriously of frailty. Researchers in Taiwan, China used CFS as a model and developed a CFS telephone version in order to screen elders in community.

iv. Edmonton Frail Scale

Edmonton frail scale (EFS) is developed by Rolfson in 2006 after investigating 364 elders over 65 in Edmonton a Canada city. The EFS has 9 domains, cognition, general health status, functional, social support, medication use, nutrition, mood, continence, and functional performance. The maximum score is 17 and represents the highest level of frailty. As the author said, EFS appeared to be valid, reliable and feasible for routine by non-geriatricians.

v. Tilburg Frailty Indicator

Based on integrated frailty model, Gobbens et al. developed a self-report questionnaire named Tilburg frailty indicator (TFI) to assess frailty, which included three domains, physical, psychological and social part. There are 15 items in TFI. The score for frailty and the 3 domains of frailty are determined by adding the responses to the items belonging to each scale. The maximum score is 15 and represents the highest level of frailty. Study demonstrated that the psychometric properties of the TFI are good, when performed in community-dwelling older people.

III. Management of Frailty

The development of frailty is a dynamic process which indicates that it is possible to postpone or reverse frailty and to prevent adverse outcomes. A number of therapeutic approaches have been used; their aim being to slow down the processor at least to avoid the adverse clinical consequences of frailty. And it is still worth exploding the most effective method. Different countries and regions have some consensus and guidelines on intervention for frailty. Multifaceted intervention contents of various guidelines can be summarized as physical

（三）临床衰弱水平量表

临床衰弱水平量表是 Rockwood 等在 2005 年加拿大全民健康与老龄化调查后开发的，对于 70 个月内老年人死亡发生有较高预测能力。该量表是在临床医生对老年人全面健康评估的基础上，根据老年人日常生活功能分为 7 个级别，级别越高衰弱程度越重。在 CFS 的基础上，有中国台湾学者开发了电话版本的 CFS 量表，以电话调查的方式，对社区老年人的健康状况进行筛查。

（四）Edmonton 衰弱量表

Edmonton 衰弱量表是 Rolfson 等 2006 年在加拿大城市爱特蒙特调查了 364 名 65 岁以上老年人后开发的量表。EFS 包括了认知、一般健康状态、情绪、功能独立性、社会支持、营养、失禁、药物使用和功能表现等 9 个维度，总分为 0~17 分，分数越高衰弱程度越高。该量表最大的优点在于调查者不需要有老年专业背景，且信效度良好。

（五）Tilburg 衰弱评估量表

Tilburg 衰弱评估量表是荷兰学者 Gobbens 等在整合衰弱模式的概念框架基础上开发的，用于社区老年人衰弱状况自评。该量表包括生理、心理和社会三个维度，共计 15 个条目。计分范围从 0 分到 15 分，分数越高衰弱程度越重。研究表明，在社区居住的老年人中进行调查，TFI 的心理测量性能良好。

三、衰弱的管理

对于衰弱进行干预包括 2 个目的：一是延缓或逆转衰弱的发生；二是对已经不能逆转的衰弱，主要目标是预防或减少衰弱带来的不良预后。为改善衰弱老年人的临床结局，研究者做出了许多尝试。不同国家和地区已有一些针对老年人衰弱干预的共识和指南。综合各类指南的干预内容，可归纳为运动锻炼、营养支持、心理咨询、慢性病管理、药

exercise, nutritional support, psychological consultation, chronic disease management, medical therapy and comprehensive geriatric assessment. Early holistic interventions are important. Nurses need to provide comprehensive geriatric assessment and rehabilitation care to the elderly and their families.

i. Physical Exercise

Physical exercise therapy may not only be important in the treatment of frailty, but also in the prevention. Elders with declines in strength are suggested to join in exercise programs aim at increasing the ability of mobility, muscular power, balance and endurance. Because frailty results from reaching a threshold of decline across multiple organ systems, an approach to prevent frailty is supposed to act on multiple systems. A study protocol showed that it is better to provide individual intervention for different level of frailty elders.

ii. Nutrition Support

Complete daily nutrition intake should be assessed and diet consultation should be made in combine with physical exercise for frailty intervention. Home delivered meals will be recommended if it is necessary. In addition, if the participant's body mass index (BMI) is ＜ 18.5, or mid upper arm circumference is ＜ the 10th percentile, nutritional supplementation will be offered using commercially available, high energy, high protein supplements.

iii. Psychological Consultation

If the depression symptoms are serious, consideration will be given for referral to a psychiatrist or psychologist for professional consultation. When elder is found socially isolated, options will be identified to encourage greater social engagement, e. g. participation in day activity groups and telephone contact with a volunteer. When the older person's family carer is noted to be experiencing significant distress due to the carer role, a supportive intervention will be provided to the carer.

iv. Chronic Disease Management

If the elder is in poor general health status, chronic disease management programs will be put in place or reinforced with the assistance of currently available health services. Medications will be reviewed by elder's general practitioner. Healthcare staff will encourage elders to comply with medications by education about the reasons for the medication and mediation taking techniques in case of forgetting.

物治疗和多学科团队的医疗护理。其中早期的全面干预（如老年综合评估、康复护理等）很重要。护士需要为老年人及其家人提供全面的老年医学评估和康复护理。

（一）运动锻炼

运动锻炼不仅可用于治疗衰弱，也是预防衰弱的重要手段之一。对于力量下降的老年人，建议其加入运动项目，通过各种针对性练习，从行动力、肌肉力量、平衡度、耐力等方面进行锻炼。衰弱是多个系统达到一定受损程度而出现的，因而针对衰弱的干预也要考虑多个系统，即多角度的整合干预。

（二）营养支持

评估每日完整的营养摄入量，并结合饮食咨询和体育锻炼，进行衰弱老年人的营养支持干预。必要时建议老年人选择家庭送餐服务。如果参与者的体重指数（BMI）＜18.5，或者上臂围小于第10百分位的老年人，将提供营养补充剂。

（三）心理咨询

对于自诉疲乏，且抑郁评分较高的老年人，建议其转诊到心理科或精神科。对于存在社交孤独的老年人，鼓励其参加社交活动，如参加每日的活动小组，与志愿者电话联系。必要时也应该为老年人家庭照护人员提供支持。

（四）慢性病管理

若老年人的总体健康状况较差，将在现有卫生服务的帮助下实施或加强慢性病管理计划。干预团队需评估老年人的用药情况，并与老年人的全科医生讨论药物选择情况。此外，干预团队将鼓励老年人提高用药的依从性。

v. Medical therapy

Medical therapy for frailty is still in the stage of clinical research. At present, studies suggest that angiotensin converting enzyme inhibitors can improve skeletal muscle structure and biochemical function, and stop or slow down muscle strength decline in the elderly. Sex hormone and growth hormone can increase muscle content and strength, and have potential effect on improving motor function. Low concentration of vitamin D is associated with the decline of the body.

vi. Comprehensive Geriatric Assessment

The British geriatrics society (BGS) has produced guidance to help. "Fit for Frailty" is a consensus best practice guidance for the management of frailty in community and outpatient settings. The gold standard for the management of frailty in older people is the process of care known as comprehensive geriatric assessment (CGA). CGA involves a holistic, interdisciplinary assessment of an individual and has been demonstrated to improve outcomes. It can be time consuming so it is not feasible for everyone with frailty in community settings to undergo a full multidisciplinary review with geriatrician/old age psychiatry involvement. Summary of BGS recommendations is provided in box 9-4.

Box 9-4　Summary of BGS Recommendations (in part)

- Provide training in frailty recognition to all health and social care staff.

- Carry out a comprehensive review of medical, functional, psychological and social needs based on the principles of comprehensive geriatric assessment.
- Ensure that reversible medical conditions are considered and addressed.
- Consider referral to geriatric medicine where frailty is associated with significant complexity, diagnostic uncertainty or challenging symptom control.

- Consider referral to old age psychiatry for those people with frailty and complex co-existing psychiatric problems, including challenging behavior in dementia.

- Use clinical judgment and personalized goals when deciding how to apply disease-based clinical guidelines to the management of older people with frailty.

- Generate a personalized shared care and support plan (CSP) outlining treatment goals, management plans and plans for urgent care. In some cases, it may be appropriate

（五）药物治疗

针对衰弱的药物治疗尚处于临床研究阶段，目前研究认为血管紧张素转化酶抑制剂可改善骨骼肌肉结构和生物化学功能，可停止或减缓老年人肌肉力量减退。性激素和生长激素可增加肌肉含量和力量，对于改善运动功能有潜在的效果。低浓度的维生素 D 与衰弱相关。

（六）老年综合评估

英国老年医学会（BGS）为老年人衰弱管理提供了帮助指南，并将老年综合评估（CGA）纳入了衰弱的管理实践指南中。老年综合评估涉及对个体进行全面、跨学科的评估，并已被证明能够改善结果。然而老年综合评估耗时较长，且此后可能还需进一步评估。此外，CGA 在实际开展过程中对于团队成员的合作性要求较高。BGS 衰弱管理指南的部分推荐内容见 box 9-4。

Box 9-4　BGS 衰弱管理指南的部分推荐内容

- 为所有的健康和社会保健人员提供衰弱识别的培训。

- 基于老年综合评估原则的需要，开展医疗、心理和社会功能的全面评估。

- 确保考虑和解决不良的医疗条件。

- 当患者的衰弱状况具有显著的复杂性、诊断的不确定性或症状控制的挑战性时，考虑将患者转诊到老年医学科。

- 当患者同时存在衰弱和复杂的精神问题时，如具有精神行为的痴呆，考虑将其转诊到老年精神科。

- 当决定如何运用以疾病为基础的临床指南对老年人的衰弱进行管理时，需将临床判断和个体化的目标相结合。

- 形成个性化的共同关心和支持计划（CSP），该计划包括了治疗目标、管理计划和紧急护理计划。在特定情况下，还需包含

to include an end of life care plan.

- Where an older person has been identified as having frailty, establish systems to share health record information (including the CSP) between primary care, emergency services, secondary care and social services.

- Recognize that many older people with frailty in crisis will manage better in the home environment but only with appropriate support systems.

Frailty state in elder people is preventable and reversible. It is very important for nurses and families to understand frailty and apply early interventions. The international frailty research is moving from the analysis of frailty concept, model and instrument development into clinical application. For example, frailty symptom management, comorbidity and frailty management and preventive strategy, all aimed to promote healthy aging. Introduction of theory and measurement of frailty will help nurses and families understand frailty and identify frail elders in earlier stage and design effective interventions to prevent or postpone individual adverse outcomes, maintain self-independence, reduce the use of health care resource and family burden, and finally reach the goal of health promotion and disability prevention among elder people.

(XI Xing)

Key Points

1. Geriatric syndromes are groups of specific signs and symptoms that share many common features and highly prevalent in older adults, especially the frail elderly.

2. Geriatric syndromes are multifactorial in cause. In geriatric syndromes, the leading symptom is linked to a number of etiological factors or diseases in other organs, and there is a large overlap between the etiological factors of different geriatric syndromes.

3. Geriatric syndromes present a challenge to the health professionals because they are associated with disability but typically lack a single underlying cause that may be cured.

4. Frailty is a syndrome which results from a multi-system reduction in reserve capacity to the extent that a number of physiological systems are approach to the threshold of symptomatic clinical failure.

临终关怀计划。

- 当老年人被确诊为衰弱，需建立系统以共享健康档案信息（包括 CSP），即包括了初级保健、急救服务、二级医疗和社会服务之间的信息共享。

- 在适当的支持系统下，许多存在衰弱危机的老年人是可以在家庭环境中正常生活的。

老年人的衰弱状态是可以预防和逆转的。对护士和家属来说，识别衰弱并及早采取干预措施是非常重要的。当前国际上对衰弱的研究已由衰弱概念的分析、理论模型的建立，衰弱评估工具的开发评价，转为衰弱概念在临床上的应用，如衰弱症状的管理、合并疾病的衰弱状态管理、预防策略的具体实施等，而这些对于减少衰弱，促进健康老龄化具有现实的指导意义。因此，在护理工作中可以引进已发展的衰弱评估工具，早期发现衰弱高危患者，进而设计并实施干预措施，以预防或延缓老年个案发生不良健康结局，维持其独立与自主性，减少健康照护资源使用和家庭照顾负担。

（奚 兴）

本章要点

1. 老年综合征是一组特殊的体征和症状，在老年人有许多共同的特征，且在老年人中发生率高，尤其是衰弱老年人。

2. 老年综合征由多方面的原因造成。在老年综合征中，主要症状与其他器官的病因或疾病有关，不同老年综合征的病因有很大的重叠。

3. 对健康专业人员来说，老年综合征是一个挑战，因为它们与残疾有关，但通常缺乏一个可以治愈的潜在病因。

4. 衰弱是一种由于多个系统储备能力降低而形成的综合征，在衰弱状态下，多个生理系统的功能都接近于临床功能耗竭的极限。

5. Markers of frailty include age-related weakness, weight loss, declines in strength and endurance, progressive functional worsening as well as psychological, emotional and social problems, resulting in adverse health outcomes.

6. Frail older people have increased risk of morbidity, institutionalization and death, resulting in burden to individuals, their families, health care services and society.

7. Frailty develops slowly in a stepwise process, with increments of decline precipitated by acute events. It is manifested as loss of skeletal muscle mass (sarcopenia), abnormal function in inflammatory and neuro-endocrine systems, and poor energy regulation.

8. Frailty may be initiated by disease, lack of activity, inadequate nutritional intake, stress, and/or the physiologic changes of aging. Once the elderly become frail, there is often a rapid, progressive, and self-perpetuating downward spiral toward failure to thrive and death.

9. Frailty determinants are complex and multiple. There are several measurements of frailty, but there is no gold standard instrument yet. Early screening of modifiable frailty risk factors allows to set up a plan for a personalized and optimal patient care.

Critical Thinking Exercise

Geriatric syndrome and frailty as an evolving concept have been developed very fast in the past three decades. However, its clinical application has been limited.

1. How would you increase the awareness of geriatric syndrome and frailty among elder people and health professionals?

2. What strategies need to be implemented to prevent frailty among elderly people?

5. 衰弱的标志包括老年期的虚弱、体重下降、力量和耐力的下降，以及生理、心理功能的进行性恶化、情感和社会问题，最终导致不良健康结局。

6. 衰弱老年人的患病、入住机构和死亡的风险增加，最终将造成对个人、家庭、医疗保健服务和社会的负担。

7. 衰弱是一个循序渐进的过程，发展缓慢，但在急性事件下加速恶化。衰弱表现为骨骼肌质量损失（肌少症），炎症和神经内分泌系统功能异常，能量调节障碍。

8. 衰弱可以由疾病、缺乏运动、营养摄入不足、压力，以及衰老的生理变化引起。一旦老年人变得衰弱，往往有一个快速的、渐进的和自我延续的螺旋下行过程，并最终走向耗竭和死亡。

9. 衰弱的影响因素繁多。有多种方法用于评估衰弱，但目前尚无金标准。早期筛查衰弱，有助于针对可改变的危险因素建立个性化、最优化的护理计划。

批判性思维练习

在过去的三十年里，老年综合征和衰弱的概念都在迅速发展。然而，目前老年综合征和衰弱的临床应用尚不多。

1. 如何提高老年人和健康专业人员对老年综合征和衰弱的认识？

2. 哪些策略可用于预防老年人衰弱的发生？

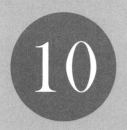

Chapter 10 Care of Elderly with Perception Impairment

第十章 感知觉障碍老年人的护理

Learning Objectives

On completion of this chapter, the reader will be able to:

- Describe age-related changes in sensory function;

- Compare and contrast common eye conditions and associated nursing interventions;

- Identify nursing interventions for older adults with low vision;

- Describe the proper method for instilling eye medications;

- Describe proper methods for removing impacted cerumen;

- Identify safety measures for older adults with vertigo;

- Describe aural rehabilitation methods for older adults with hearing impaired;

- Describe potential hazards for older adults with diminished senses of taste, smell, and touch;

- Identify nursing interventions for older adults with xerostomia.

学习目标

学完本章节，应完成以下目标：

- 描述老化对感觉功能的影响；

- 比较常见眼部疾病及其相关护理措施；

- 确认对低视力老年人的护理干预；

- 描述滴眼液的正确方法；

- 描述清除盯聍的正确方法；

- 描述老年眩晕患者的安全护理措施；

- 描述听力障碍老师人的听力康复方法；

- 描述味觉、嗅觉和触觉减退对老年人的潜在危害；

- 确认老年口干患者的护理措施。

The sensory systems connect human body to the environment. They allow individual to be aware of and interpret various stimuli, thus enable the individuals to interact with the environment. All of the sensory systems-eyes (vision), hearing, taste, smell, and touch (pressure, heat, and pain) change with human aging process. But the time of onset and rate of decline differ markedly from one to another. Dramatic ranges in degradation from minor impairments to major sensory losses influence daily living and the quality of life of older adults. Sensory changes can influence the way people see, hear, taste, smell, and respond to touch and pain. This in turn affects how people experience the world and react to things. It is very important for nurses to understand age-related sensory changes so that they can help old people adapt and function as independent as possible. This chapter discusses major sensory changes and impairments during older age and nursing interventions to assist older adults.

感觉器官联系着人体与外界环境，使个体能够意识到不同刺激的作用，并与环境相互作用。所有的感觉器官，包括视、听、味、嗅和触觉（压力、热和疼痛）等器官，均随衰老而发生变化，但变化程度因人而异。较轻微的变化对个体不会产生影响，但严重变化则可能影响老年人的日常生活和生活质量。感觉器官的变化会影响人们视、听、味、嗅的方式，以及对触觉和疼痛的反应。反过来，也会影响人们对世界的体验和对事物的反应。因此对护士而言，理解与年龄相关的感觉器官变化可让他们更好地帮助老年人适应老化并尽可能地保持功能。本章主要讨论感觉器官的老化改变和障碍对老年人的影响及相应的护理干预。

Box 10-1　Case Study

A 68-year-old man presents to the local community health center. He states that he has been having troubles with his eyes, and was diagnosed as close-angle glaucoma ten years ago. The vision screening indicates his vision is 20/200 in both eyes. He has to stay at the center for a week because his daughter and son-in-law are going to have a short visit abroad.

Questions:

1. What is the main nursing problem you would diagnose to this patient?

2. What strategies would you recommend to his caregivers regarding safety measures in the center?

Box 10-1　案例

一位 68 岁男性到社区医疗服务中心就诊，他表示他的眼睛出现了问题。10 年前他被诊断为闭角型青光眼。视力检查提示双眼视力均为 20/200。因为原来照顾他的女儿夫妇将短期出国，他不得不在社区中心住院一周。

问题：

1. 你认为这位患者的主要护理问题是什么？

2. 你会建议社区中心的照顾者对这位患者考虑哪些安全措施？

Section 1　Vision Impairment

第一节　视觉障碍

Vision impairment among the elderly is a major health care problem. Approximately one in three elderly persons of 65 years or older has some kinds of vision-reducing eye disorders. Vision impairments are connected with a decreased daily living ability and an increased risk for physical hazards and psychological issues.

视觉障碍是老年人常见的健康问题，65 岁以上老年人中约 1/3 存在视力相关问题。视觉障碍与老年人日常生活能力下降、身体损伤危险增加和心理问题均有关。

I. Common Age-related Changes

The visual system consists primarily of the eye, optic nerve, and occipital cortex (figure 10-1) and plays an integral role in a person's ability to function in the environment. Visual acuity (the ability to see clearly) is an important part of performing activities of daily living (ADLs); dressing, grooming, cooking, sewing, driving, and reading are all tasks that involve the use of eyesight. Therefore, changes in vision are particularly important because they can affect a person's ability to function in the physical environment and may lead to isolation.

一、一般老化改变

视觉系统包括眼、视神经和大脑皮层的视束（图10-1），对个体在环境中执行功能的能力起着重要的作用。视力（看清楚的能力）对于完成日常生活能力（ADL）具有重要意义，穿衣、梳妆、烹饪、缝纫、驾驶和阅读等任务全都需要良好的视力。因此，视力的改变对个体来说尤为重要，因为可影响个体在环境中行使正常功能的能力，甚至导致孤立。

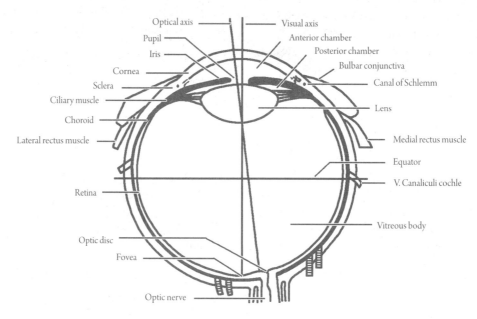

Figure 10-1 Anatomy of the eye

As people age, most will inevitably encounter some changes in their vision that may be attributed solely to the aging process. These processes are distinct from age-related pathological eye conditions, although the visual changes they produce may be similar. The natural quality of vision gradually declines with the anatomical and physiological processes that occur with aging of human eyes and visual system, including presbyopia, changes in the eyelids and tear film, and changes in the various intraocular structures contributing to the visual function.

i. Presbyopia

Presbyopia, a natural age-related change, results from the gradual decrease in accommodation of crystalline lens expected with aging and refers to light does not focus on retina for near vision. Presbyopia usually manifests after 40-45 years of age. Patients usually complain of blurred near vision, i. e. increasing difficulty with near visual

视力随年龄增长而不可避免地逐渐退化，这些变化与老年相关的病理性改变不同，尽管眼部疾病也会引起类似的变化。自然的视力衰退主要包括老视、眼睑和泪膜的变化和眼内器官的改变。

（一）老视

随年龄增长，进入眼内的光线聚焦于视网膜前的变化称为老视，多见于40～45岁人群。主要表现为视物模糊，视近物困难，视物时将物品移到离眼睛更近的距离才能看清。平均而言，青少年可轻松地调节到14D，到

tasks and may attempt to obtain clear vision by holding objects further from the eyes. The average teenagers can comfortably accommodate up to 14D, and by age 45 this drops to about 4D and is completely gone by the age of 50-55. Presbyopia can have multiple effects on quality of vision and quality of life if uncorrected.

ii. Eyelids

The eyelids lose tone and become lax, which contribute to the etiology of several eyelid disorders such as entropion (lower lid inversion), ectropion (lower lid eversion) and aponeurotic ptosis of the upper lid. These conditions usually need surgical correction.

iii. Lens

The lens increases in density and rigidity. This is accompanied by a gradual yellowing of the lens and a change in the refractive index. These changes affect the eye's ability to transmit and focus light, as well as the sensitivity of the eye to shorter blue wavelengths of light and the ability to discriminate blues and blue-greens becomes reduced. As an elderly, peripheral vision decreases, night vision diminishes, and sensitivity to glare increases.

iv. Cornea

With aging, the clarity of the cornea is maintained throughout life, but the density of the endothelial cells decreases and their morphology changes, rendering the aged cornea more vulnerable to the stress of injury or intraocular surgery. The cornea yellows and develops a noticeable surrounding ring, made up of fat deposits, called the arcus senilis. Also aberrations of the corneal surface increase with age, resulting in refractive error, glare and reduced contrast. And dry eye manifests frequently due to diminished aqueous tear production.

v. Vitreous

Progressive liquefaction of the vitreous gel occurs with aging, manifesting as the occasional floater. These tend to be more of an annoyance than a visual impairment. However, the age-related separation of the vitreous gel from the retina, called posterior vitreous detachment (PVD), may also manifest with floaters and may be complicated by retinal tears and retinal detachment.

vi. Retina

Aging causes a general decline in retinal function (color and contrast). Some changes can usually be found by ophthalmoscopic examination of the retina, such as blood vessels narrow and straighten; arteries seem opaque and gray; and drusen localized areas of hyaline macula.

45 岁时只能调节到 4D，而到 50～55 岁时这种调节能力完全丧失。老视若不校正，可对视功能和生活质量造成多重影响。

（二）眼睑

眼睑失去弹性而变得松弛，导致睑内翻、睑外翻和上睑下垂等，通常需要手术纠正。

（三）晶体

晶体变硬，密度增加，使其屈光度发生变化。晶体变黄，屈光指数发生变化。这些变化影响光线进入眼内的能力和聚焦能力，以及眼对较短的蓝色光的敏感性和分辨蓝光的能力，眼对蓝色和蓝绿色的区别能力下降。老年人的外周视力和夜视力降低，对眩光敏感性增强。

（四）角膜

尽管角膜的清晰度可保持终身，但随年龄增长，角膜内皮细胞的密度降低，生态学发生改变，使老年人的角膜容易受损。老年人的角膜变黄，可由于脂肪沉积形成老年环。角膜表面变得不规则而导致屈光不正、眩目和对比度降低。由于泪液生成减少，容易发生眼干燥症。

（五）玻璃体

由于老化，玻璃体液化的发生增加。表现为眼前偶见的漂浮物。这种变化通常对个体只带来些许烦恼，而不影响视力。但是，此症状也可能为玻璃体液化导致玻璃体后视网膜脱离（PVD）的表现，应与飞蚊症相鉴别，也需考虑视网膜撕裂或视网膜脱离的并发表现。

（六）视网膜

老化也使视网膜的功能（视物颜色和对比度）减弱，眼底检查的常见变化有视网膜上的血管变窄、变直，动脉不透明呈灰色，脉络膜疣多见，常位于黄斑处。飞蚊症和眼

Floaters and dry eyes are two common complaints of older adults and are discussed as follows.

II. Common Complaints

i. Floaters

Floaters appear as dots, wiggly lines, or clouds that the old adults may see moving in the visual field. They become more marked when an individual is looking at a plain background. It is more often for the people aged over 50 years old to develop floaters because they are usually caused by degeneration of the vitreous gel and are more common in aged people who have undergone cataract operations or laser surgery. Generally floaters are normal and harmless, but they may be a warning sign of a more serious condition, especially when patients find the increasing in number of floaters, changes in the type of floater, light flashes, or visual hallucinations.

ii. Flashers

Flashers occur when the vitreous fluid inside the eye rubs or pulls on the retina and then produces the illusion of flashing lights or lightning streaks. Flashers are present in both eyes and appear as jagged lines, last 10-20 minutes. In general, these flashers occur with advancing age; however patients should be suggested to see a doctor when they increase in number, numbers of new flashers appear, or partial loss of side vision is noted.

iii. Dry Eyes

Dry eye syndrome or keratoconjunctivitis sicca, is a deficiency in the production of any of the aqueous, mucin, or lipid tear film components; lid surface abnormalities; or epithelial abnormalities related to systemic diseases (e. g., thyroid disorders, Parkinson's disease), infection, injury, or complications of medications (e. g. , antihistamines, oral contraceptives, phenothiazines). The most common symptom is a scratchy or foreign body sensation. Others include itching, excessive mucus secretion, inability to produce tears, a burning sensation, redness, pain, and difficulty moving the lids. Aging, arthritis and the use of certain medications are likely factors associated with dry eyes. Instillation of artificial tears during the day and an ointment at night is the usual option of treatment. In serious cases of dry eye syndrome, surgical treatment are options including punctal occlusion, grafting procedures, and lateral tarsorrhaphy (i. e. , uniting the edges of the lids).

干燥症是老年患者最常见的主诉，将在下文讨论。

二、常见主诉

（一）漂浮物

视野中移动的漂浮物常表现视野中移动的点、扭曲的线或云块，这种情况在个体盯着一个简单背景时尤为明显。50 岁以上者由于玻璃体液化可发展为飞蚊症，做过白内障手术或激光手术者更常见。漂浮物的表现一般无害，但如果漂浮物数量增多、形式改变或伴有眩光或视物模糊时，提示问题加重，应予以重视。

（二）眩光

当液化的玻璃体进入或牵拉视网膜时可表现为眩光，常伴有视直线变形。眩光多累及双眼，持续 10~20 分钟。通常随年龄增长，个体可出现眩光，但若患者发生次数增多、出现新的眩光表现、一侧或双侧视力丧失，应及时就诊。

（三）干眼

干眼综合征或干燥性角膜结膜炎，常见原因有眼内液生成减少，眼睑异常，系统性疾病（如甲状腺疾病、帕金森病）、感染、损伤引起的上皮功能异常，某些药物的不良反应（抗组胺药、口服避孕药、吩噻嗪类药物）。最常见的表现为眼内刺痒感或异物感。其他表现包括瘙痒、黏液分泌过多、泪液生成减少、烧灼感、眼红、疼痛和眼睑活动障碍。年龄增长、关节炎和使用某些药物是眼干燥症的常见原因。常用治疗包括白天使用人工泪液、夜间使用眼药膏。重度眼干燥症常需手术纠正，包括封闭泪小管、移植和单侧睑缘缝合术（即缝合一侧睑缘）。

III. Common Problems and Conditions

Age-related eye conditions include ectropion and entropion, blepharitis, cataract, glaucoma, age-related macular degeneration and the retinal complications of vascular diseases.

i. Ectropion and Entropion

Ectropion is an external eye disorder of the eyelid in which it turns outward (inside out). Entropion is a disorder of the eye-lid (usually the lower) in which it curls inward toward the eye. Both conditions are due to tissue laxity and scarring of the eyelids from infection. Ectropion prevents normal eye-closure, affects tear drainage and production, and causes redness and tearing of eyeball. Entropion results in the eyelashes rubbing against the eye, causing corneal abrasion.

1. Etiology Ectropion is associated with several factors, including weakening of the muscles and tissues that normally support the lid against the eye, paralysis of the nerve going to the eyelid muscles and shrinking of scar tissue from burns, wounds, or surgery near the eye. Entropion is developed with the relaxation of the eyelid's supporting tissue along with the inward pull of the eyelid muscles and chronic eye inflammation (including allergy), which creating scar tissue in the eyelid.

2. Nursing assessment Frequent signs and symptoms of ectropion include turning out of the eyelid (usually the lower), pain, redness, and swelling in the affected eyelid, and poor eye lubrication when the patient with lubricating tears run down the cheek instead of into the eye. Most possible complications of ectropion may be corneal damage caused by dryness. The common signs and symptoms produced by entropion include swelling, redness, pain, and excessive tears of the eye. Entropion many cause blister of the cornea from eyelash and eye-lid irritation.

3. Nursing management Ectropion and entropion cannot be prevented at present and usually curable with surgery. The prognosis for complete recovery and cessation of symptoms is excellent. Artificial tears may help with symptoms relief before surgery. If infection is present, antibiotics may be prescribed. Nurse should teach home care tips to patient and family such as wearing protective glasses or goggles if exposed to wind or pollutants and applying warm compresses to the eyelids several times a day for swelling and pain. To prepare compresses, patient or caregivers should pour warm water into a clean bowl, soak a clean cloth in the water, wring it

三、常见健康问题及护理

年龄相关眼病包括睑外翻和睑内翻、眼睑炎症、白内障、青光眼、年龄相关性黄斑变性和血管性疾病的视网膜并发症。

（一）睑外翻和睑内翻

睑外翻是眼睑向外翻出所致的眼病，睑内翻是眼睑（多为下睑）向眼球方向翻转所致的眼病。均因眼睑组织松弛或瘢痕形成所致。睑外翻影响正常的眼睑闭合、泪液引流，可导致红眼和溢泪。睑内翻可使睫毛向内刺激眼球导致角膜损伤。

1. 病因 睑外翻的病因包括眼睑肌肉松弛，神经瘫痪和因烧伤、损伤或手术损伤引起的瘢痕挛缩。睑内翻的主要原因是眼的支持组织松弛和慢性炎症（包括过敏）所致瘢痕所致。

2. 护理评估 睑外翻的主要症状和体征有眼睑外翻（多见于下睑）；患眼疼痛、发红、肿胀；溢泪，眼液的润滑作用减弱。其主要并发症为眼干燥症。睑外翻的主要症状和体征包括肿胀、发红、疼痛和眼泪过多。睑内翻可因倒睫刺激角膜而引起眼刺激症状。

3. 护理措施 睑外翻和睑内翻通常需手术纠正。手术前可用人工泪液。有感染者可用抗生素。护士应教育患者及其家人当暴露于大风或污染环境时，可戴保护性眼镜或防护镜，若有眼痛和肿胀，可每天湿热敷眼睑数次。湿敷时，患者或照顾者应在干净容器中倒入热水，将干净的敷料浸入，将其拧干，敷在眼上 10～15 分钟。

out until it is almost dry, and then apply the warm, moist cloth to the closed eye for 10-15 minutes.

ii. Blepharitis

Blepharitis is a chronic inflammation of the eyelid margins that is commonly found in aged people.

1. Etiology Blepharitis can be caused by seborrheic dermatitis or infection. Because of the drying effects of the medications, the use of antihistamines, anticholinergics, antidepressants, and diuretics can exacerbate this condition. Infection is also associated with the deficiency in tear production with aging.

2. Nursing assessment Blepharitis can be classified as three main types: staphylococcal, seborrhoeic (frequently associated with seborrhoea of the scalp, eyebrows and ears) and contact dermatitis (due to cosmetics). The lid margins of the patient appear raw and red, with irritation, burning and itching. If contact dermatitis is the cause then there is generally a history of atopy, and other areas of skin may be affected. Scars are frequently seen on the lashes of both upper and lower lids, which tend to be dry in staphylococcal infections and greasy in seborrhoeic blepharitis. The lids become deformed in staphylococcal blepharitis due to ulceration. Lashes are frequently lost or may be distorted, turn inwards and rub on the cornea; this in turn can cause conjunctivitis.

3. Nursing management Treatment is aimed at removing the bacteria and healing the affected areas. Mild seborrhoeic blepharitis can often be managed with eyelid hygiene without prescribed medication. However, it should be diagnosed firstly because the condition may not respond to over-the-counter treatment. Topical antibiotics or steroids are common options to be prescribed. The nurse plays a remarkable role in the management of this condition by providing hygiene and medication using guidelines. If the patient can comply with these notes, hygienic practices, the inflammation and the patient's comfort level may improve after a week. The tips must be taught to patients include good hand washing habits (mild soap should be used) to keep eye hygiene, good contact lens cleaning and storage techniques to prevent contamination of eyes, regular replacement of eye makeup products (every 3-6 months) to avoid bacterial growth, appropriate use of makeup with cotton balls and cotton-tipped applicators, appropriate choosing and use of mascara products (water-resistant, free of lash-extending fibers, and not applied to the base of the lashes), appropriate choosing and use of eyeliner products (a medium-hard pencil and not be applied to the inner

（二）眼睑炎症

眼睑炎症是一种老年人常见的慢性眼睑炎症。

1. **病因** 脂溢性皮炎或感染所致。使用某些药物，如抗组胺药、抗胆碱能药、抗抑郁药和利尿剂，可加重损害。感染亦与老化所致泪液生成不足有关。

2. **护理评估** 可分为葡萄球菌感染、脂溢性（通常与头皮、眉毛和耳脂溢性皮炎有关）和接触性皮炎（与化妆品有关）3种类型。患者睑缘粗糙发红，有刺激感、烧灼感和痒感。如为接触性皮炎，一般有接触史及其他部位皮肤表现。葡萄球菌所致感染者常因溃疡至眼睑变形。常有睫毛缺失或朝向眼球，可进一步导致结膜炎。

3. **护理措施** 治疗目的是控制感染和修复受损部位。轻度脂溢性感染者可仅清洁眼部，而不需用药，但前提是在用药前应明确诊断，因为患者可能对非处方治疗无反应。严重感染者可用抗生素和糖皮质激素类眼液。护士应教育患者正确的清洁方式和用药护理。若患者能够坚持正确的护理措施，炎症和症状可在一周内控制。健康教育要点包括养成良好洗手习惯（应使用温和的肥皂），正确使用和保存角膜接触镜，定期更换眼部护肤品（每3~6个月）以避免细菌滋生，正确使用化妆棉、睫毛膏（防水，不涂在睫毛根部）和眼线笔（中等硬度的铅笔，不能涂在眼睑的内部边缘），避免使用喷雾式发胶（因为它们会刺激眼睛）。

margin of the eyelid), and avoiding the use of aerosol hairsprays (as they can irritate the eyes).

iii. Age-related Cataract

Cataract refers to opacity of the crystalline lens of the eye and is the most common disorder causing visual impairment in the aging adult. The role of the lens is focusing light on the retina to produce a sharp image. When a cataract forms, the lens can become too opaque to transmit light to the retina. As a result, the patient's vision is gradually impaired.

1. Etiology　Cataract results from changes in the chemical composition of the lens which can be caused by aging, eye injuries, certain diseases (e. g. diabetes), and heredity. Other risk factors include ultraviolet exposure, nutrition, steroid use, and smoking.

2. Nursing assessment　Cataracts can be classified different types. Senile cataracts refer to those associating with the normal aging process. This kind of cataracts can occur as early as age 40. Eye injuries (e. g. , a hard blow, cut, puncture, or burn) can damage the lens and result in a traumatic cataract. Also cataracts can be classified as primarily (e. g. senile or congenital cataract) and secondary types which can be caused by certain infections, drugs, or diseases.

Symptoms differ from person to person. The size and location of a cataract determine the amount of interferences with clear sight. In age-related cataract, there can further be classified three morphological types, named nuclear sclerosis (progressive yellowing of the center of the lens), cortical cataracts (peripheral spokes and radial water clefts), and posterior subcapsular cataract (opacity just beneath the posterior lens capsule). A cataract located near the center of the lens produces more noticeable symptoms, including dimmed, blurred, or misty vision, the need for brighter light to read, glare and light sensitivity, loss of color perception, and recurrent eyeglass prescription changes. These symptoms develop slowly with aging and at different rates in each eye. Signs of the cataracts include loss of the red reflex or the presence of opacities in the red reflex and an untreated mature white cataract is easily visible through the pupil.

3. Nursing management　The treatment option for the patient with cataract depends on the extent of his or her visual disability. Most age-related cataracts are treated by surgical removal. Cataract surgery improves vision, mental outlook, ability to function, and quality of life. The consideration of cataract surgery is complex and intricate, and surgery should be recommended when evidence indicates effectiveness in enhancing quality of

（三）年龄相关性白内障

白内障指晶体混浊所致的眼病，是影响老年人视觉功能的最常见眼病。晶状体的作用是将光线聚焦在视网膜上以产生清晰的图像。由于晶体混浊会影响进入眼内的光线到达视网膜，因此会影响视力。

1. 病因　老化、眼损伤、某些疾病（如糖尿病）和遗传因素所致的晶体化学成分发生变化。其他危险因素主要有暴露于紫外线、营养缺乏、应用激素类药物和吸烟。

2. 护理评估　有多种类型。老年性白内障是指与正常老化过程有关的白内障，多发于40岁之后。眼的损伤（拳击、割伤、刺伤或烧伤）可致外伤性白内障。白内障还可分为原发性（如老年性或先天性白内障）和继发性（由某种感染、药物或疾病所致）两类。

白内障的症状因人而异。临床症状与晶体混浊的部位和大小有关。根据混浊部位，老年性白内障在形态学上又可分为3类，即核性（进行性晶体中心部位变黄）、皮质性（晶体外围部分辐射状混浊）和后囊下（混浊只发生于晶体后囊下）白内障。白内障越靠近晶体中心，视力影响越明显。主要症状包括视物模糊，需在强光下阅读，出现眩光，对光敏感、对色彩的感知力下降，眼镜度数的改变等。这些症状会随着年龄的增长而缓慢发展，并且每只眼睛的发生率都不同。体征包括红反射消失，部分患者可在瞳孔区看到白内障。

3. 护理措施　治疗措施的选择基于患者视力受损的程度。多数白内障患者需手术治疗，手术可改善视力、精神状态、功能和生活质量。如果证据提示可改善生活质量，当与其他治疗方法相比，手术具更好成本－效益比时或应推荐手术。手术治疗的决策应基

life and its cost-effectiveness is indicated comparing with that of other accepted treatments. The decision-making of surgery should be also based on consideration of such factors as visual acuity, visual impairment, and potential for functional benefits.

Cataract surgery generally takes less than a quarter under local or topical (applied directly on the eye) anesthesia. In surgery, ultrasonic waves are used to break down the affected lens and suck it out through a small incision. An artificial lens is then put in place. Most patients can have their cataracts removed and a new lens inserted in the same procedure, on an outpatient basis.

Cataracts may be managed without surgeries if they are mild and do not greatly affect vision or quality of life. In this case, eyeglasses, contact lenses, and other aids for low vision may improve vision. Steps should also be taken to prevent or slow down the cataracts from progressing, including controlling blood sugar in people with diabetes and wearing sunglasses to protect the eyes against ultraviolet light. Studies suggest that the intake of antioxidants (e. g. , vitamin C, beta-carotene, and vitamin E) may slow cataract progression. Reducing glare with proper light and appropriate lighting can facilitate reading.

Nursing management for the elderly with cataracts focuses mainly on preoperative and postoperative surgical care since surgery is the only intervention for treating cataracts. In general, the patient can be performed a cataract surgery on an outpatient basis with the administration of a local anesthetic; this makes preoperative teaching difficult because the patient arrives just hours before surgery. Thus, nurses should make an arrangement to conduct preoperative assessment and patient teaching before surgery. Preoperative care focuses on administering eye drops and a sedative as ordered. And postoperative care involves teaching the patients and their family home care tips for the postoperative period, including avoiding rubbing or pressing on the eye, avoiding bending at the waist or lifting heavy objects within one month, avoiding straining with bowel movements (stool softener may be necessary), avoiding taking showers and shampooing hair (soap may irritate eye) for the specified time as instructed, and limiting reading (back and forth movement may loosen stitches).

The patients and their family should also be educated for the methods and tips for instilling eye medications. The elderly or caregiver should remember to wash hands thoroughly before and after the procedure and ensure adequate light and assume a comfortable position.

于以下因素，包括患者的视力、视损害程度、潜在的功能改善益处。

白内障手术一般在局麻下进行。术中常用超声粉碎混浊的晶体，并通过一个小切口将其吸出，然后置入人工晶体。多数情况下摘除白内障和置入新的人工晶体可在同一次手术中实现。

若白内障患者视力受损不严重或未影响生活质量，也可接受非手术治疗。对此类患者，眼镜、角膜接触镜或其他辅助方法可用于提高视力。预防白内障病情发展的措施包括控制血糖和戴太阳镜防止紫外线损害。研究发现摄入抗氧化剂（例如维生素 C，β- 胡萝卜素和维生素 E）可能减缓白内障进展，使用适当的照明可有助于阅读。

手术前后护理是重点。由于患者往往是在门诊进行手术，使术前教育的实施较为困难，因此护士应提前安排时间对患者进行术前评估和教育。术前护理的重点是遵医嘱使用眼液和镇静药。术后护理的重点是对患者及其家人进行术后护理的健康教育，具体包括避免揉或压迫术眼，术后一个月避免弯腰或提重物，避免用力排便，遵医嘱术后特定时间内避免沐浴或洗头发以免洗发液刺激术眼，减少阅读。

护士还要教会患者及其家人正确使用眼液的方法。要点包括操作前后均应充分洗手，确保光线充足和患者处于舒适体位。滴药前，应先充分摇匀药液。注意不要让药瓶尖端碰

Before instilling, shaking suspensions or "milky" solutions is necessary. Note indicates that not touch any part of the eye or face with the tip of the medication container, hold the lower lid down, and not press on the eyeball. The caregiver should apply gentle pressure to the patient's cheek bone to anchor the finger holding the lid. Usually eye drops should be instilled before applying ointments. Immediately after instilling eye drops, keep the eyelids closed, and apply gentle pressure on the inner canthus (punctual occlusion) near the bridge of the nose for 1 to 2 minutes. It should wait for 5-10 minutes before using another eye medication.

The home care instructions also need to include special precautions recommended by the ophthalmologist based on the type of surgery performed. There are several surgery types performed for cataract patients including intracapsular cataract extraction (ICCE), extracapsular surgery, and phacoemulsification. Before removal of the lens, the patient should make a decision about lens replacement options because he or she will be as aphakic (i. e. , without lens) after cataract surgery. There are three options: aphakic eyeglasses, contact lenses, and intraocular lens (IOLs) implants. Aphakic glasses are effective but heavy. Objects are magnified by 25%, making them appear closer than they actually are. Objects are magnified unequally, creating distortion. Peripheral vision is also limited, and binocular vision is impossible if the other eye is normal. Contact lenses provide patients with almost normal vision, because they need to be removed occasionally, the patient also needs a pair of aphakic glasses. Contact lenses are not advised for the elderly who have difficulty inserting, removing, and cleaning them. Frequent handling and improper disinfection increase the risk for infection. Insertion of IOLs during cataract surgery is the usual approach to lens replacement. In general, the surgeon implants an IOL in front of or behind the iris after removal of the lens in cataract surgery. IOLs are associated with a relatively low incidence of complications, but they are contraindicated in patients with recurrent uveitis, proliferative diabetic retinopathy, neovascular glaucoma, or rubeosisiridis. IOLs can also malfunction and cause complication. Nurses should help patient to choose the appropriate lens placement option before cataract surgery.

iv. Glaucoma

Glaucoma refers to a group of eye diseases characterized by optic nerve damage and is the leading cause of world blindness after cataracts. The optic nerve damage is commonly related to the elevated intraocular pressure (IOP) caused by congestion of aqueous humor

到眼或脸的任何部位，使瓶口向下，不要压迫眼球。一般在先滴眼液再用眼膏。滴好眼液后立即关闭眼睑，轻压泪点1～2分钟。若需要用另一种眼药，应间隔5～10分钟。

根据不同手术方式向患者提供针对性的术后教育。常用手术方式有白内障囊内摘除术（ICCE）、白内障囊外摘除术和超声乳化术。患者应在手术前做出替代晶体的决策，纠正手术后无晶体眼的方法有戴无晶体眼镜、角膜接触镜和置入人工晶体，无晶体眼镜可提供有效视力，但重量较重，所视物体被放大25%，看上去比实际更近，有视物变形、外周视力受限、双眼视觉不协调的缺点。角膜接触镜可提供接近正常的视力，但在摘除时需要另配一副无晶体眼镜，并且老年人在置入、移除或清洁镜片时可能存在困难，且容易发生感染。置入人工晶体可提供较好视力，其并发症较少，但反复发作的葡萄膜炎、增殖性糖尿病视网膜病变、新生血管性青光眼或虹膜新生血管为其禁忌证。护士应帮助患者选择合适的晶体替代方法。

（四）青光眼

青光眼是一组以视神经损害为特征的眼病，是世界范围内导致眼盲的第二大原因（除白内障）。视神经损害与房水排出不畅所致眼内压升高（IOP）有关。部分患者眼压未

in the eye. There is a range of pressures that have been considered "normal" but it may be associated with vision loss in some patients. Glaucoma can occur at any age; however, those most at risk are older adults than age 60. The most common form has few, if any, symptoms may cause partial vision loss before it is detected.

1. Etiology　IOP is determined by several factors and maintained between 10 to 21 mmHg when aqueous fluid production and drainage are in balance. When aqueous fluid is inhibited from flowing out, pressure builds up within the eye. Fluctuations in IOP occur with time of day, exertion, diet, and medications. It tends to increase with blinking, tight lid squeezing, and upward gazing. Systemic conditions (hypertension) and intraocular conditions (uveitis and retinal detachment) can be associated with elevated IOP. Risk factors for glaucoma include family history of glaucoma, African American race, older age, certain diseases (e. g. diabetes, cardiovascular disease, and migraine syndromes), nearsightedness, eye trauma, and prolonged use of topical or systemic corticosteroids.

2. Nursing assessment　Glaucoma is often called the "silent thief of sight" because most patients are unaware that they have the disease until they have experienced visual changes and vision loss. The patient may not seek health care until he or she experiences blurred vision or "halos" around lights, difficulty focusing, difficulty adjusting eyes in low lighting, loss of peripheral vision, aching or discomfort around the eyes, and headache. Glaucoma can be primary or secondary, depending on whether associated factors contribute to the rise in IOP. When the drainage angle is damaged by eye injury or certain conditions, such as medication use (e. g. , steroids), tumors, inflammation, or abnormal blood vessels, secondary glaucoma develops. The two common clinical types of glaucoma encountered in older adults are open-angle glaucoma and closed-angle glaucoma. Whether glaucoma is known as open-angle or closed-angle glaucoma depends on which mechanisms cause impaired aqueous outflow.

Chronic open-angle glaucoma, the most common type which makes up 90% of all primary glaucoma, develops gradually. Increased IOP occurs because degenerative changes in Schlemm's canal obstruct the escape of aqueous humor. This type of glaucoma can damage vision so slowly and painlessly that the patient is unaware of a problem until his or her optic nerve is deadly damaged. Visual loss begins with deteriorating peripheral vision.

升高但也有眼底损害。青光眼可发生于任何年龄，但更多见于 60 岁以上老年人。除少数患者有部分视力缺损外，此病在确诊前常无明显症状。

1. **病因**　眼压的正常范围是 10～21mmHg，它主要由房水生成和排出的平衡决定的。当房水排出不畅时，眼压即升高。眼压在一天内可发生波动，用力、饮食、药物也可能引起眼压波动。瞬目、压迫上睑和仰望都可使眼压升高。某些全身性疾病（如高血压）和眼内疾病（如葡萄膜炎和视网膜脱离）也与眼压升高有关。眼压升高发展为青光眼的危险因素主要有家族史、非洲裔美国人、年龄增长、某些疾病（如糖尿病、心血管疾病和偏头痛综合征）、近视、眼外伤、长期局部或全身应用类固醇激素等。

2. **护理评估**　青光眼常被称为视力的无声杀手，因为大多数患者在出现视力改变、失明前并未意识到自己已患病，发现视物模糊或出现晕轮、聚焦困难、暗光下调节困难、周围视力丧失、眼睛疼痛或不适以及头痛等症状时，才去就医。根据眼压升高的原因，青光眼可分类原发型和继发型。根据影响房水循环的机制，青光眼可分为开角型青光眼和闭角型青光眼。

慢性开角型青光眼发展缓慢，是最常见的青光眼类型，90% 的原发性青光眼为此型。眼压升高是由于 Schlemm's 阻塞所致。此型青光眼可缓慢地、无痛地损害视力，患者常不能意识到问题，直至出现视神经的损害。视力的损害从外周视力受损开始。

Closed-angle glaucoma is acute glaucoma that occurs suddenly as a result of complete blockage. It requires prompt medical intervention to avoid severe vision loss or blindness. Symptoms of closed-angle glaucoma occur rapidly, including severe eye pain, redness in the eye, clouded or blurred vision, nausea and vomiting, bradycardia, rainbow halos surrounding lights, pupil dilation, and steamy appearance of cornea.

Assessment for the elderly with glaucoma should include complaints that may relate to glaucoma which mentioned above, and the onset, duration, location, and severity of symptoms should be noted as well. Health history should also be asked about family members with glaucoma. A comprehensive eye exam should be taken to diagnose glaucoma in its open or closed angle forms, and to evaluate its severity. Core examinations include visual acuity, refractive error, pupils, anterior segment, IOP, angel structures, optic nerve, fundus, and visual field.

3. Nursing management The aim of all glaucoma treatment is prevention of optic nerve damage through medication, laser trabeculoplasty or non-laser surgery, or a combination of these approaches. Lifelong therapy is almost always necessary to prevent or decrease further optic nerve damage. The treatment goal is to maintain an IOP within a range unlikely to cause further visual field deterioration. Treatment recommendations, risks, options, and consequences of no treatment, should be discussed with the elderly patients or caregivers.

In open-angle glaucoma, unless the pressure is very high, treatment is not usually needed if high pressure in the eye is the only sign. Treatment is usually started only when there is evidence of damage to the eye. First option is usually eye drops either to increase the drainage of fluid or to decrease the production of fluid. Oral medications are also available, such as beta-blockers and carbonic anhydrase inhibitors, but the older adults must be carefully monitored because these medications may cause confusion, drowsiness, poor appetite, numbness in the hands and feet, and kidney stones.

In closed-angle glaucoma, emergency treatment is required to reduce the eye pressure promptly. If medication fails to control increased IOP, surgical intervention may be necessary, such as trabeculoplasty and trabeculectomy. Trabeculoplasty is usually performed on an outpatient basis. It requires an IOP check 3-4 hours after surgery. A sudden rise in IOP can occur immediately after surgery. The effectiveness of the procedure can be determined after 4-8 week post operation. However, it is necessary for the patient to continue using glaucoma medications.

闭角型青光眼可因房水循环完全阻塞急性发作。此型患者需要紧急治疗以避免严重的视力损害或失明。症状发生迅速，包括严重眼痛、眼红、视物模糊、恶心和呕吐、心动过缓、虹视、瞳孔放大和等角膜表面出现雾气。

老年青光眼患者的评估除以上内容外，还需要关注眼部症状的发作情况、部位和严重程度。护士应了解有无青光眼家族史，进行全面眼科检查判断青光眼是开角型还是闭角型，及其严重度。主要检查包括视力、屈光度、瞳孔、眼前节、眼内压、眼角结构、视神经、眼底和视野等。

3. 护理措施 治疗目的是通过药物、激光小梁成形术或非激光手术及综合措施预防视神经损害。患者往往需要终身治疗，将眼压控制在不造成进一步损害的范围内。治疗的目标是将 IOP 控制到合理的范围内，以免引起进一步视野损害。应与老年患者或其照顾者讨论治疗的建议、风险、选择和不治疗的后果。

对于开角型青光眼，若仅有眼压升高而无视神经损害，则不需降眼压。只有当存在眼部受损的证据时才开始治疗。治疗的第一选择是滴眼液，作用主要是增加房水的排出或减少房水生成。如需要也可用口服药，如β-受体阻滞剂和碳酸酐酶抑制剂，但老年人有使用这些药物时需严密监测药物不良反应，如精神错乱、疲乏、食欲减退、手足麻木和肾结石。

对于闭角型青光眼，应迅速用药以降低眼压。如药物无效，则需要手术治疗，如小梁成形术和小梁切除术。小梁成形术一般可在门诊进行，术后患者 IOP 可能突然升高，因此术后 3～4 小时需进行眼压检查。手术效果一般需等 4～8 周后才可确定。术后患者仍需使用抗青光眼药物。小梁切除术需住院进行，对行小梁切除术患者的术后护理包括常

Trabeculectomy requires hospitalization. Postoperative nursing care for the patient who has had a trabeculectomy includes routine post-anesthesia care, protection of the operative eye with an eye patch or a shield, proper positioning of the patient on the back or on the side of the inoperative eye, administration of pain medications and cold eye compresses to maintain comfort monitoring of the eye for increased IOP, bleeding, or infection, and assistance and teaching of safe, independent performance of ADLs.

The aim of nursing management is to teach patient that glaucoma is a chronic condition and requires lifelong medical treatment. The nurse should help patient and family understand that glaucoma can lead to blindness if not treated in the early stages and it is importance to perform eye pressure examination annually. Also the patient and family should be aware that further vision loss can be prevented although any current visual loss is permanent. The tips of care guidelines includes keeping regular and lifelong medical follow-up and eye medication administration, understanding IOP measurement and the desired range and keeping a record of IOP and visual field test results to monitor progress, being aware of continue eye drops even in the absence of symptoms, avoiding driving for 1-2 hours after administration of miotics, pressing lacrimal duct for 1 minute after eye drop insertion to prevent rapid systemic absorption, having a reserve bottle of eye drops at home and carrying eye drops on person (not in luggage) when traveling, carrying card or war Medic-Alert bracelet identifying glaucoma and the eye drops solution prescribed, reporting any reappearance of symptoms immediately to the doctor, remembering to alter staff of continued need to use prescribed eye drops if admitted to the hospital for a different medical condition, and avoiding the use of mydriatic or cycloplegic drugs (e. g. atropine) that dilate the pupils.

v. Age-related Macular Degeneration

Age-related macular degeneration (AMD) is defined as central vision loss attributable to degenerative atrophic and/or neovascular changes in the macula. It is characterized by tiny, yellowish spots called drusen beneath the retina which usually damage the macula and make reading, writing and driving very difficult. Most of older adults have at least a few small drusen which is normal with advancing age. However, if there are presence of larger and more numerous drusen in the macula, it is a common early sign of AMD. AMD is the most common cause of visual loss in people older than age 60 and often results in loss of close vision. AMD does not cause total

规麻醉后护理，用眼垫或眼盾保护手术眼，使用止痛药和手术眼冷敷，监测眼压，和协助患者日常生活的活动。

护理干预的目的是告诉患者青光眼是一种慢性疾病，需要终身治疗。护士应帮助患者及其家庭了解若早期不进行治疗，青光眼可导致失明，让其了解定期进行眼压检查的重要性。患者和家属应知道已有视力损害无法恢复，但进一步的视功能损害却可预防。健康指导内容包括坚持规律随访，理解 IOP 监测的重点性，坚持使用药物（即使无明显症状），使用缩瞳剂 1~2 小时内避免开车，滴眼液后立即压迫泪点 1 分钟，随身携带眼液，发生异常症状立即报告医生，到不同医疗机构就诊时应提醒医生患有青光眼及其用药情况，避免使用散瞳剂或睫状肌麻痹剂（如阿托品）。

（五）年龄相关黄斑变性
年龄相关黄斑变性（AMD）指因黄斑萎缩和/或新生血管生成所致的中心视力受损。特征性改变是视网膜下出现细小黄色斑点，称脉络膜疣，多累及黄斑，造成读写等功能困难。随着年龄增长，多数老年人会有少量脉络膜疣，但不会影响功能。但如数量增多或面积变大，则可有临床表现。AMD 是导致60 岁以上老年人视力丧失特别是近视力丧失的最常见原因，一般不会导致完全失明，可保留外周视力。

blindness. It mainly affects central vision and most patients retain peripheral vision.

1. Etiology The exact etiology of AMD is not clear but the primary risk factors have been identified in some studies including increasing age, ethnicity, and genetic factors. Cigarette smoking is found as a main modifiable risk factor for the development of AMD. Patients tend to cluster in families. Compelling evidence is emerging that the innate immune system and the complement factor H gene play a vital role in the pathobiology of AMD.

2. Nursing assessment Patient in early stage of AMD may have a few symptoms or a mild visual impairment. Early AMD denotes the risk of progression to late stage AMD. There are two types of late AMD, commonly known as the dry type (non-neovascular) and wet type (neovascular), based on the clinical appearance of the macula.

Dry AMD, also known as involutional macular degeneration, is most common and accounts for 85%-90% of all patients of late AMD. It develops slowly and causes gradual loss of central vision. It is characterized by geographic atrophy of the retinal pigment epithelium (RPE). Patients generally have no symptoms when the drusen occur outside of the macular area; while the drusen occur within the macula, there is a gradual blurring of vision that patients may notice when they try to read. There is no known treatment that can slow or cure this type of AMD and patients usually require vitamins and low-vision aids.

Wet AMD, also known as exudative macular degeneration, is less common and accounts for 10%-15 % of all patients of late AMD. This type of AMD results when abnormal blood vessels form and hemorrhage on the retina. Patients complain that straight lines appear crooked and distorted or that letters in word appear broken up. Vision loss may be rapid and severe with an acute drop in central vision and distortion (metamorphopsia). Wet AMD is characterized by the development of new vessels beneath the retina (choroidal neovascular membranes, CNV), serous elevation (detachment) of the neurosensory retina and/or pigment epithelium and macular hemorrhages. Macular scars are seen in end-stage disease. Some patients can be treated with the laser to stop the leakage from the abnormal blood vessels. This treatment is not ideal because vision may be affected by the laser treatment and abnormal vessels often grow back after treatment.

Main symptoms of AMD include difficulty

1. **病因** 不明，已知老化是主要的危险因素。其他危险因素包括吸烟、种族、营养因素。吸烟被发现是 AMD 发生的主要危险因素。此病常有家族聚集倾向，目前有力证据提示固有免疫系统和补体因子 H 在 AMD 的发病中起重要作用。

2. **护理评估** AMD 患者早期常无症状或仅有轻度视力损害。早期 AMD 常提示有发展为晚期 AMD 的风险。临床分干性（非渗出性）和湿性（渗出性）两种类型。

干性 AMD，约占 85%～90%，发展缓慢，引起进行性中心视力损害。特征是视网膜色素上皮层（RPE）的萎缩。早期当脉络膜疣局限于黄斑外时，患者常无症状；但当发展至黄斑区域时，患者可在阅读时出现明显的渐进性视物模糊。目前尚无方法缓解或治愈此型 AMD，患者常需服用维生素和使用低视力辅助设备。

湿性 AMD，是由于视网膜上异常血管形成和出血所致。此型较少见，仅占晚期 AMD 患者的 10%～15%。当视网膜血管变形并出血时导致此型 AMD。患者主诉视直线变形和扭曲，字母变形或断裂，视力丧失快且严重，伴有严重的中心视力下降和视物变形症。此型 AMD 的特征是视网膜下新生血管形成，血浆涌出导致视网膜感觉神经层和 / 或色素上皮层剥离，黄斑区出血。疾病晚期可见黄斑瘢痕。部分患者可用激光治疗异常血管，但此方法对受损视力影响不大，并且异常血管在治疗后可再次出现。

AMD 的主要症状包括需要近视力的操作

performing tasks that require close central vision (such as reading and sewing), decreased color vision (i. e. colors look dim), dark or empty area in the center of vision, straight lines appearing wavy or crooked, and words on a page looking blurred.

3. Nursing management There is neither a cure nor a means to prevent AMD. However, research suggests that oral vitamin supplements that contain high levels of beta-carotene (25, 000 IU), vitamin E (400 IU), vitamin C (500 mg), and zinc (80 mg) may slow the progression of visual loss. Beta carotene is contraindicated in smokers because it confers a higher risk of lung cancer to them. Therefore smokers are strongly advised to stop smoking before taking above administration. Early detection is crucial as all interventions are largely palliative and directed purely at minimizing the vision loss associated with AMD and the older adults with the macular degeneration should have periodic eye examinations. Nursing interventions of AMD also includes using aids for low vision, such as magnifying lenses and adequate lighting.

Other treatment options for AMD include Argon laser (thermal laser), photodynamic therapy (PDT), vascular endothelial growth factor (VEGF) inhibitors, and macular translocation. However, these treatments usually only postpones visual loss, rather than preventing it. Factors influencing the choice of regimen include the angiographic lesion type, the lesion composition and location and the patient affordability. PDT has been developed in an attempt as a treatment of AMD and is a two-step process. Verteporfin, a photosensitive dye, is infused intravenously over 10 minutes. Fifteen minutes after the start of the infusion, a diode laser is used to treat the abnormal network of vessels. The dye within the vessels take up the energy of the diode laser, but the surrounding retina does not, avoiding damage to adjacent areas. Retreatment may be necessary over time. Because Verteporfin is a light-activated dye, the patient should be instructed to bring dark sunglasses, gloves, a wide-brimmed hat, long-sleeved shirt, and slacks to the PDT setting.

Caution: Patient with PDT treatment must be aware of avoiding exposure to direct sunlight or bright light for 5 days after treatment as the dye within the blood vessels near the surface of the skin could become activated with exposure to strong light. This would include bright sunlight, tanning booths, halogen lights, and the bright lights used in dental offices and operating rooms. Ordinary indoor light is not a problem. Inadvertent sun exposure

困难（如阅读和缝纫），色觉减退，视野中出现暗影或暗区，视直线变形，视物模糊。

3. 护理措施 目前尚无方法治愈或预防 AMD，但研究提示口服维生素合剂包括高剂量 β– 胡萝卜素（25 000IU），维生素 E（400IU），维生素 C（500mg），锌（80mg）可减缓疾病进展。吸烟者禁用 β– 胡萝卜素，因可能增加罹患肺癌的风险。建议老年人经常进行眼部检查以早期发现。护理包括帮助老年人使用低视力辅助设备，如放大镜、充足的光线等。

其他治疗包括激光治疗、光动力治疗（PDT）、血管内皮生长因子（VEGF）阻滞剂和黄斑移位。但这些治疗通常只能延缓视力丧失，并不能起到预防作用。影响治疗选择的因素包括血管造影性损害类型、损害的成分和部位和患者的负担能力。PDT 已成为 AMD 治疗的主要选择，PDT 分两步，Verteporfin，一种感光性染料，在 10 分钟内被注入静脉。15 分钟后，可用二极管激光治疗异常血管网。血管内的染料可吸收激光能量，而周围的视网膜却不吸收，从而避免损伤。过一段时间须再次治疗。Verteporfin 是一种光激活性染料，应教育患者在行 PDT 治疗前戴太阳镜、手套、宽边帽、穿长袖衬衫和裤子。

注意：治疗后 5 天内避免阳光直射。皮肤内附近血管内的染料可被强光激活，包括明亮的阳光、制革间用灯、卤素灯和用于手术室和牙医的明亮灯光。通常室内光线不是问题。若因疏忽造成阳光暴露可导致严重的皮肤起疱和晒伤，需行整形手术。若患者必须在术后 5 天内外出，应穿着紧密织物做成的长

can lead to severe blistering of the skin and sunburn that may require plastic surgery. If a patient must go outdoors within the first 5 days after treatment, he or she should wear long-sleeved shirts and slacks made of tightly woven fabrics. Gloves, shoes, socks, sunglasses, and a wide-brimmed hat should also be worn if the patient has to go outdoors during daylight hours.

vi. Diabetic Retinopathy

Age-related systemic vascular diseases are important risk factors for the development of ischemic retinal diseases and the associated complications. Diabetes is the most common presenting diseases and loss of visual function is one of the most common complications of diabetes. The medical term for eye disease caused by diabetes is diabetic retinopathy (DR). DR is the specific microvascular complication of diabetes mellitus and affects appropriately 1 in 3 patients. The changes include defects in the small blood vessels and sometimes new blood vessel formation, which lead to bleeding within the eye, accumulation of fluid around the macula, and possibly retinal detachment. Severe levels of DR are associated with patient's poorer quality of life and poor physical, psychological, and social well-being.

1. Etiology In diabetic patients, those who have had diabetes for a long time or whose diabetes is poorly controlled are most likely to develop DR. After 10 years, 70% of people with type 2 diabetes have some form of retinopathy. Other risk factors include poor kidney function, high cholesterol, and high blood pressure.

2. Nursing assessment Altered circulation of the diabetics affects the retinal capillary circulation and then results in retinal edema, degeneration, or detachment. Further, ballooning of those tiny vessels may lead to hemorrhaging, scarring, and blindness. Symptoms of DR may be absence even when the retinopathy is advanced. Early detection requires a complete ophthalmoscopic examination; therefore patients with diabetes should have an annual examination by an ophthalmologist.

Detailed patient assessment should include the taking of health history and a complete ophthalmic examination. The nurse should ask the elderly about duration of diabetes, past glycemic control, medications (such as insulin, oral hypoglycemic, antihypertensive, and lipid-lowering drugs), and systemic diseases (e. g., renal disease, systemic hypertension, serum lipid levels, and pregnancy). Core ophthalmic exams include visual acuity, measurement of IOP, gonioscopy (when neovascularization of the iris is indicated or in eyes with

袖衬衫和长裤。若在白天，还同时应着手套、鞋子、袜子、太阳镜和宽边帽。

（六）糖尿病视网膜病变

年龄相关全身性血管疾病是缺血性视网膜疾病及其并发症的重要危险因素，糖尿病是其中最常见的原因。糖尿病所致眼病称为糖尿病视网膜病变（DR），为糖尿病的微血管并发症，影响大约 1/3 的糖尿病患者，病变包括小血管病变和新生血管形成，可导致眼内出血，黄斑液体潴留和视网膜脱离。严重 DR 可影响患者的生活质量和身心社会健康。

1. 病因 患病时间较长或血糖控制不理想的患者容易发生糖尿病视网膜病变。患者 10 年后，大约 70% 的 2 型糖尿病患者可发展为某种形式的视网膜病变。其他危险因素包括肾功能不良、高血脂和高血压。

2. 护理评估 糖尿病所致的循环变化影响视网膜毛细血管的循环，导致视网膜水肿、退化或脱离。小血管的破裂可致出血、瘢痕形成和失明。早期症状可不明显，眼底检查有助于早期发现病变。因此糖尿病患者应每年进行一次眼底检查。

系统的病情评估包括健康史和眼科检查，护士应了解患者糖尿病病史、既往血糖控制、用药（如胰岛素，口服降糖药，降压药和降脂药）和全身疾病情况（如肾脏疾病，系统性高血压，血脂水平和妊娠）。眼科检查主要包括视力、眼内压测量、前房角镜检查（如有虹膜新生血管形成）、裂隙灯检查和眼底检查。

increased IOP), slit-lamp biomicroscopy, and fundus examination.

3. Nursing management The common interventions for diabetes management are important in preventing DR, including proper diet, exercise, and blood sugar management. Controlling cholesterol, blood pressure, and other risk factors may also be beneficial. All people with diabetes but without DR should be encouraged to have screening eye exams annually. The care tips (summarized in box 10-2) should be educated to patient having been diagnosed DR to prevent further damages.

Box 10-2 Education Tips for Patient with DR

- Discuss with the patient about results or exam and implications.

- Inform the patient effective treatment for DR depends on timely intervention.

- Educate the patient about the importance of maintaining near-normal glucose levels, near-normal blood pressure and controlled serum lipid levels.

- Inform the patient what kinds of professional support can be provided if necessary, including offering referrals for counseling, vision rehabilitation and social services as appropriate.

vii. Visual Impairment

Visual impairment is the most common sensory problem faced by old people. The incidence of blindness has increased as the number of adults age 65 or older. The visually impaired population includes those with low vision and those with blindness. Low vision and blindness have a remarkable impact on the physical and psychosocial well-being of the elderly. Compared to the elderly with normal visual function, those with impaired vision are less able to perform activities of daily living, are less mobile, are more isolated, are more depressed and have a reduced level of quality of life. And the elderly with low vision are more prone to falls and injuries and have higher mortality rates.

1. Etiology Low vision and blindness are not caused by a single disease. They can result from some ophthalmologic and neurological diseases, such as AMD, glaucoma, cataracts, DR, central retinal vein occlusion, corneal damage, stroke, atherosclerosis, trauma, tumors and so on. Among the elderly, the most prominent causes

3. **护理措施** 糖尿病常规治疗措施对预防视网膜病变非常重要，包括合理饮食、运动和血糖管理。控制血脂、血压和其他危险因素对患者也有益处。糖尿病患者应每年进行一次眼科检查。对患者进行健康教育可预防进一步视力损害（box 10-2）。

Box 10-2 糖尿病视网膜眼病患者健康教育要点

- 与患者讨论检查结果和并发症。

- 告知患者DR治疗的有效性依赖于及早干预。

- 教育患者保持血管、血压和血脂处于接近正常水平的重要性。

- 告知患者可获得的专业帮助，包括转诊咨询、视力康复和社会服务。

（七）视力损害

视力损害是老年人面对的最常见的感觉功能问题，视力损害包括低视力和盲，均严重影响老年人的身心健康。与视力正常的老年人相比，伴视力损害的老年人日常生活能力较低、活动能力下降、更孤独、更易发生抑郁，生活质量更低。他们更容易发生跌倒和其他损伤，死亡率更高。

1. **病因** 导致视力损害的疾病多为眼病或神经疾病，如AMD、青光眼、白内障、DR、视网膜血管阻塞、角膜损伤、卒中、动脉粥样硬化、创伤、肿瘤等。对老年人而言，最常见的原因是AMD、青光眼、DR和白内障。

are AMD, glaucoma, DR and cataract.

2. Nursing assessment Low vision is defined as a best corrected visual acuity (BCVA) of 20/50 to 20/200 and blindness is defined as a BCVA of 20/400 to no light perception. Low vision is a general term describing visual impairment that requires patients to use devices and strategies in addition to corrective lenses to perform visual tasks. Legal blindness is a condition of impaired vision on which an individual has a BCVA that does not exceed 20/200 in the better eye or whose widest visual field diameter is 20 degrees or less. This definition does not equate with functional ability, nor does it classify the degrees of visual impairment. Legal blindness ranges from an inability to perceive light to having some vision remaining.

The complete health history should be taken include the elements summarized in box 10-3 and the patient may be asked to have a family member or caregiver present during the assessment to confirm or provide information.

Box 10-3 The Elements of Health History for the Elderly with Visual Impairment

● The elderly understanding of the diagnosis of visual impairment.

● The duration of vision impairment.

● How the life has changed after the onset of visual impairment?

● What bothers the elderly most about the current vision?

● Difficulty with tasks depending on near vision, such as using a telephone, mobile-phone or computer, reading, paying bills and managing finances, shopping and counting money, preparing and eating meals, seeing faces, etc.

● Difficulty with tasks depending on distant vision, such as seeing signage in community environments, watching TV, a movie, or a theater performance, seeing traffic signals or road signs when driving or walking, etc.
● Current use of magnifying glasses and purpose for use.
● Driving status and use of public transportation.
● Concerns about safety in the home and community, including history of falls, fear of falling, bumping into objects, and cuts.
● Complaint of glare, or visual hallucination.
● Psychosocial issues, such as depressed mood, suicidal intention, fear of dependence, participation in activities that are valued or enjoyed, impact of vision

2. 护理评估 视敏度 20/50～20/200 被定义为低视力（BCVA），视敏度 20/400 至无光感被定义为盲。低视力的患者常需借助辅助设备和策略完成需要视功能的任务。盲是指视力较佳眼的视力＜20/200 或者最大视野 ≤ 20°。

详细的病史评估见 box 10-3，在评估时可考虑让患者的家人或照顾者在场，以便提供必要的信息。

Box 10-3 视力损害老年患者的健康史采集要点

● 老年人对视力损害诊断的认识。

● 视力损害的发展过程。

● 视力损害对目前生活的影响？

● 视力损害造成的最大困惑是什么？

● 依赖于近视力的任务完成有无困难，如打电话、用电脑、阅读、付账单和理财、购物和点数现金、准备食物和进餐、看面孔等。

● 依赖于远视力的任务完成有无困难，如看社区环境中的标志，看电视、电影或戏剧，开车或走路时看交通信号或道路标志等。
● 当前使用放大镜的情况及使用目的。
● 驾驶和使用公共交通的情况。
● 在家中和社区中的安全问题，包括跌倒史、害怕跌倒的心理、碰撞物品或割伤。
● 有无视物闪光或模糊情况。
● 心理社会状况，如抑郁、自杀倾向、害怕丧失独立性，参加活动的情况，视力损害对兴趣爱好、志愿活动、度假休闲和社会地

loss impairment on hobbies, volunteering, or vocational activities, and social history (i. e. living situation, family responsibilities, social support, and employment).

- Living setting, stairs.
- Medical and surgical history, medications.
- Goal and priorities with vision rehabilitation.

The nurse should assist ophthalmologist to conduct a comprehensive assessment of visual function. Components of the visual impairment include visual acuity and refraction, contrast sensitivity, and visual field. The elderly ability to perform visual tasks and cognitive or psychological status should also be included. Based on the above information, the nurse should assess whether there are some risks for the elderly patient, including medication errors, label misidentification or product misuse, risk of mismanaging some diseases by the elderly (e. g. diabetes), nutritional compromise, injury from accidents (e. g. , falls, cuts, burns, fractures, and other injuries), errors in financial management, social isolation, depression, and driving safety.

3. Nursing management Sudden vision loss is considered a medical emergency and should be evaluated immediately. It may be caused by retinal detachment or an eye injury. How to treat a patient with vision loss depends on the type, cause, and amount experienced. Any patient with a visual disability that cannot be improved by corrected lenses or surgery should be referred to a low-vision specialist or center. Nurse should recommend appropriate assistive devices for patient, including glucose monitoring instruments, large-print books, talking clocks, and computer accessories.

It is important for nurses to understand the elderly response to vision loss, especially when it occurs suddenly; in such case, the patient usually has a harder time adjusting to the disability than a person who was born blind. Studies have indicated that loss of vision may result in a self-esteem disturbance, leading to social isolation. Further, self-esteem disturbance leads to decreased self-confidence, which can affect interactions with other people, the ability to carry out normal daily activities, job performance, and the desire to engage in familiar hobbies. Also grief and mourning occur after the loss of vision and result in reactions similar to those experienced with death, such as denial, anger, guilt, hopelessness, and depression. It is important for nurses to identify patient's emotional reactions so that provide assistance in identifying his or her strengths and resources. Problem solving can lead to alternative ways to complete

位（如生存状态、家庭责任、社会支持和工作）的影响。

- 居住环境，楼梯。
- 疾病史、手术史和药物史。
- 视力康复的目标和优先选择。

护士应协助眼科医生进行全面的视功能评估，包括视力和屈光度，视敏度和视野。老年患者完成视功能的能力和认知或心理状态也应了解，护士还应评估老年人是否存在一些危险，如用药错误、误读标签或误用药物、糖尿病管理不良、营养不良、损伤的危险、财务管理失误、社会孤立、抑郁和驾驶安全等。

3. **护理措施** 突然的视力丧失为眼科急症，需要立即处理。如何处理取决于视力丧失的类型、原因和经历。无法通过矫正镜片或手术来改善视力的患者，应转诊至低视力专家处进一步诊治。护士应为患者提供适当的辅助设备，包括血糖监测设备、大字体的读物、报时钟和电脑附件。

理解老年人对突然丧失视力的反应非常重要，患者在这种情况下往往需要一个艰难的适应过程。研究提示突然丧失视力可引起患者自尊紊乱，导致社交孤立。自尊紊乱还使患者的自信下降，从而影响其人际沟通、日常生活、工作表现等能力。视力丧失后的悲伤可引起一些与死亡经历类似的反应，如拒绝、愤怒、罪恶感、无望和抑郁等。对护士而言，能够及时识别患者的情感反应并提供帮助是非常重要的。对低视力的护理包括使用低视力辅助设备和策略、转诊至社会及社区相关服务机构。

tasks of everyday living and participate in recreational activities.

Managing low vision involves magnification and image enhancement through the use of low-vision aids and strategies, and through referrals to social services and community agencies serving the visually impaired. The goals are to enhance visual function and assist patients with low vision to perform customary activities. Low-vision aids include optical and nonoptical devices. The optical devices include convex lens aids, such as magnifiers and spectacles; telescopic devices; anti-reflective lenses that diminish glare; and electronic reading systems, such as closed-circuit television and computers with large print. Continuing advances in computer software provide very useful products for patients with low vision. Scanners teamed with the appropriate software enable the user to scan printed data into the computer and have it read by computer voice or to increase the magnification for reading. Magnifiers can be head-held or attached to a stand with or without illumination. Telescopic devices can be spectacle telescopes or clip-on or hand-held loupes. Nonoptical aids include large-print publications and a variety of writing aids. The internet continues to expand, and a telephone system has been developed that allows access to the internet and e-mail using voice commands. Strategies that enhance the performance of visual tasks include modification of body movements and illumination and training for independent living skills. Head movements and positions can be modified to place images in functional areas of the visual field. Illumination is an added feature in magnifiers. Light adjustment can help patients' reading and other activities. Simple optical and nonoptical aids are available in low-vision clinics.

Referrals to community agencies may be necessary for low-vision patients living alone who are unable to self-administer their medications. Community agencies offer services to low-vision patients that include training in independent living skills, and the provision of occupational and recreational activities and a wide variety of assistive devices for vision enhancement, orientation and mobility.

低视力辅助设备包括光学和非光学设备，光学设备包括凸面镜、望远镜、防反光眼镜和电子阅读系统。计算机软件的不断进步为视力低下的患者提供了巨大帮助。如计算机语音和扫描仪配合使用，可将信息进行语音读取或录入。非光学辅助设备包括大字印刷读物和辅助手写设备。互联网信息技术的发展，可以实现使用语音命令访问互联网和电子邮件。辅助策略包括身体行为、照明的调整和独立生活技能的训练。护士在护理视力损害患者时应学会综合使用多种技术和方法。

应将独居且无法自理的低视力患者转诊到社区机构，社区机构可为其提供生活自理能力训练、职业和休闲活动及增强视力的辅助设备、导盲服务。

Section 2　Hearing and Balance Impairment

Hearing impairment is a common but under-reported condition among the elderly. It estimates that between 25% and 40% of elderly aged 65 years and older have some degrees of hearing loss. The problems of hearing function in the elderly may be associated with depression, withdrawal from social life, loneliness, anger, decreased personal safety, cognitive decline, and poor health. Balance disorders are also common and are a major cause of falls among elderly persons, thus they are associated with increased morbidity and mortality, as well as reduced level of function.

I. Common Age-related Changes

The organs of hearing and balance (also called the auditory system) are composed of the peripheral auditory system and the central auditory system. The peripheral auditory system can be divided into three parts: the external ear, the middle ear, and the inner ear. This system is concerned with reception and perception of sound. The external ear consists of the auricle and the external auditory canal, a passageway from the outside to the eardrum. The middle ear is an air-filled space that contains the tympanic membrane, the eardrum, and the auditory ossicles. They are involved only in hearing. The inner ear contains the sensory organs for hearing and balance. It is made up of inter-connecting, fluid-filled tunnels and chambers in the petrous portion of the temporal bone and functions in both hearing and balance. The central auditory system integrates and assigns meaning to what is heard (figure 10-2).

Age-related changes in the external ear can be seen in the auricle, include seemly larger ear (because of continued cartilage formation) and loss of skin elasticity. The lobule of the auricle becomes elongated, with a wrinkled appearance. Coarse, wire-like hairs cover the periphery of the auricle. In general, men have larger tragi compared with women, which are laterally situated in the external canal. These tragi become larger and coarser with age. Inward collapsing of the auditory canal make itself narrower. The hairs lining the canal become coarser and stiffer. Cerumen glands also atrophy, causing the cerumen to be much drier. In the middle ear, age-related changes in the tympanic membrane lead to its having a dull, retracted, and gray appearance. Also degeneration of ossicular joints

第二节　听觉和平衡障碍

据估计 25%～40% 的 65 岁及以上老年人伴有某种程度的听觉障碍。听觉问题与老年人抑郁、社会退缩、孤独、愤怒、个体安全性下降、认知功能减退和健康受损等有关。平衡功能障碍在老年人中也很普遍，是老年人跌倒的主要原因，与老年人发病率和死亡率增加和功能水平降低均有一定关系。

一、一般老化改变

听觉和平衡器官（又称听觉系统）包括外周和中枢两部分。外周系统可分为外耳、中耳和内耳三部分，负责接收和感觉声波。听觉系统负责声音的接收和感知。外耳包括耳郭和外耳道，是声音从外部进入中耳的通道。中耳是一个充满气体的空间，包括鼓膜、耳鼓和听小骨，只负责听觉。内耳包含听力和平衡感觉器官，是由相互连接的、充满液体的通道和鼓室组成，负责听觉和平衡觉。中枢听觉系统统合听觉的内容（图 10-2）。

老化相关的外耳变化包括耳郭变大（由于不断形成的软骨），表面皮肤失去弹性，耳郭小叶变长变皱。男性的耳毛较女性多且硬，并随年龄增长更加粗硬。外耳道变狭窄，腺体萎缩导致耵聍变干。中耳的鼓膜随年龄增长变成灰色，听小骨之间的关节退化。内耳的老化变化使平衡敏感性下降。

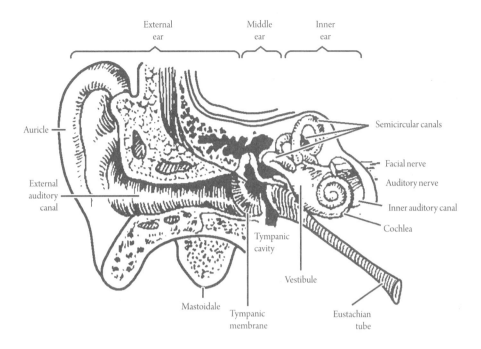

Figure 10-2 Anatomy of the ear

in the middle ear can be noted. Last, changes within the inner ear result in decreased vestibular sensitivity.

The function of balance is declined with aging caused by a combination of decreased sensory input, slowing of motor responses, and musculoskeletal limitations. Older adults have been reported an increase in postural sway comparing healthy younger people. Despite this increase, most healthy older adults have enough sensory function reserve to maintain postural control. However, the ability of maintain balance likely decreases when deprivation in more than one system occurs. In addition, under conditions in which balance is maximally stressed, such as climbing up, down steps, or curbs and getting in and out of a bathtub, maintaining balance becomes more difficult for the aged people.

II. Common Problems and Conditions

i. Cerumen Impaction

Cerumen (or earwax) is made by the glands in the outer third of the ear canal. It protects the skin of the ear canal, assists in cleaning and lubrication, and also provides some protection from bacteria, fungi, insects and water. Cerumen and old skin of the ear canal can make its way out of the ear canal, taking with it any dirt, dust, and particulate matter that may have gathered in the canal. Jaw movement assists this process and increase the likelihood of its expulsion. Cerumen impaction is an accumulation of

老化所致的平衡功能减退与感觉输入减少、运动反应迟缓和肌肉活动受限等有关。与年轻人相比，老年人常发生身体姿势不稳，但多数健康老年人能够保持身体的平衡。维持平衡的能力减退与很多系统有关，在某些情况下，如向上攀爬、下台阶、急停和出入浴缸时，对老年人而言维持身体平衡就变得更为困难。

二、常见健康问题及护理

（一）耵聍嵌顿

耵聍（或耳垢）由外耳道腺体分泌形成，可保护耳道皮肤、起清洁和润滑作用，避免细菌、真菌、昆虫和水进入耳道。耵聍和耳道内老化脱落皮肤一起，将耳道内的任何灰尘和微粒粘住并排出外耳道。下颌运动可有助于耵聍脱落，同时将耳道内的脱落皮肤及其他物质带出。耵聍嵌顿指耵聍积聚并引起

cerumen causing symptoms and usually reversible, often overlooked cause of conductive hearing loss.

1. Etiology　The Etiology involves a variety of factors. Some people form more cerumen than others, presumably as a result of genetic factors. Older men are showed more susceptible because atrophic changes in the sebaceous and apocrine glands lead to less but drier cerumen with aging. These changes coupled with a narrowed auditory canal and stiffer, coarser hairs lining the canal may likely cause cerumen impaction. Other risk factors for cerumen impaction include instrumentation of the ear canals with cotton-tip applicators and the repeated insertion of a hearing aid. Excess or impacted cerumen can press against the eardrum and/or occlude the external auditory canal and even impair hearing.

2. Nursing assessment　Common signs and symptoms of cerumen impaction include tinnitus (ringing in ear), earache (otalgia), a feeling of fullness in the ear, itching, decreased hearing, obstruction of the auditory canal by cerumen, dizziness and buzzing sounds. The cerumen blockage may interfere with the passage of sound vibrations through the external auditory canal to the middle and inner ear, affecting the older adult's ability to hear and communicate. Then the impaired communication may lead to social isolation and depression.

3. Nursing management　Identification and removal of the impaction can restore hearing acuity and relieve symptoms associated with cerumen impaction. Intervention may include manual removal, irrigation, or use of cerumenolytic agents, or a combination of these modalities. The advantages and disadvantages of therapeutic options are summarized in table 10-1.

症状，多为可逆性，是一种常被忽视的传导性听力丧失的原因。

1. 病因　涉及多种因素，有些人由于遗传的原因，比其他人更容易产生耵聍。老年人由于老化所致腺体萎缩、耳道变窄、耳毛增生等，更容易产生耵聍。其他危险因素有耳道内使用一些器具，如棉签和反复置入助听器。耵聍过多可压迫鼓膜，和／或阻塞外耳道，甚至影响听力。

2. 护理评估　耵聍嵌顿的常见症状和体征包括耳鸣、耳痛、耳内充胀感、瘙痒感、听力下降、耳道阻塞、头晕和耳内嗡嗡声。耵聍堵塞可影响声波从外耳道传导到中耳和内耳，影响老年人的听力和人际沟通。进而导致社交孤立和抑郁。

3. 护理措施　识别和去除耵聍可帮助恢复与耵聍嵌顿有关的听力障碍和缓解症状。护理措施包括手法取出、灌洗、使用耵聍清除剂或综合以上方法，这些方法的优缺点比较详见表10-1。

Table 10-1　Advantages and Disadvantages of Therapeutic Options of Cerumen Impaction

Options	Advantages	Disadvantages
Irrigation	• Effective	• Tympanic membrane perforation • Pain, vertigo • Trauma of external auditory canal • Otitis externa • Failure of impaction removal • Severe audio-vestibular loss
Cerumenolytic agents	• Easy application • Effectiveness superior to saline or water	• Otitis externa • Allergic reactions • pain, vertigo if tympanic membrane is injured • Transient hearing loss

Options	Advantages	Disadvantages
Manual removal	• Effective	• Requirement of special skills • Skin laceration, pain • Cooperation of patient needed

表 10-1　耵聍嵌顿治疗方法的优缺点比较

方法	优点	缺点
耳道灌洗	• 有效	• 鼓膜穿孔 • 疼痛，眩晕 • 外耳道受损 • 外耳炎 • 失败 • 听觉 – 平衡功能严重受损
耵聍清除剂	• 方便使用 • 有效性优于盐水或水	• 外耳炎 • 过敏反应 • 疼痛，眩晕（若鼓膜受损） • 一过性听力受损
手法取出	• 有效	• 需特殊技术 • 皮肤撕裂伤，疼痛 • 需患者配合

The nurse can provide patient and family information about discharge instructions. If the patient has been instructed to put mineral oil into his or her blocked ear (s), the nurse should ask the elderly to cooperate as following instructions. Firstly, to place the drops, the elderly turnshis or her head to the opposite side of the affected ear. The nurse then place 2 to 3 drops of mineral oil or baby oil inside the ear. Keep the elderly head tilted for 5 minutes and allow the oil to dissolve the wax. And finally the nurse plugs the ear with a cotton ball. The procedure is usually repeated 3 to 4 times per day for 3 days. Then, fill the ear canals with 3% hydrogen peroxide allowing the fluid to bubble out the wax. Turn his or her head over to the other side and allow the peroxide to run out. The elderly should be told Togo to see an ophthalmologist if signs of discharge, buzzing in the ears, and pain. The nurse also needs to remind the patient that these techniques should not be performed if he or she has a perforation, or hole, in the eardrum. If above procedures are not successful, it is necessary to refer patients to an otorhinolaryngologist to seek professional assist.

ii. Tinnitus

Tinnitus is a subjective sensation of noise in the ear, defined as a ringing, buzzing, or hissing. People at any age may experience tinnitus, but its prevalence increases with

护士应向患者及其家人提供耳道分泌物的知识，并教会患者如何配合护士使用矿物油清除耵聍。首先患者应将头转向患耳对面，护士将 2～3 滴矿物油滴入耳道内，患者保持此姿势约 5 分钟，然后护士将棉球塞入耳道。一般每天重复 3 次，持续 3 天。然后用 3% 过氧化氢溶液冲洗耳道，嘱患者将头转向患耳方向，将耵聍排出。应告知患者，如有耳道分泌物、耳内嗡嗡声或疼痛，应及时就诊。如果上述方法不奏效，护士应指导患者转诊到耳鼻咽喉科就医。

（二）耳鸣

耳鸣是一种耳内有声音的主观感觉，声音可以类似于铃声、嗡嗡声或嘶嘶声。耳鸣可发生于任何年龄人群，但老年人多发。对

aging. For many older adults it is a chronic condition with which they must cope. For others it is an indication of permanent hearing loss or a tumor.

1. Etiology　　There are many different causes of tinnitus. For many, the cause is unknown. The most common cause is noise exposure. Factors contributing to noise induced tinnitus include the noise level, the duration of noise exposure, and the presence of impulsive sounds. Tinnitus can be a side effect of taking medications. It can even occur as part of the normal aging process. It can also co-exist with various ear problems, such as Meniere's disease.

2. Nursing assessment　　Tinnitus is commonly described as ringing, whistling, buzzing or hissing, but more complex sounds and many different noises can also be described. It can be constant, intermittent, or transient and it may be perceived in one or both ears or in the head. The tinnitus can be pulsatile in nature or continuous. A targeted health history and audiologic examination should be performed to identify whether tinnitus is unilateral, associated with hearing difficulties, or persistent (i. e., 6 months or longer). Some self-report tinnitus questionnaires were developed to gather necessary subjective data from the patient with tinnitus, and those popularly used are summarized in table 10-2.

许多老年人，耳鸣是一种他们必须学会应对的慢性疾病。对其他人，耳鸣可能提示永久性听力丧失或肿瘤。

1. 病因　　耳鸣有很多种原因，但大多原因不明。最常见的原因是噪声暴露。相关因素有噪声水平、暴露的持续时间和脉冲音的存在。药物不良反应可引起耳鸣，正常老化过程也与耳鸣有关。一些耳部疾病，如梅尼埃病常伴有耳鸣。

2. 护理评估　　耳鸣常被描述为铃声、哨音、嗡嗡声或嘶嘶声等，但也有人描述为更为复杂的声音。耳鸣可以是持续的、间歇的或瞬间的，可单耳或双耳受累。耳鸣可以是脉动的或连续的声音。应通过有针对性的健康史评估和耳部检查识别耳鸣是否为单侧的，是否伴有听力困难，是否是长期的（如6个月或更长）。一些自陈式问卷可用于评估耳鸣患者的主观感受，表10-2总结了常用耳鸣评估问卷。

Table 10-2　　Comparison of Tinnitus Assessment Questionnaires

Questionnaire and authors (year)	Description
Tinnitus Handicap Inventory (THI)	<ul><li>Aim to identify difficulties the patient with tinnitus may be experiencing</li><li>25 items with 3 level category scale of yes (4 points), sometimes (2 points), or no (0 points)</li><li>3 subscales addressing the patient's functional, emotional, and catastrophic effects caused by tinnitus</li><li>Total score ranging of 0-100 points</li><li>Indicating of handicap, 0-16 points, slight; 18-36, mild; 38-56, moderate; 58-76, severe; 78-100, catastrophic</li><li>High internal consistency (Cronbach's alpha 0. 93) and high test-retest reliability</li></ul>
Tinnitus Handicap Inventory—Screening Version (THI-S)	<ul><li>Aim to identify the patient's problems caused by tinnitus</li><li>10 items with 3 level category scale of yes (4 points), sometimes (2 points), or no (0 points)</li><li>Total score ranging of 0-40 points</li><li>High test-retest reliability and good comparability with THI</li></ul>
Tinnitus Handicap Questionnaire (THQ)	<ul><li>Aim to identify handicap related to tinnitus</li><li>27 items with responses from strongly disagrees (0 points) to strongly agrees (100 points)</li><li>3 factors to reflect physical/emotional/social consequences, hearing ability and view on tinnitus</li><li>Total score ranging of 0-100 points</li><li>High internal consistency and high test-retest reliability for factor 1 and 2</li></ul>

Questionnaire and authors (year)	Description
Tinnitus Reaction Questionnaire (TRQ)	<ul><li>Aim to assess psychological distress associated with tinnitus</li><li>26 items with 5-point scale from not an all (0 points) to almost all of the time (4 points)</li><li>4 factors including general distress, interference, severity, and avoidance</li><li>Total score ranging of 0-104 points</li><li>High internal consistency (Cronbach's alpha 0. 96) and high test-retest reliability</li></ul>
Tinnitus Functional Index (TFI)	<ul><li>Aim to evaluate negative tinnitus impact on the patient</li><li>25 items with 11-point scale (0 to 10 points)</li><li>8 subscales addressing intrusive, sense of control, cognitive, sleep, auditory, relaxation, quality of life, and emotion.</li><li>Overall score within 0-100 points range</li><li>High internal consistency (Cronbach's alpha 0. 97) and test-retest reliability</li></ul>

表 10-2 耳鸣评估问卷的比较

问卷	描述
耳鸣致残量表（THI）	<ul><li>目的：识别耳鸣患者所经历的困难</li><li>25 个条目，3 级评分，即是（4 分）、有时（2 分）和否（0 分）</li><li>3 个因子：患者的功能，情感和耳鸣所致严重后果</li><li>总分为 0～100 分</li><li>残疾程度：0～16 分，轻微；18～36 分，轻度；38～56 分，中度；58～76 分，严重；78～100 分，灾难性</li><li>内部一致性和重测信度均较高</li></ul>
耳鸣致残量表筛查版（THI-S）	<ul><li>目的：识别患者经历的困难，筛选听力障碍患者</li><li>10 个条目，3 级评分，即是（4 分）、有时（2 分）和否（0 分）</li><li>总分 0～40 分</li><li>重测信度高，与 THI 相关性较好</li></ul>
耳鸣残疾问卷（THQ）	<ul><li>目的：识别耳鸣相关残疾</li><li>27 个条目，0 分（强烈同意）至 100 分（强烈不同意）评分</li><li>3 个因子：躯体 / 情感 / 社会影响，听觉能力和对耳鸣的看法</li><li>总分为 0～100 分</li><li>前 2 个因子的内部一致性和重测信度均较高</li></ul>
耳鸣反应问卷（TRQ）	<ul><li>目的：评估耳鸣相关的心理困扰</li><li>26 个条目，5 级评分，从一点儿也不（0 分）至几乎总是（4 分）</li><li>4 个因子：一般困扰，干扰，严重度，逃避</li><li>总分为 0～104 分</li><li>内部一致性和重测信度均较高</li></ul>
耳鸣功能指数（TFI）	<ul><li>目的：耳鸣对患者的负性影响</li><li>25 个条目，11 级评分（0～11 分）</li><li>8 个因子：干扰，控制感，认知，睡眠，听力，放松，生活质量，情感</li><li>总分为 0～100 分</li><li>内部一致性和重测信度均较高</li></ul>

3. Nursing management There is no cure for tinnitus. The objectives of the nursing management are helping the patient follow tinnitus prevention practices, use home masking measures and a hearing aid to relieve tinnitus, and cope with anxiety independently by using relaxation techniques. Nurses should teach patient and

3. 护理措施 此病尚无确定性的治疗方法。护理目的是帮助患者遵循预防策略、使用家庭防护措施、使用助听器和学会运用放松技术应对焦虑。护士应教会患者家庭预防措施，例如处理引起耳鸣的可纠正问题、改

family prevention practices, such as treating correctable problems that cause tinnitus, softening loud sounds through improved acoustics, using protective ear plugs, and avoiding ototoxic substances in foods, drinks, and drugs. Nurses need to provide patient education and consultation on coping strategies that help relieve anxiety and stress such as relaxation training and biofeedback. Nursing interventions are summarized in box 10-4.

Box 10-4　Chronic Tinnitus Interventions

For Mild Tinnitus (Dose Not Affect ADLs):

● Reassure the older people that tinnitus is not life threatening.

● Instruct patient to avoid ototoxic substances in foods/drinks (e. g. caffeine, sodium, chocolate, tea, and alcohol), and drugs (e. g. quinine, aspirin, and anti-inflammatory drug compounds).

For Moderate Tinnitus (Interferes with Sleep and ADLs):

● Teach simple home masking measures to relieve tinnitus, including radio tuned between stations, clocks that tick, soft, pleasant, distracting music, and semi-elevated head position to sleep.

● Recommend evaluation for properly fitted hearing aid and tinnitus masker.

● Use habituation therapy (exposing patients to low-level broad-band noise produced by wearable noise generators).

● Medications may be used, but with caution, because they may cause drowsiness and mental confusion.

For Severe Tinnitus:

● Refer patient for extensive counseling and education.

● Apply all moderate tinnitus interventions.

● Teach relaxation methods combined with biofeedback to cope with stress and promote sleep.

● Perform electrical stimulation and/or acupuncture.

● Perform surgery for patients with indications (e. g. those patients with objective tinnitus or those who have no auditory function and perceive tinnitus as originating from the nonfunctioning ear).

● Contact local self-help tinnitus support groups.

善声学环境使声音变柔和、使用保护性耳塞和避免使用耳毒性物质。应对焦虑和压力的措施包括放松训练、生物反馈和咨询。护理措施的总结见 box 10-4。

Box 10-4　慢性耳鸣的干预

对于轻度耳鸣患者（不影响 ADLs）：

● 消除疑虑，告知老年患者耳鸣不是致命的。

● 指导患者避免饮食中的耳毒性物质（例如咖啡因，盐，巧克力，茶和酒精）和一些药物（例如奎宁，阿司匹林和抗生素）。

对于中度耳鸣患者（影响睡眠和 ADLs）：

● 教会患者在家中缓解耳鸣的简单预防措施，包括避免调电台的噪声、嘀嗒嘀嗒的钟声，而选择柔和、悦耳、舒缓的音乐和睡眠时采取半抬头体位。

● 推荐使用合适的助听器和耳鸣罩。

● 采用习惯疗法（患者暴露于由可穿戴噪声发生器产生的低水平宽频噪声中）。

● 可使用药物，但要小心，因为药物可能引起疲乏和精神错乱。

对于严重耳鸣患者：

● 将患者转诊至相关咨询和教育机构。

● 采用所有中度耳鸣患者适用的措施。

● 教会患者综合使用放松和生物反馈方法，以应对压力，促进睡眠。

● 采用电刺激和 / 或针灸疗法。

● 如有适应证则实施手术治疗（如存在客观性耳鸣或已无听觉功能和感知到耳鸣源于无功能耳的患者）。

● 联系当地耳鸣自我帮助支持团体寻求帮助。

iii. Hearing Loss

Hearing impairment affects every fifth adult worldwide. The prevalence of severe hearing loss in general population rapidly increases with age from 25%-60% over 65 years of age to approximately 80% in those aged over 85 years. Hearing loss is one of the most prevalent chronic conditions in the aged not amenable to medical treatment. It has negative effects on the ADLs and socializing, and also has some psychological effects in the elderly such as cognitive decline, depression, social withdrawal, loss of self-esteem and strained interpersonal relationships.

1. Etiology　Hearing loss is classified as two main types, conductive and sensorineural. Conductive hearing loss is caused by blockage or damage in the outer and/or middle ear and leads to a loss of loudness and is often treatable. Sensorineural hearing loss is acquired or congenital and is caused by damage, malfunction or aging of the cochlea or the hearing nerve and often leads to a loss of clarity and loudness and may limit the benefit of a hearing aid. Mixed hearing loss is a problem of both the outer or middle ear and the inner ear, for example, an ear infection combined with hearing loss associated with aging.

Presbycusis is an increasingly prevalent condition which results in deterioration in quality of life, communication problems and, subsequently, affects socio-economic status. It is a sensorineural hearing loss, the most common type of hearing loss among elderly, which caused by degenerative changes in the cochlea, as a result of multifactorial extrinsic and intrinsic contributions. The condition is characterized by bilateral, symmetrical changes leading from an initial high to low frequency sensorineural hearing loss. It affects men more than women. At present, presbycusis is known as a complex disorder caused by environmental and genetic factors. However, it is still unclear how these factors contribute to the etiology of the disease, how they interact with each other and what their individual contribution is. Extrinsic factors thought to contribute to presbycusis include noise exposure, exposure to chemicals (e. g. toluene, trichloroethylene, styrene and xylene), smoking and alcohol, ototoxic medication (aminoglycoside antibiotics, cisplatin, salicylate and loop diuretics), definite medical conditions (e. g. diabetes, CVD, Renal failure), diet (i. e. , poor nutritional status), hormones, and socioeconomic status (i. e. lower social class and a low level of education).

2. Nursing assessment　Signs and symptoms displayed by the patient may include increasing the

（三）听力丧失

听觉功能障碍影响全球五分之一的人口。严重听力丧失的发生率，在 65 岁及以上老年人中为 25%～60%，85 岁及以上老年人中约为 80%。听力丧失是老年人群中最常见的且很难纠正的慢性疾病。听力丧失可影响老年人的日常生活能力和社交，还可导致认知功能减退、抑郁、社交退缩、自尊下降和人际关系紧张等不良心理后果。

1. 病因　听力丧失分为传导性和感觉神经性两类。传导性听力丧失是由于外耳或中耳道阻塞或损害引起的，通常可以治疗。感觉神经性听力丧失可为后天获得，也可为先天发生，是由于耳蜗或听神经的损害、功能障碍或老化所致，通常可引起对声音清晰度和音量听觉的丧失，此种患者使用助听器效果不佳。混合性听力丧失是指既有外耳或中耳的问题，又有内耳的问题所致者，如耳的感染同时合并老化相关的听力丧失。

老年性耳聋是一种发病率逐渐增高的疾病，导致患者生活质量的下降、人际沟通问题，继而影响社会经济水平。老年性耳聋属于感觉神经性听力丧失，是老年人中最常见的听力障碍原因。主要是由于耳蜗老化所致。疾病的特征是一般为双侧、对称发病，先影响高频音听觉，逐渐影响低频音听觉。男性多于女性。目前认为老年性耳聋是环境和遗传因素共同作用的结果。但是，目前尚未清楚这些因素是如何致病的。环境因素包括噪声暴露、暴露于某些化学物（甲苯、三氯乙烯、苯乙烯和二甲苯）、吸烟和酗酒、耳毒性药物（氨基糖苷类抗生素、铂化合物、水杨酸盐和袢利尿剂）、某些疾病（糖尿病、心血管疾病、肾衰）、饮食（如营养不良）、激素和社会经济地位（如社会阶层低和教育层次低）等。

2. 护理评估　症状和体征包括开大电视或收音机的音量，向说话人的方向转头，看

volume on the television or the radio, tilting the head toward to person speaking, watching the speaker's lids, speaking loudly, and not responding when spoken to. The characteristic presbycusis hearing loss is sensorineural, sloping and ranging from mild to moderately severe intensity according to WHO classification (table 10-3).

说话人的嘴唇，大声说话和与其说话时无反应。表10-3总结了WHO对听力丧失和语音听力困难的分类标准。

Table 10-3　WHO Classification of Hearing Loss and Difficulty in Hearing Speech

Hearing threshold in better ear (average of 500 Hz, 1000 Hz, 2000 Hz) (in Decibels)	Degree of impairment	Ability to understand speech
0-25 dB	Not significant	No significant difficulty with faint speech
26-40 dB	Mild	Difficulty with faint speech
41-55 dB	Moderate	Frequent difficulty with normal speech
56-70 dB	Moderately severe	Frequent difficulty even with loud speech
71-91 dB	Severe	Can understand only shouted or amplified speech
Above 91 dB	Profound	Usually cannot understand even amplified speech

表10-3　WHO 听力丧失和语音听力困难分类标准

听力较好耳的听阈	受损程度	语音理解能力
0～25分贝	不明显	对小声说话，理解无明显困难
26～40分贝	轻度	对小声说话，理解有困难
41～55分贝	中度	对正常音量说话，理解经常出现困难
56～70分贝	中重度	即便大声说话，理解也经常出现困难
71～91分贝	重度	只有在大声喊叫或用扩音器时才能理解
91分贝以上	极重度	即使用扩音器一般也不能理解

Nurses can use the hearing handicap scales to evaluate the subjective effects of hearing loss on various aspects of the ADLs. The most used questionnaires for the assessment of the restriction on auditory function among elderly were the hearing handicap inventory for the elderly screening version (HHIE-S). It is a 10-item questionnaire (box 10-5) assessing effects of hearing impairment on emotional and social adjustment. There are 5 items used to assess emotional effects (item 1, 2, 4, 7, and 9) and other items (item 3, 5, 6, 8, and 10) to social effects. The elderly person is asked to check "yes" (4 points), "sometimes" (2 points) or "no" (0 point) in response to each item. The total score calculated as sum of the points assigned to each of the items. Possible scores range from 0 (no handicap) to 40 (maximum handicap). Score of 0-8 suggests no handicap; score of 10-24 suggests mild-moderate handicap; and score of 26-40 suggests severe handicap.

护士可使用听力障碍量表评估听力丧失对患者影响的主观感受及对 ADLs 各方面的影响。最常用的问卷是老年听力障碍筛查量表（HHIE-S），见 box 10-5。量表包含 10 个条目，用于评估听力障碍对老年人的情感和社会适应的影响，选项设置为是（4分）、有时（2分）和否（0分），总分范围为 0～40 分。8 分以下提示无障碍，10～24 分提示轻至中度障碍，26～40 分提示严重障碍。评分 10 分以下的老年人应进行进一步的听力检查。

The elderly person with a score of 10 points or above is considered to refer for additional hearing evaluation. The sensitivity and specificity of the questionnaire ranges from 70% to 80% for identification of moderate to severe hearing loss.

Box 10-5 The Hearing Handicap Inventory for the Elderly Screening Version (HHIE-S)

- Does a hearing problem cause you to feel embarrassed when meeting new people?

- Does a hearing problem cause you to feel frustrated when talking to members of your family?

- Do you have difficulty hearing when someone speaks in a whisper?

- Do you feel handicapped by a hearing problem?

- Does a hearing problem cause you difficulty when visiting friends, relatives, or neighbors?

- Does a hearing problem cause you to attend religious services less often than you would like?

- Does a hearing problem cause you to have arguments with family member?

- Does a hearing problem cause you difficulty when listening to TV or radio?

- Do you feel than any difficulty with your hearing limits or hampers your personal or social life?

- Does a hearing problem cause you difficulty when in a restaurant with relatives or friends?

3. Nursing management For age related hearing loss there is no medical or surgical treatment to improve the hearing. Management goals are to address any underlying, influencing, or comorbid disorders and optimize hearing. Actually the only intervention available for patients with presbycusis is a hearing aid that can improve the hearing ability. However, problems remain in improving speech understanding, especially in noisy environments. Possible medications are antioxidants and growth factors. The nurse should pay more attention on the patient education about the prevention of presbycusis, and teach them to identify those predisposing factors and avoid them as possible as they can. The education should focus to raise elderly awareness of the consequences of noise exposure and ototoxic medications. The elderly

Box 10-5 老年听力障碍筛查量表（HHIE-S）

- 当您遇到初次见面的人时，是否会由于听力问题感觉到尴尬？
- 在和家人交谈时，您会由于听力问题而感到沮丧吗？
- 有人对您低声耳语时您会觉得听起来困难吗？
- 您觉得听力方面的问题给您带来很大障碍吗？
- 在您探亲访友时，听力方面的问题会给您带来困难吗？
- 您是否由于听力的问题不像以往那样经常出席正式的场合了（比如会议、仪式等等）？
- 听力方面的问题会引起您与家人争吵吗？
- 听力方面的问题给您看电视或听广播带来困难吗？
- 您是否觉得听力的困难限制或者阻碍了您的个人生活或社会交往？
- 在餐饮与亲戚朋友聚餐时听力问题会给您带来困难吗？

3. 护理措施 对年龄相关性听力丧失目前尚无有效治疗方法。对于老年性耳聋的唯一有效方法是使用助听器。老年人也存在语言理解能力的问题，尤其是在嘈杂的环境中。可能的药物有抗氧化剂和生长因子。护士在教育患者预防老年性耳聋方面起着重要的作用，护士要教育患者识别那些加重病情的因素并在生活中避免这些因素。教育策略包括使患者意识到噪声暴露的危害，在医生开药时提醒避免使用耳毒性药物或者加用保护剂，加强对糖尿病和心血管病病情的控制。

should be told to remind the doctor when have a usage of ototoxic medications and combine these medications with protective agents, for example antioxidants and free radical scavengers combined together. The nurse should also provide optimization of the care of those aged patients with diabetes and cardiovascular disease.

Management of hearing aids. The hearing aid is an instrument that amplifies the sound, thus allowing the sound waves to reach the inner ear and be decoded. A variety of hearing aids are available with various advantages and disadvantages (table 10-4).

助听器的管理。助听器的种类繁多，各有优缺点（表 10-4）。护士应帮助使用助听器的患者学会管理助听器。对每个患者都需要详细了解病史，给予全面的咨询指导、在家中测试及听力训练。

Table 10-4　Comparison of Different Types of Hearing Aids

Type of aid	Description	Advantages	Disadvantages
Behind the ear (BTE)	Body of aid sits behind ear and connects to ear mould	Widely available, good range of amplification	Sometimes unacceptable cosmetically. Mould may predispose to external ear infection
In the ear (ITE) / In the canal (ITC)	Aid sits in conchal bowl (ITE) or ear canal (ITC)	Cosmetically better, provides better speech discrimination in noisy environment	Expensive. Limited range of amplification because of feedback problems caused by proximity of microphone and speaker. Has to be customized as per canal size
Body worn (BW)	Body of aid worn on strap around patient's chest or waist	Permits very high amplification for profound hearing loss & useful in limited manipulative skills	Cumbersome. May pick up rustling of patient's clothes
Bone conduction (BC)	Body of aid either on headband or body worn feeds to bone conductor worn on skull	Bypass the conductive mechanism of ear in patients with chronically discharging ears or ear canal stenosis	Poor cosmetic appearance. Bone conductor can be uncomfortable
Bone anchored (BAHA)	Osseointegrated percutaneous titanium abutment screwed into bone of mastoid connects to body of aid	As for bone conduction aids	Requires surgical implantation
Spectacle	Modification of standard spectacle frame to incorporate standard or bone conductor aid	Permits contralateral routing of signal in those with one profoundly deaf ear	Only suitable for glasses wearers. Require glasses to be worn constantly

表 10-4　不同类型助听器的比较

类型	描述	优点	缺点
耳背式（BTE）	助听器置于耳后，连接耳模	应用广泛，放大效果好	不美观，耳模可能导致外耳道感染
耳内式（ITE）/ 耳道式（ITC）	助听器置于耳甲腔或耳道内	美观，嘈杂环境中语音区别度好	费用高，放大倍数有限，需定制以适应耳道大小

类型	描述	优点	缺点
盒式（BW）	置于患者胸部或腰部衣袋中	声音放大倍数高，适用于极重度听力障碍及操作技术较差者	体积大，笨重，需用口袋存放
骨传导式（BC）	置于靠近颅骨位置处	适用于慢性耳部炎症分泌物多或耳道狭窄患者	不美观，骨传导可能伴有不适感
耳锚式（BAHA）	植入乳突处经骨传导	同 BC	需手术植入
眼镜架式	将标准眼镜架与标准助听器或骨传导助听器整合	允许双耳信号对传，适用于极重度耳聋患者	仅适用于戴眼镜者，需经常佩戴眼镜

Patients with hearing impairment should not only be prescribed a hearing aid, but also be properly taught about the hearing aids orientation. This kind of educations needs to be performed individually. Each patient requires a detailed history review, comprehensive counseling, a phase of testing at home and concomitant acoustic training. During the first few days and weeks, patients who are naive to hearing aids may experience many new sounds and stimulus. They need reassurance and need to be trained to get used to a whole new way of living. Besides amplifying the auditory signal, auditory and listening skills and training to use the accessory listening devices is also important. Aural rehabilitation should be taught to the elderly with hearing impaired and their caregiver about the techniques to improve communication skills, such as to ensure adequate lighting and use corrective devices for vision to maximize the usage of visual clues, to be aware of the importance of face to face communication, to reduce background noise when attempting to communicate, and to state the context early to provide supportive information to aid the hearing impaired.

The older adults need sufficient time to become accustomed to the idea that a hearing aid is necessary for them. They must be trained in how to place it inside the ear and how to remove it, how to change batteries and to handle the control system. Thus nurses can play a crucial role in implementing rehabilitation programs for hearing disabled adults. The support of family is also important in determining whether the new user succeeds in wearing the hearing device or not.

Most elderly accept hearing impairment as part of the aging process thus only one in five with hearing impairment seek assistance. Still only 50% report back for further audiometric evaluation they are identified with the hearing impairment. Further, only 10%-20% of this population subsequently obtains hearing aids in most circumstances. Being poor access to audiological

护士还应指导患者如何适应助听器的使用。应根据每位患者的具体病史和咨询结果进行个性化指导和训练。在使用助听器的最初几天，患者可能经历许多新声音的刺激，需指导他们适应戴助听器的新生活，学会调节和使用助听器。听力康复重点包括指导戴助听器的老年患者及其照顾者提高沟通技巧，如确保充足的光线、应用视力线索、面对面进行交流、减少环境噪声、提供支持性信息等。

老年患者需要充足时间习惯助听器，护士需要训练他们学会如何置入和移除助听器，如何换电池和如何调节助听器。护士在老年患者听力康复中起着重要作用，家庭的支持也不可或缺。

多数老年人认为听力障碍是老化过程的正常表现，因此仅 1/5 的听力障碍患者会寻求帮助，仅 50% 会接受进一步的听力检查，仅 10%～20% 的患者最终会使用助听器。不知道如何寻求专业帮助和对助听器的负面认知是老年人不愿意寻求帮助的主要原因。另外，

services and negative attitudes towards hearing aids use are addressed as the most common reason. Many elderly adults face difficulties in using hearing aid. Other reasons for non-use of hearing aid may be excessive cost, poor maneuverability, ear discomfort, lack of appeal and embarrassment. Therefore, nurses should address these reasons so as to improve the compliance of hearing aids among the elderly.

Nurses can help to refer the elderly people with the hearing loss to an audiologist to receive aural rehabilitation, such as hearing aid orientation, auditory training, speech-reading, and counseling. As mentioned above, hearing aid orientation can be provided by nurses, which help patient overcome problems that interfere with the successful use of the aid. Auditory training teaches patient to use those sound clues to supplement his residual hearing. Patient learns to recognize and differentiate sounds by practicing with live or recorded sounds and benefit from this kind of training. Speech-reading is the use of visual cues to facilitate the understanding of speech and can be particularly effective for the elderly who have only partial hearing loss. The patient is taught some common techniques to recognize lip, facial, throat, and body positions and movements involved in speech production. Counseling can help the older adults with hearing impaired overcome negative attitudes that interfere with rehabilitation and develop strategies to manage listening situations. Counseling can be effective if addressing the elderly individual problems, such as physical conditions (e. g. poor vision, arthritis, limited manual dexterity, and limited mobility), lacking of motivation and a sense of hopelessness, and cost factors. The role of the nurse is to encourage patient to seek aural rehabilitation services and improve the ADLs and wellness.

iv. Dizziness and Disequilibrium

Dizziness and dysequilibrium are common complaints causing the elderly to visit a doctor. However, the symptoms of dizziness or imbalance should not be considered a normal part of aging. Balance conditions contribute to deficits in ambulation that may interfere with an older adult's ability to carry out normal ADLs.

1. Etiology The most common causes associated with dysequilibrium in the elderly include benign paroxysmal positional vertigo (BPPV), ampullarydysequilibrium, macular dysequilibrium, vestibular ataxia of aging, and Meniere's disease. Meniere's disease is an uncommon disease but most often occurred in older women, characterized by severe vertigo accompanied and usually preceded by tinnitus

认为费用高、操作能力差、耳部不适等是老年人不愿使用助听器的原因。因此，护士应针对这些因素进行干预以提高听力障碍老年人使用助听器的依从性。

护士应将有耳聋的老年人转诊给听觉专家以接受听力康复，包括助听器介绍、听力训练、语言阅读和咨询。如上所述，护士应向老年人介绍助听器的使用方法，帮助患者克服使用中的困难。听力训练帮助患者学会使用声音线索补充其听觉功能。在此类训练中，患者通过听现场的声音或录制的声音，学会识别和区分不同的声音。口唇阅读是使用视觉线索帮助患者理解语言，对于那些丧失部分听力的老年人尤为有效。要教会患者常用的技术，如识别在语言产生中的口唇、面部、喉咙和身体位置和运动。通过心理咨询可帮助有听力损害的老年人克服影响听力康复的负性态度，学会管理倾听环境的策略。咨询应聚焦于老年个体自身的问题，如身体问题（如视力差，关节炎，动手能力受限，身体活动度受限），动机不足和无望感，以及费用问题。护士的角色是鼓励患者寻求听力康复服务，提高日常生活能力和幸福感。

（四）头晕和平衡失调

头晕和平衡失调是老年人就诊的常见主诉，但并不是正常老化过程的变化。平衡失调导致步态不稳而影响老年人的日常生活能力。

1. 病因 与老年人平衡失调有关的疾病有良性阵发性位置性眩晕（BPPV）、壶腹性平衡失调、黄斑性平衡失调、老年性前庭性共济失调和梅尼埃病。梅尼埃病并不是一种常见病，但在老年妇女中较常见，特征性表现是严重的眩晕伴有耳鸣和进行性低频感觉神经性耳聋。引起头晕和平衡失调最常见的原

and progressive low-frequency sensorineural hearing loss. The most common source of dizziness and imbalance disorders is the vestibular system of the inner ear, however, other factors may be considered such as visual disturbances, musculoskeletal disorders, neurologic dysfunctions, metabolic abnormalities, cardiovascular disease, and medications.

2. Nursing assessment Signs and symptoms of dizziness and dysequilibrium may vary for each disorder, but commonly should include whirling dizziness when the head is moved to a certain position, dizziness or imbalance when the head is moved quickly to the certain orientation (i. e. right, left, up, or down), or constant feeling of imbalance when walking. The nurse should ask the elderly describe the symptoms, and check whether he or she experiences three major symptoms of Meniere's disease (i. e. vertigo, tinnitus, and hearing loss). Other symptoms may include loss of balance, nausea and vomiting, and spasmodic eye movements.

3. Nursing management Treatments involve medications, vestibular rehabilitation and surgery intervention. Pharmacologic treatment includes anti-vertiginous drugs such as meclizine (Antivert) or diphenhydramine (Benadryl). Nurses should alert patient and family about the side effects of these medications. Meclizine may cause drowsiness; patients should avoid alcoholic beverages while taking this drug. While taking meclizine and a diuretic (e. g. hydrochlorothiazide), because of its anticholinergic action, patients with a history of certain conditions (i. e. asthma, glaucoma, or enlargement of the prostate gland) must be monitored carefully. Diphenhydramine, as an antihistamine, is likely to cause dizziness, sedation, and hypotension in older clients. HCTZ and a low-sodium diet help remove excess endolympha fluid. Other patients undergoing diuretic therapy need to be monitored for evidence of fluid or electrolyte imbalance.

Nurses may help refer patient with dizziness and dysequilibrium to a physical therapist (PT) if vestibular rehabilitation therapy is considered necessary. The PT designs an exercise program consisting of oculomotor and postural tasks and teaches patient to incorporate these exercises into daily living.

Surgery may be performed for patient with Meniere's disease to prevent further damage and sensorineural hearing loss. Local anesthetic is normally applied for ear surgery. Preoperative care includes giving instructions for postoperative care and sedation, such as positioning the operative ear up for at least 4 hours after surgery, releasing

因是内耳前庭系统的疾病，其他危险因素包括视力障碍、骨骼肌肉疾病、神经失调、代谢异常、心血管疾病和药物。

2. 护理评估 头晕和平衡失调的症状和体征可因病因不同而不同，但通常包括眩晕（当头偏向某一特定位置时）、头晕或失去平稳（当头迅速移向某个方向时）和持续地感到走路时失去平衡。梅尼埃病以眩晕、耳鸣和听力丧失为主要特征。其他症状还包括平衡障碍、恶心和呕吐以及痉挛性眼部运动。

3. 护理措施 治疗包括药物、平衡康复和手术。药物包括抗眩晕药如美克洛嗪、苯海拉明，护士应提醒患者及其家人此类药物的不良反应。美克洛嗪可致嗜睡，应避免与酒精同服。对于同服利尿剂的患者，如伴有某些特定疾病应加强监测。苯海拉明有致头晕、镇静和血压升高的作用，可建议患者采用低钠饮食。

如果需要进行前庭功能的康复，护士可将患者转诊给理疗专家。理疗包括动眼神经和姿势动作相关的练习，需都会患者如何协调日常行动。

梅尼埃病患者可采用手术治疗以避免进一步损害和听力丧失。手术护理包括术后健康指导和镇静。术后护理包括保持术耳向上的位置（至少4小时），药物止痛和控制眩晕，安全护理，患者听力、眩晕及神经症状的监测，指导患者打喷嚏或咳嗽时张口。

pain and vertigo by medications, following safety instructions (e. g. side rails up, call light in reach, and assistance with ambulation), monitoring the patient for changes in hearing, vertigo, neurologic symptoms (e. g. headache), or facial paralysis, and instructing the patient to keep his or her mouth open when sneezing or coughing.

At present no treatment cures vertigo completely. Therefore patients must be taught how to reduce dizziness. Self-care tips include to move slowly, avoid of bright, glaring lights (a quiet, darkened room is best), and lie down immediately and hold the head still if vertigo occurs during ambulation. Nurse must teach patient the causes of vertigo, as well as medications, vestibular exercises, measures to reduce vertigo, and promote safety during an acute attack.

目前对于眩晕尚无有效治疗。因此必须教育患者缓解眩晕症状的方法。自我照顾的要点包括缓慢移动、避免明亮刺眼的光线（最好是在安静、昏暗的房间）、在眩晕发作时立即躺下并保持头部位置不动。护士应教会患者发现眩晕的原因，了解药物使用和前庭运动，了解减少眩晕发作，以及保证急性发作时的安全等。

Section 3　Taste, Smell, or Touch Impairments

第三节　味觉、嗅觉和触觉障碍

I. Common Age-related Changes

一、一般老化改变

It is natural to lose some of ability to taste and smell with aging. Although most of older adults can still identify sweet, sour, bitter, or salty foods, especially when these flavors are concentrated, loss of smell and taste may affect their food choices and intake and subsequently impair nutritional and immune status, even exacerbate disease states. A decreased sensitivity to odors puts the elderly at risk for noxious chemicals and poisonings.

Changes in taste and smell are related to alterations in the oral mucosa and tongue and the pathologic state of the nasal cavity. During aging, anatomic and physiologic changes occur, such as reductions in cell number, damage to cells, and diminished levels of neurotransmitters. Even in healthy elderly, some factors and conditions (e. g. medications, viral infections, long-term exposure to toxic fumes, and head trauma) may affect and result in olfactory losses. In addition, recognition of odors declines dramatically with age. Why taste changes occur in normal aging is unclear. Possible factors include disease states of the nervous and endocrine systems, nutritional and upper

随着年龄增长味觉和嗅觉功能会逐渐减退。尽管大多数老年人仍能识别甜、酸、苦或咸味的食物，特别是这些味道比较浓时，但失去嗅觉和味觉可影响老年人对食物的选择和摄入，继而影响其营养和免疫状态，甚至使疾病恶化。对气味的敏感性下降使老年人对有毒化学物的感知能力下降。

味觉和嗅觉的改变与口腔黏膜、舌和鼻腔的病理学改变有关。随着老化，解剖和生理上的变化，包括细胞数的减少，细胞的破坏和神经传导物质水平下降。即使在健康老年人中，某些因素和疾病（如药物，病毒感染，长期暴露于有毒废气和头部创伤）可影响并导致嗅觉的丧失。此外，随着年龄增长，察觉有害气味的能力逐渐下降。味觉随增龄发生改变的机制尚未阐明，可能因素包括神

respiratory conditions, viral infections, and medications. A decreased sense of taste is often noticed at beginning of 60s and a severe loss is typical by the age of 70s.

The skin is the largest organ of the body and has millions of nerve endings. People thrive on stimulation through touch. Touch is the most developed sense at birth. Touch involves tactile information on pressure, vibration, and temperature. Although touch, pressure, and vibration are commonly classified as separate sensations, they are detected by the same types of receptors. Sensitivity to light touch diminishes in elderly and may be related to a decreased density of cutaneous receptors for touch sensation.

II. Common Problems and Conditions

Xerostomia, or dry mouth, is the subjective feeling of oral dryness. It is not a diagnosis, but a symptom with multiple possible causes.

1. Etiology Although dry mouth is most frequently associated with altered salivary gland function, there are other causes for this oral issue. The frequent causes are from systemic diseases, side effects of medical therapy and medications, and physiologic or psychogenic causes (summarized in table 10-5).

经和内分泌系统的病变、营养性和上呼吸道疾病，病毒感染和某些药物。味觉的显著减退多开始于 60 岁左右，70 岁左右一般呈现严重的味觉丧失。

皮肤是人体最大的器官，含有无数神经末梢。个体通过触觉感知刺激，触觉在出生时大多已经发育。触觉涉及对压力、振动和温度的感知。尽管触觉、压力觉和振动觉一般被认为是不同的感觉，但其实是由同一类感受器感知的。由于皮肤上触觉感受器的密度降低，老年人对轻触觉的敏感性逐渐退化，对振动和温度的感知阈值随年龄增长而增加。

二、常见健康问题及护理

口干燥症又称口干，是对口腔干燥的主观感受。口干并非疾病诊断，是可能由多种病因导致的一种症状。

1. 病因 多与唾液腺功能改变有关，其他常见原因有系统性疾病、药物不良反应和生理或精神因素（表 10-5）。

Table 10-5　Etiological Factors of Xerostomia

Systemic diseases	● Autoimmune and inflammatory conditions (e. g. , Sjögren's syndrome, primary biliary cirrhosis) ● Graft-versus-host disease ● Immunoglobulin G4-related sclerosing disease ● Degenerative disease (amyloidosis) ● Granulomatous disease (sarcoidosis) ● Infections (e. g. , human immunodeficiency virus/AIDS, hepatitis C) ● Salivary gland aplasia or agenesis ● Lymphoma
Side effects of medical treatment	● Radiation therapy to the head/neck region ● Chemotherapy

continued

Medication	• Anticholinergics drugs
	• Antihistamines
	• Antihypertensive agents (e. g. , angiotensin-converting enzyme inhibitors, angiotensin receptor blockers, alpha- and beta-adrenergic blockers, diuretics)
	• Opioids
	• Psychotropic agents (e. g. , antidepressants, antipsychotics)
	• Skeletal muscle relaxants
Physiologic or psychogenic causes	• Dehydration
	• Mouth-breathing
	• Neurological or psychological disorders (e. g. , depression, anxiety)

表 10-5　口干的病因总结

全身性疾病	• 自身免疫性疾病（如 Sjögren 综合征，原发性胆汁性肝硬化） • 移植物抗宿主病 • 免疫球蛋白 G4 相关硬化病 • 退行性病（如淀粉样变性） • 肉芽肿病（结节病） • 感染（如人免疫缺陷病毒 /AIDS，丙型肝炎） • 唾液腺发育不全 • 淋巴瘤
治疗的不良反应	• 头颈部的放射性治疗 • 化疗
药物	• 抗胆碱能药物 • 抗组胺药 • 抗高血压药（如血管紧张素转换酶抑制剂，血管紧张肽受体阻滞剂，α- 和 β- 肾上腺素能阻滞剂，利尿剂） • 阿片类药物 • 抗精神病类药（如抗抑郁药，抗精神病药） • 骨骼肌松弛剂
生理或心理原因	• 脱水剂 • 经口呼吸 • 神经或心理疾病（如抑郁、焦虑）

2. Nursing assessment　A detailed health history taking and patient assessment are essential for the nurse to understand the status of the elderly patient with xerostomia. The nurse can ask several questions to check whether the patient has the risk of reduced saliva, such as whether the amount of saliva seems to be too little, whether the elderly mouth feels dry when eating a meal, whether the elderly sips liquids to aid in swallowing dry food, and whether the elderly has difficulty swallowing. A positive response to any of the above questions may provide a possible cue for dry mouth.

2. 护理评估　详细的健康史和患者评估可帮助护士理解老年患者的口干问题。护士通过以下几个问题了解患者有无唾液分泌减少的危险，如唾液量是否太少，在进餐时是否感觉口干，进食较干的食物时是否需要喝水以帮助吞咽，老年人是否存在吞咽困难等。若有一个问题给予肯定答案，提示可能存在口干。

Patient with xerostomia due to reduced salivary gland function usually has obvious signs of mucosal dryness. Common complaints consist of abnormal taste sensations, burning of the oral tissues and tongue, and cracking of the lips. The oral mucosa is dry, thin, and smooth, and the tongue may have a thick, white, foul-smelling coating. The decrease in salivary flow interferes with chewing and swallowing. Patients with dentures may complain of sore gums and tissues and denture slippage from the loss of salivary flow, which forms a mechanical barrier. Patient may complain of dry and raspy voice and difficulty articulating words. Dry mouth in the elderly can lead to an increased risk of serious respiratory infection, impaired nutritional status, and reduced ability to communicate.

A comprehensive head and neck examination is important for the nurse to identify the presence or absence of dry mouth, and to provide evidence of the quantity and quality of saliva.

3. Nursing management　Treatment is aim to alleviate dry-mouth symptoms, and should involve multi-facet of care. The physician and the nurse should discuss with the elderly patient about management of systemic conditions and medication use, as well as preventive measures to reduce oral disease and related complications. If it is necessary, pharmacologic treatment with salivary stimulants should be prescribed to the patient. However, palliative measures such as sugar-free stimulants (e. g. , chewing gum) may be considered to improve salivary output if the patient cannot tolerate the medication. To prevent secondary infections in mouth, the nurse should educate the elderly to maintain adequate hydration and smoking cessation.

A patient-centered education is a key to prevention and treatment of xerostomia. The nurse should emphasize daily oral hygiene and importance of effective plaque removal and regular dental visits to promote oral health. The elderly patient needs to remember useful tips to maintain oral hygiene, such as tooth-brushing twice per day, using floss regularly, and using alcohol-free mouth rinse. Nurses also need to help patients increase their awareness of the importance of maintaining moisture and hygiene of the oral cavity. If not contraindicated with other health conditions, patients need to intake 2-3 L of fluid per day, and foods need to be prepared with gravy or sauces contain moisture.

(ZHANG Jing)

由于唾液腺功能受损所致的口干患者通常有明显的黏膜干燥体征，常见主诉包括味觉异常、口腔和舌组织的烧灼感和口唇裂开。口腔黏膜变干、变薄和平滑，舌变厚、色白和舌苔异味。唾液减少会干扰咀嚼，可有吞咽困难、声音粗哑。患者可能会因口干而感到牙龈疼痛或义齿脱落，从而造成咀嚼障碍。老年人口干可导致严重呼吸道感染的危险、营养状态受损和沟通能力下降。

详细的头颈部检查可帮助护士识别是否存在口干及唾液分泌质、量的证据。

3. 护理措施　干预的目的是缓解口干症状。医生和护士应与老年患者讨论有无系统性疾病和用药因素，及减少口腔疾病和相关并发症的预防措施。如需要，提供必要的药物治疗，以促进唾液分泌。其他措施如无糖刺激（如嚼口香糖）可刺激唾液分泌。为预防继发感染，护士应教育老年人保持足够水分摄入和戒烟。

以患者为中心的健康教育对预防和治疗口干非常重要，护士应强调日常口腔卫生、清除牙菌斑和定期口腔检查的重点性。老年患者应学会保持口腔卫生的要点，包括每天 2 次刷牙，定期用牙线，应用不含酒精的漱口水。护士还需教育患者保持口腔湿润和卫生的重要性。如无其他健康问题，患者每天应摄入 2～3L 水。

（张　静）

Key Points

1. Active screening for visual loss in the elderly should become routine.

2. Presbyopia usually presents adults over 40 years of age and is easily treated with reading glasses.

3. A cataract is opacity of the lens and needs surgery for successful treatment.

4. Glaucoma is caused by raised IOP and needs life-long medication administration to lower the pressure.

5. Wet AMD is not curable or preventable and current treatments are largely directed at minimizing visual loss.

6. Diabetic retinopathy can be treated successfully with laser surgery.

7. Certain communication and caring techniques and methods can help visually impaired older adult maintain independence.

8. Prevention and treatment of cerumen impaction is an important nursing role in the care of older adults.

9. Tinnitus is a common complaint affecting the older adult and requires a management program that addresses both the audiological and psychological issues.

10. Hearing loss affects an older adult's ability to communicate and may lead to depression, social isolation, and loss of self-esteem.

11. Patients with hearing loss should receive comprehensive aural rehabilitation including hearing aid orientation, auditory training, speech-reading, and counseling.

12. Proper safety measures and methods can relief discomfort from dizziness and dysequilibrium and facilitate daily functioning.

13. Xerostomia may lead to an increased risk of serious respiratory infection, impaired nutritional status, and reduced ability to communicate.

本章要点

1. 老年人应定期进行视力障碍普查。

2. 40岁以上成年人可能存在老视，可用阅读眼镜纠正。

3. 白内障为晶体混浊，需要手术治疗。

4. 青光眼是由眼内压升高所致，需要终身药物治疗以降低眼内压。

5. 湿性黄斑变性不可治愈或预防，需早发现以降低视力损害。

6. 糖尿病视网膜病变可经激光手术成功治愈。

7. 特定的沟通和护理技术可帮助视力受损老年人保持独立性。

8. 护士可在耵聍嵌顿的预防和治疗发挥作用。

9. 耳鸣是老年人常见的主诉，需要听力和心理干预。

10. 听力丧失影响老年人的沟通能力，可致抑郁、社会孤立和自尊下降。

11. 听力丧失的老年人应接受全面听力康复，包括助听器指导、听力训练、语言阅读和咨询。

12. 合适的安全措施可缓解头晕和平衡失调症状，维持日常生活功能。

13. 口干燥症可增加呼吸道感染、营养状态受损和沟通能力下降的危险。

Critical Thinking Exercise

1. A 74-year-old woman from countryside was referred for cataract evaluation by a primary care physician for complaints of blurred vision. The patient has a history of hypertension and type-2 diabetes. She has had no prior ocular surgeries and takes no eye drops. She has undergone multiple laser procedures in both eyes for diabetic retinopathy.

批评判性思维练习

1. 患者，74岁，女，因视物模糊到乡医院就诊，疑诊白内障，转至本院。有高血压和2型糖尿病史。无眼手术史，未使用眼液。双眼刚接受激光手术以治疗糖尿病视网膜病变。

Questions:

(1) What is the main nursing problem you would consider for this patient?

(2) What strategies would you use to improve post-operational self-care of this patient?

2. A 75-year-old man complains of decreased hearing in his left ear for the past 2 weeks, associated with a full feeling in that ear. He noticed sudden onset of these symptoms on awakening. He has a history of working as a coal miner for 30 years and has been wearing hearing aids for the past 9 years. He changed the battery in the hearing aid but his symptoms persisted. Physical examination shows a cerumen impaction filling the entire left ear canal. Only a minimal amount of cerumen is present in the right ear canal.

Questions:

(1) As a nurse, what do you suggest to do next?

(2) Can you introduce some assistive devices to promote the independent function of elderly with hearing loss?

3. A 65-year-old woman complains of decreased salivation in the mouth for the past 4 months. She was diagnosed with Sjögren's syndrome six years ago and suffered a characteristic symptom of this condition—dry mouth.

Question: She asks you how to relieve this uncomfortably symptom, what's your suggestion?

问题：

（1）对这位患者而言，主要护理问题是什么？

（2）如何促进这位患者手术后的自我护理？

2. 患者，75岁，男，主诉左耳听力下降2周，伴耳内充实感。症状于晨起突然发生。他曾从事煤矿工作30年，戴助听器9年。更换助听器电池后症状未改善。体格检查发现左耳道内充满耵聍，右耳少量耵聍。

问题：

（1）作为护士，你认为下一步应做什么？

（2）你会为听力障碍的老年人推荐何种辅助设备以提高独立性？

3. 患者，65岁，女，主诉口腔干燥4个月。6年前因口干症状被诊断为 Sjögren 综合征。

问题：患者向你询问如何缓解口干的不适症状，你的建议是什么？

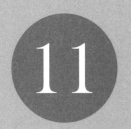

Chapter 11 Elderly Safety Issue

第十一章　老年常见安全隐患的预防与处理

Learning Objectives

On completion of this chapter, the reader will be able to:

- Delineate risk factors that increase the risk for fall;
- Describe the methods of assessing the risks for fall;
- Use interventions to control risk factors of fall;
- Teach the elderly how to cope with accidental fall;
- Define the scalding;
- Describe the risk factors of scalding;
- Define the aspiration;
- Describe the risk factors of aspiration;
- List the main nursing interventions on aspiration;
- Define the falling bed;
- List the main nursing interventions on falling bed.

学习目标

学完本章节，应完成以下目标：

- 描述增加跌倒的危险因素；
- 描述评估跌倒风险的方法；
- 提供干预措施预防跌倒；
- 教会老年人预防意外跌倒；
- 说出烫伤的定义；
- 描述烫伤的危险因素；
- 说出误吸定义；
- 描述误吸的危险因素；
- 列出误吸的预防护理措施；
- 定义坠床；
- 列出坠床的护理措施。

Older persons confront threats to their lives and well-being, such as acts of nature, pollutants, communicable diseases, accidents, and crime as any adult, but their risks are compounded by age-related factors that reduce their capacity to protect themselves from and increase their vulnerability to safety hazards. Such as age-related changes, altered antigen–antibody response, and the high prevalence of chronic disease cause older persons to be highly susceptible to infections. Based on common limitations found among older people, most of older adults also need an environment that is safe, functional, comfortable, personal, and normalizing and that compensates for their limitations. It is particularly important for older adults, many of whom spend considerable time in their homes or in a bedroom of a facility. So gerontological nurses need to identify safety risks when assessing older adults and provide interventions to address existing and potential threats to safety, life, and well-being.

老年人和年轻人一样，会面对许多影响生活和健康的威胁，例如自然行为，污染物，传染病，事故和犯罪，但随着年龄增长，机体的老化使得老年人自身保护能力下降，抗原－抗体反应的改变以及慢性疾病的高发，导致老年人对感染高度敏感，在面对影响健康的危险因素时则较年轻人显得更加脆弱。基于老年人常见的各种限制，大多数老年人同样也需要一个安全的、功能性的、舒适的、个体化的环境，以利于和促进其健康，因此居家环境的设置对老年人的来说也显得尤为重要。因此护士对老年人进行评估时，需要识别威胁老年人安全的危险因素，提供干预措施，以解除现有的和潜在的威胁老年人安全、生活和健康的危险因素。

Section 1　Fall and Injury

第一节　老年人跌倒的护理

As the graying population grows, falls and fall-induced injuries are common worldwide. Falls are not only associated with morbidity and mortality in the older population, but are also linked to poorer overall functioning. Globally, unintentional injuries are the fifth leading cause of death in aged people (after cardiovascular disease, cancer, stroke, and pulmonary disorders), and falls constitute two thirds of these deaths. According to WHO report, approximately 28%-35% of people aged of 65 and over fall each year, the rate increases to 32%-42% for those over 70 years of age. In China, fall is the fourth leading cause of injury death, and people aged 65 and over are main victims. Falls in older people are an important public health concern because of their frequency and adverse consequences in terms of morbidity, mortality and quality of life, as well as their impact on health service system and costs. Therefore, the prevention of falls is very important. When working with older adults, it is crucial for the nurse in geriatric department to recognize the person at risk and to provide a standard of care that prevents fall and promotes safety.

随着老年人口数量的增加，跌倒已成为威胁老年人健康、生命和生活质量的重要问题。在全球范围内，意外伤害在老年人死因中居第 5 位，而 2/3 的老年人意外死亡是由跌倒所致。世界卫生组织报道：目前全球老年人跌倒发生率已经由 28%～35%（≥ 65 岁）增加到了 32%～42%（≥ 70 岁）。在我国，跌倒是意外伤害导致死亡的第 4 位原因，特别是在 65 岁及以上的老年人中，跌倒则为导致死亡的首位原因。因此，跌倒的预防和救护非常重要。对从事老年护理工作的护士来说，识别跌倒的高危人群并提供预防跌倒和促进安全的措施尤为重要。

Box 11-1　Case Study

An 81-year-old man, hospitalized on a medical unit. You observe him sitting on the edge of his bed with his feet dangling about half a meter from the floor. He has one intravenous line and a Foley catheter. You see his Foley catheter is hanging on the floor beneath his feet as he sits on the edge of the bed. He always walks barefoot to the bathroom at night, which is about 6 meter saway. He tells you he steadies his balance by hanging onto his intravenous pole. You see he not only do that as he tells you but also drags his Foley catheter bag alongside.

Questions:

1. What environmental hazards can you identify?

2. What environmental modifications could you make to improve his safety?

I. Definition of Fall

The World Health Organization defines fall as "inadvertently coming to rest on the ground, floor or other lower level, excluding intentional change in position to rest in furniture, wall or other objects". Falls are in ICD-10, which include a wide range of falls those on the same level, upper level, and other unspecified falls. But in epidemiological and interventional studies of falls, the definition used for fall may vary. Most studies have required the fall to be 'unintentional' and for the some form of contact with the ground. Most studies have also excluded falls caused by road accidents and violence. Some studies have excluded falls caused directly by syncope or an acute major intrinsic event such as a stroke, although other definitions have included such falls. It is significant for the gerontological nurse to recognize that older people define falling in variable ways. For example, older people tend to describe a fall as a loss of balance, whereas health care professionals generally refer to events leading to injuries and illnesses. Therefore, the operational definition of a fall with explicit and exclusive criteria is highly important.

Falls can also be classified in several ways. A fall can be explained (for example a simple trip or an intrinsic event such as syncope) or unexplained, where no apparent cause has been found. A fall can be intrinsic, where some

Box 11-1　案例

一位 81 岁的老年男性患者，现于内科病房住院治疗。据你的观察发现，他坐在床边时双脚悬空距地面约半米。患者目前状态为有一条静脉通路进行输液治疗并携有留置导尿管。当患者坐在床边时，导尿管就悬在他的脚旁。患者半夜经常光脚走到距离床大约 6m 远的浴室。老人告诉你说，为了保持身体的稳定和平衡，他在走路时会扶住输液架，据你的观察，他不仅那样做而且还拖着集尿袋行走。

问题：

1. 上述案例中有哪些环境危险因素？

2. 可以进行哪些改进来确保和增加患者的安全性？

一、跌倒的定义

WHO 将跌倒定义为："不自主的、非故意的体位改变，倒在地上或更低的平面上，不包括靠在家具或者墙壁上的情况。"按照《国际疾病分类》（ICD-10）对跌倒的分类，跌倒包括同一平面的跌倒和从一个平面至另一个平面的跌倒。但是在有关跌倒的流行病学研究和干预措施研究中，不同研究者对跌倒的定义有所不同。大部分研究把跌倒定义为非故意地倒在地上，不包括道路交通和暴力导致的跌倒。

老年护理人员应认识到不同的个体对跌倒有不同的认识，如一些老年人易把跌倒理解为身体失去平衡，而卫生保健人员则特别

event or condition affects postural control, or extrinsic, where an environment factor is the main contributing reason for the fall, or unclassified.

关注跌倒导致受伤或不良健康后果的跌倒，因此，明确跌倒的定义非常重要。跌倒也可以进行分类。根据是否有明确的原因，分为可以解释的（例如，晕厥）或无法解释的。跌倒可能是内在的，如疾病影响，也可能是外在的，其中环境因素是导致跌倒的主要外在原因。

II. Actual and Potential Impacts of Fall on Elderly's Life

二、跌倒对老年人的影响

1. Physical injury Falling, particularly falling repeatedly, increases risk of injury, hospitalization, and death, particularly in elderly people who are frail and have preexisting disease co-morbidities and deficits in activities of daily living. In older people, falls account for 14% of emergency admissions and are the leading cause of injury-related deaths. People who fall suffer from minor trauma such as skin bruises, lacerations, abrasions or swollen joints to major injuries such as hip fractures, internal bleeding, or subdural hematomas. Of these injuries, skin bruises and soft-tissue damage are the most common. About half of elderly people who fall cannot get up without help. Remaining on the floor for more than 2 hours after a fall increases risks of dehydration, pressure ulcer, rhabdomyolysis, hypothermia, and pneumonia. Although not all falls lead to injury, about 20% need medical attention, 5% result in fracture, and other serious injuries arise in 5% -10% of falls, for example, severe head injuries, joint distortions and dislocations, soft-tissue bruises, contusions, and lacerations. These percentages can be more than doubled for women aged 75 years or older. Importantly, fall-induced injuries represent one of the most common causes of longstanding pain, functional impairment, disability, and death in elderly populations. The major underlying causes for fall-related hospital admission are hip fracture, traumatic brain injuries and upper limb injuries. The way of falling often determines the type of injury. Wrist fractures usually result from forward or backward falls onto an outstretched hand and hip fractures typically occur from falls to the side, whereas backward falls directly onto the buttocks have much lower rates of related fractures.

Hip fracture is the most common serious consequence of fall, and 92% of all proximal hip fractures are the results of fall. Half of people with hip fracture suffer

1. 身体损伤 跌倒所引起的损伤是导致老年人持续性疼痛、功能损害、残疾和死亡的最重要的原因。跌倒可以造成轻微损伤（如皮肤擦伤或关节肿胀），也可能造成严重损伤（如髋部骨折、内部出血或硬膜下血肿），其中皮肤擦伤和软组织损伤最常见。约有一半跌倒的老人在没有帮助的情况下无法起床。跌倒后在地板上停留超过 2 小时会增加脱水、压疮、横纹肌溶解、体温过低和肺炎的风险。虽然跌倒不一定会导致损伤，但约有 20% 的跌倒还是需要进行医疗处理的，约有 5% 跌倒可造成骨折，5% ~ 10% 造成其他严重外伤（包括头部创伤；关节积血、脱位和扭伤；软组织淤伤、撞伤和撕裂等）。对于 75 岁及以上的女性，这些百分比可以增加一倍以上。重要的是，跌倒引起的受伤是老年人中长期疼痛，功能障碍，残疾和死亡的最常见原因之一。损伤的类型决定于跌倒的方式。因跌倒而住院的主要原因是髋部骨折、创伤性脑损伤和上肢损伤。

跌倒损伤中最严重的是髋部骨折，92% 的髋部骨折发生与跌倒有关。髋骨骨折使 50%

functional losses which may lead to increased dependence. A large proportion of fall death are due to complications following a hip fracture. One out of five hip fracture patients dies within a year of their injury. Research have found that cognitive impairment, low body mass, gait and balance impairment, and at least two chronic conditions were factors independently associated with serious injury during a fall. Serious injury from fall is more likely to occur among those with osteoporosis. Bones weakened by osteoporosis, particularly weight-bearing bones like femur, are more susceptible to breakage.

2. Psychological trauma　Many old persons experience psychological trauma directly related to fall. Among these psychological consequences are fear of falling (FOF), loss of self-efficacy, activity avoidance and loss of self-confidence. An elderly person may become more worried about future, especially about his ability to remain independent, because of the functional loss. For elderly persons, the post-fall trauma can lead to depression and withdrawal. Many factors influence the development of post-fall trauma, including personality, depression, anxiety, and stress-related syndromes. Meanwhile, fear of falling (FOF) is a significant consequence of fall, and has been researched more extensively than other psychological injuries. However, FOF is also commonly found among elderly persons who never experienced a fall.

　　Since the identification of the post-fall syndrome and use of the term "ptophobia" (the phobic reaction to standing or walking) in the early 1980s, FOF has gained recognition as a health problem for older adults. FOF appears to occur variably in the older adult population. Prevalence of FOF appears to increase with age and to be higher in women. Fear can positively motivate some seniors to take precautions against falls such as practice gait adaptations to increase stability. For others, fear can lead to a decline in overall quality of life and increase risks of falls through a reduction in the activities needed to maintain self-esteem, confidence, strength and balance. In addition, fear can lead to maladaptive changes in balance control that may increase the risk of falling. The main consequences of FOF described are physical, functional, psychological and social changes. Studies have shown FOF to be associated with negative consequences such as falling, less physical activity, restriction or avoidance of activities, depression, decreased social contact and lower quality of life (figure 11-1) .

的老年人功能丧失，无法恢复原有的独立生活。20% 的老年人在骨折后 1 年内死亡。研究发现，认知功能障碍，低体重，步态和平衡障碍以及至少两个慢性病，是与跌倒时严重受伤的独立相关因素。患有骨质疏松症的人更容易发生跌倒从而造成的严重伤害。骨质疏松导致的骨骼脆弱，特别是像股骨这样的承重骨骼更容易断裂。

　　2. 心理损伤　跌倒会给老年人带来心理创伤，表现为害怕跌倒、自我效能降低、不敢活动和自信心下降。跌倒后的心理创伤导致老年人出现抑郁和与社会的隔离。其中，跌倒恐惧症（FOF）是跌倒后常见的心理创伤，但是没有跌倒史的老年人中也存在害怕跌倒的心理。

　　自从 1980 年代初发现跌倒后综合征并使用术语"恐惧症"（对站立或行走的恐惧反应）以来，FOF 已被公认是老年人的健康问题。FOF 严重影响老年人健康，其发生率随着年龄的增加而升高，且女性高于男性。可以指导一些年长者采取预防措施，例如通过调整步态以增加稳定性来预防跌倒。跌倒的严重后果使老年人产生恐惧心理并限制其自身活动，导致他们自理能力信心的下降及功能状态的进一步衰退，这样又增加了跌倒的风险，形成恶性循环（图 11-1）。

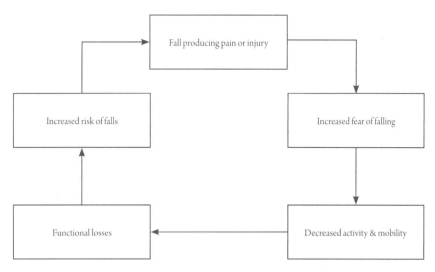

Figure 11-1　Consequences of falls – a viscous cycle

Box 11-2　Measurement Tools of FOF

The tools that have been developed over the past decades to measure FOF use different definitions and premises. The simple question "Are you afraid of falling?" was used initially with a "yes/no" or "fear/no fear" response format, and this format has the advantages of being straightforward and easy to generate prevalence estimates. This measure was later criticized for its limited ability to detect variability in degrees of fear and because it may express a generalized state of fear that does not directly reflect FOF. Various authors have expanded the answer choices to this question to provide a hierarchy of responses (e. g., "not at all afraid" "slightly afraid" "somewhat afraid" "very afraid") to better reflect the degree of fear. Others have continued to advocate use of the simple question only as a screen for FOF of older adults. Fear of falling has been operationally defined by some researchers as "low perceived self-efficacy at avoiding falls during essential, nonhazardous activities of daily living". The falls efficacy scale (FES) was developed to examine older adults, listing 10 questions, with questions related to how confident the person is during activities such as walking or cleaning the house.

III. Factors Contributing to Fall

The causes of fall are also known as risk factors. Normally, falls are caused by multiple risk factors, the more risk factors people exposed to, the more chance of fall, and the more threats to d to person's independence. Many fall risk factors are preventable. As obvious as it may sound, a lack of knowledge about risk factors and risk prevention contributes to many falls. Some people believe that falls

Box 11-2　跌倒恐惧评估工具

用于测量跌倒恐惧心理的工具在过去的几十年中不断发展。通过简单的问题"你害怕跌倒吗？"最初使用"是／否"或"恐惧／不恐惧"作为问题回答的选项，这种格式的优点是简单，结果容易估计。这种方法后来被认为无法检测跌倒恐惧的程度，因为它并不直接反映跌倒恐惧的心理程度。于是这个问题的答案选项逐渐形成层次结构（如："不害怕""轻微害怕""有点害怕""非常担心"），以更好地反映恐惧的程度。也有人提倡继续使用简单的问题对老年人跌倒恐惧进行筛查。跌倒恐惧的定义为"为避免跌倒而限制自己正常的日常活动"。跌倒效能量表主要是用于老年人，共列出 10 个关于个体在活动（如：散步或打扫房子）时的自信程度。

三、老年人跌倒的危险因素

跌倒的原因又称为危险因素。跌倒并不是由单一的原因引起的，个体暴露的危险因素越多，发生跌倒的可能性就越大。然而，许多危险因素是可以预防的。因此，了解老年人群跌倒的危险因素，可以为预防跌倒制订措施提供参考依据。

are a normal part of aging, and as such are not preventable. Lack of knowledge leads to lack of preventive action. Identifying risk factors, followed by timely and appropriate interventions, is the key to a successful program of fall prevention.

Over the past 20 years, researchers have assessed risk factors and grouped them in various ways to facilitate comparisons in research studies. Typically, risk factors have been grouped into two main categories: intrinsic factors that lie within the individual and include both demographic and health factors, and extrinsic factors that lie within either the physical or socio-economic environment. According to WHO Global Report on Falls Prevention in older age, risk factors are categorized into four dimensions: biological, behavioral, environmental and socioeconomic factors. Risk factors and the interaction of them on falls and fall-related injuries are demonstrated in the Figure.

1. Biological risk factors Biological factors embrace characteristics of individuals that are pertaining to the human body. For instance, age, gender and race are non-modifiable biological factors (figure 11-2). These are also associated with changes due to ageing such as the decline of physical, cognitive and affective capacities, and co-morbidity associated with chronic illnesses.

目前，已有许多不同的危险因素分类体系。通常，危险因素被分为内在原因（健康因素）和外在原因（社会经济环境）。WHO 在《全球老年人跌倒预防报告》把有关老年人跌倒的危险因素分为生物因素、行为因素、环境因素和社会经济因素四类。这四类因素相互作用，对老年人而言，暴露的危险因素越多，发生跌倒以及与跌倒有关的受伤可能性就越大。

1. **生物因素** 生物因素指年龄、性别、种族等对个体而言不可改变的因素（图 11-2），它们往往与机体的衰弱、认知能力的下降以及疾病等密切相关。

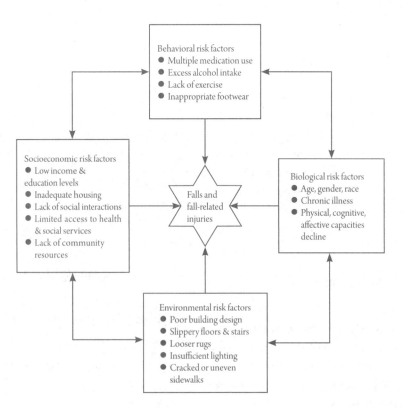

Figure 11-2　Fall risk factor model in older age

Interaction among biological, behavioral and environmental risk factors can increase the risk of fall. For example, loss of muscle strength can lead to loss of function and higher levels of frailty, which intensifies the risk of fall when there are environmental hazards exist.

(1) Age: The rates of falls and their associated complications rise steadily with age. It increases markedly among group aged 75 and older, and reaches a peak among group aged 80 to 89.

(2) Gender: Gender is a key factor as women fall more often than men and sustain more injuries when they fall. However, fall-related mortality is higher among old men. The difference between the two groups may stem from the gender-related factors, such as women being inclined to make great use of multiple medications and living alone. In addition, biological difference also contributes to greater risk. For instance, women's muscle mass declines faster than that of men, especially in the immediate few years after menopause. To some extent, women are less likely to engage into muscular building physical activity through the life. Health seeking behavior differs according to gender. Culturally-oriented expectations to gender roles affect behavior when seeking medical care. Higher fatality rates among men may be related to the tendency of reluctant medical care seeking behavior until conditions become severe, resulting in substantial delay to the access to prevention and management of diseases. Further, men are more likely to be engaged in intense and dangerous physical activity and risky behaviors and ignoring the limits of their physical capacity–such as climbing high ladders, cleaning roofs. Various fall prevention strategies for men and women based on gender differences are needed.

(3) Age-related changes: Numerous age-related changes can predispose older people to fall. Normal aging inevitably brings physical, cognitive and affective changes that may contribute to the risks of fall. Most observations for risk relate to gait and balance change, sensory deficits, central nervous system changes, decreased muscle strength, osteoporosis, and nocturia. For the elderly population, quantifying the age-related changes in physical functions that are independent of disease is difficult.

(4) Gait and balance changes: Impaired control of balance and gait is a factor leading to instability and falls for the elderly. As a person age, lean muscle mass

生物、行为和环境因素之间的相互作用会增加跌倒发生的危险。例如，肌肉力量的减弱会导致功能的下降和机体更高程度的虚弱，当存在环境危害时，导致跌倒发生的风险增高。

（1）年龄：跌倒及并发症的发生随着年龄的增长逐渐增加，75岁显著增加，80~89岁达到最高。

（2）性别：女性跌倒发生率大于男性，且更易于受伤。但是，跌倒所导致的死亡率男性高于女性。两组之间的差异可能源于与性别相关的因素，例如女性频繁用药并独自生活的可能性增大。此外，生物学差异也导致更大的风险。例如，女性的肌肉质量下降速度快于男性，尤其是在绝经后。女性体育锻炼不如男性多。寻求健康的行为也因性别而异。男性死亡率高可能与不愿寻求医疗护理有关，从而导致病情加重。此外，男性更有可能从事高风险的体育活动和危险行为，而忽视身体能力的限制，如爬高梯子、清洁屋顶。故而需要基于性别差异制订预防跌倒的策略。

（3）退行性改变：老化使机体功能下降，导致步态和平衡能力改变、感觉功能减退、中枢神经系统改变、肌力减弱、骨质疏松和夜尿，使老年人容易发生跌倒。

（4）步态和平衡的改变：平衡功能和步态稳定性下降，易导致老年人跌倒。为弥补活动能力的下降，女性老年人会采取短步幅的

decreases, and tendons and ligaments begin to calcify, causing increased rigidity and decreased flexibility, especially in the legs and back. Postures tend to become stiff because of degenerative changes in the spine, causing a change in the center of gravity. These changes affect gait. Women develop a narrow base of support and a waddling gait, whereas men tend to have a wider base and a short-stepped, shuffling gait.

Degenerative changes in the cerebellum and the vestibular system, slowed neurologic response times, and an altered center of gravity all affect an older individual's ability to main balance.

(5) Sensory deficits: A sensory system consists of vision, hearing, touch, vestibular sensation, and proprioceptive sensation. Sensory system is responsible for processing sensory information, and then affects the balance of body functions. Accompanying the aging process, changes in structure of eye shape and crystalline lens flexibility can induce visual deficits such as reduced acuity or contrast sensitivity, declined accommodation to light and darkness, or altered depth perception. Elderly people are more likely to slip or trip when hazardous items are outside their visual field or when their depth perception has been compromised. Sidewalks, grass, other uneven surfaces, and brightly patterned floors are also visual hazards and are particular difficult to maneuver. Loss of color perception can make it difficult to distinguish objects in a pathway such as a blue footstool on a gray carpet.

Age-related conductive hearing loss, presbycusis or accumulation of earwax can affect hearing. Hearing impairment can influence safe mobility, particularly when old people are in unfamiliar or institutional environments. Hearing loss can impair an older person's ability to distinguish sounds that ordinarily signal danger, such as verbal warnings from another person, alarms, traffic noise, and so on.

The vestibular system monitors directions of motions during turning, moving forward-backward, side-to-side, and up-and-down. The proprioceptive system tells what part of the body is down and touching the ground as well as what parts of the body are moving. Diminished of one of these systems can create instability. For example, changes vestibular system can result in a sensation of dizziness. Similarly, variations in proprioception can change people's awareness in three dimensional spaces.

蹒跚步态，男性老年人形成步幅变宽、摆动腿抬高程度降低、行走拖拉的步态。

小脑和前庭系统的退行性改变，使反应时间延长，重心改变，从而影响老年人的平衡能力。

（5）感觉功能减退：感觉系统包括视觉、听觉、触觉、前庭感觉和本体感，通过处理感觉信息影响机体的平衡功能。老年人表现为视力、视觉分辨率、视觉的空间／深度感及视敏度下降，增加跌倒的危险性。

老年性传导性听力损失、老年性耳聋甚至耳垢堆积也会影响听力，有听力问题的老年人很难听到有关跌倒危险的警告声音，增加了跌倒的危险性。

前庭功能对维持机体的立体定向有重要作用。本体感觉系统与维持体位的稳定性有关。老年人前庭功能和本体感觉功能减退，可导致眩晕和平衡能力降低。

(6) Changes of nervous system: Age-related changes of the nervous system affect cognition, gait, balance, body sway, reaction ability and reaction time, which in turn, increase the risk for falls. Maintenance of balance in an upright position is a complex skill that is affected by the following age-related changes: a decline in the righting reflex; impaired proprioception, and diminished vibratory sensation and joint position sense in lower extremities. Age-related decreases in reaction time and speed of performance can influence mobility and safety. Therefore, old adults are at increased risk for falls in unfamiliar environments or when encountering the unexpected.

(7) Changes of musculoskeletal system: Changes of structure and function in musculoskeletal system including bones, joints, muscles, and tendons can contribute to activity intolerance and impaired physical mobility, leading to weakness and increased risk of falls. Loss of muscle strength, balance, flexibility and coordination can contribute to difficulty accomplishing activities of daily living. The bones of aging individuals, particularly the weight-bearing joints, undergo "wear and tear", which causes bones thin and more sponge-like. When the bones are weak and do not support the body structure, there is an increased risk for fractures, falls, and gait problems.

(8) Changes of cardiovascular system: Age-related change affecting the elasticity of arteries. Lack of elasticity leads to decrease in tissue recoil, and results in changes in blood pressure with position changes. Older individuals who get up quickly from supine position are likely to experience lightheadedness resulted from blood pressure drops, which is an effect of lack of tissue elasticity.

(9) Medical conditions: In addition to the age-related changes, common pathologic conditions can also increase the risk for falls (table 11-1 for further information). These two factors often interplay and contribute to falls. Chronic illness has been associated with increased risk of fall. Arthritis is a major contributor, and senior women experience more arthritis than men. Osteoporosis, characterized by low bone mass and the deterioration of bone tissue, does not affect the risk of fall per se, but does increase the risk of fractures from fall, particularly those of the hip, spine and wrist. Many neurologic, cerebrovascular, cardiovascular, and musculoskeletal conditions cause seizures, drop attacks, and syncopal episodes that result in falls. Other frequently implicated chronic conditions include urinary and bladder dysfunction. Older adults with acute disease are at a high risk for falls and injuries as a result of weakness, fatigue

（6）神经系统的变化：中枢神经系统的退变往往影响认知、反应能力、反应时间、平衡能力、步态及协同运动能力，使跌倒的危险性增加。老化导致翻正反射能力降低、本体感觉障碍以及振动感和下肢关节的位置感消失，从而影响直立位置平衡的维持。老年人在陌生的环境中或遇到意外时更易发生跌倒。

（7）骨骼肌肉系统的变化：老年人骨骼、关节、韧带及肌肉的结构、功能损害和退化使老年人的活动能力、力量和耐受性下降，导致跌倒危险性增加。老年人骨质疏松，尤其负重关节的骨头，会使与跌倒相关的骨折危险性增加。

（8）心血管系统的变化：老化使动脉壁弹性下降，体位改变时血压变化较大，老年人易出现直立性低血压。

（9）病理因素：除了退行性变化外，疾病也会增加跌倒的危险（表11-1），而且这两个方面相互作用相互影响。慢性疾病中的关节炎是跌倒的常见疾病。老年女性关节炎更多见。骨质疏松对跌倒本身不产生影响，但是会增加跌倒后骨折的风险，尤其是髋部、脊柱和手腕的骨折。神经系统疾病、脑血管疾病、心血管疾病和骨骼肌肉系统的疾病可以引起短暂的头昏、眩晕，因站立不稳而跌倒。患有急性疾病的老年人常因虚弱、眩晕而跌倒。

or dizziness. Even the short periods of immobility, often associated with an acute illness, are known to contribute to reduce reduction of bone density and muscle mass.

Table 11-1 Disorders that Contribute to Risks of Fall

Functional impairment	Disorder
● BP regulation	● Anemia ● Arrhythmias ● Cardio inhibitory carotid sinus hypersensitivity ● COPD ● Dehydration ● Infections (e. g. , pneumonia, sepsis) ● Metabolic disorders (e. g. , thyroid disorders, hypoglycemia, hyperglycemia with hyperosmolar dehydration) ● Neurocardiogenic inhibition after micturition ● Postural hypotension ● Postprandial hypotension ● Valvular heart disorders
● Central processing	● Delirium ● Dementia
● Gait	● Arthritis ● Foot deformities ● Muscle weakness
● Postural and neuromotor function	● Cerebellar degeneration ● Myelopathy (e. g. , due to cervical or lumbar spondylosis) ● Parkinson's disease ● Peripheral neuropathy ● Stroke ● Vertebrobasilar insufficiency
● Proprioception	● Peripheral neuropathy (e. g. , due to diabetes mellitus) ● Vitamin B_{12} deficiency
● Otolaryngologic function	● Acute labyrinthitis ● Benign paroxysmal positional vertigo ● Hearing loss ● Meniere's disease
● Vision	● Cataract ● Glaucoma ● Macular degeneration (age-related)

表 11-1 导致跌倒发生的疾病

功能障碍	疾病
● 血压调节	● 贫血；心律失常；心脏抑制性颈动脉窦过敏；慢性阻塞性肺疾病；脱水；感染（如：肺炎、脓毒血症）；代谢紊乱（如：甲状腺疾病、低血糖、高血糖伴高渗性脱水）；神经源性尿频；直立性低血压；餐后低血压；心脏瓣膜疾病
● 中枢处理	● 谵妄；痴呆

功能障碍	疾病
● 步态	● 关节炎；足畸形；肌无力
● 姿势及神经运动功能	● 小脑变性；脊髓病变；帕金森病；周围神经病变；脑卒中；椎－基底动脉供血不足
● 本体感觉	● 周围神经病变；维生素 B_{12} 缺乏
● 耳鼻喉功能	● 急性迷路炎；良性阵发性位置性眩晕；耳聋；梅尼埃病
● 视力	● 白内障；青光眼；老年黄斑变性

(10) Psychological status: Psychological function also increases the risk for falls in older adults. Older adults who are frustrated, depressed and anxious, are at increased risk for falls secondary to gait change, medication effects, and a diminished ability to concentrate on and respond to environment factors. Cognitive impairment, such as confusion due to dementia and delirium, can also increase the risk of fall.

2. Behavioral risk factors Behavioral risk factors include those concerning human actions, emotions or daily choices. They are potentially modifiable. For example, risky behavior such as take multiple medications, excess alcohol use, and sedentary behavior. These behaviors can be modified through strategic interventions for behavioral change.

(1) Fall history: A history of previous falls is one of the best predictors for future fall. Any previous fall increases the risk for another fall threefold. A previous fall may reduce mobility in older people, resulting in loss of strength, balance and reflexes. Feeling of fear and helplessness may also ensure restrictions on participation activity.

(2) Fear of falling: Fear of falling has been identified relatively as a risk factor in the fall prevention literature. Both recent fallers and those not reporting recent falls acknowledge their fear of falling. Specific fears vary but often include fear of falling again, being hurt or hospitalization, unable to get up after a fall, social embarrassment, loss of independence, and being moved away from home. Reduced physical and functional activity is associated with fear and anxiety about falling. Up to 50% of people who are fearful of falling restrict or eliminate social and physical activities because of that fear. Strong relationships have been found between fear and poor postural performance, slower walking speed and muscle weakness, poor self-rated health and decreased quality of life.

（10）心理因素：沮丧、抑郁、焦虑以及认知障碍均增加跌倒的危险。

2. 行为因素 行为因素与个人行动、情感或日常选择有关，行为因素是潜在的和可改进的，恰当的干预可以使老年人改变危险的行为。

（1）跌倒史：跌倒史是老年人跌倒的危险因素之一，可使再次跌倒的风险增加 3 倍。

（2）害怕跌倒：有跌倒史和无跌倒史的老年人都有害怕跌倒的心理。害怕跌倒使老年人活动减少，行走速度慢、肌肉力量减弱和生活质量下降，最终导致身体能力的丧失。

(3) Medications: Numerous studies over the years have revealed the number and types of medication consumed by seniors as contributors to risk of falls and subsequent injuries. We know medication use increases with advancing age due to prevalence and severity of health problems among the elderly. Mechanisms for digesting and metabolizing drugs change with age. Both half-life and active levels of a given dose increase with age, making the cumulative effects of medication use unpredictable. Also, age-related losses of gastrointestinal, hepatic or renal function predispose older persons to adverse drug reactions.

Polypharmacy, defined as taking five or more prescribed medications, is shown to be a significant factor in many falls. The variety of medication prescription is increasing and they are used in greater numbers and in new combinations. Drug-herb interactions may also be implicated in falls. As supplements, herbs and vitamins can react with each other or with prescription medications. The effects of various drug combinations are not yet clearly understood, especially the possible risks for falls in elderly individuals.

Agents that have been associated with falls, include anticonvulsants, antidepressants, antipsychotic, benzodiazepines, class IA antiarrhythmics (e. g. , procainamide, quinidine), digoxin, diuretics, narcotic analgesics, and sedative/hypnotics. Medications can affect one's risk of fall in several ways. They can reduce mental alertness, judgment and coordination. Certain drugs increase postural hypotension -a significant drop in blood pressure with a change in position (lie to sit or stand) -resulting in dizziness. Drugs can also alter the balance mechanism and the ability to recognize and adapt to obstacles. Finally, drugs may impair mobility by causing increased stiffness or weakness. Table 11-2 summarizes adverse drug effects that may contribute to the risk of falls in older persons.

（3）药物：老年人服用药物的数量和种类是导致跌倒和受伤的危险因素。老年人药物代谢动力学改变，如半衰期和有效剂量都随年龄增长而增加，使得药物使用的累积效应不可预测。此外，与年龄有关的胃肠道、肝或肾功能的老化也使老年人易发生药物不良反应。

多重用药，定义为服用五种或更多的处方药，是导致跌倒的重要因素。复方药物及草药的使用也与跌倒有关。

能够引起跌倒的药物包括抗惊厥药、抗抑郁药、镇静/安眠药、苯二氮䓬类、IA类抗心律失常药物（例如，普鲁卡因，奎尼丁）、地高辛、利尿剂及麻醉性镇痛药等（表11-2）。这些药物使老年患者出现意识模糊、定向力障碍、头晕、直立性低血压及步态不稳等不良反应，而引起跌倒。

Table 11-2 Potential Adverse Effects of Medications Contributing to Falls in Elderly

Medication (s)	Adverse drug reaction
Antidepressants, caffeine, neuroleptics, stimulants	Agitation
Antiarrhythmics	Arrhythmias
Benzodiazepines, narcotics, neuroleptics, any drug with anticholinergic effects	Cognitive impairment, confusion
Anticonvulsants, antidepressants, antihypertensives, benzodiazepines, narcotics, neuroleptics	Dizziness, orthostatic hypotension
Antidepressants, metoclopramide, neuroleptics	Gait abnormalities, extrapyramidal reactions

continued

Medication (s)	Adverse drug reaction
● Diuretics	● Increased ambulation
● Anticonvulsants, benzodiazepines, neuroleptics	● Postural disturbances (e. g. , problems with balance)
● Anticonvulsants, antidepressants, benzodiazepines, narcotics, neuroleptics	● Sedation, drowsiness
● Beta-blockers, nitrates, vasodilators (e. g. , alpha1-adrenergic blockers such as doxazosin)	● Syncope
● Neuroleptics, any drug with anticholinergic effects	● Visual disturbances (e. g. , blurred vision)

表 11-2　可能导致跌倒的药物

药物	不良反应
● 抗抑郁药、咖啡因、抗精神病药、兴奋剂	● 烦躁不安
● 抗心律失常药物	● 心律失常
● 苯二氮䓬类、麻醉药、抗精神病药、具有抗胆碱能效果的药物	● 认知功能障碍，意识模糊
● 抗惊厥药物、抗抑郁药、降压药、苯二氮䓬类、麻醉药、镇静剂	● 头晕、直立性低血压
● 抗抑郁药、甲氧氯普胺（止吐药）、抗精神病药	● 步态异常，锥体外系反应
● 利尿剂	● 排尿增加
● 抗惊厥药物、苯二氮䓬类、抗精神病药	● 姿势障碍（如平衡障碍）
● 抗惊厥药物、抗抑郁药、苯二氮䓬类、麻醉药、抗精神病药	● 镇静、嗜睡
● β 受体阻滞药，硝酸酯类，血管扩张剂（如 α1 肾上腺素能受体阻断药——多沙唑嗪）	● 晕厥
● 抗精神病药，具有抗胆碱能效果的药物	● 视力障碍（如视物模糊）

(4) Inactivity and sedentary lifestyle: Regular participation in moderate physical activity is integral to good health and maintaining independence. It prevents onset of multiple pathologies and functional capacity decline. Moderate physical activities and exercise also lower the risk of falls and fall-related injuries in older age through controlling weight as well as contributing to healthy bones, muscles, and joints. Exercise can improve balance, mobility and reaction time. It can increase bone mineral density of postmenopausal women and individuals aged 70 years and over. Moreover, it should be noticed that participation in vigorous physical activities – for instance intensive running in older age may increase the risk of falls. Undoubtedly, bed rest and restricted physical activity lead to accelerated deconditioning and

（4）体力活动：参加剧烈的体育活动可能会产生跌倒，同时卧床和限制体力活动可以加速身体功能的减弱，增加跌倒的风险。适度的体育活动和锻炼有利于老年人对体重的控制，进而促进骨骼、肌肉和关节的健康，降低老年人跌倒和跌倒相关损伤的风险。

loss of function and characterize the sequelae of injurious falls.

(5) Inadequate diet: A low body mass index suggesting malnutrition is associated with increased risk for fall. Eating a healthy balanced diet is central to healthy ageing. Adequate intake of protein, calcium, essential vitamins and water is essential for optimum health. If deficiencies do exist, it is reasonable to expect that weakness, poor fall recovery and increase risk of injuries will ensure. No dairy and fish consumption was associated with a higher risk of fall. Growing evidence supports dietary calcium and vitamin D intake improves bone mass among persons with low bone density and that it reduces the risk of osteoporosis and falling. Vitamin D deficiency is particularly common in older people in residential care facilities and may lead to abnormal gait, muscle weakness, osteomalacia and osteoporosis. Older persons with low dietary intake of calcium and vitamin D may be at risk for falls and therefore fractures resulting from them.

(6) Excessive alcohol: Use of excessive alcohol has been shown to be a risk factor of falls. Consumption of 14 or more drinks per week is associated with an increased risk of falls in older adults. Alcohol may also interact with certain drugs to increase the risk of falls by producing changes in awareness, balance and gait. Alcohol used in moderation has not been associated with increased fall rates.

(7) Inappropriate footwear, clothing and handbags: Footwear, clothing and handbags can contribute to falls, although clear research evidence is lacking. Footwear that fits poorly, has worn soles, is not laced or buckled when worn, or is of an unusual heel height for the individual, can contribute to falls. As people age, their height and posture change and long dressing gowns or trousers, which may have fit well at one time, can cause tripping hazards resulting in a fall and related injury. Many older people report falling or sustaining a fall-related injury, as a result of carrying an object such as a handbag, laundry basket or a grocery bag. Suspected mechanisms relate to altered balance, altered recovery mechanisms upon a trip or stumble, and altered means of protection as the senior lands on the ground or floor. Holding an object, for example, has been shown to impede ability to recover balance as it prevents one from rapidly grasping a handrail or other object for support.

3. Environmental risk factors Factors related to physical environment are the most common cause of falls in older adults. A number of hazards in the home and public environment that interact with other risk factors, such as poor vision or balance, contribute to falls and fall-

（5）营养不良：低身体质量指数是老年人跌倒的危险因素。充足的蛋白质，钙，必需的维生素和水的摄入对于保持最佳健康至关重要。身体虚弱、跌倒后恢复能力差以及受伤风险增加与营养不良有关。钙和维生素D缺乏可导致肌肉无力和骨质疏松，使老年人跌倒后容易出现骨折。

（6）过量饮酒：过量饮酒（老年人每周饮酒14个或以上标准饮酒单位）可以增加跌倒的危险。酒精也可能与某些药物发生相互作用，从而通过改变意识，平衡和步态而增加跌倒的风险。

（7）不合适的衣着：鞋子不合适、鞋子磨损严重、高跟鞋、过于宽松的衣服都易导致跌倒。穿鞋时未系鞋带，或者鞋跟过高可能会导致摔倒。老年人身高和形态会发生变化，穿着长礼服或长裤可能会导致绊倒。携带大号手提包，洗衣篮或购物袋也会增加跌倒的风险。

3. 环境因素 环境因素是指个人与周围环境间相互作用，包括居住环境中的危害和公共环境中的危害。环境本身并不会导致跌倒发生，但暴露在环境中的人与其相互作用

related injuries for seniors.

(1) Stairs: Stairs can be problematic – hazardous characteristics include uneven or excessively high or narrow steps, slippery surfaces, unmarked edges, discontinuous or poorly-fitted handrails, and inadequate or excessive lighting. Unsafe features identified most frequently were no contrast markings for stair edges, non-uniform risers, stair dimensions that differ from the recommended seven-inch maximum height or rise and eleven-inch minimum run (toe to heel allowance), open risers and lack of handrails. Handrails that are securely mounted at an appropriate height and shaped correctly allow a functional grip to be established. Stair surfaces and floors that are slippery, excessively patterned, glare-producing or uneven also have been implicated in falls.

(2) Factors in and around the home: Since nearly half of falls among seniors occurs at home, the home environment is critical for avoiding them. High risk factors found in the home include absence of night lights; an absence of accessible light switches at room entrances; slippery floors; loose or uneven rugs; appliance cords or other obstacles in walking routes; hazardous bathrooms or kitchen; lack of grab bars or handrails; items stored in high cupboards; and low furniture such as beds or chairs. Outside the home hazards can be found in such features as garden paths and walks that are cracked or slippery from rain, snow or moss. Entrance stairs and poor night lighting can also pose risks. Even pets can be a tripping hazard.

(3) Factors in the public environment: Factors in the public environment can also trigger falls. Even walking on a familiar route can lead to falls as a result of poor building design and inadequate consideration. Most problematic factors are cracked or uneven sidewalks, unmarked obstacles, slippery surfaces, poor lighting and lengthy distances to sitting areas and public restrooms.

(4) Assistive devices: Assistive devices can promote independence and mobility and may prevent falls if properly used and safely maintained. However, when used improperly these aids are also associated with an increased risk of falls. Cane tips can become worn, making them unsafe. Walkers with wheels or wheelchairs may lack a functioning locking mechanism posing a hazard. Moreover, the use of canes and walkers can interfere with the ability to maintain balance in certain situations, and the demands of using these devices can be excessive for older adults. Having an assistive device does not necessarily

是造成跌倒的重要原因。

（1）楼梯：楼梯的台阶面不平或边缘不明显、台阶过高、楼梯过窄、扶手不连续或不牢固以及照明不足等可导致老年人跌倒。

（2）室内环境：1/2 的跌倒发生于室内，室内常见的危险因素包括光线不良、地面光滑、地毯松脱、过道有障碍物、无扶手、储藏物位置过高、床和座椅过低等。室外的危险因素包括台阶和人行道缺乏修缮，雨雪天气路面湿滑。饲养宠物增加了绊倒的风险。

（3）公共环境：建筑设计差和维护不当、人行道凹凸不平、障碍物不明显、路面光滑、照明差、距离休息的地方和公共厕所的距离过远等因素常导致老年人跌倒。

（4）辅助器具：正确使用辅助器具可以提高生活自理能力，增加活动的安全性并预防跌倒。但是使用不当就会增加跌倒的风险，如拐杖磨损、轮椅缺乏刹车装置等。有些老年人可能拥有辅助器具但不一定使用，因为他们将使用辅助工具视为年老和脆弱的象征而不愿意使用。

guarantee its use. Many older people see such aids as symbols of their old age and advanced frailty, and they may be reluctant to use them because of this stigma).

(5) Restraints: The use of physical restrains such as belts and bed rails is based on the belief that restricting a body part will prevent movement that could lead to falls and injuries. However, medical research has produced strong evidence that restraints do not prevent falls, and may in fact represent a safety hazard for the senior. People, especially the elderly are often at risk for falling and restraints used to be applied in a regular manner to prevent these accidents that often lead to hip fractures. A research has shown likelihood of serious injury actually decreased after restraint removal and hip fracture rates did not increase.

4. Socioeconomic risk factors Socioeconomic risk factors are those related to influence social conditions and economic status of individuals as well as the capacity of the community to challenge them. These factors include low income, low education, inadequate housing, lack of social interaction, limited access to health and social care especially in remote areas, and lack of community resources.

(1) Social factors: Isolation and loneliness are commonly experiences by older people particularly among those who lose their spouse or live alone. They are much more likely than other groups to experience disability and the physical, cognitive, and sensory limitations that increase the risk of falls. Isolation and depression triggered by lack of social participation increase fear of falling, and vice versa. Fear of falling can increase the risk of falls through a reduction in social participation and loss of personal contact -which in turn increase isolation and depression. Providing social support and opportunities for older people to participate in social activities to help maintain active interaction with others may decrease their risk of falls.

(2) Economic factors: Lower income is associated with increased risk of falling. Older people, especially those who are female, live alone or in rural areas with unreliable and insufficient incomes face an increased risk of falls. Poor environment in which they live, their poor diet and the fact of not being able to access health care services even when they have acute or chronic illness exacerbates the risk of falling. The negative cycle of poverty and falls in older age is particularly evident in rural areas and in developing countries. The fall-related burden to health system will keep increasing unless resources and money are allocated in order to provide proper primary health care and opportunities to older

（5）身体约束：身体约束常被用来保护患者的安全。然而越来越多的研究表明，身体约束并不能预防跌倒，会对老年人的安全造成威胁。对有跌倒危险的老年人应用身体约束会导致髋部骨折的发生。

4. 社会经济因素 社会经济因素是指影响个人的社会状况和经济状况等因素，包括低收入水平、低教育水平、住房不足、缺少社会互动、缺少保健和社会照护以及缺乏社会资源等。

（1）社会因素：失去配偶或独居的老年人易产生孤独和被隔离感，其身体、认知和感觉能力下降，容易发生跌倒。为老年人提供社会支持，增加人际交往，可以降低他们跌倒的风险。

（2）经济因素：低收入会增加跌倒的风险。老年人尤其是女性、独居、农村地区的、没有稳定和足够的收入，其跌倒的风险会增加。生活环境差、饮食习惯不良、患病时不能获得医疗保健服务会加剧跌倒的产生。

people for social participation. It is never too late to break this vicious cycle.

IV. Nursing Assessment

While the statistics on falls are staggering, falls are not a natural part of aging. Furthermore, most falls are predictable and preventable. Research has identified the key risk factors for falling and many are modifiable. Research has further shown that the incidence of falls in older adults can be reduced by targeting modifiable risk factors using proven interventions. So conducting a falls risk assessment is a critical step in falls prevention. Fall risk assessment is multidimensional and includes: focused history, physical examination, functional assessment, laboratory, and environmental assessment.

1. Focused history

(1) History of falls: Some falls are promptly recognized because of an obvious fall-related injury or concern about a possible injury. However, because elderly people often do not report falls, they should be asked about falls at least once per year. An older person should be asked whether they have fallen in the last year. If a fall has occurred, ask about the context and circumstances of the fall, symptoms he experienced at the time of or just before the fall, the frequency of falling, and severity or injuries sustained from the fall. Many people will minimize or even forget falls if no injuries resulted. They may also be reluctant to share this information if they perceive a threat to their independence or the possibility of having to undergo uncomfortable or costly diagnostic procedures or treatment. The fall diary (table 11-3) helps to monitor fall occurrences, injuries and patterns. Older adults can use the fall diary to jot down all the important information that led to the fall, occurred during the fall, or followed the fall. This information is extremely useful in determining antecedents and consequences of falling.

(2) Medication review: Medications are well-recognized as a contributing factor to falls in older adults. A careful medication review is valuable for any patient but particularly so for older adults, who tend to take more medications, have more co-morbid illnesses, and suffer more adverse drug reactions. A number of studies have shown after medication review the risk of falls decreases significantly. The first critical step in the medication review process is to accurately identify all the patient's current

四、护理评估

通过对危险因素的评估，可以及早识别可以改变的危险因素并给予干预措施，从而减少跌倒的发生。跌倒危险性的评估包括健康史评估、体格检查、功能评估、实验室检查和环境评估等多个方面。

1. 健康史评估

（1）跌倒史：向所护理的老年人询问有关跌倒的情况，每年至少应询问一次。如发生过跌倒，进一步了解跌倒的环境、跌倒前身体状况和跌倒时的症状、跌倒的次数以及受伤的严重程度。跌倒日记可以监测跌倒发生的情况及带来的伤害，有助于确定跌倒原因及带来的后果（表11-3）。

（2）用药史：药物是导致老年人跌倒的因素。仔细的药物审查对老年人非常重要。回顾所使用过的处方药和替代药物治疗情况，有否改变或者调整用药。

Table 11-3 Fall Diary

Date	Time	
● Where did you fall?		
● What happened?		
● Did you trip?	☐ Yes	☐ No
● Did you have any of the following symptoms before you fell?	☐ Dizziness	☐ Palpitations
	☐ Legs gave away	☐ Blacked out
● Did you hurt yourself?	☐ Yes	☐ No
● Could you get up from the floor?	☐ Yes	☐ No
● If no, how did you get up?		
● Did you see a doctor?	☐ Yes	☐ No

表 11-3 跌倒日记

日期：	时间：	
● 是在哪里跌倒的？		
● 发生了什么事情？		
● 是被绊倒的吗？	☐ 是	☐ 否
● 发生跌倒前是否有以下症状？	☐ 头昏眼花	☐ 心慌
	☐ 下肢麻木	☐ 晕厥
● 是否受伤？	☐ 是	☐ 否
● 跌倒后能从地上站起来吗？	☐ 是	☐ 否
● 如果不能站起，最后是怎样起来的？		
● 是否就医？	☐ 是	☐ 否

medications-what medications the patient is taking, either from the patient himself or, if that isn't possible, from his caregiver.

A variety of tools are available to assist the medication review process. The Beers criteria lists medications considered potentially problematic in older adults that should generally be avoided. The criteria, based on expert opinion, were introduced in 1991 and most recently updated in 2003. The criteria are commonly used in the literature to assess quality of prescribing in older adults. While the Beers list is a useful starting point, the Beers criteria cannot be applied universally or exclusively.

可以使用一些工具进行用药史的评估，如比尔斯标准，纳入了与疾病无关的，应避免在老年人中使用的药物。

Consideration should be given to a wide variety of issues, including appropriateness of each medication for the individual patient, potential and current side effects, and compliance issues.

One common sense approach to the medication review process is called ARMOR (assess, review, minimize, optimize, and reassess). Assess each medication as well as the total number of medications with focused attention towards side effects, safety, and fall risk. Review for possible drug/drug and drug/disease interactions, and weigh risk versus benefit. Minimize nonessential drug use by discontinuing those that lack evidence of efficacy or are not indicated. Optimize by addressing therapy goals and appropriate geriatric and renal dosing. Reassess vital signs, cognitive status, clinical status, and medication compliance.

A second and similar common sense approach uses a patient-centered visual grid to classify each medication according to its purpose (cure, prophylaxis, or symptom relief) and its importance (vital, important, optional, or not indicated). This approach involves the patient in the decision-making process and initiates the important conversation to assess the patient's understanding of each medication's purpose, perceived importance, dosing, and administration instructions as well as the level of adherence. When a medication has been classified as optional or not indicated, discontinuation should be considered. If the medication is classified as vital or important but may also increase the risk of falls, it may be possible to switch to a safer alternative or to attempt a dosage reduction. Another tool, presented in figure 11-3, shows a simple algorithmic approach to the medication review process.

(3) Medical history: The medical history should include outcomes of past events. Chronic diseases, such as Parkinson's disease, arthritis, osteoporosis, heart disease and stroke, bowel and bladder incontinence, blood pressure problems and other diseases, as well as short-term illnesses such as flu and infections can cause increased frailty and physical impairment. Knowledge about medical history can help you identify risk factors and plan preventive interventions.

(4) Social History: A social history is important in identifying risk factors. Data collected include living arrangement, presence of caregiver, home access and level of social connectedness. A senior who lives alone, has experienced significant losses, and has few social support is at greater risk than average for depression and cognitive

药物审查过程中的一种常见方法称为ARMOR（评估、审查、最小化、优化和重新评估）。评估每种药物以及药物总数，重点关注副作用、安全性和跌倒风险。审查药物间的相互作用，并权衡使用风险。尽量减少非必需药物的使用。根据治疗目标优化用药。用药后重新评估生命体征、认知状态、临床表现和药物依从性。

另一种审查方法是以患者为中心的表格化判断法，根据其目的（治疗、预防或缓解）及重要性（非常重要的、重要的、可选的或不明确的）对每种药物进行分类。这种方法让患者参与决策过程，以评估患者对每种药物的用途、重要性、剂量、给药说明以及依从性的理解。当一种药物被归类为可选择的或不明确的时，应考虑停药。如果药物被归类为重要药物，但也可能增加跌倒的风险，则可改用更安全的药物。

（3）疾病史：了解老年人的患病史，是否患有慢性疾病（如帕金森病、关节炎、骨质疏松、心脏病、脑卒中、大小便失禁、血压异常等）或急性疾病（如流行性感冒和感冒）。

（4）社会状况：了解老年人的居住安排、是否有照顾者以及老年人与社会联系的水平。独居老年人获得的社会支持较少，易产生抑郁和认知障碍。

impairment, which can lead to functional losses.

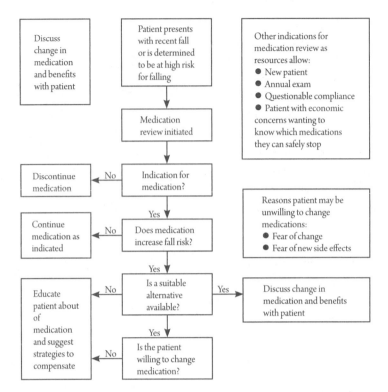

Figure 11-3　Medication review algorithm

2. Physical examination　The physical examination should be comprehensive enough to exclude obvious intrinsic causes of falls. A physical examination should include a thorough review of systems with emphasis on the musculoskeletal, neurological and cardiac systems, as well as assessment of gait, balance, mobility, orthostatic vital signs, and cognition.

(1) Cardiovascular assessment: Evaluating the cardiovascular system helps to exclude arrhythmia, valvular heart disease and heart failure. Measurement of orthostatic vital signs is very important. Postural hypotension was defined as a 20 mmHg or greater drop in systolic blood pressure and/or a 10 mmHg or greater drop in diastolic blood pressure over 3 minutes and/or a history of symptoms consistent with postural hypotension. Blood pressure and pulse are measured with the patient supine, then immediately after standing and after at least two minutes of standing to check for orthostatic hypotension.

(2) Musculoskeletal assessment: Musculoskeletal assessment includes muscle strength, range and motion and lower extremities. Manual muscle testing is a very important clinical tool used to assess a patient's muscle strength and determine the extent and degree of muscular weakness. In this form of testing, the individual is asked

2. 体格检查　体格检查应全面。体格检查应包括对肌肉骨骼系统、神经系统和心脏系统的全面检查，以及对步态、平衡、认知能力等的评估。

（1）循环系统的评估：检查老年人是否患有心律失常、心脏瓣膜病、心脏衰竭等疾病，是否存在直立性低血压。分别于仰卧和站立至少两分钟后测量血压。若收缩压下降 20mmHg 以上，舒张压下降 10mmHg 以上和 / 或出现与直立性低血压相关的症状即可判定直立性低血压。

（2）骨骼肌肉系统的评估：包括肌力、肢体活动范围以及四肢末梢的情况。徒手肌力检查可以评估肌力、确定肌无力的程度和范围（表 11-4）。

to hold a limb or other body part at the end of its available range or at another point in its range of motion while the clinician provides manual resistance. Manual Muscle Test Grades is in table 11-4.

Examination of the lower extremities includes an inspection of leg joints and the feet for deformities, pain, arthritis and podiatric problems that could impair gait. Footwear should be checked for appropriateness; the sole wear pattern may provide insight into abnormal weight distribution while walking.

同时应观察腿关节和双脚是否存在畸形、疼痛、炎症等问题，这些可能影响步态。此外，还应检查鞋和袜子是否合适。

Table 11-4　Manual Muscle Test Grades

Numerals	Letters	Description
Against gravity test:		The patient is able to move through:
5	N	● The full available range of motion (ROM) against gravity and against maximal resistance, with hold at the end of the ROM (Hold for about 3 seconds)
4	G	● The full available ROM against gravity and against moderate leading resistance
4-	G-	● Greater than one half of the available ROM against gravity and against moderate resistance
3+	F+	● Less than one half of the available ROM against gravity and against moderate resistance
3	F	● The full available ROM against gravity
3-	F-	● Greater than one half of the available ROM against gravity
2+	P+	● Less than one half of the available ROM against gravity
2	P (poor)	● The full available ROM gravity eliminated
2-	P-	● Greater than one half the available ROM; gravity eliminated
1+	T+	● Less than one half of the available ROM; gravity eliminated
1	T (trace)	● None of the available ROM; gravity eliminated and there is palpable or observable flicker contraction
0	0 (zero)	● None of the available ROM; gravity eliminated and there is no palpable or observable muscle contraction

Note: N –normal; G-good; F-fair; P-poor.

表 11-4　徒手肌力检查分级指南

分级	名称		评定标准
5	N	（正常）	正常范围抗阻
4	G	（良）	能抗较大阻力
4–	G–	（良 –）	能抗较弱阻力加重力
3+	F+	（好 +）	与 4– 只是阻力大小的区别

分级	名称		评定标准
3	F	（好）	抗重力完成全范围的运动
3-	F-	（好 -）	抗重力完成全范围 50% 以上的运动
2+	P+	（差 +）	抗重力完成全范围 50% 以下的运动
2	P	（差）	解除重力的影响，可完成全范围的运动
2-	P-	（差 -）	解除重力的影响，可完成全范围 50% 以上的运动
1+	T+	（微 +）	解除重力的影响，可完成全范围 50% 以下的运动
1	T	（微）	可触及肌肉收缩，但不能引起关节活动
0	0	（零）	不能触及肌肉收缩

(3) Neurological assessment: A formal neurological assessment includes assessment of muscle strength and tone, sensation (including proprioception), coordination (including cerebellar function) and station and gait. Neurological findings may suggest cerebrovascular disease, Parkinson's disease, myelopathy, peripheral neuropathy or proximal myopathy. Proprioceptive and cerebellar function can be tested with a group of gross balance tests (Chapter 11 Section 1 Assessment of gait and balance.)

The mental status examination is a series of detailed but simple questions designed to test mood state and cognitive ability. Mood state especially depression can impact mobility functioning and potentially increase falls risk. The geriatric depression scale was developed as a basic screening measure for depression in older adults. The original version (GDS-30) consisted of 30 questions in the form of yes / no and was designed for self-administration.

Impairments in cognitive functioning have been demonstrated to increase falls risk. The mini-mental state examination (MMSE) is a brief 30-point questionnaire test that is used to screen for cognitive impairment. The MMSE facilitates the detection of mental status changes, particularly in the elderly, and thereby enhances patient care. In the time span of about 10 minutes, it samples various functions including arithmetic, memory and orientation. The MMSE test includes simple questions and problems in a number of areas: the time and place of the test, repeating lists of words, arithmetic such as the serial sevens, language use and comprehension, and basic motor skills.

(4) Assessment of gait and balance: Postural control is a complex task that involves balance, ambulation capability, endurance, range of motion, sensation and strength. Informal assessment begins with observation. Does the patient require assistance walking down the

（3）神经系统的评估：包括肌力、感觉、协调能力和步态评估。通过神经系统的检查，判断患者是否患有脑血管疾病、帕金森病、脊髓病及周围神经病变。本体感觉和小脑功能可以通过平衡测试检查（见第十一章第一节"步态和平衡能力的评估"）。

通过情绪状态和认知能力的测试对精神状况进行评估。情绪状态尤其是抑郁会影响运动功能，并可能增加跌倒风险。使用老年抑郁量表进行抑郁的筛查。

简易精神状态检查（MMSE）是一种简短的 30 分问卷测验，用于筛查认知障碍。MMSE 评估需要大约 10 分钟，测试内容包括一些简单的问题，如回答正确的时间和地点、复述单词、简单计算、语言的使用和理解，以及基本的运动技能。

（4）步态和平衡能力的评估：姿势控制是一项复杂的技能，涉及身体的平衡、行走能力、耐力、活动范围、感觉和肌力。首先直接观察步态和平衡状况，观察患者步态是连

hall or getting from the chair to the examination table? Is the gait continuous and fluid, or is it halting and unsteady?

Formal screening begins with tools or assessment instruments. Many tools or assessment instruments such as timed up and go test, one-leg balance, performance-oriented assessment of mobility problems (Tinetti scale), functional reach, dynamic gait index, Berg balance scale are used to measure gait and balance. One-leg balance is tested by having the patient stand unassisted on one leg for five seconds. The patient chooses which leg to stand on (based on personal comfort), flexes the opposite knee to allow the foot to clear the floor and then balances on one leg for as long as possible. The physician uses a watch to time the patient's one-leg balance. This test predicts injurious falls but not all falls.

The timed "Up & Go" test evaluates gait and balance. The patient gets up out of a standard armchair (seat height of approximately 46 cm), walks a distance of 3m, turns, walks back to the chair and sits down again. The patient wears regular footwear and, if applicable, uses any customary walking aid (e. g., cane or walker). No physical assistance is given. The physician uses a stopwatch or a wristwatch with a second hand to time this activity. A score of 30 seconds or greater indicates that the patient has impaired mobility and requires assistance (i. e., has a high risk of falling). This test has been shown to be as valid as sophisticated gait testing.

(5) Sensory assessment: Vision and hearing impairment, although not routinely assessed, are important risk factors for falls in older people. Hearing and vision assessment and referrals have been a component of successful multi-factorial falls prevention programs. Measurement of visual functions such as visual acuity, contrast sensitivity and depth perception may identify older people at risk of falls.

(6) Elimination assessment: Getting to and from the bathroom and transferring to and from the toilet have been identified as major factors of falls, so be sure to document the patient's usual patterns of bowel and bladder elimination along with any related ongoing problems.

(7) Nutritional assessment: Consider the patient's overall appearance, and include measures of height and weight at first. Assessment including a record of the patient's usual eating and drinking patterns can provide valuable information. Additionally, in evaluating a patient's nutritional status, pay particular attention to hydration status and protein values. Dehydration can cause hypovolemia, which can cause light-headedness or orthostatic hypotension, a primary cause of falls. Depleted

续的、流畅的，还是停顿的、不稳定的。然后使用评估工具进行测评。

单腿平衡测试要求受试者单腿站立并保持平衡 5 秒，但该测试不能预测所有的跌倒事件。

计时起立行走测试要求受试者从靠背椅上站起（座椅高度大约 46cm），站稳后，按照平时走路的步态，向前走 3m 后转身，走回到椅子前，转身坐下，靠到椅背上，通过计算完成此项任务所花费的时间测评受试者的稳定功能。完成时间超过 30 秒，表明受试者活动能力有障碍。

（5）感官评估：对老年人的视力和听力进行检查。视功能检查包括视力、对比敏感度和深度觉等。

（6）排泄系统的评估：老年人跌倒易发生于沐浴和如厕过程中。应注意记录老年人的排泄习惯及其排泄相关的问题。

（7）营养状况的评估：注意评估老年人的营养状况。测量老年人的躯体健康，如身高、体重；评估内容应包括老年人的日常饮食记录；注意评估老年人体内的水分和蛋白质的水平。脱水会导致血容量不足，而导致头昏眼花或直立性低血压，这是跌倒的主要原因。蛋白质水平下降（特别是白蛋白）会增加药

protein stores (especially albumin) increase the incidence of drug interactions and adverse reactions, which also increase the incidence of falls.

3. Functional assessment　Overall physical function should also be assessed. This is accomplished by assessing the patient's ADLs and instrumental activities of daily living (IADLs). An alternative is the physical performance test (PPT). This performance-based test includes seven usual daily activities. The patient is asked to write a sentence, lift a book, put on and take off a jacket, pick up a penny, turn 360 degrees and walk about 15 m. The physician evaluates the performance of these activities to determine whether the patient is at increased risk for recurrent falls. Additionally, many older people, whether or not they have fallen, develop a fear of falling. This fear can cause them to limit their activities, which in turn leads to reduced mobility and physical fitness and subsequently to an increased risk of falls. This fear can lead to deteriorating health, a decline in physical and social functioning, and increased likelihood of admission to a nursing home. Therefore, fear of falling in elderly should be assessed. Falls efficacy scale (FES) (box 11-3 Falls Efficacy Scale), developed by Tinetti et al, is an instrument to measure fear of falling. The FES is a questionnaire that measures an individual's perceived confidence in avoiding falls while completing 10 activities of daily living. Individuals are asked to rate each item on a scale from 1 to 10, with total scores ranging from 10 to 100. Higher scores indicate less perceived confidence.

物的不良反应，这也会增加跌倒的发生率。

3. 功能评估　功能评估包括对日常生活功能（ADL）、工具性日常生活功能（IADL）的评估及身体能力测试（PPT）。身体能力测试包括7种常见的日常活动，受试者被要求写一句话，举起一本书，穿上并脱下一件夹克，捡起一枚硬币，身体转360度，走大约15m。通过对这些活动的评估判断受试者是否有跌倒的危险。此外，评估老年人是否存在害怕跌倒的心理，测评老年人在进行日常活动时对跌倒的自我效能和对不发生跌倒的自信程度。由 Tinetti 等人开发的跌倒效能量表（FES），测量一个人在完成10项日常生活活动时避免跌倒的自信程度（box 11–3）。每个人被要求在1到10分的范围内对每个项目进行评分，总分在10到100分之间。分数越高，人们的自信度越低。

Box 11-3　Falls Efficacy Scale

On a scale from 1 to 10, with 1 being very confident and 10 being not confident at all, how confident are you that you do the following activities without falling?

<table>
<tr><td align="center">Activity</td><td align="center">Score
(1 very confident, 10 not confident at all)</td></tr>
</table>

- Take a bath or shower.
- Reach into cabinets or closets.
- Walk around the house.
- Prepare meals not requiring carrying heavy or hot objects.
- Get on and out of bed.
- Answer the door or telephone.
- Get on and out of a chair.
- Getting dressed and undressed.
- Personal grooming (i. e. washing your face).

- Getting on and off of the toilet.

Total Score:

* A total score of greater than 70 indicates that the person has a fear of falling.

Box 11-3　跌倒自我效能量表

请从1到10进行打分（1代表非常自信，10代表完全不自信），请用1~10描述在进行下列活动时，你确保不跌倒的自信程度：

<table>
<tr><th>活动</th><th>分值
（1为非常自信，10为完全不自信）</th></tr>
</table>

- 沐浴。
- 从橱柜或衣柜内拿东西。
- 在房间里走动。
- 准备简单的饭菜。
- 上下床。
- 应门或接电话。
- 从椅子上起落。
- 更衣。
- 洗漱（洗脸）。
- 如厕。

总分：

* 总分数大于70分表明个体害怕跌倒。

4. Laboratory assessment There is no standard diagnostic evaluation. Laboratory assessment is based on the history and physical examination and helps rule out various causes. A comprehensive metabolic panel (electrolytes, kidney function, and liver function tests) and complete blood count should be considered to assess for metabolic abnormalities, anemia, and nutritional deficiencies. Vitamin D adequacy can be measured by the 25-hydroxyvitamin D level. Serum thyroid-stimulating hormone (TSH), Uitamin B_{12} and folate levels should be obtained if there is evidence of neuropathy or cognitive impairment. Bone mineral density assessment should be performed to assess for osteoporosis and increased fracture risk. An electrocardiogram is usually not necessary in the absence of syncope or suspected cardiac cause of falls (e. g. , an arrhythmia). Spinal x-rays and cranial CT or MRI are indicated only when the history and physical examination detect new neurologic abnormalities.

4. 医学检查 当病史或体格检查提示有导致跌倒的潜在原因时，建议进行彻底的医学检查。如行电解质、血常规、肝肾功能检查来诊断代谢异常，贫血和营养缺乏。如有认知障碍，应进一步检测血清促甲状腺素（TSH），维生素 B_{12} 和叶酸水平。检查骨密度以评估骨质疏松症和骨折风险。如果存在晕厥或疑似心脏病而发生跌倒（如心律失常），需行心电图检查。神经系统异常时，须行脊柱 X 线和颅 CT 或 MRI。

5. Environmental assessment　A significant proportion of falls in community-dwelling older people occur in the home and immediate vicinity. Because such environmental variables are implicated in the majority of falls, removing potential hazards in the home environment is intuitively sensible. An assessment of the home environment aims to enhance accessibility, safety, and performance of daily living activities.

Environmental assessments inquire about home hazards of people at risk of falling, including external and internal ways, the general environment, and specific rooms such as bathroom. A home safety checklist (table 11-5), which can be completed by seniors themselves or together with volunteers or health care workers can help identify potential hazards in and around the home and recommends ways to reduce risk.

5. 环境评估　家庭环境的评估旨在提高老年人日常活动的便利性和安全性。

老年人可自己或与卫生保健人员、志愿者共同使用居家危险因素评估表来识别判断环境中的潜在危险（表 11-5）。

Table 11–5　Home Safety Checklist

Items	Contents
● Illumination and color contrast	● Is the lighting adequate but not glare producing? ● Are the light switches easy to reach and manipulate? ● Can lights be turned on before entering rooms? ● Is color contrast adequate between objects, such as a chair and the floor?
● Hazards	● Are there highly polished floors, throw rugs, or other hazardous floor coverings? ● If area rugs are used, do they have non-slip backing, and are the edges tacked to the floor? ● Are there cords, clutter, or other obstacles in pathways? ● Is there a pet that is likely to be running underfoot?
● Furniture	● Are chairs the right height and depth for the person? ● Do the chairs have armrests? Are tables stable and of the appropriate height? ● Is any furniture placed well away from pathway?
● Stairways	● Is lighting adequate? ● Are there light switches at the top and bottom of the stairs? ● Are there securely fastened handrails on both sides of the stairway? ● Are all the steps even? ● Are the treads nonskid? ● Should colored tape be used to mark the edges of the steps, particularly the top and bottom steps?
● Bathroom	● Are grab bars placed appropriately for the tub and toilet? ● Does the tub have skid-proof strips or rubber mat in the bottom? ● Has the person considered using a tub seat? ● Is the height of the toilet seat appropriate? ● Has the person considered using an elevated toilet seat? ● Does the color of the toilet seat contrast with surrounding colors? ● Is toilet paper within easy reach?

continued

Items	Contents
● Bedroom	● Is the height of the bed appropriate? ● Is the mattress firm at the edges to provide enough support for sitting? ● If the bed has wheels, are they locked securely? ● Would full or partial side rails be a help or a hazard? ● When side rails are in the down position, are they completely out of the way? ● Is the pathway between the bedroom and bathroom clear of objects and adequately ● illuminated, particularly at night? ● Would a bedside commode be useful, especially at night? ● Is a lisht near the bed, and does the person has sufficient physical and cognitive ability to turn it on before getting out of bed? ● Is furniture positioned to allow safe use of assistive devices for ambulation? ● Is a telephone situated near the bed?
● Kitchen	● Are storage areas used to the best advantage? ● Are appliance cords kept out of the way? ● Are nonslip mats used in front of the sink? ● Are the markings on stoves and other appliances clearly visible? ● Does the person know how to use the microwave safely?
● Temperature	● Is the temperature of the room (s) comfortable? ● Can the person read the markings on the thermostat and adjust it appropriately? ● During cold months, is the room temperature high enough to prevent hypothermia? ● During hot weather, is the room temperature cool enough to prevent hyperthermia?

表 11-5　居家危险因素评估表

项目	内容
● 照明与色彩的搭配	● 照明是否良好不刺眼? ● 电灯开关是否容易触及和控制的? ● 房间内的灯是否可在进入房间前打开? ● 房间内物体是否有合适的颜色对比,如椅子和地板之间?
● 危险	● 地板是否非常光滑或上面有小块地毯或其他的覆盖物? ● 小块地毯是否是防滑的? 其边缘是否已固定在地板上? ● 地面是否有绳子、杂物或其他障碍物? ● 是否可能有宠物在脚下跑过?
● 家具	● 椅子的高度和深度是否合适? ● 椅子是否有扶手? 桌子是否稳定,高度是否适合? ● 家具的摆放位置是否合理?
● 楼梯	● 照明是否良好? ● 楼梯的顶部和底部是否都有电灯开关? ● 楼梯的两边是否有坚固的扶手? ● 是否所有的台阶都很平坦? ● 每一级楼梯的边缘是否安装了防滑踏脚? ● 每个台阶的边缘是否(尤其是最上面和最下面的一层台阶)使用彩色胶带进行标记?

项目	内容
● 卫生间	● 浴缸和马桶旁是否装有扶手？ ● 浴缸底部是否有防滑条或垫有橡胶垫？ ● 是否考虑使用带座位的浴缸？ ● 马桶的高度是否合适？ ● 是否考虑抬高马桶座圈的高度？ ● 马桶的颜色是否与周围颜色形成对比？ ● 厕纸是否容易拿取？
● 卧室	● 床的高度是否合适？ ● 床垫边缘是否坚固，可以为坐姿提供足够的支撑？ ● 如果床脚有轮子，是否已被安全固定？ ● 全部或部分护栏是否有益于安全？ ● 护栏的位置是否过低，已起不到保护的作用？ ● 卧室和浴室之间的通路是否通畅无障碍物，且照明良好（尤其是夜间）？ ● 是否使用便盆（尤其夜间）？ ● 床边是否安装有照明的装置，个体是否能够在起床前先将床头照明打开？ ● 家具的位置是否不会影响需助行器辅助的人在室内行走？ ● 床旁是否安装了电话？
● 厨房	● 厨房用品的放置是否便于拿取？ ● 过道上是否无任何电线？ ● 水槽前是否使用防滑垫？ ● 炉灶及其他电器上的标记是否清晰可见？ ● 是否能够安全使用微波炉？
● 温度	● 室内温度是否舒适？ ● 个体能否看清恒温器上的标记线，并将恒温器调节至合适的温度？ ● 最寒冷的时节，室内是否足够暖和，以避免受凉？ ● 最炎热的时节，室内是否足够凉爽，以避免中暑？

V. Nursing Management

Management of falls is challenging to the nurses, especially when older adults experience multiple or recurrent falls. The goals of interventions are to identify the underlying cause, to reduce the incidence of recurrent falling, and to prevent serious injury.

1. Fall prevention When the cause of a fall is not determined or a patient remains at high risk for falls, referral to a falls prevention program may be warranted. There has been a substantial increase in the past decade in research on the prevention of falls among older persons. Considerable evidence now exists that most falls among older persons are associated with identifiable and modifiable risk factors and that targeted prevention efforts are shown to be cost-effective. There is compelling evidence to support the use of multidisciplinary, multifactorial, health and environmental approaches to fall

五、护理措施

实施老年跌倒的干预具有挑战性，尤其是对有跌倒史的老年人。其护理目标是明确原因、减少跌倒的发生，并减轻跌倒所致伤害的严重程度。

1. 跌倒的预防 老年跌倒的发生是由许多危险因素引起的，采取针对性的预防措施能在较大程度上降低跌倒的发生。已有证据支持使用多学科、多因素、健康和环境方法来预防跌倒。预防老年人跌倒的综合方法通常包括评估和干预相结合。

prevention. A comprehensive approach to fall prevention among seniors typically includes a combination of assessment and interventions. The interventions are as followings:

(1) Providing education and information: Education is an important and fundamental component of most successful falls prevention strategies. It can build an awareness of the importance of falls within all sectors of society that are impacted by falls and fall-related injuries. Education of patients and caregivers can be considered as primary and secondary prevention measures and is also important for the implementation and sustained use of fall prevention strategies. In many cultures, falling is considered to be a normal, unavoidable consequence of growing older. By applying such an approach to educating old adults about falls and fall prevention, not only would old adults become more aware of the importance of paying close attention to fall-related risk factors and determinants but they would also be more likely to take action to correct these challenges to their health and independence. Both informal and formal caregivers have a critical role to play in building awareness about the importance of falls and falls prevention. It is especially important to provide family members, peer counsellors and other informal caregivers with information and training on how to identify risk factors for falls and how to take action to decrease the likelihood of falling among those at greatest risk. It is also critical to ensure that formal caregivers are fully familiar with the latest evidence related to the assessment, prevention, and treatment of falls.

Key aspects of education include: information about data on fatal and nonfatal fall injuries and healthcare costs, information about fall risk factors among older adults, information about effective fall prevention intervention, information about where can go for further help and advice and information about how to cope if a fall happens.

Effective education may take many forms, including printed materials as handouts, discussion groups or the use of the media. Trained peer volunteers are well received by other seniors as reliable sources of information. Timing is also an important aspect of effective education programs. A senior who has had a recent fall is more likely to be receptive to learning about prevention than someone who has never fallen.

Education for older adults and their caregivers can be delivered to individuals or to groups. Individual education sessions may work better for people who are hearing or

（1）健康教育：在社区内向公众开展健康教育，是预防跌倒发生的有效措施。开展健康教育，可以增强公众对老年跌倒的预防意识，提高知晓率并引导大家采取健康行动。

健康教育的内容可包括老年跌倒的危险因素、跌倒可导致的后果和医疗费用、预防跌倒的措施及跌倒后的自我处置与他人救助。

健康教育可以采用不同的形式，如发放宣传手册、进行媒体宣传或者组织小组讨论等。同伴教育也是健康教育的有效方式。与从未摔倒的人相比，近期摔倒的老年人更容易接受预防方面的知识。

可以向老年人及其照顾者开展个体化或团体的健康教育。对于听力或视力障碍或有

vision impaired or have special needs. Sessions should be tailored to the attention span and cognitive ability of older adults. Visual aids such as brochures, fact sheets, and checklists will help facilitate the education session. Group sessions provide the benefits of social interactions. Informal group discussions that include sharing personal experiences may reduce anxiety and increase motivation to adopt new behaviors. Group teaching saves time and helps spread the information more quickly to more people.

(2) Exercise programs: Exercise can improve balance, mobility and reaction time. It can increase bone mineral density in post-menopausal women in people age 70 and over. The falls exercise programs typically involved cardiovascular endurance, muscle strength, flexibility and balance. Research studies have supported both general physical activities, such as walking, cycling, mild aerobic movements or other endurance activities, and specific exercise regimes that are geared towards balance, strength or flexibility.

Evidence confirmed showed programs of muscle strengthening and balance retraining, individually prescribed by a trained health professional, was likely to be beneficial. Moreover, it should be noticed that participation in vigorous exercise activities for instance intensive running in older age may increase the risk of falls. Promoting appropriate exercises to improve strength, balance, and flexibility is one of the most feasible and cost-effective strategies to prevent fall among older adults in the community. Exercise interventions must be developed and adopted with careful consideration to the individual's abilities because optimal levels of intensity are unclear and some programs may actually increase the risk of falls.

Activities such as outdoor walking or mall walking indoors are the most feasible and accessible way of exercising that improves strength, balance and flexibility leading to a reduction on the risk of falling. Recently, Tai Chi has drawn more and more attention within the rehabilitation/geriatric community. Tai Chi is an ancient Chinese martial art consisting of a series of slow but continuous movements of every body part. Tai Chi movements incorporate elements of strengthening, balance, postural alignment, and concentration, and then benefit older people for fall prevention. Additionally, there are some other balance trainings. Standing on one leg is an exercise that can be practiced anywhere you have a chair or counter to hold on to. This exercise will strengthen your ankles and hips,

特殊需求的人，个体化教育更适宜。教育内容应针对老年人的感觉和认知能力进行量身定制。健康宣传册有助于简化教育过程。小组讨论是一种高效的健康教育方式，可分享个人经验，并提高行为改变的动力。

（2）锻炼：坚持进行有规律的体育锻炼，可以增强肌肉力量，提高身体的柔韧性、协调性、平衡能力、步态稳定性和灵活性，从而减少跌倒的发生。

锻炼时应避免参加剧烈活动，运动量应以老年人自身的健康状态为基础，量力而行，循序渐进，以防止社区内老年人发生跌倒。

适合老年人的运动包括太极拳、散步等。其中，太极拳是我国优秀的传统健身运动，研究发现，太极拳可以有效预防跌倒。此外，平衡训练有利于帮助老年人保持稳定性。

which are vital in keeping us stable.

(3) Medication management: Many older adults are unaware that their daily medications may increase their fall risk. Aging affects the absorption, distribution, metabolism, and elimination of medications. Age can also increase sensitivity to potential side effects. Older adults may get prescriptions from multiple doctors. Fall risk increases with the total number of prescription and over-the-counter medications. Medication review and management is to identify and eliminate medication side effects and interactions, such as dizziness or drowsiness, which can increase the risk of falls.

Medication reviews can be done by a pharmacist or physician. Coordinated medication management that involves changing or reducing types or dosages of medications, should be done by the older adult's healthcare provider. When medications are routinely assessed in patients with falls risk, their use will be minimized whenever possible. Pharmacist involvement assists prescribers in determining whether a lower dose of a medication or an alternate drug has less falls risk potential, considering laboratory test results (i. e. , renal and hepatic function) and side effects. Further, pharmacists can assist prescribers with medication selection for patients known to be at high risk for falls. Pharmacists also review medications for increased falls risk when prescriptions orders are being filled. If providers are not knowledgeable about the contraindications for patients at high risk for falls, then the pharmacy staff may provide information to prescribers about which medications have fewer side effects. Targeted warnings to seniors taking these drugs are needed, to alert them to the heightened risk of falls. Examples include drugs taken to treat acute infections, such as lung and bladder infections. Drugs taken to treat diabetes and cardiac disease are also more highly associated with a risk of falling, pointing to the role of these chronic conditions in increasing the risk of falling.

Additionally, medication review and management may include assessing the need for vitamin D and calcium supplements as well as osteoporosis treatment. Vitamin D deficiency is common in older people and when present impairs muscle strength and possibly neuromuscular function. Older persons with suspected vitamin D deficiency should be routinely offered supplementation to reduce fall risk. Moreover, vitamin D supplementation at appropriate levels should also be considered for all older adults.

(4) Vision improvement: Aging is often associated with changes in visual acuity, development of cataracts,

（3）合理用药：老年人可能服用多种药物。跌倒风险随用药种类的增加而增加。有些药物存在头晕或嗜睡的副作用而导致老年人跌倒，要注意识别和避免此类药物。

请医生检查老年人服用的所有药物。有跌倒风险的患者使用能增加跌倒危险的药物时，应尽可能减少用药剂量。可根据实验室检查（如肝肾功能）和药物副作用，评估患者使用药物后跌倒的风险。避免同时服用多种药物，应了解药物的不良反应并注意用药后的反应。此外，药剂师可协助医生开处方。例如某些抗感染药、治疗糖尿病和心脏病的药物与跌倒风险的高度相关，使用时应当注意。

还应注意补充适量的维生素 D 和钙剂，预防和治疗骨质疏松。

（4）改善视力：视力改变、白内障、黄斑变性、青光眼与跌倒有关。应评估其视力，

macular degeneration, glaucoma, and other conditions that would suggest an effect on risk of falling. If patients report problems or concerns, their vision should be formally assessed, and any remediable visual abnormalities should be treated, particularly cataracts. Some vision problems can be corrected with corrective lenses. Progressive lenses may give better quality vision of surroundings; however, it is not recommended that older patients be switched from bifocal to progressive lenses or vice versa.

Opticians can warn older persons that it takes time to adjust to new lenses, particularly multi-focal lenses and that during this period they may be at high risk for a fall or associated injury, particularly on stairs. Simple suggestions include making sure the environment is well-lit, avoiding neutral colors, avoiding clutter and remembering to remove reading glasses when moving around.

(5) Assistive devices and other protective equipment: Assistive and protective devices such as canes, walkers, safety poles or bathroom grab bars are often recommended to reduce the risk of falling. For those elders with gait and balance disorders, canes and walkers can be used to maintain or improve mobility. Ambulation devices, such as a cane or walker, increase the elder's standing and walking base of support and stability. Furthermore, their use can play an important role increasing senior's confidence and encouraging independence. If assistive devices are inappropriate for the physical impairment of elderly, they may actually increase the risk of falls. The specific device should be selected and fitted to the needs of older person with the help of a physical therapist or prosthetist. It's very important to make sure the cane is the right height and that the rubber tips are checked every once in a while to ensure they are still in good shape.

Hip protectors can significantly reduce the risk for hip fracture in people at risk for falls. A wide variety of hip-protectors are now on the market, most of which feature a plastic or foam oval shaped shield that covers the hip area. Worn over the hip in a pair of undergarments or exercise shorts, the shield absorbs the impact of a fall or disperses the energy of the fall over a wider area, therefore decreasing the likelihood of a bone fracture.

(6) Managing foot and footwear problems: Foot problems are common in older population and are related to impaired balance and performance in tests of function. The type and condition of footwear may also contribute to the risk of falling. Comfortable shoes that provide good support can help to prevent falls. Lower heels are easier on your feet and back, and are more stable for walking. Elastic laces are available to make laced shoes easier to get on and

并治疗或纠正视觉异常。有视力障碍的老年人应佩戴矫正视力的眼镜。

在佩戴老视镜，尤其多焦点眼镜时要逐渐适应，在行走或爬楼梯过程中要注意安全。确保环境光线充足，走动时记得摘下老花镜。

（5）辅助工具和其他保护性装置：根据个人需要选择适当的辅助工具。使用的拐杖长度要合适，要经常检查橡皮底垫是否磨损。

有针对性地使用髋部保护器能有效预防跌倒后引起的髋部骨折。

（6）选择合适的鞋袜：舒适的鞋可以提供良好的支撑作用来预防跌倒。老年人应该尽量不穿高跟鞋、拖鞋，不宜穿鞋底过于柔软、容易滑倒的鞋。

off. Beware: easy-on shoes or slippers (without heels) can be dangerous; shoes with smooth, slippery soles can cause a fall; and composition soles, such as crepe soles, can stick to carpets and trip you.

(7) Environment modification: Environmental hazards are any objects or circumstances in the environment that increase an individual's risk of falling and may be within the home and grounds (commonly termed home falls hazards) or away from the home (public falls hazards). Identification and mitigation of environmental hazards has been a recommended component of many successful fall prevention programs.

In and around home: Environmental factors play a part in approximately half of all falls that occur at home. Modifications include removing clutter and securing electrical cords and loose carpets to prevent tripping; installing grab bars and handrails; improving lighting and keeping a working flashlight nearby; and improving shower and tub safety. An important aspect of successful home modifications is ensuring that the identified hazards are actually corrected. When modify home environment, there are some considerations (box 11-4).

In public spaces: The project of reducing public fall hazards need pull together government officials, seniors, city maintenance workers, and building owners to examine and reduce fall hazards in the community. A telephone hotline enabled people to report falls and hazards, leading to a repair or spray-painting of the hazard until the repair could be done. Public awareness campaigns can also educate the community about fall hazards – municipal workers, seniors, caregivers, letter carriers, and others are well situated to observe and report on fall hazards in need of repair.

Box 11-4 Considerations for Modifying Home Environment

When modify home environment, should consider the followings:

- Keep all areas of the home, including hallways and stairs, well-lit, but free from glare.

- Remove scatter rugs, or attach a nonskid backing to them.

- Reduce the risk of falling on uncarpeted floors by ensuring that they are not slippery. Do not use any gloss polish.

- Use night lights in the bedroom, hall-ways, kitchen and bathrooms.

（7）环境改造：环境危害来自室内和室外。识别并减少环境中的危险因素对预防跌倒非常重要。

超过半数的老年人跌倒是在家中发生的，因此家庭内部的环境改造非常重要。改进措施包括移走可能影响老年人活动的障碍物，固定好电线和地毯，安装好牢固的扶手，改善照明条件，把手电筒放在触手可及的地方，提高卫生间安全性（box 11-4）。

政府官员、城市和社区管理人员、老年人群体应共同关注社区公共环境安全。群众也可以利用热线电话举报公共环境中的危险因素，从而使其得到整治。

Box 11-4 家庭环境改造的注意事项

对家庭环境改造时，应考虑以下方面内容：

- 确保家中，包括走廊和楼梯所有区域的良好照明，但不要刺眼。
- 除去所有的小块地毯，或者在后面贴上防滑地垫。
- 地面（板）不宜光滑，不要抛光。

- 在床旁、过道、厨房和卫生间安装夜明灯。

- Keep the stove area in the kitchen free of towels, paper towels, napkins, curtains, and other things that might catch fire.

- Remove all newspapers & magazines from the kitchen counter areas.

- Keep a fire extinguisher in the kitchen, and teach everyone of age to use it.

- Inspect electrical cords for fraying or cracking; be sure they are placed away from walking paths, but not under carpet or furniture, where they could present a fire hazard.

- Set the hot water temperature at 46℃ or below on the water heater.

- Use slip-resistant decals or non-skid mats in the tub or shower.

- Install grab bars in the bathtub and by the toilet; be sure the screws go directly into the wall studs, so they stay securely in place.

- Check to be sure that extension cords are not overloaded & are clear of walkways.

- Install smoke detectors on every floor of the home and test them monthly.

- Destroy out-of-date medications and those which are no longer being used.

- Place a telephone in the bedroom.

- Post emergency numbers by all telephones.

- Keep space heaters away from flammable materials, and be sure the room is well ventilated.

- A three-pronged plug should be used in a three hole outlet, or an adapter should be used.

- Always turn off heating pads before an older person goes to sleep.

(8) Addressing fear of falling: When older people have falls-even if the fall is not serious-they often become fearful of falling again. This can lead to inactivity that can cause additional health problems. Any interventions that reduce the risk for falls are likely to reduce a person's fear of falling, but some people need additional interventions to address this problem. Building confidence or fall-related efficacy is crucial and important to decrease FOF.

- 厨房炉灶旁不要放置毛巾、纸巾、餐巾、窗帘和其他可能会着火的物品。

- 报纸和杂志不可放在厨房的台面上。

- 厨房应备家用灭火器，教会所有人如何使用。

- 检查电线是否磨损或破裂，不可放置于过道，也不可放于地毯或家具下，以免成为火灾隐患。

- 热水器的水温设置在46℃以下。

- 沐浴时使用防滑贴或防滑垫。

- 浴缸和马桶旁安装扶手，确保螺丝固定牢固。

- 电线延长线不可超载，不可放在过道上。

- 在每层安装烟雾探测器，每月进行一次功能测试。

- 销毁过期的及不再使用的药物。

- 卧室内应安装电话。

- 在每一部电话旁贴上紧急电话的号码。

- 暖气旁边不可放置易燃的材料，并确保房间内通风良好。

- 三线插头应使用三孔插座，或配有适配器。

- 老年人入睡前应关掉电热垫。

（8）克服害怕跌倒的心理：老年人跌倒后常产生害怕跌倒的心理，从而减少正常活动。应通过增强老年人的自信心、自我效能提供社会支持以减少老年人对跌倒的恐惧。

Intervention to reduce fear of falling through group sessions is also effective for participants who are less physically impaired, have greater concern about falling and have greater self-efficacy in making changes. Also, increased social support is needed as a means to lessening fear.

2. Coping with falls Although some falls can be preventable, some falls cannot be avoided. Lying on the floor or ground for some time can lead to additional problems, such as pressure sores, dehydration or going without usual medicines. An experience like this can also be quite distressing, both at the time and afterwards. If an old person lives alone, or is alone for long periods, he or she needs a plan to get help quickly. A good plan will involve how to call for help and how to get up.

(1) Calling help: Personal emergency response systems (PERS) are electronic devices designed to provide frail older persons with a means to summon assistance in the event of a fall, and thus prevent a lengthy lie time. While they do not prevent people from falling, they can reduce the seriousness of injury complications by ensuring prompt treatment and reduced harm. They increase the elder's feeling of security and confidence as well as allay family fears regarding the safety of their loved one. These devices are worn on the person's body or clothing. When a person falls, he or she can press the button that signals an emergency call center. Help can then be obtained quickly. The effectiveness of alerting system depends on the ability of the fallen person to signal for help and on the availability of a helping person. A major limitation of such devices is that cognitively impaired people may not be able to learn to use them.

(2) Getting up: Teaching elderly knowing how to get up by themselves is very important. The instructions are as followings. Calm down and take some deep breaths. Check the body for any injuries. Can the person move their legs and arms? Is the person in pain? Is there any obvious deformity? Are bones sticking out, swelling, bleeding, and unusual position of the limbs? Has the person hit their head? Does the person appear grey in color? Is the person unconscious?

If he or she has not been seriously injured and can get up, he or she can follow these six steps for getting up (figure 11-4):

a. Roll onto his side, and push up into sitting position.

b. Turn onto his hands and knees, and crawl to the nearest stable furniture, e. g. bed, chair, stool, toilet.

2. 跌倒后的处理 虽然部分跌倒可以预防和避免，但是有些跌倒却是不可预知、无法避免的。跌倒后，如果长时间躺在地上不能起来，可以导致压疮、脱水，甚至死亡。要使老年人学会并正确使用在无人帮助的情况下求救和安全起身的方法。

（1）寻求帮助：紧急呼救系统（PERS）是一种电子设备，可以帮助老年人在跌倒后寻求救助。跌倒后，按动呼叫按钮，就可以与急救中心联系，并获得救护。但认知障碍的老年人可能无法使用这类设备。

（2）跌倒后起身：教会老年人跌倒后如何起身非常重要。如果在家中或室外无人的地方跌倒后不要紧张，先放松，深呼吸。检查身体有无损伤，能否移动，头部有无撞伤，肢体有无疼痛、畸形等。

如果受伤不严重，能够自行爬起，可以采用下面6个步骤站起来（图11-4）：

a. 转至侧身，用手推起身体坐下来。

b. 转身用手和膝盖按着地面，然后爬向离身体最近的家具或其他容易借力的物体，

c. Place his hands on the seat.

d. Place one foot flat on the floor.

e. Lean forward and push up with the other foot.

f. Sit, rest, and then tell someone he has fallen.

For elderly, It is important to talk to doctor about the fall and the possible causes and to tell someone else (family, friend or neighbor) that he or she has fallen.

例如床、椅子、搁脚凳、马桶、树木、长椅、假山等。

c. 用双手按着座椅或其他固定物。

d. 单膝跪地，将一只脚平放在地板上。

e. 身体向前倾斜，然后用平放的脚支撑站起来。

f. 坐下休息，然后向他人汇报跌倒的情况。

对老年人而言，非常重要的是要告知医生自己跌倒的相关情况以及可能的导致跌倒的原因，并通知其他人（家人、朋友或邻居）自己摔倒了。

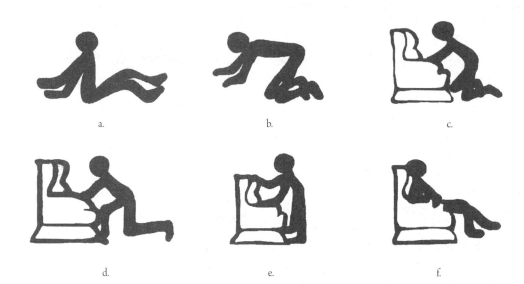

Figure 11-4　Steps for getting up

If a person is seriously injured, he can't get up. He should:

a. Call for help.

b. Keep warm. Use anything that is near, such as bedding, a coat, even a tablecloth. If he is wet, move away from the damp area to keep warm.

c. Move his limbs. Gently moving his arms and legs will help his circulation, and reduce pressure areas.

如果受伤严重，不能自行爬起来，则应采取以下措施：

a. 求救。

b. 保持温暖，用任何可随手拿到的物品保暖，如床单、衣服、台布等。如果跌倒在有水的地方，则需设法挪动身体离开潮湿处，尽量保暖。

c. 活动手脚，轻轻摆动，以助血液循环，防止身体局部过度受压。

Section 2　Scalding

Scalding usually occurs in the home environment and the problem of scald injuries also sustained in the home environment. Scalds are among the most distressing injuries as they can affect a person's physical and mental well-being. About fifty percent of all burn injuries concern scalds. Scald injuries always carry a high burden of disease and subsequent scarring. Due to their frequency and high admission rates, scald injuries are also associated with high economic costs. A survey in Guangdong shows that the main causes of injury include traffic accident, falling and scalding. They are also the main injury causes of death. Scald burns regarded as being preventable. So prevention of scald injuries is very important especially in elderly person.

Box 11-5　Case Study

A 71-year-old woman with a dense right hemiplegia who lived in home presented. She had been lowered into a hot bath by families who had not checked the temperature of the water. Her scalds were estimated to be 37% of her body surface area. She was rushed to nearby hospitals for treatment. She was resuscitated and the burns managed conservatively. She developed cardiac failure and died seven days after admission.

Questions:

1. What information is relevant to this case?

2. What are the current problems for home care?

3. What's your suggestion about improving the present situation of this private nursing home?

I. Definition of Scalding

Scalding (from the Latin word calidus, meaning hot) is a form of heat burns (thermal burn) resulted from heated fluids such as boiling water or steam. A survey in the Netherlands shows that from the analysis of injury data already presented, three risk groups appear: young children (0–4 years), young adults (15–24 years) and the elderly (55 years and older). And for the elderly, the incidence of fatal burn injuries is higher than for younger persons. The injury mortality rate of the elderly is the

第二节　老年人烫伤的护理

烫伤常常发生于居家环境中，烫伤不仅给老年人的机体组织带来损伤，也同样影响老年人的心理健康，从而影响其生活质量。降低导致烫伤发生危险因素，减少老年人烫伤的发生十分重要。

Box 11-5　案例

老年女性，71 岁，左侧肢体偏瘫。现居住于家中。家属帮助她进行淋浴时，并没有事先检查和确认水温。导致其体表皮肤约 37% 被烫伤，被紧急送往附近的医院。入院后已苏醒，并进行保守治疗。但入院后第 7 天因心力衰竭死亡。

问题：

1. 从以上案例中你可以获取哪些相关的信息？

2. 该家庭照顾中目前可能存在的问题有哪些？

3. 你认为应如何改善？

一、烫伤的定义

烫伤是指由于热液（如沸水）、蒸汽等所引起的组织损伤，是热力烧伤的一种。相关研究表明，55 岁以上的老年人是烫伤的多发人群之一。老年人群中致死性烫伤的发生率要高于年轻人，老年人的伤害死亡率是所有年龄组中最高的。热的液体导致的烫伤是老年人最多发的烫伤形式。

highest of all age groups. Scald burns from hot liquids are the most common burns to older adults.

II. Factors Contributing to Scalding

1. Age Older adults are at a higher risk for scalding, mostly scald burns from hot liquids. It has been well documented that an older aged population is at higher risk for burn injury as a result of several predisposing factors that are associated with increased age. These factors include reduced reaction time, poorer dexterity, decreased flexibility, inaccurate assessment of risks, impaired senses, and higher incidence of premorbid conditions, such as chronic disease, alcoholism, medications, senility, and neurological and psychiatric disorders.

2. Gender Men have burn injuries more often than women.

3. Age-related change The function of the nervous system declined with aging. The sensory systems include touch (pressure, heat, and pain) and eyes (vision) change with human aging process. Loss of skin elasticity, peripheral circulation undesirable can decrease the skin heat tolerance. Redness, swollenness, blister, ulcer may appear on the heated area easier. Burns of different depth may occur when this last for a long period. The elderly suffer from a higher instance of burn injury as a result of their thinner skin, poorer microcirculation, and increased susceptibility to infection.

4. Thermal application Most scalds result from exposure to high-temperature water, such as tap water in baths and showers, hot foot bath or cooking water boiled for the preparation of foods. Another common cause of scalds is spilled hot drinks, such as coffee. Scalds are typically far more severe when caused by steam, because it has absorbed a great amount of latent heat, and is therefore far more effective at heating objects. Moreover, thermotherapy such as for pain relief and health that can take the form of hot compresses, hot water bags, hot lamps, sits bath, electric heating pads, and others. Improper use of thermotherapy also can lead to scalding.

III. Nursing Assessment

1. General situation Before applying thermotherapy, it's important to assess the elderly people's physical condition for signs of potential intolerance to heat and the skin area including its integrity and local

二、烫伤的主要危险因素

1. **年龄** 烫伤的发生随年龄增长而逐渐增加。老年人由于反应力、灵活性下降，对危险因素的估计不足，判断力下降及其自身原因，如慢性疾病、酗酒、药物、衰老和神经精神疾病，均可增加其发生烫伤的危险。

2. **性别** 男性烫伤的发生率高于女性。

3. **老化因素** 老年人感觉神经系统的生理性老化，触觉、温痛觉减退，视力下降，皮肤组织衰老，末梢循环功能下降，使老年人对热的耐受力下降，受热后皮肤容易发生红肿、水疱及破溃等不同程度的烫伤。

4. **热应用因素** 大部分烫伤由于盆浴、淋浴、泡脚时水温过高或烹饪时的沸水所致。导致烫伤的另一个常见原因是溢出的热饮料，如咖啡。由蒸汽导致的烫伤通常更严重。热疗法具有缓解疼痛的作用，有益于健康，热疗法的形式可以有热敷，热水袋，烤灯，坐浴，电热毯等。热疗法使用不当也会导致烫伤。

三、护理评估

1. **一般状况的评估** 在进行热疗之前，应当了解老年人的身体状况、局部皮肤的完整性、肢体感觉、末梢循环情况及其对热疗

circulation to which the heat will be applied. In addition, it is also necessary to determine the elderly people's ability to tolerate the therapy and identify conditions that might contraindicate treatment, such as bleeding, circulatory impairment. Prior to the application of heat, the elderly people's level of sensation should be assessed in the same way.

2. Thermal application Assessing whether the elderly people use the heat application and whether or not in a right way, for example hot-water bags, hot lamps, electric blankets, hand warmerset, etc.

3. Estimation of burn depth Burns injure the skin layers and can also injure other parts of the body, such as muscles, blood vessels, nerves, lungs, and eyes. Burns are defined as first-, second-, third-, or fourth-degree, depending on how many layers of skin and tissue are burned. The deeper the burn and the larger the burned area, the more serious the burn is. The seriousness of a burn is also determined by several things, including depth, size, cause, affected body area, age, and health ofthe burn victim (figure 11-5).

的耐受情况。识别可能的禁忌证，如出血、循环障碍。

2. 热应用的评估 了解老年人是否应用热水袋、电热毯、护手宝、烤灯等，及应用时是否能够正确地使用。

3. 烧烫伤程度的评估 烧伤会伤害皮肤，还可能伤害身体的其他部位，如肌肉，血管，神经，肺部和眼睛。烧伤的严重程度取决于深度、面积、年龄和烧伤患者的健康状况（图 11-5）。

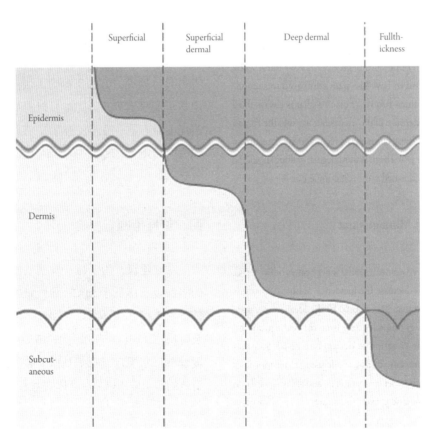

Figure 11-5 Diagram of the different burn depths

(1)First-degree burns are burns at the epidermis of skin. With only a red but intact epidermis, the functions of the skin are preserved. First-degree burns are obvious to everyone and require no treatment.

(2)Second-degree burns are a spectrum that can be arbitrarily divided into superficial and deep:

a. Superficial second-degree burns extend into superficial (papillary) of skin. With deeper but still superficial partial-thickness injury, the outer skin is gone but the contour of the skin is preserved. When providing the proper environment in this type of burn wound, healing should occur with little or no scar formation in 10 days or less. These wounds manifest severe pain as a result of exposure of the nerve endings in the wound, particularly during dressing changes.

b. Deep second-degree burns extend into deep (reticular) dermis. These burns have a more homogenous, but still red, appearance in the dermal bed. The area may even be covered with a white eschar for the first 10 days that eventually thins and disappears. The healing process takes from 10 to 21 days for epithelial coverage and may leave a significant scar.

(3) Third-degree burns (full-thickness burns) injure all the skin layers and tissue under the skin. There are no epidermal cells left to resurface the wound. These burns extends through entire dermis and even into underlying fat, muscle and bone third-degree burns have thick, white eschar and tend to have less pain compared to second-degree burn injury. Brown or black eschar is always third degree with extension of the thermal injury into the fat and deeper tissues. These burns always require medical treatment. Once it is clear that a burn is third degree, grafting should be planned and performed as expeditiously as possible.

IV. Nursing Management

Experts recommend setting water heaters below 50°C. Approaches to decrease the incidence of hot water scalds have suggested that 50°C would be the ideal temperature for tap water, giving adequate time for realization and retrieval of the situation to occur (box 11-6). So other measures to prevent scalds include using a thermometer to measure bath water temperatures, and splash guards on stoves. The specific prevention strategies are showed in table 11-6.

（1）Ⅰ度烧伤：损伤限于表皮浅层。症状是伤处皮肤发红，疼痛不剧烈。可自然愈合，无瘢痕。

（2）Ⅱ度烧伤：分为浅Ⅱ度烧伤和深Ⅱ度烧伤。

a. 浅Ⅱ度烧伤：损伤至真皮乳头层，症状是伤处红肿、起水疱，可有剧烈疼痛和灼热感。可自然愈合，无瘢痕或轻微瘢痕。

b. 深Ⅱ度烧伤：损伤为表皮和真皮深部，症状是患处发红、起白色大水疱，由于神经末梢部分受损，疼痛较浅Ⅱ度要轻。可自然愈合，会留下瘢痕。

（3）Ⅲ度烧伤：全层皮肤损伤。伤处呈皮革状黑色焦痂或苍白。可有流液现象。由于大部分神经末梢损坏，此类烧伤者经常无患处疼痛感。Ⅰ度和浅Ⅱ度烧伤为轻度烧伤，伤者可自行处理，方法正确则很快痊愈。严重烧伤可能导致死亡，如能及时得到专业烧伤治疗（而不是一般医院治疗），存活的可能和预后情况会大大改善。

四、护理措施

专家建议，为了减少烫伤的发生，理想的水温设置应低于50℃。研究证实，当水温低于50℃时，个体可以对所发生的情况做出及时反应（box 11-6）。因此，诸如沐浴时用温度计测量水温以及在炉灶前安装防溅罩都是有效的预防烫伤措施。具体措施见表11-6。

Box 11-6　Relationship between Water Temperature and Scalding

From classical experiments on human and porcine skin, it has long been known that a partial thickness bum is sustained within 5 seconds if the water temperature exceeds 65 ℃ . Below 44 ℃ this time would be 6 hours, rising exponentially until at 50℃ it would take 2-3 minutes.

Box 11-6　水温与烫伤的关系

人们很早便从对人和猪的皮肤进行相关的实验而知，如果持续接触水温超过 65℃的热水 5 秒钟，便可造成局部较深程度的烫伤，如果水温在 44℃以下则为 6 小时，随水温上升造成皮肤损伤所需的时间则越短，当水温上升到 50℃时，2～3 分钟即可造成皮肤的损伤。

Table11-6　Burn Prevention Strategies

Activity	Recommendations for burn risk reduction
● Bathing and showering	● Supervision while bathing ● Liquid crystal thermometer in tub, do not enter tub if temperature exceeds 50°C ● Run cold water first then add hot water to reduce risk of burn by falling into tub while its being filled ● Test water with a fully sensible body part before entering ● Clearly label hot and cold valves ● For single valve units, turn valve to cold after tub is filled ● Thermostat on water heaters limiting maximum water temperature to 50°C ● Tighten or remove hot water valve after tub is filled ● Install a tempering valve in bathroom (commercially available) to limit maximum water temperature to 50°C ● Install 'push and turn' valves to reduce risk of accidental valve opening or closing ● Install an anti-scald safety device (commercially available) which reduces water flow when temperature exceeds a set temperature ● Minimize bathing and showering duration and frequency
● Cooking	● Supervision ● Hot foods prepared by others ● Use of microwave ovens ● Install fitted guards on hot elements ● Use of self-sealing deep fat fryers instead of chip pans ● Use of insulated plastic kettles (commercially available) ● Use of stoves with controls and supplies at front to reduce reaching across hot stove ● Avoid wearing loose clothing such as night gowns when cooking ● Avoid wearing synthetic clothing (e. g. polyester) while cooking ● Minimize number of hot dishes prepared
● Therapeutic heating devices	● Lie under heating pad instead of on top of it ● Avoid use in areas of compromised blood supply ● Use heating pads with thermostats ● Avoid areas where skin is thinnest ● Flame-retardant furniture ● Minimize frequency and duration of use (12-20 consecutive hours at 42-43°C has been shown to cause partial skin thickness burns)
● Resting in front of fireplace or heaters	● Supervision ● Keep adequate distance from heat source ● Keep insensible body parts farthest from heat source

Activity	Recommendations for burn risk reduction
• Smoking	• Allow others to light cigars/cigarettes • Allow others to refill lighters with lighter fluid to avoid spills onto clothing Caution with prescribing sedatives to patients who smoke • Flame-retardant apron covering front and back • Flame retardant furniture and wheelchairs • Smoke detectors • Sprinkler systems • Advise to quit
• Home oxygen therapy	• Caution with prescribing if patient continues to smoke

表 11-6 烫伤的防护策略

活动	降低烫伤风险的建议
• 洗澡和淋浴	• 洗澡时监护 • 用水温计对浴缸内水温进行测量和显示，如果水温度超过 50℃，则不要进入 • 先打开冷水然后向内添加热水调节温度，以防意外落入满是热水的浴缸而被烫伤 • 进入浴缸前，选择身体的一部分先进入水中进行水温适宜度的测量 • 冷热水阀门上应有明显清楚的标志 • 若是单阀门，使用完毕后一定将其旋转至冷水方向处 • 恒温热水器内水的最高的温度应设定在 50℃ • 浴缸接满水后，及时拧紧或移开热水的出水阀 • 浴室应安装调温阀，以限制水温不可超过 50℃ • 选择推动式控制（非旋转式）的阀门 • 安装防烫伤安全装置，当水温超过了预先的设定温度时，可以使水流减少 • 缩短洗澡时间、减少洗澡的频率
• 烹饪	• 监护 • 避免接触热的食物，尽量由他人准备 • 使用微波炉 • 热的装置上安装合适的防护装置 • 用饼铛代替平底锅 • 使用外层绝缘的塑料水壶 • 避免跨越烤箱或火炉 • 烹饪时不要穿宽松的衣服，如睡衣 • 烹饪时不要穿涤纶之类合成纤维质地的衣服 • 减少过热菜品的数量
• 热疗装置的使用	• 不可直接躺在加热垫上 • 不可用于血液供应不足的区域 • 选用带恒温器的电热毯 • 避开皮肤较薄的部位 • 选择阻燃家具 • 减少使用频率和持续时间（已证明，在 42~43℃ 条件下，连续使用 12~20 小时将导致局部皮肤深度的烫伤）
• 在壁炉或加热器前休息	• 监护 • 与热源保持合适的距离 • 无知觉的身体部位应远离热源

续表
活动	降低烫伤风险的建议
● 吸烟	● 请其他人帮助点烟 ● 请他人帮助充打火机，避免打火机液洒在衣服上 ● 前后围好能阻燃的围裙 ● 使用阻燃的家具和轮椅 ● 配备烟雾探测器 ● 配备喷洒灭火系统 ● 建议戒烟
● 家庭氧疗	● 如果患者一直吸烟，则应谨慎开具处方

Section 3　Falling Bed

第三节　老年人坠床的护理

To the sick and elderly, falling bed can mean injury and possible worsening of their conditions. Among the elderly individuals, the main causes of accidental deaths in bed are head injuries caused by falls from bed and asphyxia caused by pressure to the neck when wedged against a bed rail. Patient falls from bed are a source of constant concern to hospital and nursing service administrators. They occur at an alarmingly regular rate and have significant impact on liability insurance premiums and on the general quality of patient care. The best source of information on falls from bed is the mandatory hospital incident report, completed by the examining physician and a registered nurse on the unit in which the fall occurred. Many assumptions are made regarding the cause of falls from bed, but the literature is relatively devoid of research. Prevention of falls is thus a matter of great concern in the healthcare industry.

对于老年人而言，坠床的发生往往意味着伤害或是使其健康状态受损。由于坠床所导致的头部受伤和窒息是老年人群床上意外死亡的主要原因。因此，老年人的坠床问题应受到医院和护理服务管理员的关注。如何有效地预防老年人的坠床问题，也是医疗保健行业极为关注的问题。

Box 11-7　Case Study

A 72-year-old man is hospitalized for management of his hypertension. He has a history of functional urinary incontinence and cataract. The nursing staff observes him climbing over the side rails on numerous occasions at night on route to the bathroom. He is quite agitated during this time. The nursing assistant requests that you obtain an order for a body restraint at night to prevent him from falling out of bed.

Questions:

1. Should this client be restrained to prevent injury?

Box 11-7　案例与思考

患者，男，72岁，因患高血压住院治疗。既往有功能性尿失禁、白内障史。护理人员观察发现其晚间经常在去洗手间的途中翻爬栏杆。患者近期表现烦躁不安。护理助理要求你向医生申请医嘱，即夜间给予患者约束以防止其发生坠床。

问题：

1. 是否应该对该患者进行约束以防止其发生损伤？

2. Would you request the order for a body restraint? Why or why not?

3. What nursing interventions could be tried before considering a restraint?

2. 你是否会申请医生下医嘱对其采取约束？请说明原因。

3. 对该患者采取约束前，可以尝试给予哪些护理干预？

I. Definition of Falling Bed

Falling bed is defined as fall from bed. Relevant researchers found poor room and floor design the major contributing factors in all patient accidents, including falls. In a nursing home environment, people found that most accidents occur in patient rooms, during the evening hours when it is most difficult for the elderly to distinguish between light and dark.

A related survey shows that gender did not appear to be a significant factor of the patients who fell from bed, 47.2 percent were male and 52.8 percent were female. However, 83 percent of patients who fell from bed were over age 65, while this age group represented only 22 percent of the entire patient population. Slightly over one-third of the patients who fell were ambulatory. A cross-tabulation of age with level of activity showed that over 50 percent of patients over age 65 were non-ambulatory. Most patients (83 percent) fell from bed between the hours of 3 p. m and 7 a. m. When comparing the relationship between age and time of fall, it was noted that more patients age 76 and older fell from bed during the evening shift than during the day or night shifts.

II. Factors Contributing to Falling Bed

1. Environmental factors The home environment is critical for avoiding the elderly people falling from bed. High risk factors found in the home include items such as telephone, cup and light switch placed not reasonable that is not convenient for the elderly to reach; poor stability of the bed; unsuitable height, width and hardness of the bed; and absence of bedrails.

2. Physiological factors The rates of falling bed rise steadily with age. It increases markedly among group aged 75 to 85. Normal aging inevitably brings physical, cognitive and affective changes that may contribute to the risk and the injury of falling bed. Delayed response and reaction time can increase the risk of injury related to inability to respond in timely manner.

3. Morbidity Morbidity contributes to falling

一、坠床的定义

坠床是指从床上掉落在地上。在养老院里，大多数的坠床事故发生在患者的房间里，且多发生于老年人视线较差的房间。夜间的坠床发生率明显高于白天。

相关调查显示，性别似乎并不是导致患者坠床的重要因素。83% 的坠床患者，其年龄在 65 岁以上。

二、坠床的主要危险因素

1. **环境因素** 安全的居家环境可避免坠床的发生。常见居家环境危险因素包括，物品摆放不合理，不便于拿取，如电话、水杯、电灯开关等未放置于随手可取处；床的稳固性差，高度、宽度及床的硬度不合适，缺少床挡等。

2. **生理因素** 坠床的发生率与年龄有关，75 岁至 85 岁年龄组老年人坠床率明显增高。老年人的反应时间延长和反应能力下降会增加坠床的风险。

3. **疾病因素** 常见的老年性疾病可增加

bed of the elderly, like geratic diseases. Chronic illness has been also associated with increased the risk of falling bed, arthritis, Parkinson's disease, cardiovascular and cerebrovascular diseases, age-related cataract and glaucoma, orthostatic hypotension, epilepsy, mental disease, and Meniere's disease, etc.

4. Medications Altered pharmacokinetics, self-administration problems, and the high volume of drugs consumed by older individuals can also lead to considerable risks to safety. Risks include adverse effects and accidents resulting from effects such as drowsiness or dizziness. So the agents that have been associated with falls were also found to be associated with falling bed. It is also estimated that 5% to 30% of geriatric admissions to hospitals are associated with inappropriate drug administration.

5. Others Most of the older adults complain of difficulty sleeping. Sleep disorders and use of improper body mechanics are associated with falling bed of the elderly. It is possible that nocturnal hallucinations in the sleep-wake transition may have contributed to sleep-related falling out of bed. In addition, muscle weakness, obesity, alcohol abuse, disturbance of consciousness, and cognitive dysfunction can also lead to falling bed of the elderly.

III. Nursing Assessment

1. General condition The nurse should assess the elderly people regarding history of present illness, past medical history, medication review, history of falling bed, cognitive function, state of consciousness, functional status, life style and whether the elderly is obese.

2. Environmental risk factors When nurses conduct the assessment of the elderly people's risk factors for falling bed, they need to consider all the possible treats, which include hazards in their immediate environment. Sometimes, the family needs to be included to conduct an accurate assessment. Within health care facilities and home, nurses should assess the hazards in their unit. For example, is it easy for them to reach items on a bedside table? Whether use the restraints, side rails, bed-exit alarms, etc. The assessment of nurses and transfer tools is also very important.

IV. Nursing Management

1. Comprehensive assessment Evaluate the

其坠床的危险，如关节炎、帕金森病、心脑血管疾病、眼科疾病、直立性低血压、癫痫、精神病、梅尼埃病等。

4. 药物因素 老年人药物代谢动力学的改变及用药不当导致老年人发生困倦、眩晕进而导致坠床的发生。据估计，5% 到 30% 的老年住院患者坠床与用药不当有关。

5. 其他 各种原因引起的睡眠障碍、肌无力、肥胖、酗酒、意识障碍、认知功能障碍均可导致坠床。

三、护理评估

1. 一般状况的评估 评估老年人现病史、健康史、用药情况及有无坠床史，老年人的认知功能、意识状态、自理活动能力、生活习惯以及是否肥胖等。

2. 环境危险因素评估 评估老年人时应考虑到所有可能的危险因素，包括目前所处环境及内在的危险因素，并邀请老年人的家属参加评估活动。护士应注意评估老年人床单位安全性，如卧床期间，床旁物品是否易于拿取；是否使用约束带、床挡、离床报警器等。评估搬运人员及搬运工具情况。

四、护理措施

1. 综合评估 评估老年人发生坠床的危

elderly fall risk factors of falling bed. Determine the high-risk groups and give them focused protection. Shorten the round time interval, especially for the inpatient at night. To ensure that the hidden dangers can be discovered in time, such as whether the patients with restlessness have been restrained and sleep in the middle of the bed, etc.

2. Safety of the bed A recent study in an acute care hospital in Michigan found that 51.4% of the adult inpatient fall incidents and 56.0% of the adult inpatient injurious falls occurred while the patient was getting out of or back to the bed. One family member emphasized that hospital beds were so high that patients' feet dangled when they were getting out of bed. The researchers claimed that the bed height that is too high (> 120% of lower leg length) can result in unsafe transfer and bed-related falls because of foot placement instability. In addition, recently discharged older adults claim that hospitals should provide lower patient beds. The review study on interventions designed to prevent healthcare bed-related injuries in patients concluded that the effectiveness of the two interventions designed to prevent patient injuries from their beds (low height beds and bed exit alarms) remains inclusive. Therefore, for the elderly the bed should be stable or have been braking. The height and width of the bed should be suitable for the elderly such as the width of the bed should be appropriate widened. Moderate hardness of the mattress is also very important. Do not choose too soft mattress. Bedrails and bedside chairs are commonly used as safety devices to prevent people falling from bed. Both of them are most likely to be used with older. Bedrails are safety devices designed to prevent patients accidentally slipping, sliding, rolling or falling out of bed. If bedrails are designed a safety devices but can also compromise individual patient safety, dignity and autonomy, their use should be explored using these concepts. Their use is often considered a benign, routine, even essential, safety measure. In addition, when change the position, slow action and small activities should keep in mind to ensure their own safety.

3. Safety of the night Pay attention to the security of the elderly at night. Do not go to the bathroom as far as possible when need to urinate at night, especially for the elderly with orthostatic hypotension, or who are taking blood pressure drug. Required items and bedpan should be placed beside the bed. Calling device should be prepared for unaccompanied elderly. It is important for them to get first aid.

险因素，确定高危人群，做好重点防护。对住院的老年人应增加巡视次数，尤其应加强夜间巡视，以随时发现安全隐患问题，如躁动患者是否已给予约束、患者是否睡在床的中央。

2. 床的安全 床应稳固或处于制动状态。床的高度、宽度及床垫硬度适合。适当加宽床的宽度，高度适合于老年人上下床，床垫不可过软。根据情况适当使用床挡或者床旁椅挡护，有条件的应配备离床警报器。此外，告知老年人变换体位动作要缓慢、动作幅度应小一些以确保安全。

3. 夜间安全 直立性低血压及服用镇静催眠或降压药的老年人，夜间尽量不要去卫生间排尿，可将其所需物品及便盆放于床旁。无人陪伴的老年人应配备呼叫装置，对于保证急救护理而言非常重要。

4. Safety education Provide health education and information by distributing brochures, explanation and individual conversation should be used to illustrate the necessity of safety measures. Make the elderly and caregivers know that the importance and the specific operation method of safety precautions. Supervise the implementation of effective safety measures to the elderly in actual work.

4. 安全教育 以宣传手册、讲解、个别交谈等方式对老年人及其照顾者进行宣教与指导，使其清楚了解安全防范措施的重要性及其实施方法。并在实际工作中督导有效措施的实施。

Section 4　Aspiration and Asphyxia

第四节　老年人误吸的护理

Aspiration can cause serious complications, and its occurrence in various diseases can seriously affect the prognosis and quality of life of the elderly. The etiology of aspiration is multifactorial. Oropharyngeal aspiration increases in older adults, which can lead to lung infection and pneumonia. The latter is a major cause of morbidity/mortality and is a leading cause of death among elderly residents in nursing homes. Hospitalizations for aspiration pneumonia have doubled among the elderly. More than 50% of healthy adults aspirate during sleep, and in a previous study, silent aspiration was demonstrated in 71% of patients with pneumonia compared with 10% in control participants.

误吸可引发严重的并发症，伴发于其他多种疾病的误吸严重影响了老年人疾病的预后及生活质量。误吸的原因是多方面的。老年人经口咽部发生的误吸在逐年增加，易导致肺炎的发生。肺炎是造成老年人住院和死亡的主要原因。超过 50% 的误吸发生于睡眠中。

Aspiration is a common occurrence, and in most cases it resolves spontaneously without clinical manifestations. Clinically significant aspiration can range from acute pneumonitis and respiratory failure caused by a single massive aspiration to chronic symptoms of respiratory disease caused by recurrent small-scale aspiration. These syndromes may overlap with pneumonia that occurs when the lungs are exposed to bacteria from the gastrointestinal tract.

大多数情况下，发生误吸后个体可以自发的缓解，而不伴随任何临床表现。一次大量误吸或反复误吸可引起胃肠道细菌侵入呼吸道，引发急性肺炎和呼吸衰竭。

A recent study of food/foreign body asphyxia revealed that observers were present in 63% of the choking events. The fatal incident was correctly identified in only 8% of cases by emergency personnel. Common misdiagnoses were cardiovascular failure; epileptic seizures; and intoxication from medication, drugs, or alcohol. The fatal event of food/foreign body asphyxia may be preventable. Prevention depends on understanding the nature and frequency of food/foreign body asphyxia and its specific causes.

关于食品或异物导致窒息的一项研究显示，63% 的窒息事件中有他人在场。但只有 8% 获得了正确的识别和紧急的救援。由于食物或异物所导致的窒息事件是可以预防的。预防取决于对导致窒息的食物性质及相关其他特殊原因等的了解。窒息常容易被误诊为心力衰竭、癫痫发作、药物或酒精中毒。

Box 11-8　Case Study

A 72-year-old woman, at a fashionable restaurant, is partaking of broiled lobster. At the same time, she is conversing with companions at dinner. Suddenly, she ceases to eat and talk. The dinner companions are perplexed but not alarmed for there is no indication of distress. Then, the old woman suddenly collapses at the table. Attempts at resuscitation are made by the waiters, and her friends. The ambulance arrives and the person is rushed to the nearest hospital emergency room where she is dead on arrival.

Questions:

1. What might have happened on the old woman?

2. How to avoid the occurrence of such events in the elderly?

Box 11-8　案例

一位72岁的老妇人，与同伴一起在餐厅共同进食晚餐，并边吃边聊。在享用红烧龙虾的时候，她突然停止了进食和说话，但并没有痛苦的迹象和表现，因此其同伴虽感到迷惘，但没有感到惊慌。但接下来，她突然间晕倒在地。服务员和她的朋友们尝试对她进行复苏。救护车到来后将其送往最近医院的急诊室，但到达时医院时已死亡。

问题：

1. 这位老妇人发生了什么？

2. 如何避免老年人发生此类事件？

I. Definition of Aspiration and Asphyxia

Aspiration is defined as the misdirection of oropharyngeal or gastric contents into the larynx and lower respiratory tract. There are two types of aspiration, silent aspiration and overt aspiration. Silent aspiration is defined as aspiration without overt symptoms such as choking, coughing or throat clearing.

Asphyxia in a broad sense is a condition in which an abnormality in the arterial blood gases (hypoxemia or hypercapnia) occurs due to a disruption in breathing mechanics. So the host can no longer maintain normal activities. The resultant death is called asphyxial death. The main function of the lungs is to exchange gases. They extract oxygen from the air and supply it to the arterial blood while they eliminate carbon dioxide from the venous blood.

II. Factors Contributing to Aspiration and Asphyxia

1. Factors contributing to aspiration

(1) Aging: Advanced age (variably defined as greater than 60 to 5 years of age) is consistently identified as a risk factor for aspiration. Elder patients tend to have a reduced swallowing ability and are more likely to have neurologic disorders (such as stroke and Parkinson's disease) and other medical conditions (such as long-

一、误吸与窒息的定义

误吸是指进食或非进食时，有数量不一的食物、口腔内分泌物或胃食管反流物随着吞咽动作进入了声门以下的气道。误吸可以分为显性误吸与隐性误吸两大类。隐性误吸则是指不伴有咳嗽等明显临床症状的误吸，可在毫无知觉的情况下发生。

窒息是指由于某种病因使机体呼吸过程受阻，氧气吸入、利用及二氧化碳排出发生困难，肺组织不能进行气体交换，导致机体严重缺氧及二氧化碳潴留，各种代谢活动相继停止，很快致人死亡的过程。

二、误吸与窒息的危险因素

1. 误吸的危险因素

（1）年龄：衰老是导致老年人发生误吸的危险因素之一。老年人吞咽能力的下降且可能患有神经系统疾病（如脑卒中、帕金森病）及其他慢性疾病（如糖尿病），都使得老年人发生误吸的风险增加。

standing diabetes mellitus) that increase aspiration risk. There is also a strong association between advanced age and the probability of developing pneumonia once aspiration has occurred.

(2) Hypofunction: For the elderly the degenerative changes of organizational structure occur gradually, such as the oral cavity, pharynx, throat, esophagus and so on. Mucosa atrophy and thinning and the reflection of nerve endings receptor function become slow gradually. The peristalsis ability of pharyngeal and esophageal weakened. These age-related degenerative changes can lead to swallowing dysfunction and aspiration.

Aspiration status in older adults was associated with decreased tongue strength and pharyngeal pressure, likely due to age-related atrophy of swallowing muscles. Muscle atrophy and associated functional decline with aging (sarcopenia) has been widely studied in muscles of the extremities. However, oropharyngeal muscle atrophy and loss of balance among different muscle groups during aging are poorly understood, which may explain the lack of effective treatment for oropharyngeal dysphagia, swallowing deficits with aging, and other age-related neurological diseases. Decreased pharyngeal strength and decreased posterior tongue strength are associated with aspiration status in healthy older adults. However, aspiration status could also be associated with decreased pharyngeal closure, a process for airway protection in which the precise timing of the elevation of hyoid bone is important. A decreased range of motion and velocity of movement in the hyoid bone occurs in older adults compared with younger adults. Several suprahyoid muscles play a similar role in the raising, protracting, and stabilizing of the hyoid bone during swallowing. For example, the geniohyoid (GH) muscle connects the posterior aspect of the mandible in the midline and anterior surface of the body of the hyoid bone. The GH muscle's contraction drives the hyoid bone upward and forward together with the mylohyoid, stylohyoid, and anterior belly of the digastric muscles. Sarcopenia of these muscles may play an important role in reducing hyoid bone movement during aging and the resultant increased risk of aspiration in older persons. In addition, age-related increase in fatty infiltration into the muscle is correlated with decreased muscle mass and strength in the elderly population.

（2）组织结构衰老、功能减退：老年人的口腔、咽、喉与食管等部位的组织结构发生退行性改变，黏膜萎缩变薄，神经末梢感受器的反射功能逐渐迟钝，咽及食管的蠕动能力减弱。这些衰老性的退行性变化会导致吞咽功能障碍，易导致老年人误吸的发生。

老年人的误吸发生与舌活动和吞咽能力降低有关。人们对骨骼肌老化认识较深入。但是，由于对吞咽肌肉老化的机制和吞咽肌协调运动的认识不足，导致缺乏治疗吞咽障碍的有效方法。吞咽动作虽可随意开始，但此动作的完成过程是复杂的反射活动。当食物团进入咽腔时，腭咽肌能反射性地封闭通往口腔、鼻咽腔的通路，以防止食物向口腔、鼻腔逆流，而老化导致上述腭咽闭合的反射减弱。吞咽过程中，舌骨上提的精确时间非常重要。与年轻人相比，老年人舌骨运动范围和运动速度降低。这些老化改变增加了误吸的风险。

(3) Related disease

a. Decreased level of consciousness: The strong relationship between a decreased level of consciousness (LOC) and aspiration is indisputable. Whether it is defined as an altered mental status (such as being unable to respond to simple commands) or as a low Glasgow coma scale score （<9）, a decreased LOC has consistently been identified as a significant risk factor for aspiration. A decreased LOC also increases the risk for aspiration by causing impaired function of the lower esophageal sphincter (LES) and delayed gastric emptying. The almost continuous sedation used in many critically ill patients increases aspiration risk by adversely affecting gastric emptying and cough and gag reflexes.

b. High-risk disease: Neurologically impaired patients are at especially high risk for aspiration. Patients with degenerative neurologic diseases such as stroke and Parkinson's disease usually have long-standing dysphagia, thus increasing their risk for aspiration. In addition, patients with Parkinson's disease often have impaired gastric motility. Spinal cord-injured patients must be maintained in a supine position, which significantly increases their aspiration risk.

In addition to having risk factors such as a decreased LOC, tracheal intubation mechanical ventilation, and nasogastric intubation, the critically ill are often the recipients of medications (such as morphine, meperidine, and barbiturates) that predispose to aspiration by worsening the LOC and lowering lower esophageal sphincter pressures. Low-dose dopamine can adversely affect gastroduodenal motility.

(4) Iatrogenic factor

a. Supine position: There is evidence that a sustained supine position (with the head of the bed flat) increases gastroesophageal reflux (GER). Related study suggests that although aspiration is significantly more likely when patients are supine, it also occurs when they are semirecumbent. The effect of a continuous supine position on aspiration was demonstrated in a recent study that tested for the gastric enzyme pepsin in 136 tracheal secretions collected from 30 critically ill patients. Fourteen of the 136 tracheal secretions contained pepsin (a proxy for the aspiration of gastric contents). Thirteen of the 14 pepsin-positive specimens were collected from patients whose bed was continuously flat because of spinal cord injury (p<0.001).

（3）疾病因素

a. 意识水平下降：误吸的发生与意识水平（LOC）下降有明显的相关性，尤其是精神状态的改变（如无法应对简单的命令）或格拉斯哥昏迷评分得分较低（<9分）。意识水平下降可导致食管下括约肌功能受损和胃排空延迟而增加误吸的风险。临床许多危重患者的持续镇静状态，影响了胃排空和咳嗽和呕吐反射，而导致误吸的风险增加。

b. 疾病因素：神经受损的患者发生误吸的风险增高。患有神经系统退行性疾病，如脑卒中和帕金森病的患者通常会长期存在吞咽困难，从而增加了误吸发生的可能性。此外，帕金森病的患者经常有胃动力受损。脊髓损伤的患者必须保持仰卧位，也大大增加了他们发生误吸的风险。

此外，除了意识水平降低，气管插管，机械通气和鼻饲，危重患者往往需接受将导致其意识水平和食管下括约肌压力降低的药物治疗，增加其发生误吸的风险，如吗啡、哌替啶、巴比妥类药物。低剂量的多巴胺也会影响胃与十二指肠的功能。

（4）医源性因素

a. 仰卧位：持续的仰卧位会增加胃食管反流和误吸的可能性。虽然仰卧位时患者发生误吸的可能性更大，但处于半卧位状态的患者也可发生误吸。

b. Presence of a nasogastric tube: Because a nasogastric tube transgresses the esophagus and thus presumably interferes with the lower esophageal sphincter, it is a frequently cited risk factor for GER and aspiration. Obviously, aspiration risk is increased when a feeding tube's ports are positioned in or near the esophagus. In addition, the speed of nasogastric fluid infusion is too fast or too much infusion quantity also can make force of gastric internal pressure.

c. Tracheal intubation/mechanical ventilation: A tracheal device (either a tracheostomy or an endotracheal tube) is a frequently cited risk factor for aspiration and pneumonia. Possible mechanisms whereby tracheal intubation might predispose to aspiration include reduction in upper airway defense related to ineffective cough, desensitization of the oropharynx and larynx, disuse atrophy of laryngeal muscles, and esophageal compression by an inflated cuff. Positive abdominal pressure generated during mechanical ventilation predisposes to the aspiration of gastric contents, probably by increasing GER. Also, swallowing dysfunction has been demonstrated in patients receiving long-term mechanical ventilation. There is evidence that the risk for ventilator associated pneumonia increases by about 1% for each day a patient needs mechanical ventilation. Aspiration risk also exists in the first 48 hours after extubation; possible reasons include sedation after-effects and decreased pharyngeal sensation. Presence of a nasogastric tube aggravates the situation by further desensitizing the pharynx. The need for reintubation has been identified as a highly significant risk factor for the development of pneumonia in mechanically ventilated patients.

2. Factors contributing to asphyxia Food / foreign body asphyxiation is common in the elderly. Related study demonstrates old age, poor dentition, neurologic disorders, certain types of foods, and the intake of sedatives as risk factors for food/foreign body asphyxia. Prevention of these fatal events requires neither special diagnostic facilities nor highly sophisticated knowledge, but merely a simple awareness of predisposing factors. Rapid feeding rates may overload marginally functional deglutition, resulting in life-threatening bolus misdirection into the airway. Semisolid dysphagia diets significantly increase the risk of fatal food/foreign body asphyxia in the elderly. The literature suggests that for dysphagic patients, food should not be semisolid, but instead limited to a particle size of 1cm combined with careful patient monitoring at mealtimes.

b. 鼻胃管的置入：因为胃管使食管下括约肌关闭受阻，引起胃食管反流而导致发生误吸。当胃管的端口未插入胃内而位于食管内时，吸入风险会增加。鼻饲液输注速度过快或输注量过多都会影响胃内压力，导致胃食管反流，引发误吸。

c. 气管插管、机械通气：气管切开和气管插管是发生误吸和肺炎的危险因素。气管插管时，咳嗽、口咽及喉的敏感度、上呼吸道的抵御能力均下降，易发生喉部肌肉萎缩、吞咽功能障碍等，容易诱发误吸。机械通气可使腹内压增加，造成误吸。机械通气中的药物使用造成镇静后遗症和咽部感觉的不敏感，增加了反流的机会。

2. 窒息的危险因素 由食品／异物所致的窒息在老年人窒息事件中较为常见。相关研究表明，高龄、牙列不齐、神经系统疾病、某些特殊类型的食物和使用镇静剂都是导致食物／异物窒息发生的危险因素。具备相关的诊断设施和掌握专业知识，是有效预防窒息事件的前提条件。进食过快可能导致机体无法顺利下咽，导致误吸的发生，危及生命。半固态、较难以咽下的食物会明显增加老年人致命性窒息的发生。

Box 11-9　Classification of Asphyxia

1. Obstruction of the air passage by aspiration of a foreign body and resultant constriction of the airway from inside.

This type of asphyxia occurs when solid objects (e. g. , a lump of viscous food, such as a rice cake and peanuts, a piece of candy, peas, meat or other chunks of food, a denture, and a rubber balloon) becomes lodged in and blocks the airway. When a small piece of food or other foreign body is accidentally aspirated into the airway, it is normally expelled by coughing (about 2%of all foreign bodies are expelled in this manner), unless the airway is completely occluded.

2. Presence of fluid in the airway or aspiration of fluid. It is most often attributable to aspiration of gastric contents associated with underlying illness or intoxication.

3. Asphyxia due to compression and obstruction of the naso-oral region (smothering). Smothering is a type of asphyxia caused by simultaneous compression and closure of the external nares and mouth with a soft and wide object that does not permit airflow (such as the palms of the hand, clothes, and bedding). Include positional asphyxia where respiration is compromised by abnormal positioning of a body.

4. Sputum or throat edema or smoke caused by various reasons blocked respiratory tract.

Box 11-9　窒息的分类

1. 由于误吸导致异物阻塞气道　这种类型的窒息多因固体物质阻塞气道而致（如年糕、花生、糖果、豌豆、肉类或其他大块的食物，义齿，气球）。当小块食物或其他异物意外吸入气道，通常可通过咳嗽清除（约2%的异物以这种方式从气道内清除），除非气道完全闭塞。

2. 因液体误吸导致的窒息　通常是疾病或中毒导致胃内容物反流所致。

3. 堵住口鼻所致窒息　这种类型的窒息是指同时被质地较软的物品（如手掌、衣服、床上用品）堵住口鼻，而导致无法呼吸。其包括与体位相关的窒息，因个体的体位导致呼吸受限。

4. 由于液痰堵塞、喉头水肿、烟雾等不同原因造成的呼吸道阻塞。

III. Nursing Assessments

1. Swallowing functional assessment and the risk of aspiration　In clinical practice, a screening test for oropharyngeal dysphagia has three goals:

a. Determine the likelihood that aspiration is present.

b. Need to have a formal swallow evaluation.

c. Determine when it is safe to recommend resumption of oral alimentation.

In clinical practice, a screening test has two kinds of tests:

a. Simple tests: Water-swallowing test, repeated spectrum swallowing test, repetitive saliva swallowing test and simple swallowing provocation test (table 11-7).

b. Thorough tests: Plain X-ray, radiography for swallowing, nasal and pharyngolaryngeal fiberscope, and scintigraphy.

三、护理评估

1. 吞咽功能的评估　临床对个体进行吞咽困难筛查的主要目标包括：

a. 确定误吸存在的可能性。

b. 确定其接受正式评估的必要性。

c. 确定恢复口服营养的时间。

临床对个体进行吞咽困难筛查有两种方法：

a. 简单的测试：洼田饮水试验，反复唾液吞咽试验和简易吞咽激发试验（表11-7）。

b. 全面的测试：普通X射线，吞咽造影检查，纤维鼻咽镜和放射性核素显像。

Table 11-7   Water Swallowing Test

	The patient drinks 30 ml warm water at rest state	
Numerals	●	Description
1	●	Swallow the water well in one gulp (in 5 seconds)
2	●	Swallow the water in twice without bucking (in 5 seconds)
3	●	Swallow the water in one gulp with bucking
4	●	Swallow the water in twice or more times with bucking
5	●	Coughing frequently and can't swallow all of the water

*level 1 and level 2, oral feeding is allowed; level 3 and level 4, swallowing restriction; level 5, serious swallowing dysfunction, oral feeding is forbidden.

表 11-7   洼田饮水试验及评估标准

	患者放松自然，不知是在给自己做实验的情况下进行。取坐位或半卧位，按习惯喝下 30ml 温水
分级	评定标准
1级（优）	能顺利一次将水饮下（五秒钟内）
2级（良）	分 2 次以上，能不呛咳的咽下（五秒钟内）
3级（中）	能 1 次咽下，但有呛咳
4级（可）	分 2 次以上咽下有呛咳
5级（差）	频繁咳嗽，不能全部咽下

* 测试结果：2 级以上者可经口进食；3 级及以下，说明患者存在吞咽功能障碍；5 级则存在严重的吞咽功能障碍，应禁止经口进食。

2. Airway secretions block the respiratory tract   The artificial airway is not like the nose and pharynx has the effect of air clean, heating and humid, when patient was given a tracheotomy. It makes the mucous membrane of lower airway obstruction dry. Respiratory secretions easier to become dry and scabby and then blocked the respiratory tract leading to the occurrence of asphyxia. In addition, pulmonary infection occurred due to the airborne dust enter the respiratory tract directly. So it is important and necessary to evaluate the sputum viscosity.

2. 分泌物痂块堵塞呼吸道   气管切开术后，由于人工气道缺少鼻腔和咽部对空气的清洁、加温及湿化的作用，导致下呼吸道的黏膜干燥，分泌物容易干燥进而结痂而堵塞呼吸道。此外，由于空气中的尘埃直接进入了呼吸道，因此易继发肺部感染。因此，应注意评估痰液的黏稠度。

IV. Nursing Management

Prevention should focus on identification of patients who are at risk for aspiration and then use of strategies to minimize the risk.

1. Head-of-bed elevation   A sustained supine position (0° head-of-bed elevation) increases gastroesophageal reflux and the probability for aspiration; for example, using a radioactive-labeled formula,

四、护理措施

误吸的预防应致力于识别误吸的高危人群，并应用相应策略以降低误吸发生的风险。

1. 提升床头高度   持续的仰卧位增加了患者发生胃食管反流和误吸的概率。因此，病情允许的情况下，建议将可能发生吸入性

endobronchial counts were higher when patients were lying flat in bed (0°) compared to when they were in a semirecumbent (45°) position. Thus, elevating the head of the bed to an angle of 30° to 45°, unless contraindicated, is recommended for patients at high risk for aspiration pneumonia (e. g. , a patient receiving mechanical ventilation and/or one who has a feeding tube in place). Although effectiveness of the reverse Trendelenberg position in minimizing aspiration has not been studied, it is likely to produce similar results to an elevated backrest position. If backrest elevation is not tolerated, consider use of the reverse Trendelenberg position to elevate the head of the bed, unless contraindicated. If necessary to lower the head of bed for a procedure or a medical contraindication, return the patient to a head-of-bed elevated position as soon as feasible.

2. Use sedatives as sparingly as feasible
Sedation causes reduced cough and gag reflexes and can interfere with the patient's ability to handle oropharyngeal secretions and refluxed gastric contents; in addition, sedation may slow gastric emptying. To reduce the risk for aspiration, it is prudent to use the smallest effective level of sedation. It is important to use an appropriate sedation scale to guide the administration of sedatives. Consider clinical situations that affect the need for sedatives.

3. Diet nursing care

(1) For the elderly receiving gastric tube feedings: The amount of each gastric tube feeding for each meal should not be too much, about 300-400 ml is advisable. Tube feeding speed should not be too fast. At the beginning of the tube feeding, the infusion speed should be 30-50 ml/h and keep a uniform infusion speed. Then adjust to 80-100 ml/h if without any adverse reaction happened. The temperature of the tube feeding liquid should be around 40° C。

Assess feeding tube placement before every gastric tube feeding. Assess for intolerance to feedings every 4 hours by monitoring gastric residual volumes, abdominal discomfort, nausea/vomiting, and abdominal girth/tension. It is important to measure residual volumes from all types of gastric tubes, including gastrostomy tubes. A 60 ml syringe is most suitable for measuring residual volumes. It is helpful to inject 30 ml of air before attempting to aspirate fluid from flexible, small-diameter tubes. Withdraw as much fluid as possible to make an accurate assessment. It may be helpful to reposition the patient to facilitate withdrawal of fluid from the tube (e. g. , turning the patient from side to side may allow the feeding

肺炎的高危患者（例如，机械通气和 / 或鼻饲患者）的床头抬高 30° 至 45° 角。

2. 慎用镇静剂　镇静药物的使用可减少咳嗽和呕吐反射，干扰患者处理口咽分泌物和胃内容物反流的能力；此外，镇静剂可能减缓胃排空。为降低误吸发生的危险，应用镇静药物应谨慎，并使用最小且有效的计量。根据患者的镇静程度评估结果适当的使用镇静剂是非常重要的。同时还应注意，患者的状态也可能影响到其对镇静药物的耐受情况。

3. 饮食护理

（1）鼻饲喂养的老年人预防误吸的护理：每餐的鼻饲液量不宜过多，一般以 300～400ml 为宜，输注的速度不可过快，开始输注的速度应为 30～50ml/h，输注速度应保持匀速，若无任何不良反应，则再将输注速度调至 80～100ml/h。营养液温度保持在 40℃左右为宜。

每次进食前均应评估胃管位置。注意监测患者的胃残余量（每 4 小时评估一次）、腹围及腹部皮肤张力，评估患者是否有腹部不适、恶心呕吐。对所有类型的胃管而言，测量残余量都是非常重要的，包括胃造口管。如果老年人能够沟通，询问其是否有腹部不适或恶心，如果发生呕吐，应立刻停止管饲饮食，并通知医生。

tube's ports to enter a pool of gastric fluid). If the elderly are able to communicate, ask if they are experiencing abdominal discomfort or nausea. If vomiting is present, feedings should be stopped, and the physician notified. Palpate the abdomen for firmness; a millimeter tape may be used to measure abdominal girth. Evaluate the significance of a single abnormal finding, such as a high gastric residual volume, in relation to other indicators of gastrointestinal intolerance to tube feedings, such as abdominal distention, abdominal discomfort, and nausea and vomiting. Although clinicians disagree about the necessity for small bowel feedings to minimize aspiration risk in all critically ill patients, small bowel feedings have been recommended when patients are intolerant of gastric feedings or when they have documented aspiration.

It is better to introduce feedings evenly over a period of hours to minimize risk for regurgitation and aspiration of gastric contents; for example, continuous infusion of nutrient by infusion pump can be used for gastric tube feedings. Avoid bolus feedings for those at high risk for aspiration.

Strengthen the management and training of the patients with gastric tube feeding. Enforce the operation process of nasogastric tube intubation strictly. Provide health education for nasal feeding patients and their caregivers to reduce complications caused by aspiration. Get ready for first aid items in order to rescue in time.

In order to avoid the happening of choke, the elderly with serious swallowing dysfunction should be early received gastric tube feedings.

(2) For the elderly receiving oral feeding: Assessment of nutritional status, hydration, and respiratory function via lab values are also important preventive measures, because they provide crucial insight into the residents' ability to fend off aspiration pneumonia.

In order to avoid the occurrence of aspiration, daily care is of the utmost importance, as follows: encourage food and fluid intake at meals. Offer between-meal snacks for the elderly with gastroesophageal reflux disease or gastrointestinal conditions that limit bulk intake. Treat gastrointestinal conditions that may hinder absorption of nutrients. Encourage the elderly to be up in chair for all meals and for 30 to 60 minutes after meals. Use an upright position for all food, beverage, and medication presentations. Elevate the head of the bed at all times for the elderly with gastroesophageal reflux disease.

最好分次输入鼻饲液，以最大程度地减少胃反流和胃内容物吸入的风险。当胃残余量过多时，还应结合其他提示胃肠道不耐受的表现（如腹胀、腹部不适、恶心和呕吐）对其进行评估。微量泵连续输注的方式可以降低胃内容物反流和发生误吸的危险。对于误吸的高危人群尽量避免喂食团状的食物。

加强对鼻饲患者的管理及培训，严格执行鼻饲的操作流程，做好鼻饲患者及其照顾者的宣教，减少因误吸引起的并发症。准备好急救物品以便及时抢救时使用。

吞咽功能严重障碍者应及早留置胃管，进行管饲饮食，避免进食时发生窒息。

（2）经口进食老年人的喂养的护理：患者的营养状况、机体的水合作用状态、呼吸功能状态（通过实验室检查结果反映）决定了个体是否具有抵抗吸入性肺炎的能力。

为了避免发生误吸的发生，日常护理至关重要，如进餐时鼓励个体摄入食物及液体。患有胃食管反流疾病或限制摄入量的老年人应少量多餐。治疗肠胃疾病期间，可能会导致营养吸收不良。鼓励老年人坐在椅子上进餐，进餐结束后在餐椅上稍坐一会儿，大概30至60分钟。摄入任何食物或饮料、药物后，均保持身体的直立，防止反流。若个体患有胃食管反流疾病，则应始终抬高床头。

Encourage sedentary elderly to stand, walk, or propel their wheelchairs.

The caregiver should be kindly to the elderly while feeding them. The food quantity of every spoon should be appropriate. The feeding speed should not be too fast so the elderly can have enough time to chew. Do not rush them and feed them gently. Encourage the elderly to eat slowly, if vomiting, nausea is present, feedings should be stopped and the aspirator should be used when necessary. For old people with visual disabilities, use food or tableware touched the elderly lips first to stimulate the consciousness and promote the movement of the tongue. And then send food to their mouth. For old people with facial paralysis, put food into the healthy side of the mouth. For the elderly people with buccinator weak contractility that cannot close their mouse tightly, put mixed food near to tongue root and then wait for swallowing reflex. For the elderly with cerebrovascular disease, Alzheimer's disease and have slight difficulty with swallowing, semi-liquid food should be prepared for them, avoided Liquid and dry out foods. Mix their intake of water in the semi-liquid food.

4. Application of fiber bronchoscope For the elderly with sticky sputum, difficulty in expectoration or inability to expectorate independently, and the effect of electric aspirator is not ideal, fiber bronchoscope should be used as soon as possible.

(MU Xiaoyun)

Key Points

1. Among those age 65 and older, falls are the leading cause of injury death. They are also the most common cause of nonfatal injuries and hospital admissions for trauma.

2. Falls can cause elderly to suffer from physical injury and psychological trauma.

3. Risk factors contributing to falls in older adults include biological, behavioral, environmental and socioeconomic factors.

4. Thorough and accurate assessment of the risk factors related to falls is essential.

5. Fall risk assessment is multidimensional and includes a focused history, a physical examination, functional assessment, laboratory and environmental assessment.

鼓励久坐不动的老年人站立、行走，或推轮椅带其活动。

喂饭时态度要亲切和蔼，每勺饭量不要太多，速度不要太快，要给老年人充足的时间进行咀嚼，不要催促老年人，动作要轻。鼓励老年人进食时要细嚼慢咽，出现恶心、呕吐反应时要暂停进食，必要时用吸引器吸出。给视觉障碍的老年人喂饭时，应先用食物或餐具触碰老年人的嘴唇，刺激知觉促进舌的运动，然后再将食物送入口腔。为一侧舌面肌瘫痪的老年人喂食时，应将食物放在口腔的健侧。对于口唇无法紧闭，颊肌收缩无力的老年人喂食时，将调拌好的食物放入到舌根附近，等待吞咽反射。对于脑血管病、阿尔茨海默病，且吞咽困难的老年人，食物应以半流质为宜，避免流质饮食和干硬的食物。尽量将水混在半流质食物中一同给予。

4. 纤维支气管镜的应用 对于痰液黏稠咳痰有困难或不能自主咳痰的老年人，以及电动吸引器的效果不理想时，应尽早使用纤维支气管镜。

（穆晓云）

本章要点

1. 跌倒是 65 岁及以上的老年人发生伤害死亡的主要原因，是导致老年人发生非致死性损伤和住院最常见原因。

2. 发生跌倒会对老年人造成身体损伤及心理损伤。

3. 老年人跌倒危险因素包括生物因素、行为因素、环境因素和社会经济因素。

4. 对跌倒的相关危险因素进行全面、准确的评估是至关重要的。

5. 跌倒的危险因素的评估是多方位的，包括健康史、体格检查、功能评估、实验室检查和环境评估。

6. A comprehensive approach to fall prevention among seniors includes providing education and information, exercise programs, medication review and modification, vision improvement, assistive and protective devices, managing foot and footwear problems, and environmental modification etc.

7. When a fall cannot be avoided, the elderly needs a plan to get help quickly. A good plan involves how to call for help and how to get up.

8. There are basically four risk factors of scalding: age, gender, age-related change and thermal application.

9. A comprehensive approach to aspiration and asphyxia prevention among the elderly includes head-of-bed elevation, use sedatives as sparingly as feasible, use sedatives as sparingly as feasible, application of fiber bronchoscope.

10. The safety of the bed is the most important factor of older people's falling bed, can lead to fatal injury.

Critical Thinking Exercise

1. What content could be included in a program to educate older adults about actions they can take to avoid accidents and injuries?

2. What changes could be made to the average home to make it user friendly and safe for the elderly people?

3. How to make the elderly and their caregivers can understand and master the daily protection strategy of burns?

4. What content could be included in education about food/foreign body asphyxia risk factors to healthcare workers and the elderly people themselves?

6. 预防老年人跌倒的护理措施包括提供教育和信息，制订锻炼计划，检查用药，改善视力，使用辅助和防护装置，选择合适的鞋以及改善环境等。

7. 发生跌倒后，老年人应计划如何尽快获得帮助；包括如何寻求帮助和跌倒后应如何起身。

8. 老年人发生烫伤的风险因素包括年龄、性别、老化因素和热疗法的应用。

9. 预防老年人发生误吸和窒息的护理措施包括提升床头高度、慎用镇静剂、饮食的护理、纤维支气管镜的应用。

10. 导致老年人发生坠床最重要的危险因素是床的安全性。

批判性思维练习

1. 为了使老年人有效地避免意外伤害的发生，向老年人进行教育时应包含的内容有哪些？

2. 为了使老年人感到亲切和安全，应该如何布置老年人的居家环境？

3. 为使老年人及其照顾者理解和掌握关于烧伤的日常保护策略，应如何对其进行健康教育？

4. 如何对护理人员和老年人进行健康教育，使其能清楚了解导致食品／异物性窒息的危险因素有哪些？

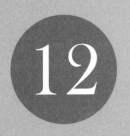

Chapter 12 Care of Elderly with Mobility Limitation

第十二章　活动受限老年人的护理

Learning Objectives

On completion of this chapter, the reader will be able to:

- Understand the concept of the elderly with limitation of mobility;

- Describe the risk factors related to the elderly with limitation of mobility;

- Summary clinical manifestations of the elderly with limitation of mobility;

- List the main nursing interventions on elders with limitation of mobility.

学习目标

学完本章节，应完成以下目标：

- 了解老年人活动受限的概念；

- 描述老年人活动受限的危险因素；

- 概述老年人活动受限的主要临床表现；

- 列出活动受限的主要护理措施。

Basic human activity refers to the activities that are necessary for survival which include walking, running, jumping, throwing, climbing, support, weight, handling, wading, etc. These activities are closely related to people's daily living. It was regarded as the foundation of human survival.

Mobility is the capacity for movement with the personally available microcosm and macrocosm. Moving about is the major mode of learning and interaction with the environment in infants, while the aged move more slowly and purposefully, sometimes with more forethought and caution. Movement remains a significant means of personal contact, sensation, exploration, pleasure, and control throughout the whole life. Movement is integral to levels of needs conceived by Maslow. Identified needs of elders include pride, maintaining dignity, social contacts, and activity, all of which are facilitated by mobility. Thus, in terms of Maslow's hierarchy and the needs identified of the elders, maintaining mobility is exceedingly important. However, the normal changes that accompany aging, and more frequent diseases attacks in the elderly tend to affect older persons, resulting in older people with reduced mobility or limited mobility. This chapter focuses on maximizing the possibility of mobility in case of obstacles in the aged, the care of gait disorders, osteoporosis, rheumatic diseases, and constraints.

Box 12-1 Case Study

Ms. Zhang, 69 years old, has a history of hypertension for 15 years, and there are many "transient ischemic attack", the day before yesterday she has found that the right side of the body was weak, could not move, and she had no disorders in communication and incontinence. Physical examination: blood pressure was 160/100 mmHg, consciousness, but crooked mouth, right limb muscle strength was 2-3 degree. Head CT examination showed a low density infarct.

Questions:

1. What are the main nursing problems of the patient?

2. What are the possible complications of the patient and what precautions should be taken?

3. How to do rehabilitation training after the recovery of the disease?

人类的基本活动是指维持人类生存所必需的活动。基本活动包括行走、奔跑、跳跃、投掷、攀登、爬越、支撑、负重、搬运、涉水等。由于这些活动与人们的日常生活息息相关，故被视为是人类赖以生存的基础。

儿童的主要活动是学习与环境相互作用的结果，而老年人的活动目的性明确，变得缓慢、谨慎。在人的一生中，活动是进行联络、体验、探索、享乐和控制的重要手段。通过活动可满足马斯洛所提出的人的基本需要。老年人的需要包括自豪感、维护尊严、参与社会交往等，这些需要均可以通过活动得到满足。由此，维持老年人活动是一个极其重要的问题。然而，伴随衰老的正常变化，发生于老年人的疾病变得频繁，这些疾病往往影响老年人的活动，造成老年人行动不便、活动受限。本章侧重于介绍老年人在存在各种障碍的情况下如何维持最佳的活动状态，包括步态失调、骨质疏松症、风湿性疾病、约束等所引起活动受限的护理。

Box 12-1 案例

张女士，69岁，有高血压病史15年，并有多次"短暂脑缺血发作"，1天前晨起发现右侧肢体无力，不能活动，并有言语不清，无大小便失禁。体格检查：血压 160/100mmHg，神志清楚，口角歪斜，右侧肢体肌力 2～3 级。头部 CT 检查可见低密度梗死灶。

问题：

1. 张女士的主要护理问题有哪些？

2. 张女士可能会发生哪些并发症，应采取哪些预防措施？

3. 在病情恢复后，如何指导该患者进行康复训练？

Section 1　Risk Factors and Impact on Body

I. Risk Factor

Adverse living factors, diseases, adverse environmental and psychological factors can cause the mobility limitation in the elderly. Nurses would take appropriate measures for prevention and care of mobility limited individual after understanding of the main risk factors.

i. Daily Living Factor

1. Inappropriate clothing may hinder mobility　Fitted, back-closing, or knee-length clothing is not comfortable for persons confined to wheelchairs, those with limited range of motion, or those who require catheters or prosthetic devices. Elders living alone have no one help them button or zip the back. This can make dressing and undressing a time-consuming and frustrating experience.

2. Inappropriate shoes　They include the shoes such as the size of the shoe is too large or too small, sole perfect or without non-slip, the heel is too high, shoes and tie too long, are likely to cause the elderly trip.

3. Others　Wheelchair or indwelling catheter devices, such as lack of a suitable wheelchair bags, catheter bags is inconvenient to move around.

ii. Health Factor

1. Fall　Fall is one of the most common and serious problems associated with aging. Fall in the elder people could lead to a series of problems, though it is just a symptom. An accidental fall in elder individual may show health problems like nervous, perception, cognition, medication, or musculoskeletal disease or weakness.

2. Gait disorder　Mobility and comparative degrees of agility are based on muscle strength, flexibility, postural stability, vibratory sensation, cognition, and perceptions of stability. Muscles and joints change with the aging produces, particularly in the back and legs. In older age, strength and flexibility of muscles decreases remarkably; endurance decreases to a somewhat lesser extent, especially if there is a diminution become more limited. Normal wear and tear reduces the smooth cartilage of joints. Degenerative changes lead to slowed tissue regeneration, muscle atrophy, gait disorders, such as slow stand up, smaller steps, slow speed and body

第一节　活动受限的危险因素及对机体的影响

一、危险因素

某些不利的生活因素、疾病、环境、心理因素等均可引起老年人活动受限。了解老年人活动受限的诱因或危险因素，有利于护理人员采取恰当的预防和护理措施。

（一）生活因素

1. 衣服穿着不适　老年人穿着过紧、背扣或过膝的上衣，尤其是坐轮椅、留置导管、有假肢的老年人，容易出现无人帮助他（她）拉开后背衣服拉链或扣纽扣，这样的服装使得穿、脱衣成为耗时和令人沮丧的经历。

2. 不适当的鞋　如鞋码尺寸过大或过小、鞋底过硬或无防滑、鞋跟过高、鞋子系带过长等，容易造成老年人绊倒。

3. 其他　对于坐轮椅、留置导管的老年人，缺乏合适的轮椅袋、导管袋等，使其不方便走动。

（二）健康因素

1. 跌倒　跌倒是与老化相关的最常见和最严重的问题之一。跌倒虽然是一个症状，但是一旦发生，便会带来一系列问题。跌倒往往表明老年人在神经、感知、认知、用药或骨骼肌肉方面存在问题。

2. 步态失调　人的活动能力和敏捷性是基于个体的肌力、姿势稳定性、灵活性、振动觉、认知觉和感知觉。老化可导致背部、腿部肌肉和关节的退行性变化，出现肌力和灵活性显著下降，耐力降低，身体重心不稳，出现活动幅度受限。随着活动生理性的磨损和老化所带来的关节及其组织退行性变化，组织再生缓慢，肌肉萎缩，出现步态失调，如起立缓慢、迈步变小、前进速度慢、身体左右摇摆等。

swing, diminished arm swing. These changes are less pronounced in those who remain active and a desirable weight.

3. Related Disease Comorbidity is common condition that accompanies the normal changes of aging. Special attention should be paid to the disorders that occur more frequently in the elderly, such as orthopedic impairments that significantly impede the aged. Severe malnutrition, osteoporosis, gait disorders, Parkinson's disease, accidents, and fear of falling must be considered. Rheumatoid arthritis, osteoarthritis, and osteoporosis markedly affect movement and functional capacities. Mobility may be limited by parenthesis; hemiplegia, neuro-motor disturbances, fractures, foot, knee, and hip problems, and illnesses that deplete one's energy. All of these conditions are likely to occur more frequently and have more devastating effects as one age. Many elders in later years have some of these afflictions, with women significantly outnumbering men in this respect.

iii. Environmental Factor

The elderly are also often limited to mobility within a certain range because of the lack of transport or loss of driving ability. The lack of walking aids such as cane, wheelchairs, etc. The elder lives in small bedroom or living room, without elevators, crowded surrounding also result in limitation of mobility.

iv. Psychological Factor

Some elderly are limited in mobility because of the bad experience of falling or fear of falling. In addition, there are some older people lack understandings of the knowledge of their own disease, worried that mobility will aggravate the health condition.

II. Impact on Body

1. Skin The impact on the skin of patients with limited activity or long-term bed, the main impact on the skin is the formation of pressure sores.

2. Motion system Effects of motion system for some patients, limit the scope of activities and strength when necessary, but if the bones, joints and muscles in the long-term sedentary state, will lead to the following situations:

a. Low back pain.

b. Muscle tension decreased and muscle atrophy.

c. Osteoporosis, and bone deformation may severe

3. **相关疾病** 与老化伴随而来的是频繁的疾病困扰。值得特别注意的是，这些疾病或损伤严重妨碍老年人的活动。严重营养不良、步态失调、骨质疏松症、类风湿关节炎、骨关节炎、糖尿病、慢性肺部疾病、心脏病、帕金森病、意外事件等显著影响老年人的躯体功能和运动。患病老年人的活动还可能会受到感觉异常、偏瘫、神经运动障碍、骨折、足、膝、髋关节问题及消耗性疾病的影响，特别是老年女性更容易受累。

（三）环境因素

老年人通常因为缺乏交通工具或失去驾驶能力而局限于一定范围内活动。缺乏助行器如拐杖、轮椅等，居室面积狭小，居住楼房无电梯，生活周边拥挤，缺乏残疾人通道等是影响老年人活动的环境因素。

（四）心理因素

部分老年人因跌倒的经历或担心害怕跌倒而活动局限。另外，还有部分老年人由于缺乏对自身疾病知识的了解、担心活动会加重病情而有意限制活动。

二、对机体的影响

1. **对皮肤的影响** 活动受限或长期卧床的患者，对皮肤最主要的影响是形成压疮。

2. **对运动系统的影响** 对某些患者来说，限制活动的范围和强度是必要的，但如果骨骼、关节和肌肉组织长期处于活动受限的状态，会导致下列情况的出现：

a. 腰背疼。

b. 肌张力减弱，肌肉萎缩。

c. 骨质疏松、骨骼变形，严重时会发生

pathological fracture occurs.

d. The joint stiffness, contracture, deformation, appear, pedal vertical wrist, hip external rotation, and joint activities to narrow the range.

3. Cardiovascular system Postural hypotension, also known as orthostatic hypotension, due to changes in posture, such as a sudden shift from supine position to upright, or long standing cerebral hemorrhage caused by insufficient blood pressure. It is generally believed that the post systolic blood pressure decreased 20 mmHg or diastolic blood pressure decreased by 10 mmHg compared with supine position.

4. Respiratory system The restriction of effective ventilation and the effect of the discharge of respiratory secretions.

5. Digestive system Loss of appetite, anorexia, intake of nutrients to reduce, cannot meet the needs of the body, and even severe malnutrition.

6. Urinary system The perineal muscles relax, while muscle pressure to stimulate urination.

7. Psychological state Having anxiety, fear, insomnia, self-esteem changes, anger, and frustration.

Section 2   Nursing Assessments

I. Health History

1. Assess adverse factors of daily life, including not fitted clothing, shoes and others.

2. Ask the elder if he has the experience of fall. To know currently taking medications, especially whether the impact of mobility.

3. Assess the elderly whether the impact of limited mobility of health factors, including gait disorders, osteoporosis, heart disease, diabetes, chronic lung disease, osteoarthritis, constraints, and fear of fall.

4. Ask the elderly living state of the environment,

病理性骨折。

d. 关节僵硬、挛缩、变形，出现垂足、垂腕、髋关节外旋，及关节活动范围缩小。

3. 对心血管系统的影响 主要有直立性低血压和深静脉血栓。直立性低血压是由于体位的改变，如从平卧位突然转为直立，或长时间站立发生的脑供血不足引起的低血压。通常认为，站立后收缩压较平卧位时下降20mmHg或舒张压下降10mmHg，即为直立性低血压。

4. 对呼吸系统的影响 可表现为限制有效通气和影响呼吸道分泌物排出，最终导致坠积性肺炎的发生。

5. 对消化系统的影响 常出现食欲缺乏、厌食、摄入的营养物质减少，不能满足机体需要量，甚至会出现严重营养不良。

6. 对泌尿系统的影响 若长时间处于站姿或坐姿时，会使会阴部肌肉放松，同时肌肉下压刺激排尿。

7. 对心理状态的影响 老年人常出现焦虑、恐惧、失眠、自尊的改变、愤怒、挫折感。

第二节　护理评估

一、健康史

1. 评估老年人生活中有无不利因素，如影响活动的着装、鞋等。

2. 了解老年人有无跌倒的经历。目前所服用药物，特别是有无影响活动的药物。

3. 评估老年人有无影响活动受限的健康因素，包括步态失调、骨质疏松症、心脏病、糖尿病、慢性肺部疾病、关节病变、约束以及对活动的恐惧和害怕等。

4. 询问老年人目前的居住环境状态，是

whether enough space, convenience, mobility aids.

II. Clinical Manifestation

Various degrees of immobility are often temporary or permanent consequences of illness. On a broader scale, elders frequently have limited environmental mobility because of lack of transportation or loss of drive license. Limitations on capacity for involvement with surrounding, and mobility, for whatever reason, have serious consequences. Clinical Manifestations of mobility in gait disorders, osteoporosis, rheumatic diseases, and constraints are described as follows.

1. Gait disorder makes one vulnerable to tripping and falling. In addition, they impede activity and increase anxiety in the elder who is aware of instability in gait. Postural reflex impairment occurs with aging, and postural sway, forward and backward, can be observed when an individual stand still. A cane or supportive device may be essential to provide a sense of security.

2. Osteoporosis (OP) is a major medical, economic, and social health problem in elderly. It results in significant pain, loss of function, suffering, and mortality. The loss of bone with OP is silent, without symptoms, until a fracture occurs. Some of the outward signs that identify a history of OP are a loss of height (perhaps 7-10 cm since young adulthood) and "dowager's hump", or kyphosis, which is curvature of the thoracic spine, usually with the presence of a bulging abdomen (all indicative of vertebral fractures).

3. Rheumatic disease of older adults. A number of rheumatic disorders occur in older adults; some of these are bursitis, polymyalgia rheumatic, gout, rotator cuff tears, tendinitis, frozen shoulder, low back pain, acute disk herniation, chronic disk degeneration, lumbar spinal stenosis, rheumatoid arthritis, osteoarthritis, and many others. Osteoporosis and chronic arthritis is the most common of the afflictions that disable elders. It is estimated that there are 100 different types of arthritis that arise from various combinations of heredity, overuse, obesity, and infections. Arthritis, though the most prevalent disorders of aging, is by no means equally distributed throughout the elderly population by age, gender, race, socioeconomic group, or geography. These disorders create pain,

否空间足够、出行方便、有无助行工具等。

二、临床表现

任何原因造成活动受限均可导致严重后果。不同程度的活动受限往往是疾病导致的暂时或永久的结局。更广定义的活动受限也包括老年人由于缺乏交通工具或失去驾照而产生的环境活动受限。无论出于何种原因，老年人参与周围环境和活动能力的限制都会对生活造成不同程度的影响。下面主要介绍步态失调、骨质疏松症、风湿性疾病、约束等所引起的活动受限的表现。

1. **步态失调** 表现为起立缓慢、迈步变小、前进速度慢、身体左右摇摆、步态不稳等。站立时，可以发生姿势反射障碍，前进和后退姿势不稳，有摇摆倾向，给人感觉需要用拐杖或支持设备才有安全感。

2. **骨质疏松症** 骨质疏松症（OP）是一个严重的医疗、经济和社会问题。它会导致老年人明显的疼痛、功能丧失、痛苦，容易发生骨折，甚至死亡。骨质疏松症患者的骨质丢失是隐性的，没有任何症状，直到发生骨折发生才发现有骨质疏松症。在某些人中发现的骨质疏松症外在症状是身高较年轻时变矮 7～10cm 或脊柱后凸、胸椎弯曲，通常伴有腹部膨隆。

3. **风湿性疾病** 老年人常患风湿性疾病，如滑囊炎、风湿性多肌痛、痛风、肌腱炎、肩周炎、腰腿痛、急性椎间盘突出症、慢性椎间盘退行性变、腰椎管狭窄症、类风湿关节炎、骨关节炎等。据估计，有上百种不同类型的关节炎，是由遗传、负荷过重、肥胖、感染等多种因素引起。关节炎是导致残障最痛苦的疾病。虽然关节炎在老年人中是较普遍的，但可因不同的年龄、性别、种族、社会经济状态及地理环境而异。关节炎患者常表现出疼痛、行动不便、抑郁症、功能失调和自我概念紊乱。

depression, immobility, and functional and self-concept disturbances.

4. Restraint has been used historically for the protection of the client and for security of the client and the staff. The constraints are generally divided into physical constraints, chemical constraints and environmental constraints.

(1) Physical restraint are devices, materials and equipment that are attached to or are adjacent to the patient's body; prevent free bodily movement to a position of choice (standing, walking, lying, turning and sitting); cannot be controlled or easily removed by the patient. Temporary immobilization of a part of the body for the purpose of treatment, such as casts, splits and arm boards, is not included in this definition.

(2) Chemical restraint has come under careful security, legal and ethical. This is the misuse of psychotropic medications and can be considered a potential form of elder abuse.

(3) Environmental restraint. Intentional environmental impediments may be effective in limiting movement and in some cases (Akathisia-induce ambulation, self-stimulatory behavior, modeling, exit-seek behavior) may avoid the more devastating alterative of applying physical restraints. Door may be locked, or chairs may be difficult to rise from. These effectively limit individual movement.

III. Experimental and Other Test

1. The get-up and go test is a practical assessment tool for elderly people and can be conducted in any setting. The client is asked to rise from a straight backed chair, stand briefly, and walk forward about 3 m, turn, walk back to the chair, turn around, and sit down. Performance is grated on a 5-point scale from 1 (normal) to 5 (severely abnormal). The quality of movement is assessed for impaired balance. A score of 3 or higher suggests high risk of falling.

2. A number of tests may need to be ordered to discover the cause of the limited mobility. These include X-ray, CT, the dual-energy X-ray absorptiometry (DEXM) scan, ECG, complete blood (CBC), electrolytes, and liver

4. **约束** 约束是为了保护患者，对患者进行干预治疗的一种简单、有效的解决方法，并且也保护照护者的安全。约束一般分为身体约束、药物约束及环境约束。

（1）身体约束：是指任何徒手或采用物理的、机械的设备、材料或者使用患者附近不易移动的设施，限制患者活动或身体自由。其定义明确了利用约束工具、材料和设备：①连接患者的身体；②选择一种体位（站立、行走、卧位、转动、坐位），防止身体自由运动；③无法被患者控制或被轻易除去。临床上身体约束是在患者出现谵妄、烦躁、不配合治疗，甚至有自伤行为时使用。

（2）药物约束：通过给药来限制患者活动自由，或用于控制意外行为。药物约束应保证患者安全，符合法律和道德规范，否则滥用精神科药物，可以认为是一个潜在的虐待老人形式。

（3）环境约束：主要针对有不能静坐、自我刺激行为、跟踪、寻找出路逃跑等精神症状的个体，采用有意的改变环境以有效地限制个体运动，避免身体约束可能的损伤。这种约束可采用锁门、固定椅子高度等方法。

三、实验室及辅助检查

1. **步态失调的评估** 可采用简单"起立－行走"试验测评，该方法可以在任何环境下进行。要求患者先坐于靠背椅——站立起来——向前步行约 3m——转身——走回椅子——转身——坐下。采用 5 点评分法，从 1 分表示"正常"至 5 分表示"严重异常"，评估其平衡受损的情况。3 分或更高分表示有跌倒的危险。

2. **其他** 为了解患者的基础疾病状态或明确诊断，有必要进行双能 X 线骨密度测定（DEXM）、血常规、心电图、CT 等检查。

function, etc.

IV. Psychosocial Aspect

Limited mobility or mobility is the psychological impact of the elderly is the impact of self-concept and self-esteem. The lack of freedom and independence to move around has negative consequences on people's autonomy and independence of consciousness. Long fixed a small and confined to the living area may lead to the perception and behavior abnormalities, signs of emotional depression, listlessness, withdrawal, and irritability or anxiety. Limitation of activity for a long time or mobility, can lead to reduced contact with others, lack of social interaction, the occurrence of the change of social roles.

四、心理社会状况

活动受限或行动不便对老年人最大的心理影响是自我概念和自尊的影响。无法自由活动和独立走动,对人的自主性和独立性意识产生消极后果。长时间固定于一个小而局限的生活区域,可能会导致感知和行为异常,出现情绪抑郁、精神萎靡、退缩、烦躁或焦虑。长时间活动受限或行动不便,可导致与他人接触减少,缺乏社会交往,发生社会角色改变。

Box 12-2 Function Evaluation: the Barthel Index

Since 1955, the chronic disease hospitals in Maryland (Montebello State Hospital, Deer's Head Hospital, and Western Maryland Hospital) have been using a simple index of independence to score the ability of a patient with a neuro-muscular or musculoskeletal disorder to care for him/her, and by repeating the test periodically, to assess his improvement. The index (BI) has also been taught to many nurses, who have been helpful in evaluating patients prior to admission to these hospitals and after discharge.

Barthel Index

	With Help	Independent
1. Feeding (if food needs to be cut up = help)	5	10
2. Moving from wheelchair to bed and return (includes sitting up in bed)	5-10	15
3. Personal toilet (wash face, comb hair, shave, clean teeth)	0	5
4. Getting on and off toilet (handling clothes, wipe, flush)	5	10
5. Bathing self	0	5
6. Walking on level surface (or if unable to walk, propel wheelchair) *score only if unable to walk	10 0*	15 5*
7. Ascend and descend stairs	5	10
8. Dressing (includes tying shoes, fastening fasteners)	5	10
9. Controlling bowels	5	10
10. Controlling bladder	5	10

Box 12-2 Barthel 指数活动能力评价

自 1955 年以来,马里兰州慢性病医院(蒙特贝罗州医院、鹿头医院和马里兰西部医院)已经使用独立的简单指数评分与神经肌肉或肌肉骨骼疾病患者自我照顾的能力,并通过重复定期测试,来评估他的进步。该指数(BI)也被用来指导护士评估入院和出院患者的活动能力。

Barthel 指数

项目	需要帮助	独立
1. 进食（如果食物需要被切碎＝帮助）	5	10
2. 从轮椅转到床上并返回（包括坐在床上）	5~10	15
3. 个人卫生（洗脸、梳头、刮胡子、清洁牙齿）	0	5
4. 如厕（松解衣裤、擦拭、冲洗）	5	10
5. 沐浴	0	5
6. 在平地行走（或不能行走、推动轮椅）	10	15
* 不能走路时	0*	5*
7. 上下楼梯	5	10
8. 穿衣（包括系鞋带、扣纽扣）	5	10
9. 大便	5	10
10. 小便	5	10

A patient scoring 100 BI means he/she is continent, feeds himself/herself, dresses himself/herself, gets up out of bed and chairs, bathes himself/herself, walks at least a block, and can ascend and descend stairs. This does not mean that he/she is able to live alone: he/she may not be able to cook, keep house, and meet the public, but he/she is able to get along without attendant care.

评估某患者若得分为 100 分，说明该患者能自己独立进食、洗漱、起居、穿衣、座椅、沐浴、步行至少一个街区和上下楼梯。这并不意味着他能够独自生活：他／她可能不能做饭、打扫房子和满足公众，但他／她可以不需要照顾地与人相处。

Section 3　Nursing Management

I. Improving Living Condition and Decreasing Hazards Related to Mobility

1. The space of the bedroom and living room for the elderly should be large enough, all the facilities and furniture should be placed in a fixed position and a height of suitability; washroom and toilet room nearby, installing toilets and handrails; flat ground, non-slip; light bright, accessible, and so on.

2. Teach and help the older people choose the right clothing and shoes, crutches, leg support device, a pain relief device, handrails, walker, and wheelchair may improve mobility status. Adaptive fashions have been designed to facilitate easy or independent dressing and

第三节　护理措施

一、减少生活中老年活动相关的不利因素

1. 老年人生活居室空间面积适宜、设施简单、定位放置；家具高度适宜，洗漱间及厕所与居室邻近，安装坐便器及扶手；地面平坦、防滑；光线充足，出入方便等。

2. 指导和帮助老年人选择合适的服装和鞋子、拐杖、腿部支撑器、疼痛缓解装置、扶手、步行器等，对坐轮椅、留置有导管等的老年人，设计适当的轮椅袋、导管袋等，

include features such as back and side openings, Velcro front openings, raglan sleeves, and cape-styled clothing. Slacks, with front flaps or extra room in back, or longer skirts are helpful. The fabric should be chosen for comfort, durability, attractiveness, and ease of laundering. Other items to facilitate moving around include wheelchair bags, catheter bags, and carefully chosen footwear.

3. One intervention that is useful in a facility is to identify those at risk for falls and make a notation or color code for them, on the chart or at the bedside. Furthermore, a bed sensor is useful for those who may try to get out of bed without the needed assistance; nurses must attend to call lights in order to prevent injury to those who would hurry to the bathroom without assistance if none is forthcoming when needed, often urgently. This is vital when elders are on diuretics.

4. Provide mobility aids enough for the elderly to have mobility.

II. Assessment and Training the Gait Timely

The nurse is responsible for the initial assessment of gait disturbance and gaining appropriate professional consultation for prostheses and gait training. Rehabilitative specialists are usually responsible for teaching gait training to patients, but nurses must understand concepts and specific methods because they will assist the patient to carry out correct procedures on a daily basis. A complete analysis of gait patterns and characteristics requires special equipment and expertise, but simple gait observation by nurses can yield valuable information. In most gait disturbances, nervousness or anxiety aggravates the condition. Nurses may assist by gently holding the arm on the unaffected side and supporting the client's efforts.

III. Treat Underlying Diseases Actively

Intervention, like prevention, should be directed toward educating clients about their medical regimen, assisting them in adapting to their disease, and preventing disease progression. Medical interventions of which the nurse should be knowledgeable include the various types of therapies used in the treatment of osteoporosis, Parkinson's disease, rheumatoid arthritis, osteoarthritis, diabetes, heart disease, chronic lung disease, etc.

尽可能方便老年人移动。老年人服装设计和选择宜简单、方便、独立可穿脱，宜前胸或侧面开口，开口用魔术贴，也可着插肩袖、斗篷风格的服装，有充足的反折空间。面料宜舒适、耐用、吸水性强和易于洗涤。

3. 对于长期卧床老年人，尽可能将必需物品放在床头柜上，给予醒目的预防跌倒、坠床标识；安装床头呼叫装置，以便呼叫得到及时援助，特别是对于使用利尿剂的老年人。

4. 保障老年人外出助行和交通工具，包括搬运和驾驶。

二、及时评估老年人的步态和加强步态训练

护士应对老年人步态失调进行初步评估，并给予适当的假肢和步态训练的专业咨询。虽然康复专家负责制订训练计划，但是护士也需要了解训练的方法和程序，因为护士是患者每日训练的协助者。尽管对患者步态的全面评估需要借助特殊设备和专业知识，但是护士简单的观察也非常重要。大部分步态失调是由于紧张或焦虑而加重的。护士可以通过扶助老年人健侧肢体来提供帮助。

三、积极治疗基础疾病

鼓励和指导老年人积极治疗基础疾病，包括骨质疏松症、帕金森病、类风湿关节炎、骨关节炎、糖尿病、心脏病、慢性肺部疾病等，遵循医疗方案，防止疾病进展。

IV. Remove Restraints as Early as Possible

Reducing environmental hazards, keeping an individual moving about to increase endurance and function, and identifying the person most at risk of falling is the method that may be used to avoid accidents and falls and maintain mobility. Thoughtful, clear communication, creative planning, and nursing skills can obviate the need for restraints. Nurses in many setting are working together to solve the problems inherent in restraint use, but there is still much to be done.

Restraint period, be taken to avoid the constraints to cause harm to the elderly, and more communication with the elderly, to explain the purpose of constraints and precautions to prevent falls and other accidents. A limited range of activities for environmental constraints elderly, help and guidance older people, increasing endurance and functional, good use of nursing skills as much as possible, lift the constraints as soon as possible, and restore the normal mobility of the elderly.

V. Mobility Aid

Mobility aid for the elder includes assistive devices, wheelchairs, transportation and automobiles. In general, the following principles should be obeyed:

1. Move the assistance device first, then the weaker leg, and finally the stronger leg; always wear low-heeled, nonskid shoes; when using with a cane on stairs, step up with the stronger leg and down with the weaker leg. Use the cane as support when lifting the weaker leg. Bring the cane up to the step just reached before climbing another step. When descending, place the cane on the next step down, move the disable leg down, and then move the healthy leg down.

2. When using a walker, stand upright and lift the walker with both hands, place all of its legs down at a comfortable distance. Step toward it with the weaker leg and then bring the stronger leg forward. Do not climb stairs with a walker.

3. Every assistive device must be adjusted to individual height; the top of the cane should align with the crease of the wrist.

4. Choose the right size and shape of cane handle that fits comfortably in the palm; like a tight shoe, it will be

四、尽早解除约束和恢复老年人的正常活动

减少环境危害,促进活动以增加耐力和功能,这也是预防摔倒的有效干预方法。清晰的沟通,周密的计划和护理技巧可以避免一些不必要的约束。约束中存在很多护理问题,护士需要及时关注和处理。

约束期间,注意避免约束对老年人造成危害,多与老年人沟通,交代约束的目的及注意事项,预防跌倒等意外。对于环境约束的老年人,帮助和指导老年人在限定范围内活动,增加耐力和功能训练,使用护理技巧,尽早解除约束,恢复老年人的正常活动。

五、合理选择和正确使用助行工具

帮助老年人选择合适的助行工具并正确使用。助行工具包括辅助设备、轮椅、运输、汽车等。在一般情况下,应遵守以下原则:

1. 首先移动辅助设备,然后移动患侧下肢,最后移动健侧下肢。穿低跟、防滑鞋。当挂拐杖上下楼梯时,上楼时帮助健侧腿,而下楼梯时帮助患侧腿。当抬患侧腿时,使用拐杖作为用力支撑。携带拐杖爬坡时,在往上爬一步之前拐杖应先支撑;而下坡时,应注意先将拐杖先下一步,然后移动患侧腿,最后移动健侧腿。

2. 使用步行器时,身体直立并用双手抬起步行器,将双腿站于步行器中一个舒适的距离,移动患侧腿向前时用步行器,然后移动健侧腿。步行器在攀爬楼梯时不能使用。

3. 每种辅助设备均必须进行调适,以符合个人的高度。拐杖的高度应与人站立时手腕高度持平。

4. 拐杖的手柄应舒适,适合手掌的大小和形状。

a constant irritant if it is not properly fitted.

5. Cane tips are most secure when they are flat on the bottom and have a series of rings. Replace tips frequently because they wear out and a worn tip is insecure.

(HUANG Jin)

5. 拐杖的底端部位是安全的保障，部分采用环状橡胶圈设计，使用越多，其磨损越快。应注意及时更换底部，以免影响安全。

（黄　金）

Key Points

1. Adverse living factor, health factors, environmental factors and psychological factors can result in mobility limitation among the elderly.

2. Most of the clinical manifestations mobility limitations are related to the temporary or permanent of illness.

3. Improving living condition and decreasing hazards related to mobility can promote mobility.

4. Remove restraints as early as possible is very critical in elderly care.

本章要点

1. 某些不利的生活因素、疾病、环境、心理因素等均可引起老年人活动受限。

2. 大多数活动受限与基础性疾病有关。

3. 改善生活条件，减少活动受限有关的危害，可促进活动。

4. 尽早去除约束对老人护理非常重要。

Critical Thinking Exercise

1. Spend 30 minutes in one public park in one day morning, please you observe what are the kind of the gait disorders of the elderly and the tools to help them walk?

2. What constraints are commonly used in the elderly?

3. How to take care of an elderly patient with indwelling catheter, unconscious and intravenous infusion?

批判性思维练习

1. 选择某天上午到公园散步 30 分钟，请观察老年人存在哪些步态障碍和使用哪些助行工具？

2. 老年人常用的约束有哪些？

3. 怎样照顾一位留置导尿管、有意识障碍并正接受静脉输液的老年患者？

Chapter 13 Care of Elderly with Nutritional Disorder

第十三章 老年人营养失调的护理

Learning Objectives

On completion of this chapter, the reader will be able to:

- Describe the changes in nutritional requirements for elderly;
- List the common nutritional problems in elders;
- Identify factors contributing to malnutrition in elderly;
- Describe the differences between a nutritional screen and a nutritional assessment;
- Identify the core data collection elements of a nutritional assessment ;
- Describe the social, cultural, and emotional aspects of food;
- Identify strategies to promote adequate nutrition for elderly;
- Discuss an interventional care plan to assist the elderly in developing and maintaining good nutritional status.

学习目标

完成本章内容的学习，应完成以下目标：

- 描述老年人营养需求的变化；
- 列出老年人常见的营养问题；
- 识别影响老年人营养的因素；
- 描述营养筛查与营养评估的不同；
- 提出营养评估需要收集的核心数据；
- 描述食物在社会、文化及情感方面的内涵；
- 提出能促进老年人合理膳食的策略；
- 制订一个干预性的护理计划，使其能够帮助老年人形成并维持一个好的营养状态。

Proper nutrition means that all the essential nutrients (e. g. , carbohydrates, protein, fat, vitamins, minerals, and fluids) are adequately supplied and used to maintain optimal health. The variance in nutritional requirements throughout the life span is not well established in the elderly. Nutritional well-being of the elderly people is influenced to a small degree by age-related gastrointestinal changes and to a large degree by risk factors that commonly occur in older adulthood such as functional impairment, social isolation, and poor economic status. Although elderly can easily compensate for age-related changes in the digestive tract, they have more difficulty compensating for factors that interfere with their ability to obtain, prepare, and enjoy food. This chapter discusses nutritional requirements, risk factors affecting nutrition, nutritional assessment, and nursing interventions to promote optimal nutrition in elderly.

营养对人的健康非常重要。拥有良好的营养状态，人体才能维持正常功能、保持充沛的体力和预防疾病，从而保证生活质量。合理营养是指所有的基本营养素（如：碳水化合物、蛋白质、脂肪、维生素以及矿物质和液体）都能充足的供应并且用于维持最佳的健康状态。老年人的营养健康受老化的影响，特别是老年期常见的危险因素，如功能障碍、社会和经济状况等。老年人可以很容易地弥补消化道中与年龄相关的变化，但是他们很难弥补那些干扰他们获得、准备和享用美食能力的因素。本章主要讨论老年人的营养需求、影响营养状况的因素、营养评估和促进老年人营养状况的护理措施。

Box 13-1　Case Study

Mr. Yang is 78-year-old who lives alone at home. His wife died one month ago. He has two sons, but they live in other cities and seldom come back to visit him. In the past, his wife prepared food for him, so he does not know how to cook. Mr. Yang only eats one meal a day and loses interests in food. He lost 5 kg weight in the past month.

Questions:

1. What are the risk factors contributing to Mr. Yang's weight loss?

2. What would you do to promote Mr. Yang's nutritional status?

Box 13-1　案例

78 岁的杨先生是一位独居的老人，他的妻子已去世一个月。他有两个儿子，但他们生活在外地，很少回来看望他。过去，是杨先生的妻子做饭，因此他不知道怎样做饭。杨先生每天只吃一顿饭并且食欲也不好，一个月瘦了 5 千克。

问题：

1. 杨先生体重减少的危险因素是什么？

2. 怎样能改善杨先生的营养状况？

Section 1　Nutritional Disorder and Related Factors

第一节　老年人的营养需求及常见营养问题

I. Nutritional Requirements for Elders

一、老年人的营养需求

The dietary reference intakes (DRIs) from the Food and Nutrition Board of the U. S. , the Institute of Medicine, the National Academy of Sciences, and Health Canada establish standards for meeting the basic nutrient needs of older adults in categories 51 to 70 years and beyond 70 years. DRIs also address the changes of nutritional

美国国家科学院医学研究所食品和营养委员会和加拿大卫生部的膳食参考摄入量（DRI）规定了 51 岁至 70 岁及 70 岁以上年龄段老年人的基本营养需求。膳食参考摄入量强调老年人的营养需要量会变化。例如：50 岁

requirements for older adults. For example, calcium increases to 1200 mg/d for those 50 years and older, vitamin D increases to 400 IU /d for those aged 51 to 70 years and 600 IU/d for those aged 70 years and older, and iron decreases to 8 mg/d in women 51 years and older. Other nutritional changes are introduced below:

1. Calories Caloric requirements are determined by a combination of factors, including gender, height, weight, body build, health status, and the level of physical activity. Caloric requirements in older adults gradually decrease because of decreased physical activity and basal metabolic rate. To meet minimal nutritional requirements, this decrease in caloric intake requires a proportionate increase in the quality of calories (nutritional density). In China, recommended daily calories intake for the elderly are 2000-2200 kcal for man, 1800-1900 kcal for woman.

2. Protein Age-related changes, including decreased lean body mass and muscle tissue, and decreased plasma albumin and total body albumin levels, may influence protein requirements in elders. As people age, their ability to utilize protein decrease, and rates of protein decomposition is greater than the synthesis. With weakened digestion and excretion system, they can not tolerate excessive protein intake. Protein supply should be determined according to the specific circumstances of the elderly, should also be preferred high quality protein, such as milk, fish, poultry, meat, eggs, seafood, and beans. It is suggested that the protein requirements for older adults should be increased to 1.0 to 1.2 g/kg for optimal muscle and bone health.

3. Carbohydrates and fiber Carbohydrates provide an essential source of energy and fiber. Carbohydrates should contribute about 65 percent of calories in the daily diet. Older adults are prone for Glucose. Compared to the simple carbohydrates, complex carbohydrates put less stress on the circulating blood glucose. Dietary guidelines for older adults suggest at least 55% of the total calories consumed derive from complex carbohydrates. Recommended daily carbohydrates intake for elder people is 50-100 g. If the intake of carbohydrates is inadequate, the body will derive energy from protein and fat, causing an increase in serum lipid levels and a depletion of water, electrolytes, and amino acids.

An adequate intake of fiber may lower blood

以后钙的需要量增加到 1 200mg/d、51 岁至 70 岁维生素 D 的需要量增加到 400IU/d，而 70 岁以后的需要量增加到 600IU/d、女性 51 岁以后铁的需要量减少至 8mg/d。其他营养的变化介绍如下：

1. 热量 热量的需要受多个因素的影响，包括性别、身高、体重、体型、健康状况和体力活动。老年人的体力活动减少、基础代谢率降低，对热量的需求逐渐减少。为满足基本营养需求，老年人应摄取高质量的热能饮食。我国营养学会推荐的老年人每日热能供给量标准（以轻度劳动为例）为：男性 2 000～2 200kcal，女性 1 800～1 900kcal。

2. 蛋白质 随年龄的变化，老年人体重和肌肉组织减少，血浆白蛋白和全身白蛋白水平降低，可能会影响其蛋白质的需求。老年人对蛋白质的利用率降低，分解大于合成，蛋白质摄入量应不低于成人需要量。但是老年人消化能力和排泄能力减弱，不能耐受过多蛋白质的摄入，应根据老年人的具体情况决定蛋白质供给量，同时应优选优质蛋白质，如乳、鱼、禽、肉、蛋、海产品、豆类等。老年人的蛋白质建议摄入量为每日 1～1.2g/kg，用于促进肌肉及骨骼的健康。建议每周吃鱼 280～525g，蛋类 280～350g。每天豆类摄入量为 25～35g。

3. 糖类及纤维素 糖类是主要的热量和纤维素来源，老年人膳食中糖类提供的能量应占总能量的 65% 左右。老年人喜食甜食。相比于单糖，多糖对循环血糖的压力较小。膳食指南推荐老年人至少 55% 的能量要来源于复合糖，每天摄入 50～100g 糖类。如果糖类摄入不足，能量就由蛋白质和脂肪提供，这样会使血脂升高，水、电解质及氨基酸丢失。但要限制可直接引起血糖波动的单糖（如葡萄糖、果糖、半乳糖）和双糖（如蔗糖、麦芽糖、乳糖），其总量不应超过糖类的 10%，以果糖为宜。

适当的纤维摄入可以降低血压，降低血

pressure, improve serum cholesterol and triglyceride levels, and play a role in prevention of diabetes, cardiovascular disease, and colorectal cancer. Increasing consuming fiber-rich foods (e. g. whole-grain and whole-wheat foods, fresh fruits and vegetables) to 14 g/1000 calories are recommended for older adults.

4. Fats   Fat should constitute no more than 10% to 30% of a person's daily caloric intake. Saturated fats are associated with the detrimental accumulation of serum cholesterol, which increase risk of heart disease. It is recommended to consume more polyunsaturated and monounsaturated fatty acids, and consume limited cholesterol and saturated fats. Consuming fewer than 10% of calories from saturated fat is recommended for older adults.

China Nutrition Society recommended that only 20%-25% of total calories should come from fat and with proportion of 1/3 of saturated fatty acids, 1/3 of monounsaturated fatty acids (aquatic animals, vegetable oil content) and 1/3 of multi-unsaturated fatty acids (except coconut oil, vegetable oil). The elderly also need to pay attention to their cholesterol intake.

5. Water   Water is often overlooked as a nutritional requirement. However, it is essential for all metabolic activities and must be consumed in adequate amounts. Reduced body water may lead to decreased efficiency of thermo-regulation, increased risk to dehydration, and increased concentrations of water-soluble medications in the body. Poor fluid intake in older adults may further diminish total body water and cause dehydration. The recommended amount of water intake is 1500-1700 ml at least.

6. Vitamins, salts and trace elements   Dietary vitamins, mineral and trace elements are essential nutrients to maintain body functions. Some vitamins also play an important role to enhance the body resistance and have anti-aging effects. The elderly should always eat food rich in various vitamins. Chinese Nutrition Society recommended the elderly daily dietary vitamin intake including vitamin A 800 μg, vitamin D 10 μg, vitamin E 12 mg, vitamin C 60 mg, vitamin B_1 1.2 mg, vitamin B_2 1.2 mg, and niacin 12 mg.

The elderly have decreased ability to absorb calcium and prone to the negative balance of calcium. Increase

清胆固醇和三酰甘油的水平，对预防心血管疾病、糖尿病和直肠癌有重要意义。老年人应多食富含纤维素的食物（如全谷和全麦食物、新鲜的蔬菜和水果）。纤维素的推荐量为每日35g。应餐餐有蔬菜，保证每天摄入300～500g蔬菜，深色蔬菜应占1/2，保证200～350g新鲜水果，果汁不能代替鲜果。谷类250～400g。

4. 脂肪   脂肪的摄入量为每日摄入热量的10%～30%。饱和脂肪酸能提高血清胆固醇水平，从而增加心脏疾病的风险。老年人的脂类供给应保证不饱和脂肪酸的摄入，限制饱和脂肪酸的摄入。建议老年人摄入的饱和脂肪要低于总热量的10%。

我国营养学会推荐的脂肪摄入量为占总热量的20%～25%，其中饱和脂肪酸、单不饱和脂肪酸（水生动物、植物油含量高）和多不饱和脂肪酸（除椰子油外的植物油）各占1/3为宜。老年人应少食胆固醇高的食物，每日胆固醇总摄入量应低于300mg。每日食用油的摄入量保证在25～30g。

5. 水   作为营养素，水经常被忽视。但是，水是所有的代谢活动所必需的。减少水的摄入会降低体温调节的效率，增加脱水的风险，并增加水溶性药物在体内的浓度。老年人通常摄入的液体量不足，进一步减少了体内的水分，容易导致脱水。推荐每日饮水量至少为1 500～1 700ml。

6. 维生素、无机盐和微量元素   膳食中的维生素、无机盐和微量元素是维持人体功能的必需营养素，其中维生素对增强机体抵抗力、延缓衰老具有重要作用。老年人应经常食用富含各类维生素的食物，我国营养学会推荐的老年人每日膳食维生素摄入量为维生素A 800μg，维生素D 10μg，维生素E 12mg，维生素C 60mg，维生素 B_1 1.2mg，维生素 B_2 1.2mg，烟酸12mg。

老年人对钙的吸收能力降低，容易出现钙的负平衡，应增加钙的摄入量。西方国家

calcium intake is important. In Western countries, the recommended amount daily calcium intake is 1000 – 1200 mg for elders and 1200-1500 mg for postmenopausal women. The elderly should eat milk, beans, and fish food. The elderly also have decreased ability of phosphorus absorption and hypophosphatemia were more common. The recommended supplement calcium and Phosphorus ratio is 1: 1.

Excessive salt intake will increase the risk of suffering from hypertension. The elderly should take strictly controlled salt intake. A daily intake of 6 g salt is recommended. Sufficient source of some trace elements are also important to the elderly. It is recommended for the elderly to take iron 15 mg, selenium 100 μg, manganese 10 mg.

II. Common Nutrition Problems

Problems in nutrition are very common in the elderly. Physiological changes with aging, functional impairment, chronic illness, depression, dementia, social isolation, and poverty are factors that affect the nutritional status of older adults.

1. Dehydration Older adults are vulnerable to fluid. Even small decreases in fluid intake can cause dehydration in an elder because the elderly people have decreased water in their body composition. Thirst sensation diminishes with aging, resulting in the decreased intake of fluids in older adults, and making dehydration a prime risk. Depression, confusion, and dementia also contribute to reduced food and fluid intake. Loss of sodium during a gastrointestinal illness and increased fluid losses from fever can also cause dehydration in older adults.

Standard indicators for dehydration among elders are not always reliable. Dry mucous membranes, diminished skin turgor (best evaluated on the forehead or sternum), and orthostatic hypotension are the general signs in mild dehydration. Other signs include sunken eyeballs, swollen tongue, elevated body temperature, diminished urine output, and electrolyte disturbances. Dry mucous membranes may be misleading because many elders breathe by mouth. Additional signs and symptoms such as oliguria or anuria, confusion, and resting hypotension will be found in moderate dehydration. Shock or near shock will be found in severe dehydration. Many of the signs and symptoms

推荐量为每日 1 000～1 200mg，对绝经后妇女的建议摄入量为每日 1 200～1 500mg。老年人应多食牛乳、豆类和鱼虾类的食物。老年人对磷的吸收能力下降，低磷血症较多见，推荐老年人按 1∶1 的比例补充钙和磷。

食盐过多会增加患高血压病的危险，老年人应严格控制食盐的摄入，食盐的摄入量以每日不超过 6g。老年人对某些微量元素的摄入量偏低，应适当补充海产品、蛋、肉、豆类和粗粮等，以获取足够的微量元素，建议每日摄入量为铁 15mg、硒 100μg、锰 10mg。

二、老年人常见的营养问题

营养问题在老年人中非常普遍。随着年龄的增长，老年人会出现生理变化、功能障碍、慢性疾病、抑郁、痴呆、社交孤立和贫穷，这些因素会影响老年人的营养状态。

1. 脱水 老年容易受到体内液体的影响。老年人体内水分含量下降，即使摄入液体量有轻微的减少也能导致脱水。老年人口渴感觉变迟钝，饮水量减少，更易发生脱水。老年人抑郁、困惑、痴呆都能减少水分及食物的摄入。另外，因胃肠疾病导致钠的丢失以及发热导致液体的丢失也可引起脱水。

老年人脱水的标准指标并不总是可靠的。黏膜干燥，皮肤张力减小（最好的评估部位是额头或胸骨）以及直立性低血压都是轻度脱水的一般体征。其他迹象包括眼球凹陷、舌头肿胀、体温升高、尿量减少和电解质紊乱。黏膜发干可能会误导人，因为许多老年人经口呼吸。另外，在中度脱水时会发现其他体征和症状，例如，少尿或无尿、意识不清和静息性低血压。严重脱水时会出现休克或接近休克。以上许多体征和症状可能存在于老年人中，但是老年人的体容量并未减少，

may be present in the elders without volume loss, which make it difficult to give a definitive diagnosis.

Dehydration can cause serious consequences such as electrolyte imbalance and altered mental status. Other consequences of dehydration include constipation, thromboembolism, pressure ulcers, orthostatic hypotension, and kidney stones. Adequate fluid intake is as important to total nutrition as food. Daily fluid needs of elders depend on general health status, medications, and activity level. A 24-hour intake of at least 2000 ml of water is recommended and should be offered hourly during the day.

2. Malnutrition Malnutrition is not only common, but also overlooked in the elderly people. Malnutrition refers to the insufficient, excessive or imbalanced consumption of nutrients. It encompasses both under-nutrition and over-nutrition. Inadequate dietary intake, impaired absorption, increased nutrient loss from body, or excessive intake of food may lead to malnutrition. Medications including digoxin, theophylline, nonsteroidal anti-inflammatory drugs, iron supplements, and psychoactive drugs are also associated with malnutrition.

Undernutrition is one of the most concerned health issues for older adults, especially those with chronic disease. Undernutrition can be defined as "Imbalanced nutrition: less than body requirements." Specific nutrients that are likely to be deficient in older adults include fiber, calcium, magnesium, potassium, and vitamins C, D, E, and K. Malnutrition in elders is associated with poor clinical outcomes and risk for increased mortality. It is important to assess and manage the nutritional problems in elders. The nutritional assessment and interventions will be discussed in the following sections.

III. Factors Related to Malnutrition

1. Physiological factors related to malnutrition Physiologic changes in aging can lead to problems with nutrition. The organ function of digestion, metabolism, absorption of nutrients, and the ability to eliminate waste products via the kidneys decline in older adults. Changes in the oral cavity including tooth loss, mouth dryness, and decreased esophageal motility influence nutritional status because they affect chewing, eating, and swallowing. Lack of teeth and inadequate dental care are two conditions common in elders that have detrimental effects on eating and nutrition. These adverse effects include malnutrition,

这使得医生难以给出确定的诊断。

脱水可能导致严重的后果，如电解质紊乱和精神状态改变。脱水的其他后果包括便秘、血栓栓塞、压力性溃疡、直立性低血压和肾结石。充足的液体摄入量与食物的总营养一样重要。老年人的每日液体的需求取决于一般健康状况、药物和活动水平。建议24小时内水的摄入量至少为2 000ml，并且白天每一小时喝水一次。

2. 营养失调 营养失调在老年人中不仅常见，而且很容易被忽视。营养不良是指营养素的摄入过度或不平衡。它包括营养不良和营养过剩。饮食摄入不足、吸收功能受损、营养物质的流失或过量摄入食物都可导致营养失调。地高辛、茶碱、非甾体抗炎药、铁补充剂和精神活性药物也与营养失调有关。

营养不良是老年人，特别是有慢性疾病老年人最关心的健康问题之一。营养不良可以定义为"营养失衡：低于机体需要量"。老年人可能缺乏的特定营养素包括纤维素、钙、镁、钾、维生素C、维生素D、维生素E和维生素K。老年人营养不良与不良的临床结局和增加死亡风险相关。评估和管理老年人的营养问题是很重要的。营养评估和干预措施将在以下部分讨论。

三、影响老年人营养的因素

1. 生理因素 随年龄的增长，生理方面的改变也能导致一些营养问题。老年人消化、新陈代谢、营养物质的吸收能力以及通过肾脏排除废物的功能都会减弱。老年人牙齿松动、唾液分泌减少，不利于食物的咀嚼和吞咽。牙齿脱落和牙齿保健不足是老年人常见的两种情况，这对饮食和营养有不利的影响。这些影响包括营养不良、脱水、牙周病、呼吸道感染、心血管疾病和卒中风险增加。胃

dehydration, periodontal disease, respiratory infections, cardiovascular disease, and increased risk of stroke. The gastrointestinal system slows with age. Delayed gastric emptying may cause bloating and discomfort. Changes in the pH of the gastrointestinal tract result in the malabsorption of B vitamins. Decreased hepatic and renal reserves make it harder to metabolize medications and alcohol, to conserve water, and excrete nitrogenous wastes.

Functional impairments are associated with malnutrition. Elderly with functional impairments may have difficulty performing activities of daily living related to eating. For example, mobility or visual impairments can interfere with the ability to procure and prepare food. Some conditions such as pain or shortness of breath can affect an elder's ability and desire to eat. Dysphagia (difficulty swallowing) is a functional impairment that can affect chewing, safe swallowing, and nutrition in older adults. Smell and taste perception generally decline with age and can become quite exaggerated with some medication, resulting in greater differences in taste or smell. Foods once cherished and enjoyed now smell very different and may be avoided by the elderly.

2. Psychosocial factors related to malnutrition Psychosocial factors are likely to affect an older adult's appetite and eating patterns. Social isolation is contributing to malnutrition. The elderly may skip meals when they live alone and have no companionship to prepare and share meals. As individuals age their loss of family members and friends can be significant and overwhelming. For the older adults, grieving over the loss of a spouse or friends may affect their diet quality and intake. When the elderly have established a long-term pattern of preparing meals for family, it is especially difficult for them to adjust to purchasing, preparing, and eating food for just one person. Similarly, elders who have never purchased or prepared foods may have great difficulty taking these tasks after the loss of a spouse or other person who assumed these tasks.

Depression is common in older adults and often accompanied with GI complaints, poor appetite, weight loss, and weight gain. Weight loss is an important concern in elders with depression. Depression influences the individual's decision to eat or not to eat and regulation of hunger and satiety. Older adults who are depressed are likely to experience anorexia and loss of interest in eating. Cognitive deficits such as confusion, memory problems, and dementia may interfere with eating patterns and the ability to prepare food. Cognitive deficits can also

肠系统的功能随年龄增长而减弱。老年人胃肠道排空延迟可能引起腹胀和不适，胃肠道pH值的变化导致B族维生素的吸收不良，肝脏和肾脏储备减少使得药物和酒精的代谢、水分保存和排泄含氮废物更加困难。

功能障碍与营养不良有关。有功能障碍的老年人很难进行与进食有关的日常活动。例如：移动性或视觉障碍可能干扰采购和准备食物的能力、疼痛或呼吸急促可影响老年人的吃饭的能力和食欲。吞咽困难是一种功能障碍，能影响老年人的咀嚼、安全吞咽和营养状况。嗅觉和味觉通常随着年龄下降，并且服用一些药物可使嗅觉和味觉功能下降得更加厉害。老年人在品尝或闻气味时与真实情况产生较大的差异，曾经喜欢的食物与现在气味非常不同，可能会避免它。

2. 心理社会因素 心理社会因素会影响老年人的食欲和饮食方式。社交孤立会造成营养不良。独自生活、没有人陪着准备或分享食物时，老年人可能会不吃饭。丧失亲人、朋友会使老年人悲伤，影响其准备食物或降低饮食欲望。对于老年人，失去配偶或朋友的悲伤可能影响他们的饮食质量和摄入量。当老年人已经建立了为家庭准备饭菜的长期模式时，他们很难适应一个人购买、准备和吃食物。同样，从未购买或准备食物的老年人失去配偶或承担这些任务的其他人后可能很难接受这些任务。

抑郁在老年人中很常见。并且有抑郁情绪的老年人经常伴有胃肠道疾病、食欲缺乏、体重减轻或体重增加。在有抑郁情绪的老年人中，体重减轻是非常需要关注的。抑郁能影响人决定吃或不吃食物以及饥饿感和饱腹感。抑郁的老年人可能有厌食和食欲缺乏。认知缺陷如混乱、记忆力出现问题和痴呆，可能会干扰老年人饮食模式和准备食物的能

lead to the loss of awareness of need to eat and therefore inadequate intake of foods. Cognitive impairment and depression are risk factors related to poor nutrition in the elderly.

3. Social cultural factors related to malnutrition

Food and dinning are culturally related. In many cultural, foods are given to the rich social and cultural connotations. Traditionally, Chinese medicine practitioners believe that some food can promote and maintain health by stimulating the yin and yang. Many herbs are used in food preparation. However, due to the lack of medicinal knowledge, herb was used abusively in some situations. Social events and religions are also factors influencing nutrition status. It is easy to break personal usual dietary routines during special events such as celebrations. In some religious, some food and drink is prohibited.

4. Socioeconomic factors related to malnutrition

Poverty is a significant problem for older adults, especially those who live in the rural areas. Low income is associated with poor nutrition. As the percentage of income required for health care rises, food may be sacrificed in elders who are poor. Food may initially be limited in quality as choosing cheaper food, followed by a limitation in quantity. Some older people eat only once a day due to financial constraints. Poor older adults are likely to reside in substandard housing. Some live in single rooms with limited space for food storage and cooking. The crowded environment may also affect food enjoyment and consumption. If food intake has been inadequate for a period, the progressive effects of poor nutrition may precipitate to new health problems in elderly individuals, especially in combination with age-related changes in nutrient intake and utilization.

Transportation may influence the purchase of food for older adults. The public transportation is crowded in big cities and not convenient in rural areas. It may become difficult to reach the supermarkets by public transportation, or to carry a bag of groceries while using a cane. Older adults fear being knocked down or falling as they walk in crowded streets, and not being able to cross the street in the time of green traffic light. They purchase their groceries at smaller convenience stores, where prices are higher and selection is limited. The additional cost and limited selection may decrease the amount of food purchased by the elders and lead to nutrient deficiencies.

Additional factors contributing to nutritional disorders include alcohol and smoking. Alcohol, which has a high caloric content but low nutrient value, interferes

力。认知缺陷也可能导致对食物需要的意识丧失，使食物摄入不足。认知障碍和抑郁是老年人营养不良的危险因素。

3. 社会文化因素 食物和餐饮与文化有关。在许多文化中，食物被赋予丰富的社会和文化内涵。在古代，中医认为一些食物可调整阴阳平衡，促进和维护健康，许多草药被用于食物的制作。但是，由于人们对食物药用知识的缺乏，民间存在药膳滥用现象。一些事件和宗教信仰是营养状况的影响因素。一些特别的事件如庆祝活动，很容易让人打破个人平时的饮食规律。在一些宗教团体中，有些食物和饮料是被禁止的。

4. 社会经济因素 由于保健水平的提高需要收入的增加，一些较贫穷的老年人在食物方面作了一些牺牲。食物最初的限制是质量上的限制，即选择较便宜的食物，其次是数量上的限制。由于经济条件的限制，一些老年人每天只吃一顿饭。贫穷的老年人可能住在不合标准的房间。有些老年人住在单间里，食物储存和烹饪空间很有限。拥挤的环境也可能影响食欲。如果一段时间内食物摄取不足，营养不良的渐进效应可能会导致老年人新的健康问题，特别是在与年龄相关的营养摄入和营养利用发生变化相结合方面。

交通可能影响老年人购买食物。在大城市公共交通是很拥挤，而在农村却不方便。利用公共交通很难到达超市，或者在拄着拐杖时还要携带一大袋杂货。老年人害怕在拥挤的街道上行走时被撞倒或跌倒，而在绿灯时也无法穿过街道。因此，老年人会在较小的便利店购买杂货。便利店里的东西价格较高且选择有限。额外的成本和有限的选择可能会减少老年人购买食物的数量，导致自身营养缺乏。

导致营养不良的因素还包括喝酒和吸烟。酒精含有很高的热量，但营养价值很低。酒精干扰维生素 B 族和维生素 C 的吸收。吸烟

with the absorption of the B-complex vitamins and vitamin C. Smoking diminishes the ability to smell and taste food and interferes with absorption of vitamin C and folic acid. Smoking and drinking alcohol are common in older adults and often unrecognized or under-treated.

Physiologic, psychosocial, and socioeconomic factors affect nutritional status in older adults. The nurse must assess these contributing factors during nutritional screening or a comprehensive nutritional assessment.

会使老年人的味觉和嗅觉下降，并干扰维生素 C 和叶酸的吸收。然而吸烟和饮酒在老年人群中比较普遍，常被忽视。

生理、心理和社会经济文化方面的因素能影响老年人的营养状况。护士在营养筛查或综合的营养评估时必须评估这些方面的因素。

Section 2　Nutrition Assessment

I. Nutritional Screening

Nutritional screening is an abbreviated assessment of nutritional risk factors. The aim of nutritional screening is to determine which clients need a more comprehensive assessment and nutritional interventions. Many tools have been developed to conduct nutritional screening. The most widely used tool for older adults is the "determine your nutritional health" screening tool developed as part of the Nutrition Screening Initiative (NSI). The NSI is a project of the American Academy of Family Physicians, the American Dietetic Association, and the National Council on the Aging. This 5-year national project began in 1990 to promote routine nutrition screening.

The "determine your nutritional health" screening tool is a checklist used by older adults or caregivers to determine risk factors associated with nutrition and health. This checklist includes 10 statements. Each statement has a score for the yes answer. The 10 statements are listed in the box 13-2.

第二节　老年人的营养评估

一、营养筛查

营养筛查是对营养危险因素的简单评估，目的是确定哪些人需要进一步的综合评估和干预。许多工具被开发出来用于营养筛查。针对老年人的、最广泛应用的筛查工具是"确定你的营养健康"，该筛查工具是由美国启动营养筛查（NSI）项目组研发的。NSI 是美国饮食协会、美国家庭医师学会和国家老龄化委员会的项目。这个为期 5 年的国家项目始于 1990 年，旨在促进常规营养筛查。

"确定你的营养健康"是用于确定老年人及其照顾者营养健康相关的危险因素的筛查工具。它包括 10 项陈述，对每一项陈述的肯定回答都有一个相应的分数。这 10 项陈述如 box 13-2 所示。

Box 13-2　Nutrition Screening Tool

1. I have an illness or condition that made me change the kind and/or amount of food I eat. (Yes, score 2)

2. I eat fewer than 2 meals per day. (Yes, score 3)

3. I eat few fruits or vegetables, or milk products. (Yes, score 2)

4. I have 3 or more drinks of beer, liquor or wine almost

Box 13-2　营养筛查工具

1. 我有一种疾病或情况，改变了我吃的食物的种类和 / 或数量。(是，2 分)

2. 我每天吃饭次数少于 2 次。(是，3 分)

3. 我吃少量的水果或蔬菜，或奶制品。(是，2 分)

4. 我几乎每天喝 3 次以上的啤酒、烈酒或葡

every day. (Yes, score 2)

5. I have tooth or mouth problems that make it hard for me to eat. (Yes, score 2)

6. I don't always have enough money to buy the food I need. (Yes, score 4)

7. I eat alone most of the time. (Yes, score 1)

8. I take 3 or more different prescribed or over-the-counter drugs a day. (Yes, score 1)

9. Without wanting to, I have lost or gained 5 kg in the last 6 months. (Yes, score 2)

10. I am not always physically able to shop, cook and/or feed myself. (Yes, score 2)

A total score of 0-2 indicates it is good and to recheck the nutritional score in 6 months. A score of 3-5 indicates moderate nutritional risk, something need to be done to improve eating habits and lifestyle, and to recheck the nutritional score in 3 months. A score of 6 or more indicates high nutritional risk, the need to see a health professional, and to ask for help to improve nutritional health. If a client has moderate to high nutritional risk, a more comprehensive nutritional assessment is needed. The level II screen also developed in the project of NSI is used to conduct a more in-depth assessment of nutritional status by health care professionals. The level II screen includes serial measurements such as anthropometrics (height, weight, body mass index, mid-arm circumference, triceps skinfold, mid-arm muscle circumference), laboratory data (serum albumin, serum cholesterol), drug use (three or more prescription drugs, over-the-counter medications, and/or vitamin and mineral supplement daily), clinical features, eating habits, living environment, functional status, and mental/cognitive status.

It is well recognized that malnutrition is related to negative clinical outcomes and increased costs of hospitalization and care. Nutrition is an integral intervention in many diseases. The importance of nutritional screening is emphasized in the standards and guidelines for the health care. The standards developed by the Joint Commission on Accreditation of Healthcare Organizations require nutritional screening of all hospitalized and home care clients who receive clinical services. They also require referral for a comprehensive nutritional assessment if the client is at moderate to severe nutritional risk.

葡酒。(是，2分)

5. 我的牙齿或嘴有一点问题，使我吃饭很困难。(是，2分)

6. 我没有足够的钱买我需要的食物。(是，4分)

7. 我大多数时间在吃饭。(是，1分)

8. 我每天服用3种或更多不同的处方药或非处方药。(是，1分)

9. 没有任何想法，我就在过去6个月中减少或增加了约5kg。(是，2分)

10. 我的身体使我不能购物、做饭和/或喂自己吃饭。(是，2分)

得分0~2分说明情况良好，6个月后复查；3~5分说明有中度的营养危险，需要改善饮食习惯和生活方式，3个月后复查；6分及以上，说明有高度危险，需要专业人员的帮助来改善营养健康。如果患者存在中到高度营养危险，就需要进行进一步的综合营养评估。在NSI项目中开发的II级筛查用于卫生保健专业人员的营养状况的深入评估。II级筛查包括一系列的测量，如人体测量（身高、体重、体重指数、中臂周长、肱三头肌皮褶厚度、中臂肌肉周长），实验室数据（血清白蛋白，血清胆固醇），药物使用（三种及以上的处方药、非处方药和/或每日维生素和矿物质补充剂），临床特征，饮食习惯，生活环境，功能状态和精神/认知状态。

营养不良与不好的临床结局和增加的住院及护理费用有关。营养对许多疾病起到综合干预作用。在卫生保健的标准和指南中强调了营养筛查的重要性。卫生保健组织鉴定联合委员会制订的标准要求所有接受临床服务的住院患者和居家的患者都要进行营养筛查。如果患者有中度到重度的营养风险，他们还需要转诊进行全面的营养评估。

II. Nutritional Assessment

Nutritional assessment is a comprehensive evaluation of a client's nutritional status. It is performed when a risk is identified on a nutritional screening or when the risk status is obvious without a preliminary screening. According to the standards published by the American Society for Parenteral and Enteral Nutrition (ASPEN, 1995), the goals of a nutritional assessment are to: a. establish baseline subjective and objective nutrition parameters; b. identify specific nutritional deficits; c. determine nutritional risk factors; d. establish nutritional needs; e. identify medical and psychosocial factors that may influence the prescription and administration of nutritional support.

A client's demographic and psychosocial data, medical history, dietary history, medications, laboratory values, anthropometrics, and a physical assessment are typically included in a nutritional assessment. The following will focus on the assessments such as dietary history, anthropometrics, and laboratory values special for nutrition:

1. Diet history Besides a complete history and physical assessment, clients who are at nutritional risk require a more specific assessment of their dietary intake patterns. A diet history usually includes the following information: number of meals and snack per day; oral health and denture use; chewing or swallowing difficulties; use of medications; gastrointestinal problems or symptoms affecting eating; appetite; activity level; need for assistance with meals and meal preparation; and food allergies, preferences, and aversions. A 24-hour food recall is included in a diet history to estimate the average number of calories and amount of protein ingested daily. Another purpose of a food recall is to detect any deleterious food intake patterns (e. g. overuse of fried foods, lack of fruit or vegetables). Older adults should be instructed about how to estimate portion sizes and should be given samples from which to estimate their intake. For example, a serving of vegetables is ½ cup and 85 g of meat is the size of a pack of cards. Days selected for recording should be typical of their intake patterns. Some elders may have poor memory and may need assistance from the caregiver to complete the food recall.

A 3 to 7 day food intake history is obtained to get a more detailed picture of a client's diet and food patterns. Clients are asked to keep a detailed record of everything they eat, the amount of each type of food consumed, and the time at which they eat. Activities and feelings

二、营养评估

营养评估是对老年人营养状况的一个综合评价，营养评估是在营养筛查评估出风险或没有初步筛查就存在明显的风险时进行的。根据美国肠外和肠内营养学会（ASPEN，1995）出版的标准，营养评估的目标是：a. 采集主、客观营养参数的基本资料；b. 找出营养缺陷；c. 识别营养的危险因素；d. 明确营养需要；e. 分析影响实施营养支持的医疗和心理社会因素。

营养评估的内容包括人口统计学资料、心理社会资料、疾病史、膳食史、用药史、实验室检查、人体测量和身体评估。下面将着重介绍膳食史、人体测量学和实验室检查等方面的评估：

1. **膳食史** 除了完整的膳食史和生理评估，有营养风险的患者需要更具体地评估他们的饮食摄入模式。评估膳食史时应包含以下信息：每日餐数和茶点数；口腔卫生和义齿的应用；咀嚼或吞咽困难；服用的药物；影响饮食的胃肠道问题；食欲；活动程度；就餐或备餐辅助；以及过敏的食物、喜欢和厌恶的食物。膳食史包括24小时食物回顾，用以估计每日饮食的蛋白质和热量，了解不良的饮食类型（如过多食用油炸食物、缺少蔬菜和水果等）。评估时，指导老年人估计所吃食物的量，并且提供估计其摄入量的样品。例如，一份蔬菜是1/2杯，85g的肉是一副纸牌的大小。选择用于记录的天数应为其摄入模式的典型值。若老年人记忆力差，可由照护者帮助回忆。

如要获得更加详细的膳食和食物类型的情况，需要收集3~7天的饮食史。详细记录所吃的每种食物的种类、数量和饮食时间；记录活动和情绪，以便保健人员确定是否有

are also recorded. The health care professional can use the information to determine whether there are activities or emotional issues that may interfere with or enhance eating pleasure. Food frequency is also a means of assessing dietary patterns. Food frequency questionnaires are used to assess a particular nutrient category (e. g. calcium intake) or the adequacy of an individual's entire diet. One of the advantages of food frequency questionnaires is that dietary data is collected without compromising the client's sense of privacy about food intake and diet. They are often recommended to new clients.

2. Anthropometrics Height, weight, body mass index, triceps skinfold and mid-arm muscle circumference are often measured or calculated to assess an individual's nutritional status. Height and weight are the mainstays of anthropometric measurements. Usually the client is weighted in the morning dressing lightly and bared feet. Height can be estimated by measuring knee height (the distance from the heel to the top of the knee) using a broad-bladed caliper if an elder is unable to stand without assistance. Chumlea developed the following formula to estimate height with knee height:

Stature for men = (2.02 × knee height in cm) – (0.04 × age) + 64.19

Stature for women = (1.83 × knee height in cm) – (0.24 × age) + 84.88

With age there is an increase of body fat and a loss of lean body mass; therefore weight alone can be misleading for assessing nutritional status in older adults. Elderly people should avoid extreme leanness.

Body mass index (BMI) is often used to determine if a person's weight is healthy for his/her height. The BMI is calculated by dividing weight in kilograms by the square of height in meters. In the U. S. , federal standard for ideal weight is BMI of 18.5-25 kg/m². In China, it is recommended that 20-26.9 kg/m². The BMI has limitations for defining health in the elderly. It is based on weight, not percent body fat. It is not a reliable measurement of obesity and health risks in the elderly as they gain fat mass and lose muscle mass with age. A higher BMI threshold is used for underweight elderly individuals. International Dietetics and Nutrition Terminology defines underweight in persons >65 years of age as a BMI of <23. This BMI value is one indicator of malnutrition in the elders (American Dietetic Association).

活动或情感问题干扰或增强食欲。进食频率是评估膳食类型的一种方式,可用进食频率问卷评估某一特定营养素(如钙的摄入)或整个膳食的合理性。食物频率问卷的优点之一是饮食数据的收集没有损害患者食物摄入和饮食的隐私。它们经常被推荐给新的患者。

2. 人体测量 身高、体重、身体质量指数(BMI)和肱三头肌皮褶厚度等常用来评估老年人的营养状况。体重和身高是人体测量的重要组成。体重通常在早晨赤脚和穿着轻便的衣服时测量。如果老年人在没有帮助的情况下不能站立,可以通过使用尺子测量膝盖的高度(从脚跟到膝盖顶部的距离)来估计身高。Chumlea 开发了以下公式来估计膝盖高度的高度:

男性身高=(2.02×膝高度厘米数)–(0.04×年龄)+64.19

女性身高=(1.83×膝高度厘米数)–(0.24×年龄)+84.88

随着年龄增加,体内脂肪增加,体重减轻,因此,单独的体重测量可能对评估老年人的营养状况产生误导。老年人应避免极度瘦弱。

我国老年人通常使用的计算理想体重公式如下:男性老年人理想体重(kg)=[身高(cm)–100]×0.9;女性老年人理想体重(kg)=[身高(cm)–105]×0.95。实际体重在理想体重的±10%以内属正常,大于10%为超重,大于20%为肥胖,大于30%为严重肥胖。身体质量指数(BMI)常用来确定一个人的体重相对于其身高来说是否健康。计算BMI的方法为:体重(kg)除以身高(m)的平方。在美国,理想体重的联邦标准是BMI为18.5~25kg/m²。中国营养学会建议老年人BMI在20~26.9kg/m²比较适宜。用BMI来评估老年人的营养健康有一定的局限性。BMI是基于体重来计算的,

Other types of anthropometric measurements such as triceps skin fold and mid-arm muscle circumference are also recommended for detecting those overweight and underweight for their height. Triceps skin fold is measured with calipers that have a known degree of accuracy. The mid-arm muscle circumference is measured at the midpoint of the distance between the tip of the acromial process of the scapula and the olecranon process of the ulna. These measurements have limited value when measured only one time. Measurements over time may reveal changes in fat stores and muscle mass.

Some new scanning devices such as dual-energy X-ray absorptiometry (DXA) have developed to assess lean tissue and bone mass. The DXA is a fast, noninvasive, and highly accurate method. The practitioner can evaluate bone density at several sites and evaluate body fat in a minimum amount of time with minimum radiation exposure by using the DXA. One of the disadvantages of DXA scanning is that the client must be mobile and able to get to a clinic site to take advantage of this equipment.

3. Laboratory values Some tests reflecting protein synthesis can also reflect nutritional status. Serum albumin that reflects the liver's ability to synthesize plasma protein is most frequently cited in reference to malnutrition. Albumin has a half-life of about 21 days, so it is not always reflective of current nutritional

而不是用身体脂肪的百分比。中国人理想身体质量指数的标准是 BMI=18.5～23.9。随着年龄的增加，老年人身体脂肪增加，肌肉组织减少，因此身体质量指数用于评估老年人肥胖和健康风险是不可靠的。低体重老年人使用较高的 BMI 阈值。国际营养与营养术语定义低体重老年人是指年龄＞65 岁、BMI＜23 的老年人。该 BMI 值是老年人营养不良的一个指标（美国饮食协会）。

其他形式的人体测量，如肱三头肌皮褶厚度、中臂肌肉周长，也用来衡量低体重或超体重。中臂肌肉周长在肩胛骨肩峰过程的尖端和尺骨的直角过程之间的距离的中点处测量。仅测量一次时，这些测量值是局限值。测量随着时间不断进行，可以揭示脂肪储存和肌肉质量的变化。皮褶厚度是指人体一定部位连同皮肤和皮下脂肪在内的皮肤褶皱的厚度。测量时使用特定的皮褶计连续测量 3 次，取平均值，单位为毫米，它反映体脂状况。肱三头肌皮褶厚度（TSF）的测量方法为：被测者站立、上臂自然下垂，取左上臂背侧肱三头肌肌腹中点，即左肩峰至尺骨鹰嘴连线中点上方 2cm 处。测量者位于被测者的后方，用左手拇指和示指，从测量点旁 1cm 处将皮肤连同皮下脂肪沿手臂的长轴提起皮褶测量。老年男性 TSF 超过 10.4mm，老年女性超过 14mm 可判断为肥胖。

一些新的扫描设备，例如双能 X 射线吸收测定法（DXA）已经开发用于评估瘦肉组织和骨量。DXA 是一种快速、无创、高度准确的方法。医生可以在几个部位评估骨密度，并以最小的辐射暴露量，在最短的时间内评估身体脂肪。DXA 扫描的一个缺点是患者必须是移动的，并且患者所在的诊所能使用这种设备。

3. 实验室检查 一些反映蛋白质合成的测试也可以反映出营养状态。血清白蛋白反映肝脏合成血浆蛋白的能力，经常用于营养不良的测试。白蛋白的半衰期为 21 天，不能反映目前的营养状况。白蛋白的值易受药物、

status. Albumin values can be influenced by medication, hydration, immune status, and disease status. Therefore, albumin levels below 35 g/L may indicate some degree of malnutrition.

Transferrin is a carrier protein for iron. It has a half-life of 8 to 10 days and is a more rapid predictor of protein depletion. Transferrin levels below 2 g/L may reflect mild-to-moderate protein depletion and below 1 g/L may reflect severe protein depletion.

Pre-albumin, also called as transthyretin, is a transport protein for thyroxine and a carrier for retinal-binding protein. It has a shorter half-life of 2 to 3 days. Therefore, pre-albumin is more sensitive to changes in protein-energy status than albumin. Its concentration closely reflects recent dietary intake rather than overall nutritional status. Pre-albumin levels that range from 15 to 5 mg/dl indicate mild to moderate protein depletion and levels below 5 mg/dl indicate severe protein depletion.

Laboratory tests based on blood and urine can be important indicators of nutritional status; however, they are affected by non-nutritional factors as well. No single laboratory test is diagnostic of malnutrition and the laboratory data should be viewed as a part of the whole.

4. Nursing diagnoses associated with nutritional problems　Problems related to nutrition may be identified through the nutritional assessment. If nutritional deficits are identified, a pertinent nursing diagnosis is imbalanced nutrition: less than body requirements, defined as "intake of nutrients insufficient to meet metabolic needs". Related factors that may affect the elderly include chewing or swallowing difficulties, medications, anorexia, social isolation, depression, and inability to prepare food. Nursing diagnoses associated with a primary nutritional problem and diagnoses commonly having a nutritional component are listed below:

(1) Primary nutritional problem

a. Imbalanced nutrition: Less than body requirements.

b. Imbalanced nutrition: More than body requirements.

c. Risk for imbalanced nutrition: More than body requirements.

血压、免疫以及疾病的影响。因此，白蛋白水平低于35g/L可说明有一定程度的营养不良。

转铁蛋白的半衰期为8~10天，是较快的反映蛋白耗竭的指标。转铁蛋白水平低于2g/L反映有轻到中等程度的蛋白耗竭，低于1g/L反映有严重程度的蛋白耗竭。

血清前白蛋白，又称转甲状腺蛋白，是甲状腺素的运输蛋白，也是视黄醇结合蛋白的载体。前白蛋白的半衰期较短，为2~3天，比白蛋白更能反映蛋白-能量状况的变化。它能反映目前的饮食情况而不是整体的营养状态。前白蛋白水平在5~15mg/dl之间显示轻到中等程度的蛋白耗竭，低于5mg/dl显示重度蛋白耗竭。

实验室检查可作为评估营养状况的重要指标，但由于受多种非营养因素的影响，单一的检查不能诊断营养失调，只能作为参考。

4. 与营养问题相关的护理问题　与营养相关的问题可通过营养评估来确定。如果发现营养缺陷，有关的护理问题是营养不均衡：小于身体的需求，定义为"摄入的营养素不能满足代谢的需求"。能影响老年人营养状况的相关因素有咀嚼或吞咽困难、药物、厌食，社交隔离、抑郁和不能准备食物。与初级营养问题相关的护理问题以及常见的危险因素列举如下：

（1）主要的营养问题

a. 营养失衡：低于机体需要量。

b. 营养失衡：高于机体需要量。

c. 有营养失衡的危险：高于机体需要量。

(2) Risk factors

    a. Risk for aspiration.

    b. Diarrhea.

    c. Dysfunctional family processes: Alcoholism.

    d. Deficient fluid volume.

    e. Feeding self-care deficit.

    f. Disturbed sensory perception.

    g. Impaired swallowing.

    h. Risk for ineffective gastrointestinal tissue perfusion.

Section 3　Prevention and Intervention of Malnutrition

Alterations in nutrition require a care plan that specifically addresses the nutritional problem. Nursing interventions to promote healthy nutrition in elders include health education about optimal nutrition and disease prevention, and direct interventions to eliminate risk factors that interfere with nutrition. In this section, general information on social, cultural, and emotional aspects of food, dietary guidelines for elders, interventions to address risk factors affecting nutrition in elders, and strategies to promote optimal nutrition and disease prevention in elders are introduced.

I. Social, Cultural, and Emotional Aspects of Food

Food not only provides energy and nutrients for the body, but also serves as alternative therapies, a social centerpiece, a symbol of celebration, and a source of comfort. The therapeutic function of food can be traced from a statement of Hippocratic Oath: "I will apply dietetic measures for the benefit of the sick according to my ability and judgment; I will keep them from harm and injustice." (Tannahill, 1988). Another example is from the traditional Chinese medicine in which certain foods are considered to stimulate the yin and the yang and prescribed for clients to keep healthy. In present societies, the public has grown increasingly interested in consumption of herbal teas and vitamin therapy. The use of these complementary and alternative therapies can affect drug or nutrient interactions. Therefore, assessment

（2）危险因素

    a. 误吸的危险。

    b. 腹泻。

    c. 家族性功能障碍：酒精中毒。

    d. 体液不足。

    e. 自我照顾不足。

    f. 感知觉障碍。

    g. 吞咽障碍。

    h. 胃肠组织灌注无效的风险。

第三节　促进老年人营养健康的护理措施

营养状况的改变需要解决营养问题的护理计划。促进老年人健康营养的护理干预包括有关最佳营养和疾病预防的健康教育和消除干扰营养状况危险因素的直接干预。在本节中，介绍了食物在社会、文化和情感方面内涵、老年人的膳食指南、针对老年人营养状况危险因素的干预措施，以及促进老年人最佳营养和疾病预防的措施。

一、食物在社会、文化及情感方面的内涵

食物不仅能为身体提供能量和营养，而且参与了替代疗法，还是社会装饰品、庆祝的象征和舒适的来源。食物的治疗功能可以追溯到希波克拉底的誓言："为了患者的利益，我将根据我的能力和判断采取节食措施，我会让患者免受伤害和不公正"（Tannahill，1988）。另一个例子来自中国传统医学，某些食物被认为能刺激阴阳，并让患者保持健康。目前，人们对草药茶和维生素治疗越来越感兴趣。这些互补和替代疗法的使用可以影响药物或与营养物相互作用。因此，评估患者的饮食和补充摄入量对了解患者整体的医疗状况非

of a client's diet and supplement intake is important in understanding the client's overall medical status.

There are many cultural meanings in food, such as celebration of life events (e. g. , birthday, marriage, and holiday), expression of caring for another, business negotiations, and validation of social, cultural, or religious ceremonial functions. In religious practices, some foods and beverages are prohibited.

Older adults usually hold strong ties to their culture, believe in a home-cooked meal with fresh food, have emotional preference to certain food, and need social interaction to enhance functional status. It is important to understand the geriatric clients' social, cultural, and emotional ties to food when developing effective nutritional interventions.

II. Nutritional Guidelines for Elders

Healthy eating is important for all people, regardless of age. A number of organizations in the US have published numerous nutritional guidelines such as the *Food Guide Pyramid* (now known as MyPyramid), *the Recommended Dietary Allowances and Dietary Intakes* (RDAs and RDIs), *the Dietary Guidelines for Americans 2010*, and *the Healthy Eating Pyramid from Harvard School of Public Health*. However, guidelines that more specifically address the aging population are less due to a lack of data. Some of older adults are at risk for malnutrition because of a number of factors noted earlier. The National Health and Nutrition Examination Survey III (NHANES III) data demonstrate that the elders' diets are insufficient in a number of macronutrients and micronutrients (vitamins and minerals). NHANES III also reported an increased prevalence of anemia, either as iron deficiency or in combination with vitamin B_{12} or folate deficiencies. The ADA advocates all elders to eat a diet rich in fruits and vegetables, whole grains, and dairy products (ADA position paper, 2005). Some nutritional guidelines are also modified to include reference intakes for older adults.

1. **Modified MyPyramid for older adults** *The Modified MyPyramid for Older Adults* has been adapted from the *Tufts University's Food Guide Pyramid for Older Adults* to correspond with the new USDA *Food Guide Pyramid* (MyPyramid). The Modified MyPyramid for Older Adults continues to emphasize nutrient-dense food choices and the importance of fluid balance. It has added additional guidance about forms of foods that could

常重要。

食物包含了许多文化内涵，如庆祝活动（生日、婚姻和假日）、关心他人、商业谈判以及各种社会、文化或宗教仪式。在宗教活动团体中，一些食物和饮料是被禁止的。

老年人的饮食习惯通常与他们个人喜好有着紧密的联系，如有的老年人喜欢新鲜食材在家烹饪的食物。老年人对某些食物有情感偏好，需要社交互动来提高其功能状态。制订有效的营养干预措施时，需要理解老年人与食物的社会、文化和情感内涵间的联系。

二、遵循老年人的营养指南

健康的饮食对任何年龄人来说都很重要。美国已经出版了许多营养指南，例如《食物指南金字塔》（现在称为 MyPyramid）、《建议饮食补贴和膳食摄入量》（RDAs 和 RDIs）、《美国 2010 版饮食指南》、哈佛公共卫生学院制订的《健康饮食金字塔》。然而，由于缺乏数据，这些指南没有具体地关注老年人群的饮食。由于前面提到的一些因素，一些老年人面临营养不良的风险。国家健康和营养第三次调查（NHANES III）的数据表明，老年人的饮食中一些大量营养素和微量营养素（维生素和矿物质）不足。NHANES III 还报告由于缺乏铁和维生素 B_{12} 或叶酸而导致老年人贫血发病率上升。ADA 倡导老年人应多吃水果和蔬菜、全谷物和乳制品（2005 年，ADA 声明）。一些营养指南也针对老年人的参考摄入量进行了指南修订。

1. **膳食金字塔** 改良版的老年人膳食金字塔是在由 Tufts 大学制订的《老年人膳食金字塔》的基础上修订，强调选择高营养食物以及液体平衡的重要性，还增加了能够更好地满足老年人特殊需要的食物指南和规律锻炼的重要性的相关内容。

best meet the unique needs of the elderly and about the importance of regular physical activity.

Adults over the age of 70 tend to need fewer calories because they are not as physically active as they once were and their metabolic rates slow down. However, their bodies still require the same or higher levels of nutrients for optimal health outcomes. *The Modified MyPyramid for Older Adults* emphasizes a higher ratio of nutrients to calories (nutrient density) and stresses the importance of consuming adequate amounts of fiber rich foods (e. g. , whole grain products, whole fruits and vegetables), fluids, and certain supplemental nutrients (e. g. , calcium, vitamin D and vitamin B$_{12}$). With proper instruction, *the Modified MyPyramid for Older Adults* is an easy and systematic way for the elders to evaluate their own nutritional intake and independently make corrective adjustments. Some examples of food patterns are listed in table 13-1.

70 岁以上的老年人体力活动和代谢率下降，热量需求减少。然而，他们仍需要相当或较高水平的营养来保持健康。该指南主张高比例的强化营养素和饮食适量的富含纤维素的食物（如全谷物产品、水果和蔬菜），以及补充一些营养素（如钙、维生素 D 和维生素 B$_{12}$）。通过恰当的指导，使老年人能评估自身的营养状况、改进饮食方案（表 13-1）。

Table 13-1　Food Pattern in *the Modified MyPyramid for Older Adults*

Level	Food Pattern
First level (Foundation)	water/liquids 8 or more servings (choose water, fruit or vegetable juice, low-and nonfat milk, or soup)
Second level	whole, enriched and fortified grains and cereals 6 or more servings (choose whole grains and fortified foods such as brown rice, 100% whole-wheat bread, and bran cereals)
Third level	bright-colored vegetables 3 or more servings ; deep-colored fruit 2 or more servings
Fourth level	low-and nonfat dairy products 3 or more servings; dry beans and nuts, fish, poultry, lean meat, eggs 2 or more servings
Fifth level (a flag on the top)	use saturated and trans fat, sugar and salt sparingly; calcium, vitamin D, vitamin B$_{12}$ supplements (not all people need these supplements, check with your healthcare provider)

表 13-1　老年人膳食金字塔食物模型

层级	食物模型
第一层（基础）	水 / 液体 8 份或更多（选择水，水果或蔬菜汁，低脂和脱脂牛奶或汤）
第二层	全谷物 6 份或更多（选择全谷物和强化食品，如糙米，100% 全麦面包和糠谷物）
第三层	颜色明亮的蔬菜 3 份或更多；深色水果 2 份或更多
第四层	低脂和非脂肪乳制品 3 份或更多；干豆和坚果、鱼、家禽、瘦肉、鸡蛋 2 份或更多
第五层（顶端）	少量使用饱和脂肪和反式脂肪、糖和盐；钙、维生素 D、维生素 B$_{12}$ 补充剂（并不是所有的人都需要这些补充剂，需保健医生制订）

Corresponding with the federal government's *2015—2020 Dietary Guidelines for Americans,* the researchers at Tufts University developed the *MyPlate* for Older Adults. *MyPlate* provides examples of foods that fit into a healthy and well balanced diet for the older adults.

根据美国政府《2015—2020 年美国人饮食指南》，塔夫茨大学的研究人员开发了用于老年人的 MyPlate。MyPlate 提供了适合老年人健康和均衡饮食的例子。

2. Recommended dietary allowances and dietary intakes The Food and Nutrition Board of the U. S. National Research Council published the tenth edition of *the Recommended Dietary Allowances (RDAs)* for nutrients in 1989. The *RDAs* list protein, vitamins, minerals, and selected trace elements with their recommended daily intake for healthy people (age 0-51). *RDAs* are being replaced by the *Recommended Dietary Intakes (RDIs)*, because the *RDIs* include reference intakes for older adults in categories 51 to 70 years and beyond 70 years, adjusting for a major limitation of the *RDAs*. *RDIs* are composed of four levels of intake: estimated requirements, *RDAs*, adequate intake, and tolerable upper intake levels.

3. Other dietary guidelines for older adults In 2008, the Federal Interagency Forum on Aging-Related Statistics published *National Dietary Guidelines for Older Adults*. According to the guidelines, older adults need to: (a) increase their intakes of whole grains, dried peas and beans, all types of fruits and vegetables (especially dark green and orange vegetables), and fat-free or low-fat milk and milk products; (b) replace solid fats with oils, including those in fish, nuts, and seeds; (c) consume less sodium and saturated fat; and (d) consume less food and beverages with added sugar, solid fats, and alcohol.

4. Servings and food group 6–9 bread, rice, pasta, and cereal; 3–4 vegetables; 2–3 fruits; 2–3 meat, fish, poultry, or legumes (dried peas and beans, lentils, nut butters, soy products); 2–3 non-fat or low-fat milk, cheese, yogurt, and dairy desserts; 8 or more 8 glasses of water or other fluids low in added sugars. Basic nutritional requirements will be met if the older adults' daily diet includes at least the minimum number of servings from each food group listed above and if it includes complex carbohydrates and high-fiber foods. It is important to know that recommended guidelines are simply guidelines. For the elderly population, individuals are in complex situations. They may consume many types of medications, have a variety of medical conditions, and take vitamins and other supplements. It is recommended to consult a dietitian when considering special dietary needs.

5. Food labeling Education in the area of reading nutritional information on labels is needed for elders. The U. S. Food and Drug Administration (FDA)

2. 推荐的膳食允许量和摄入量 1989 年，美国国家研究委员会食品与营养部发布了第十版《营养的推荐膳食允许量》(RDA)，包括了蛋白质、维生素、矿物质和一些微量元素，在健康人群（0～51 岁）中的每日推荐摄入量。RDA 已经被 RDI 膳食营养素参考摄入量 (Dietary Reference Intakes) 所取代，因为 RDI 里还包括了为 51～70 岁以及 70 岁以上老年人群制订的摄入量参照标准。在 RDI 中，包括了以下 4 个摄入量水平：预计的需求量、膳食允许量、适当的摄入量和可允许的最高摄入水平。

3. 其他老年人膳食指南 2008 年，美国老年化相关数据联邦论坛发布了《老年人膳食指南》。该指南指出，老年人应该做到：（a）增加全谷类、干果和豆类、任何类型的水果和蔬菜（尤其是青绿色和橙色蔬菜）以及脱脂或低脂牛奶和奶制品的摄入；（b）食用油类，包括鱼、坚果和种子油代替固体脂类；（c）减少食盐和饱和脂肪的摄入；（d）减少摄入加有糖、固体脂肪和酒精的食品和饮料。

4. 推荐成人每日饮食种类和最低摄入量 6～9 份面包、大米、面条和谷类；3～4 份蔬菜；2～3 份水果；2～3 份肉、鱼、家禽或豆类（干豌豆和蚕豆、扁豆、果仁奶油、大豆产品）；2～3 份脱脂或低脂牛奶、奶酪、酸乳和乳制品甜点；8 杯或 8 杯以上的水或低糖液体。如果每日膳食中包含了以上的食物类别并达到了最低量，并且包括复合碳水化合物以及高纤维食物，那么老年人的基本营养需求将会得到满足。值得一提的是，以上的膳食指南只是简单的指南，对于老年人群来说，每个人的情况都是复杂的。老年人大多身患多种疾病，使用各种药物、维生素和其他保健品，因此，特殊情况的膳食应寻求专业帮助。

5. 食品标签 帮助老年人学会阅读食品标签上的营养信息。自 1994 年，美国食品与药品管理局（FDA）要求生产商根据每日营养

has required producers of processed foods to list nutrition information based on daily values since 1994. Daily values are the maximum amounts of nutrients and fiber that are desirable in daily diets of 2000 to 2500 calories. The label law requires a label to include the amount of protein in grams, the energy as calories, the water-soluble vitamin content (vitamin C, vitamin B_6, vitamin B_{12}, thiamine, riboflavin, niacin, and folate), the fat-soluble vitamin content (vitamin A, vitamin D, vitamin E, and vitamin K), calcium, phosphorus, magnesium, iron, zinc, iodine, and selenium. The label must specify the percentage of the RDI that the product provides based on 2000 kcal a day. In addition, the label must specify calories based on a serving size and indicate the number of servings. FDA suggests a food that contains 10% to 19% of the daily value per serving as a good source.

III. Addressing Risk Factors Affected Nutrition

Nursing interventions may be needed to address functional consequences of age-related changes in elders. For example, if elders experience early satiety during meals, they may benefit from eating five smaller meals a day, rather than three meals a day. Similarly, nurses can encourage elders to maintain a sitting upright position during eating and for 1/2 to 1 hour after eating to compensate for any effects of slowed swallowing. If the food intake is inadequate to meet daily nutritional requirements due to poor appetite, the following strategies may be used to improve intake of the elders:

(1) Determine food preferences, including ethnic preferences.

(2) Ensure that the person has adequate time to eat.

(3) Provide snacks between meals and at night.

(4) Encourage family members to share mealtimes for a heightened social interaction.

(5) Encourage eating in congregate dining for a more enjoyable social atmosphere.

(6) Seat people together who have like interests and abilities, and encourage socialization.

(7) Sit while feeding a person who needs assistance, use touch, and carry on a social conversation.

(8) Provide music during dining.

(9) Recommend an exercise program.

量列出所加工食品的营养信息。每日营养量是指每日 2 000～2 500cal 摄入量所需要的最大营养素和纤维数量。标签法要求标签应包含蛋白质的克数、能量的热卡数，水溶性维生素（维生素 C、维生素 B_6、维生素 B_{12}、硫胺素、核黄素、烟酸和叶酸等）含量，脂溶性维生素（维生素 A、维生素 D、维生素 E 和维生素 K）的含量，以及钙、磷、镁、铁、锌、碘和硒的含量。标签必须详细说明产品在每日 2 000cal 基础上占每日摄入量的百分率。另外，标签还必须详细说明每份的热卡数量和份数。美国食品药品管理局提示每份量能包含每日营养量的 10%～19% 的食品是推荐食品。

三、减少影响老年人营养的不利因素

护理干预需要解决与老年人年龄相关的一些功能性变化。老年人即使少量进食也容易产生饱胀感，应选择少量多餐的进餐方式，如一日 5 次。同样，对于吞咽慢的老年人，鼓励老年人取坐位进餐，且持续 30 分钟至 1 小时，以减轻吞咽障碍。因食欲缺乏，食物摄入量不能满足日常营养需求，以下策略可用于改善老年人食物的摄入：

（1）了解老年人饮食偏好，包括种族差异。

（2）确保充足的进食时间。

（3）在两餐之间和晚上提供零食。

（4）鼓励家人与老年人共同进餐，增加人际互动。

（5）鼓励老年人参与聚餐等社交活动，享受良好的社会氛围。

（6）鼓励老年人与有共同爱好的老年人在一起，增进社交。

（7）需进餐辅助者，尽可能取坐位，恰当运用抚触、交谈等沟通方式，促进进食。

（8）进餐时播放音乐，营造良好的进餐环境。

（9）鼓励老年人参加运动锻炼，促进消化，增进食欲。

When functional limitations affect the activities involved in procuring, preparing, and enjoying food, interventions focus on improving the elders' access to palatable and nutritious meals. This may involve identifying resources that offer assistance in obtaining food. Local offices on aging may provide assistance with transportation or grocery shopping and are an excellent source of information about meal programs. When environmental barriers, such as high cupboards, interfere with elders' ability to prepare meals safely, environmental modifications can be made. When the elders have functional impairments, nurses can suggest specially adapted items for improving independence in eating and food preparation, such as assistive feeding devices help to grasp and get food.

When elders display dysphagia because of a medical condition such as stroke, the nurse can help the elders who are not totally dysphagic to ingest thickened liquids and solids. Thickeners can be added to liquids to achieve a consistency (like the consistency of mashed potatoes) that can be ingested. Thin liquids are most difficult to swallow for individuals with dysphagia. Elders with dysphagia must be assisted during meals and the nurse should carefully observe that foods are successfully swallowed to avoid aspiration. Elders with severe dysphagia require eternal tube feeding.

Medication use is common in elders. The interactions between nutrients and medicines may affect metabolism, absorption, digestion, or excretion of drugs. When medications affect nutrition, nurses, caregivers, or elders can discuss this problem with prescribing health care practitioners to identify ways of alleviating this risk or addressing the consequences. If over-the-counter medications have a detrimental effect on nutrition, nurses educate elders about medication–nutrient interactions and discuss ways of managing the negative effects. When alcohol consumption interferes with nutrition, interventions might address the potential problem of alcoholism, or compensate for the detrimental effects on nutrition. Nurses can recommend vitamin supplementation for individuals with a history of alcoholism and having underlying conditions, such as pernicious anemia.

Oral and dental health is also important factor influencing nutrition in elders. Good oral care is an essential, but often overlooked, component of daily care for the elderly people. Nurses have important responsibilities in implementing interventions to promote oral and dental health. If elders have avoided dental care because of

当老年人功能受限影响食物采购、准备和享用时，干预措施的重点是帮助老年人获得可口和营养的膳食。这可能需要有获得食物方面帮助的资源。当地的老龄办公室可以为运输或日用品购买提供帮助，并且能提供膳食计划。若出现不利的环境，如橱柜较高，可能会影响老年人安全地准备食物时，需要做环境调整。当老年人不能自行进食时，护士可推荐专门器具帮助其独立进食，如辅助进食装置，帮助老年人抓取食物。

当老年人因为卒中等出现吞咽困难时，护士可以给老年人比较黏稠的食物。可以将增稠剂加入液体中增加黏稠度（如土豆泥）。对于吞咽困难的个体，稀薄液体最难吞咽。患有吞咽困难的老年人需要辅助进食，护士应仔细观察食物成功吞咽避免吸入。有严重吞咽困难的老年人需要永久管饲。

老年人使用药物治疗非常普遍，营养物质与药物之间的相互作用可能会影响药物的新陈代谢、吸收、消化和排泄。当药物对营养状况、护理、照顾者及老年有影响时，可以与医疗保健人员讨论这个问题，确定减轻这种风险或解决后果的方法。如果非处方药物对营养有不利的影响，护士就关于药物－营养相互作用对老年人进行健康教育，并与其讨论管理不利影响的方法。当饮酒对营养状况产生干扰时，干预措施是解决有关酗酒的潜在问题或弥补酒精对营养的不利影响。护士可以为有酗酒史和有潜在疾病（如恶性贫血）的人推荐补充维生素。

口腔和牙齿健康是影响老年人营养的重要因素。良好的口腔护理是老年人日常护理的重要组成部分，却常常被忽视。护士在促进口腔和牙齿健康方面有着重要责任。当老年人因为口腔健康状况较差或对预防性牙科

resignation to poor oral health or a poor understanding of the need for preventive dental care, nurses need to educate elders to change these attitudes. Nurses need to emphasize the importance of obtaining dental care every 6 months and facilitate referrals for dental care. Nurses also need to provide elders and their caregivers the information about local resources and the dental services that are available in their community. If xerostomia interferes with nutrition, nurses may suggest or facilitate a referral for a medical evaluation to identify the contributing factors.

For health education about oral care, general information including using a toothbrush with soft nylon bristles, using toothpaste with fluoride to reduce cavities and prevent periodontal disease, diluting the mouth rinses with equal amounts of water before use, and never using lemon glycerin swabs for edentulous elders are recommended. If elders experience dry mouth, nurses need to provide measures to alleviate dry mouth. Miller (2012) summarized following evidence-based recommendations related to dry mouth care: ① drink at least 10 to 12 glasses of non-caffeinated fluid during the day, and drink sips of water at frequent intervals; ② suck on xylitol-flavored fluoride tablets or sugar-free hard candies to stimulate saliva flow; ③ chew sugar-free gum with xylitol for 15 minutes after meals to stimulate saliva flow and promote oral hygiene; ④ try using saliva substitutes available at drugstores, but avoid those that contain sorbitol because this can worsen the condition; ⑤ avoid sucking lozenges containing citric acid because of their detrimental effects on tooth enamel; ⑥ avoid alcohol, alcohol-containing mouthwashes, and highly acidic drinks (e. g. , orange or grapefruit juice) because these tend to exacerbate the condition; ⑦ avoid smoking because this exacerbates the symptoms and further irritates the oral mucous membranes; ⑧ pay particular attention to oral hygiene because a dry mouth increases the risk for gum and dental diseases; ⑨ maintain optimal room humidity, especially at night.

IV. Apply Therapeutic Diets According to the Diseases

Therapeutic diets have long been recognized as essential interventions for chronic diseases, such as diabetes and cardiovascular conditions. Therapeutic diets have been modified to include more or less than the RDAs and RDIs for a specific nutrient or nutrients to manage

护理需要的理解不足而不愿意进行牙齿护理时，护士需要对老年人进行教育，使其改变这些态度。护士需要强调每 6 个月进行牙齿护理的重要性，并促进牙齿护理的转诊。护士还需要向老年人及其照顾者提供有关当地资源和社区牙科服务的信息。如果口腔干燥对营养状况产生干扰时，护士可以建议或协助转诊，对老年人进行医学评估，以鉴别相关的影响因素。

口腔护理健康教育的内容包括使用软毛的尼龙牙刷和含氟牙膏，以减少蛀牙和牙周疾病的发生；漱口前应先用等量的水稀释漱口液；不要用沾有甘油的棉签擦拭缺齿的部位。Miller（2012）的循证护理总结出的防治口腔干燥的方法有：①日间饮用 10～12 杯不含咖啡因的液体；②吃含有木糖醇的氟化物药片或者无糖的坚硬糖果，以刺激唾液产生；③饭后嚼无糖木糖醇口香糖 15 分钟，以刺激产生唾液和促进口腔卫生；④使用唾液替代品，但要避免含山梨醇的替代品；⑤避免食用含柠檬酸的硬糖块，因为它们对牙釉质有害；⑥戒酒，避免含酒精的漱口水和酸性饮料（例如，橙汁或葡萄汁），因为它们会加剧病情；⑦戒烟；⑧注意口腔卫生；⑨保持环境湿润，尤其是夜间。

四、根据疾病的需要采用治疗饮食

治疗性饮食很早就被认为是抵抗慢性疾病，例如糖尿病和心血管疾病必不可少的干预措施。治疗性饮食的种类包括严格限制钠、胆固醇、蛋白质、总热量或脂肪的膳食；改

a chronic disease or illness. Examples of therapeutic diets include those which are restricted in sodium, cholesterol, protein, total calories, or fat; modifications in the texture of foods (e. g., low-fiber or high-fiber diet, liquid diet, semiliquid diet, or clear liquid diet); and specialized nutrition such as parenteral nutrition, eternal tube feeding, or oral supplements. Oral supplements are often prescribed for clients who cannot ingest adequate calories or protein because of early satiety or fatigue during eating. For example, the client may improve protein or overall caloric intake by adding a concentrated liquid oral supplement. Supplements are often given between meals and at bedtime so that they do not become a "meal substitute". The nurse must carefully assess the impact of the supplement on overall intake.

变食物性状的膳食（如低纤维或高纤维饮食、流食、半流食等）；特殊营养如胃肠外营养、管饲饮食或口服补剂。口服补剂通常提供给由于饱腹感或过度疲乏不能摄取足够的热量和蛋白质的老年患者。通常在两餐之间或临睡前给予，使其不会成为食物的替代品。护士必须仔细评估补剂对整体营养摄入的影响。

V. Role of Nutrients in Preventing Disease

There is increasing recognition of the role nutrients play in preventing disease. Nutritional interventions for healthy elders emphasize the inclusion of foods containing antioxidants and other nutrients that may play a protective and preventive role. Distinctions must be made between nutrients obtained from foods and those from supplements when analyzing information about nutrients as preventive interventions. For example, a high dietary intake of a particular nutrient (e. g., carotenoids) may be beneficial in disease prevention, but a dietary supplement product with the same nutrient may not have the same beneficial effects. Thus, nurses need to educate elders about the importance of obtaining nutrients from food sources.

Nurses teach elders about basic nutritional requirements using easy-to-understand educational materials. Nutrition education can be provided on an individual basis or in group settings, perhaps with registered dietitians. Healthy elders generally maintain optimal nutritional status through the daily intake of the foods according to the guidelines mentioned above. If the elderly people have any illness or take any medications that interfere with nutrition, the daily diet will have to be modified to compensate for these effects.

五、营养素在预防疾病中的作用

营养在疾病预防中的重要性越来越引起重视。健康老年人的营养干预强调食用含有抗氧化剂和其他有预防疾病和保健作用营养素的食物。护士应区分食物营养素和营养素补充剂在疾病预防中的作用。例如，摄入较多的特定营养物（如类胡萝卜素）可能有益于疾病预防，但具有相同营养物的膳食补充剂产品可能不具有相同的效果。因此，护士应教育老年人认识从食物中获取营养素的重要性。

护士用易于理解的健康教育材料帮助老年人了解基本的营养需求。营养教育的形式可以是一对一的，也可以是集体教育，或者和营养师一起进行。健康老年人按照营养指南合理饮食可以保持最佳的营养状态。如果老年人由于患病或药物治疗影响营养的摄入，则必须调整膳食以代偿不良影响。

(LIU Hongxia)

（刘红霞）

Key Points

1. Nutritional needs are changed in elders because of age-related changes.

本章要点

1. 由于年龄的变化，老年人的营养需求发生了变化。

2. Dehydration is common, but over-looked in elders.

3. Malnutrition is related to chronic illness and poor clinical outcomes.

4. Physiologic, psychosocial, and socioeconomic factors affect nutritional status in elders.

5. The JCAHO requires nutritional screening of all clients receiving clinical services, and a referral for a comprehensive assessment if the client is at risk of malnutrition.

6. Nutritional assessment is a comprehensive evaluation of a client's nutritional status.

7. Dietary history, anthropometrics, and laboratory studies are components of a nutritional assessment.

8. Understanding an elder's social, cultural, and emotional ties to food can be a great asset in working with nutrition and health issues.

9. A balanced dietary intake using *the Modified MyPyramid for Older Adults* can promote nutritional health.

10. Nutrition education and problem solving of the potential or actual nutritional deficit with the elders is the most significant intervention.

Critical Thinking Exercise

1. Mrs. Tao who is 76 years old comes to the nutritional clinic to consult about her weight loss. She states that she has a gradual unintended weight loss over the past few months. Mrs. Tao also states that food no longer appeals to her. You notice that her mouth is very dry and her teeth are in poor condition. Mrs. Tao had a stroke 3 years ago and recovered well except for some dysphagia and right-sided weakness. She takes two blood pressure medications and an antidepressant. She does not know the names of the medications.

Questions:

(1) What assessment questions you would use with Mrs. Tao?

(2) What would you ask Mrs. Tao to do to provide additional information so that you can plan some interventions?

2. Mrs. W is 72-year-old. She is 162 cm tall, weighs 72 kg. She does not walk often because of arthritis. She also has hypertension for 20 years. Her medications include citalopram (Celexa) 20 mg daily; clonidine (Catapres)

2. 脱水是常见的，但在老年人中被忽视了。

3. 营养不良与慢性病和疾病预后差有关。

4. 生理、心理社会和社会经济因素影响老年人的营养状况。

5. JCAHO 要求对接受临床服务的所有患者进行营养筛查，如果患者有营养不良的风险，则需要进行全面的营养评估。

6. 营养评估是对患者营养状况的综合评价。

7. 饮食史、人体测量和实验室检查是营养评估的组成部分。

8. 了解老人与食物的社会、文化和情感内涵间的联系，有利于处理老年人的营养和健康问题。

9. 将膳食金字塔用于老年人的饮食，可以促进营养健康。

10. 对老年人进行营养指导、解决老年人潜在或实际的营养不良的问题是最重要的护理干预。

批判性思维练习

1. 76 岁的陶女士到营养诊所咨询她的体重减轻问题。她说，她在过去几个月中体重的减少超乎了她的想象，并且食物不再吸引她。她的嘴巴很干燥，牙齿状况不好。陶女士 3 年前卒中了，但恢复良好，仅有一些吞咽困难和右侧躯体无力。她服用两种降压药和一种抗抑郁药。她不知道药物的名称。

问题：

（1）你想问陶女士哪些营养评估的问题？

（2）你想让陶女士提供哪些额外的信息，以便于制订干预措施？

2. W 女士 72 岁，身高 162cm，体重 72kg。因为关节炎，她不经常走动。她患有高血压 20 年。服用的药物有每日 20mg 西酞普兰、

0. 2 mg daily; triamterene 37.5 mg/hydrochlorothiazide 25 mg (Dyazide) daily; and levothyroxine (Synthroid) 100 μg daily. The following is her 24-hour intake:

Breakfast: 1 glass orange juice, 2 slices white wheat toast, 1 tablespoon butter.

Lunch: 1 piece of peanut butter and jelly sandwich, 1/2 cup cottage cheese, 1 cup coffee.

Dinner: 1 serving pasta, 1 cup skim milk.
Snack: 1 cup ice cream.

Questions:

(1) What conclusions can be made about Mrs. W's dietary status based on her diet?

(2) What interventions would you suggest to improve Mrs. W's nutrition?

每日 0.2mg 可乐定、每日 37.5mg 氨苯蝶啶、25mg 氢氯噻嗪以及每日 100μg 左甲状腺素。以下是她 24 小时的摄入量:

早餐:1 杯橙汁,2 片白麦面包,1 汤匙黄油。

午餐:1 片花生酱和果冻三明治,1/2 杯奶酪,1 杯咖啡。

晚餐:1 份意大利面,1 杯脱脂牛奶。

小吃:1 杯冰激凌。

问题:

(1)根据 W 女士的饮食,你对她的饮食状况可以得出什么结论?

(2)对于改善 W 女士的营养状况,你有哪些建议?

Chapter 14 Care of Elderly with Elimination Disorder

第十四章　老年人排泄障碍的护理

Learning Objectives

On completion of this chapter, the reader will be able to:

- Define the constipation;

- Describe the risk factors of constipation;

- List the main nursing interventions on constipation;

- Define the urinary incontinence;

- Describe the risk factors of urinary incontinence ;

- Define the fecal incontinence;

- Describe the risk factors of fecal incontinence.

学习目标

通过学习本章节，应完成以下目标：

- 定义便秘；

- 描述便秘的危险因素；

- 列举老年人便秘的主要护理措施；

- 定义尿失禁；

- 识别尿失禁的危险因素；

- 定义大便失禁；

- 识别大便失禁的危险因素。

Excretion is a necessary process to maintain health and life. With increasing of the age, the functions of urinary and digestive systems gradually weaken, or due to the influence of diseases, the elderly prone to much suffering, such as nocturia, dysuria, urinary incontinence, constipation, fecal incontinence, and others. Elimination disorders cannot be avoided in aging process, and have a tremendous influence on the physical and mental health of the elderly. Therefore, according to the excretion characteristics of the elderly, nurses need to properly help the elderly handle the obstacles of the elimination disorders well.

排泄是维持健康和生命的必要过程。随着年龄的不断增加，泌尿系统和消化系统的功能逐渐减弱，或因疾病的影响，老年人易发生夜尿、排尿困难、尿失禁、便秘、大便失禁等现象。排泄障碍是机体老化过程中无法避免的，对老年人的身心健康产生了极大影响。因此，临床护理工作人员要根据老年人的排泄特点，帮助老年人妥善处理好排泄障碍。

Section 1 Care of the Elderly with Constipation

Constipation refers to bowel movements that are infrequent or hard to pass，it is a decrease of defecation, 2-3 days or longer frequency of defecation, dry feces, and difficult defecation. There are 12% of the population worldwide reports having constipation. Compared with young people, the elderly are easier to have constipation. It accounts for about 30% of the elderly, and can be as high as 80% in the elderly in the long-term center. Constipation is a common cause of painful defecation. Severe constipation includes obstipation (failure to pass stools or gas) and fecal impaction, which can progress to bowel obstruction and become life-threatening. Constipation will not only cause local and systemic discomfort, but may cause complications of cardiovascular system, digestive system, and other systems, and seriously influence the old people's quality of life.

Box 14-1　Case Study

Mr. Liu, at 73 years old, could truthfully say he had never had problems about his bowel movements. He had bowel movement each morning about 20 minutes after breakfast. But after he had a hospitalization for a fractured hip last year he had never regained his reliable pattern of bowel function. He has complained of it is hard to pass, typically 3 times or fewer per week. He was greatly distressed by this because bowel function was a symbol to him of good health. Admittedly, he did not move about as much now and used a walker when he did. And he had heard that pain medications sometimes made one constipated, but he tried to use them very sparingly. He had even reestablished his

第一节　便秘老年人的护理

便秘是指排便频次减少或排便困难，排便次数减少，每2~3天或更长时间排便一次，粪便干硬，排便困难。据报道，全球有12%的人患有便秘。与中青年人比较，老年人更容易发生便秘，约占老年人群的30%，在长期卧床老年人中则可高达80%。便秘是排便困难的常见原因。严重的便秘（粪便或气体不能排出）和粪便嵌塞，可发展为肠梗阻并危及生命。便秘不仅会引起局部及全身不适，还有可能引起心血管系统、消化系统等并发症，严重影响老年人的生活质量。

Box 14-1　案例

刘先生，73岁，可以说，他从来没有排便的问题。他每天在早餐后大约20分钟后进行排便。但去年他因髋部骨折住院治疗后，再也没有规律地排便，经常出现便秘。他抱怨排便困难，通常每周3次或更少。他非常苦恼，他认为能正常排便是健康的象征。虽然他走路时使用了助行器，但他不能再像健康人一样走动。他听说止痛药有时会引起便秘，故很少使用。他努力尝试重建他每天早饭后的排便习惯。他开始非常担心他的便秘，因此，经常使用泻药。他说："便秘真的让我很

pattern of attempting a bowel movement every morning after breakfast. He began to worry considerably about his constipation and to use laxatives almost routinely. He said: "This constipation really upset me, I just don't feel like myself if I don't have a bowel movement every day."

Based on the case study, answer the following questions:

1. What is the main cause of Mr. Liu suffering from constipation?

2. What is the possible effective nursing management to improve the function of his bowel movement?

I. Etiology

i. Decrease or Disappearance of Gastric Bowel Peristalsis and Defecation Reflection

1. Due to the function decrease of the elderly digestive system, stomach acid and various kinds of digestive enzymes, atrophy of digestive mucosa and muscle, and gastric bowel flabby, those cause lack of bowel movements and decrease of bowel function, contents passing slowly, excessively absorb water to lead to constipation.

2. Those of decrease of the elderly gastrointestinal reflex, declined contraction of abdomen and pelvic muscles, and defecation fatigue, are easy to cause difficulties of defecation and constipation.

3. Loose or off teeth in elders, chewing difficulties, the cellulose content of eating too little, those can not produce effective stimulation of the gastrointestinal tract, and decrease defecation reflex.

4. Little drinking water, dry hard stool can cause constipation.

5. Bedridden or limited mobility, and lack of promoting the stimulation of the colon feces running, are prone to constipation.

ii. Lifestyle and Psychosocial Factor

1. Those changes, such as life or living environment, timetable, diets, toilet and wash facilities, can change elimination habit, and inhibit defecation and constipation by awareness.

2. Depression or excessive stress inhibits the normal defecation reflex resulting in constipation.

不舒服，我每天不排便，我感觉不舒服。"

根据该案例，回答以下问题：

1. 刘先生便秘的主要原因是什么？

2. 如何提供有效的护理措施改善其排便状态？

一、病因与发病机制

（一）胃肠蠕动及排便反射减弱或消失

1. 老年人消化系统功能减退、胃酸及各种消化酶减少，消化器官黏膜及肌肉萎缩，胃肠松弛无力，造成排便动力缺乏及肠蠕动功能减弱，肠内容物通过缓慢，粪便内水分过度吸收，致使大便秘结。

2. 老年人胃肠反射减弱，腹部和盆腔肌肉收缩力普遍下降，排便乏力，因而容易发生排便困难和便秘。

3. 老年人牙齿松动脱落、咀嚼困难，进食的纤维素含量太少，不能对胃肠道产生有效刺激，排便反射减弱。

4. 饮水过少，粪便干硬也可引起便秘。

5. 长期卧床或活动受限，缺乏引起推动结肠内粪便运行的刺激，容易发生便秘。

（二）生活习惯及心理社会因素

1. 如生活或居住环境变化，作息时间、饮食种类、厕所及洗漱设施等改变，造成排便习惯改变，产生意识性抑制排便而发生便秘。

2. 精神抑郁或过度紧张，使正常排便反射抑制，导致便秘。

3. The rectum and anal lesions, fear of defecation may cause anal pain generate awareness inhibition of defecation.

iii. Gastrointestinal Obstruction

Intestinal obstruction by variety of causes, such as eating too much difficult to digest , like glutinous rice, the Lantern, glutinous rice balls and others, can lead to intestinal obstruction, intestinal tumors, intestinal paralysis, etc. Intestinal contents can not operate normally; remaining in the intestine leading to constipation.

iv. Iatrogenic Constipation

1. Medication long-term application of laxatives, narcotics, anticholinergics, ganglion blockers, antidepressants or containing aluminum, calcium, bismuth, iron, barium preparations, etc., so that they preferred rising threshold or relaxing muscle, or intestinal loss of their own bowel function.

2. Long-term repeated enema causes defecation reliance.

3. Abdominal surgical trauma.

4. In addition to the gastro-intestinal diseases, neuropsychiatric disease, cerebrovascular disease, muscle disease, metabolic and endocrine diseases, may also cause bowel movements slow and even intestinal paralysis to cause constipation.

II. Nursing Assessment

i. Health History

Ask the elderly living habits, bowel habits, medication, activities, and whether the environment has changed, work stress, and so on; assess the elderly defecations, including time of constipation, number of defecations, with or without difficulty in defecation, stool shape, degree of the stool hardness, surface with or no blood and associated symptoms, diseases with or no causing constipation.

ii. Clinical Manifestation

1. Defecation changes　decreased number and difficulties of defecation.

Decreased natural defecation: the natural frequency of defecation less than three times a week, less stool, extended interval time of natural defecation, and gradually increased.

3. 直肠和肛门病变，畏惧排便可能引起肛门疼痛，产生意识性抑制排便。

（三）胃肠道梗阻

各种原因导致的肠梗阻，如进食过多难以消化的糯米、元宵、汤圆等导致肠梗阻、肠道肿瘤、肠麻痹等。肠道内容物不能正常运行，滞留在肠道内而发生便秘。

（四）医源性便秘

1. 药物，如长期应用缓泻剂、麻醉药、抗胆碱能药、神经节阻滞药及抗抑郁药及含有铝、钙、铋、铁、钡制剂的药物等，使便意的阈值上升或肌肉松弛，肠道丧失自行排便功能。

2. 长期反复灌肠，产生灌肠排便的依赖。

3. 腹部手术创伤。

4. 疾病，除肠道疾病外，神经精神疾病、脑血管病、肌肉病变、代谢与内分泌疾病等，也可能引起肠蠕动缓慢甚至肠麻痹等而造成便秘。

二、护理评估

（一）健康史

询问老年人的生活习惯、排便习惯、服用药物、活动情况以及有无环境改变和工作紧张过度等；评估老年人排便的情况，包括便秘发生的时间、排便次数、有无排便困难、粪便形状、粪便的干硬程度、表面是否带血及便秘的伴随症状，有无引起便秘的疾病等。

（二）临床表现

1. 排便改变　包括排便次数减少和排便困难。

自然排便次数减少：自然排便次数每周少于3次，粪便量少，自然排便间隔时间延长，并逐渐加重。

Defecation difficulties: Bowel movements that are difficult to pass, very firm, or made up of small hard pellets (like those excreted by rabbits) qualify as constipation, even if they occur every day. The forms of human stool are classified by Bristol stool chart (see figure14-1）。

排便困难：粪便非常坚硬，或呈小硬颗粒（如兔子的粪便），难以排出，此种情况即使每天都排便，也属于便秘。评估大便形状参考 Bristol 的大便评定图（图14-1）。

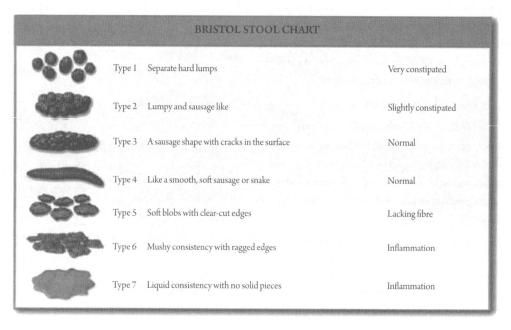

Figure14-1 Bristol stool chart

2. Associated symptoms constipation is often accompanied by abdominal pain, bloating, loss of appetite, thirst, nausea, and others; some may have dizziness, and fatigue performance.

3. Complication

(1) Fecal impaction is the state and most common complication which stool keeps in the large intestine to form a hard fecal incarcerated the intestine. Fecal impaction can cause fecal incontinence, mechanical intestinal paralysis, fecal ulcer, urinary retention or incontinence, and severe mental disorder.

(2) Increased pressure of abdominal and intestinal by severe constipation can cause hiatal hernia, gastro-esophageal reflux, abdominal hernia, colonic diverticulitis, megacolon, rectal prolapsed, hemorrhoids, etc.

(3) Forced defecation of elders can lead to blood flowing changes of coronary, cerebral causing angina, acute myocardial infarction, arrhythmias, aneurysm, or aneurysm rupture, hypertension, acute cerebrovascular disease, and even sudden death. Constipation is considered to be a common factor of death from cardiovascular diseases.

2. 伴发症状 便秘的患者常伴有腹痛、腹胀、食欲缺乏、口渴、恶心等症状，有的可有头晕、乏力等表现。

3. 并发症

（1）粪便嵌塞：粪便嵌塞是指粪便滞留在大肠中形成坚硬的粪块并嵌顿在肠道内的状态，是便秘最常见的并发症。粪便嵌塞可引起大便失禁、机械性肠麻痹、粪性溃疡、尿潴留或尿失禁、严重精神错乱。

（2）严重便秘使腹腔和肠内压力增高，可引起食管裂孔疝、胃食管反流、腹壁疝、结肠憩室、巨结肠症、直肠脱垂、痔疮等。

（3）老年便秘用力排便，可导致冠状动脉、脑血管血流改变，引起心绞痛、急性心肌梗死、心律失常、动脉瘤或室壁瘤破裂、高血压、急性脑血管疾病，甚至猝死。便秘被认为是心血管疾病死亡的常见原因。

iii. Experimental and Other Test

1. Gastrointestinal X-ray test includs barium meal exams gastrointestinal motor function, barium discharge within 72 hours, emptying delay prompts constipation; barium enemas particularly help in the diagnosis of organic constipation.

2. Endoscopy colonoscopy, sigmoidoscopy, colonoscopy for suspected patients with organic disease to make clear diagnosis.

iv. Psychosocial Aspect

1. For the elderly, long-term constipation can cause mental tension, fear, irritability, depression, anxiety and others, and even dependence with laxatives, enemas, and others aggravating constipation.

2. Chronic constipation not only causes the elderly own pain, but also need a family members' or caregivers' assistance in defecation, this will suppress the feeling of defecation, may cause aversion of family members or caregivers, also increases the time and effort of families' caring, so that increase economic burden of the family and society.

III. Nursing Management

The principles of management: eliminate the risk factors of constipation, such as constipation by disease treats the primary disease to supplement symptomatic therapy; if those of diet, habits, environment changes and mental factors cause constipation, it might always take a comprehensive intervention.

1. Help defecation Offer the commode to ambulatory patients on time, preparing the defecation environment such as using screens to shield, and maintain the natural defecation posture according to habits of defecation, or use the bedpan or bedside chair properly. If situation allowed, use portable commode at the bedside to defecate; try to head up the elderly with serious diseases, or use the commode taking a half supine in bed.

2. Abdomen massage Register nurses do or guide patients do it by themselves. Take supine position, blend knees and relax the abdominal muscles in early morning or before going to bed. With the palm massage abdomen along the ascending colon, transverse colon, descending colon, sigmoid colon direction from the right lower abdomen up to the right upper-side, and then

（三）实验室及其他检查

1. 胃肠 X 线检查包括钡餐检查观察胃肠运动功能，一般钡剂在 72 小时内全部排出结肠；若排空延迟提示便秘。钡灌肠特别有助于器质性便秘疾病的诊断。

2. 内镜检查包括结肠镜、乙状结肠镜、全结肠镜检查，对疑有器质性病变的患者能明确诊断。

（四）心理社会状况

1. 老年人长期便秘可产生精神紧张、恐惧、烦躁不安、抑郁、焦虑等情绪反应，甚至对泻药、灌肠等产生依赖性，而加重便秘。

2. 长期便秘除了引起老年人自身的痛苦外，在排便时可能还需要家人或照顾者协助，会压抑便意，也可能引起家人或照顾者的厌恶情绪，同时也增加了家庭照顾的时间和精力，使家庭和社会的经济负担加重。

三、护理措施

老年人便秘的处理原则：消除便秘的危险因素，如疾病引起的便秘则以治疗原发病为主，辅以对症治疗；若因饮食、习惯、环境改变、精神等原因引起便秘，则常需要采取综合性防治护理措施。

1. **协助患者排便** 非卧床患者按时给予便器，准备排便环境如用屏风遮挡，还可以根据患者排便习惯，维持自然排便姿势，或适当使用便盆或床边便椅。若情况允许可使用移动坐便椅在床边排便；病情较重者要尽量将床头抬高，或取半卧位，在床上使用便器。

2. **按摩腹部促进排便** 该方法是由护士操作、指导陪护或患者自己进行：①清晨或睡前取仰卧位，屈膝，放松腹肌。②用手掌沿升结肠、横结肠、降结肠、乙状结肠方向，即自右下腹向上至右上腹，再横行至左上腹，然后再向下至左下腹，沿耻骨上回至右下腹，

transverse to the left upper quadrant, and then down to the left lower abdomen, along the suprapubic back to the right lower quadrant, circularly massage the abdomen. During massaging the left lower quadrant, strengthen the pressure until not feeling pain, one circle one time. Breath when pressed, and inhale when relaxes, the frequency of massage increase gradually from 1 to 10 times, time is about 10 minutes a day.

3. Medication Prescribed medication or enemas relieve the symptoms of intractable constipation. The purpose is to promote the fecal excretion and form normal defecation. Pay attention to follow the medical principle of "less amount of medication, less frequent dosing, earlier stopping medication before regular defecation".

(1) Oral laxatives: The fundamental function of laxatives stimulates intestinal secretion and reduced absorption, and increases osmotic pressure and hydrostatic pressure. The elderly is suitable for mild laxatives. Medical staff should choose medication and dose according to the degree physical condition and constipation of the elderly，then observe the effect of medication. In generally, oral cathartic works after six or eight hours, so the elderly take medication at bedtime is more reasonable, and then defecation will be in the next morning after getting up or after breakfast. Commonly used oral laxatives include:

1) Senna: The volume is 3-5 g in every time, taking it in boiling water at night. There are anthraquinone in senna; the active ingredient is hydrolyzed by colonic bacteria to only work in the colon or distal ileum, and defecation is after taking 8 to 10 hours.

2) Phenolphthalein: Also known as "GuoDao", the volume is 0.1 g in per time, taking before bedtime at every night. Phenolphthalein forms soluble sodium salt with intestinal alkaline intestinal juice after oral administration to stimulate colon. As parts of it is excreted by gallbladder and absorbed by intestinal to form enter hepatic circulation, so the effect can maintain 3 to 4 days.

3) Cisapride: Gastrointestinal motility medications mainly promote the release of acetylcholine in my enteric plexus, and improve the peristalsis of esophagus and gastrointestinal tract, then promote gastric emptying and operation of intestinal contents. In the clinic, it is mainly used the peristalsis movement dysfunction which is caused by intestinal pseudo-obstruction and related with motor function disorder, and long-term treatment of chronic constipation., the daily dosage is 15-40 mg, 2 times per day, taking before breakfast and going to bed. After a week

环形按摩腹部。③当按摩至左下腹时，应加强指压力度，以不感觉疼痛为度，转一圈为1次。④按压时呼气，放松时吸气，按摩次数从10次开始逐渐增加，每日可作10分钟左右。

3. 遵医嘱给药物治疗 对于顽固性便秘者可遵医嘱给药物治疗或灌肠以解除症状。药物治疗的目的是促进粪便的排出，同时建立正常的排便习惯。在药物治疗过程中要注意遵循"用量尽可能小、用药次数尽可能少、建立排便规律后尽早停药"的原则。

（1）口服泻药：泻药的基本作用为刺激肠道分泌和减少吸收，增加肠腔内渗透压和流体静力压。老年人适合用温和的缓泻剂，可根据患者的体质及便秘的情况选择药物种类和药物用量，并注意观察药物的疗效，一般泻剂口服后需6～8小时发挥作用，故患者较为合理的服药时间是睡前服用，使排便时间在次晨起床后或早餐后。常用的口服泻药有：

1）番泻叶：3～5g/次，每晚泡水服，味苦。番泻叶中含蒽醌，由结肠细菌水解活性成分后发生作用仅作用于结肠或远端回肠，服用后8～10小时可能排便。

2）酚酞：又名果导，0.1g/次，每晚睡前服。酚酞口服后在肠内与碱性肠液形成可溶性钠盐，对结肠有刺激作用。由于其部分由胆汁排泄，肠内再吸收形成肠肝循环，故一次给药可维持3～4天。

3）西沙比利：胃肠道动力药，主要是促进肠肌间神经丛中乙酰胆碱的释放，增强食管、胃肠蠕动，促进胃排空及肠内容物运转。临床上主要用于与运动功能失调有关的假性肠梗阻导致的推进性蠕动不足，及慢性便秘患者的长期治疗，每日用量15～40mg，分2次服用，早餐前及睡前各服一次，1周内常可使便秘症状改善，严重便秘患者的理想治疗

of treatment, it may relief constipation, and maintains the desired effects for 2 to 3 months.

(2) Simplified method

1) Enema: Use 20 ml per plastic ampoule of 20% mannitol. Before using, cut the top of pear-shaped plastic capsule, first crush a little liquid to lubricant, and then insert into the anus to squeeze into the liquid to the rectum, tell the elderly to tolerant 5 to 10 minutes, so that it can stimulate bowel movements, softening stool, and stimulating defecation.

2) Glycerin suppository: The main components are glycerin and gelatin. Operator inserts the top into the anus of 6-7 cm with gloves. Glycerin suppository is melted by body temperature, stimulating the rectum, lubricating feces, then causes reflex defecation after using 15 to 30 minutes.

(3) Clyster: A certain amounts of solution pass the anal canal, and pour into the colon from the anus through the rectum to stimulate bowel movements and promote defecation or soften dry stool to relieving constipation. Clyster can quickly relieve constipation and fit the severe constipation which is invalid in general treatments. According to constipation extent and general condition, nurses should select and prepare with enemas of different nature and function. The common enema:

1) Saline: To take salt 9 g and dissolve it in warm water of 1 000 ml, the solution temperature is 39-41℃, and this can be used in a variety of constipation laxative.

2) Glycerol or paraffin oil: Glycerol or paraffin oil 50 ml, add equal amount of warm water, temperature is 38 ℃.

3) Enema using 1:2:3 solutions: This kind of solution consists of 50% magnesium sulfate 30 ml, glycerin 60 ml, and warm water 90 ml. Temperature of the solutions is 38 ℃ properly.

4. Take bezoars method Due to long-time constipation, lead to a lot of manure to accumulate in the rectum which cannot discharge by self, therefore need to care provider wear gloves to help patients take the bezoars out of the rectum. When taking bezoars, the patient should take the left lateral position, the operator coated with lubricant in the right hand gloves, gently index finger, middle finger insert into the anus and slowly pulled out the hard stool. Keep gentle movements during the operation, avoid forced to dig, avoid damaging the rectal mucosa and increasing the patients' suffering.

结果需 2～3 个月。

（2）简易通便法

1）开塞露：20ml/ 支。使用前，剪去梨形塑料囊尖端，先挤出少许药液起润滑作用，然后插入肛门内把药液挤入直肠内，嘱患者忍耐 5～10 分钟，以刺激肠蠕动，软化粪便，促进排便。

2）甘油栓：其主要成为甘油和明胶。操作者戴手套将其尖端插入肛门 6～7cm。甘油栓在体温作用下溶化，刺激直肠壁，润滑粪便，反射性地引起排便，用后 15～30 分钟见效。

（3）灌肠法：将一定量的溶液通过肛管，自肛门经直肠灌入结肠，刺激肠蠕动，促进排便或使干燥粪便软化，以缓解患者便秘。灌肠排便法解除便秘见效快，适应于严重便秘在一般治疗措施无效时。老年人灌肠根据便秘程度和全身状况选择和配制不同性质和作用的灌肠液。常用灌肠液有：

1）生理盐水：取盐 9g，溶于 1 000ml 温开水中，溶液温度为 39～41℃，用于各种便秘的通便。

2）甘油或石蜡油：用甘油或石蜡油 50ml，加等量温开水，温度 38℃。

3）"1：2：3" 灌肠液：50% 硫酸镁 30ml、甘油 60ml、温开水 90ml，温度 38℃。

4. 取粪结石法 由于长时间便秘，导致大量的粪块聚积在直肠内，无法自行排出，需要戴手套帮助患者从直肠内取出。在取粪结石时患者应取左侧卧位，护士用右手戴手套涂润滑油，轻轻将示指、中指插入肛门，慢慢将硬结的粪便掏出。在操作过程中注意动作轻柔，切忌强行硬挖，以免损伤直肠黏膜，增加患者痛苦。

5. Health education

(1) Guide the elderly to establish normal physiologic and well habits defecation. The elderly is suit to take seats in defecation; the frequency is 1-2 times a day. Encourage elder to defecate when they have the feeling of defecation, not inhibiting this feeling, and so as to avoid constipation or intestinal form bezoars by controlled defecation. During defecation, the elder should be concentration, do not read newspapers, novels or listen to the radio, etc.

(2) Reasonable diet. Eat more fruits, vegetables and foods which have rich fiber, such as flour, crude, crude rice bran, oats, kelp, celery, leeks, spinach and others, daily food cellulose should be increased to 30 g and reduce pungent food. Drink more water, 1 500-2 000 ml per day, keep drinking a glass of warm water every morning to ensure lubricate the intestinal tract enough. It may appropriately take honey 20–30 ml melted by warm water, fasting drink in the morning, this is nutrient-rich and laxative.

(3) Persisted activities. Encourage the elder to participate actively in suitable activities such as walking, jogging, Tai Chi, Qi Gong, gardening, painting, etc. Bedridden patients should be assisted in physical activity; regular turning and abdominal massage, if that can improve digestion and promote bowel movements.

(4) Maintained happiness. Adjust the lifestyle of the elderly to maintain an optimistic state of mind, and eliminate mental tension to improve digestive function.

(5) Avoiding forced defecation. Forced defecation can cause coronary artery, cerebrovascular blood flow change, then cause angina, acute myocardial infarction, arrhythmias, aneurysm, or aneurysm rupture, hypertension, acute cerebrovascular disease, and even sudden death. Therefore, it is recommended that the elder of cardiovascular disease should prepare such as nitroglycerin to prevent accidents in defecation.

5. 健康教育

（1）指导患者建立正常的排便生理和良好的习惯：老年人排便宜取坐位，每天排便1～2次。老年患者若有便意时，不要随意抑制便意或憋尿，及时排便，避免强制控制排便而造成便秘或形成粪结石。排便时集中注意力，不看报、小说或听收音机等，以免破坏排便习惯。

（2）合理饮食：多吃水果、蔬菜和富含纤维的食物，如面粉、粗粮、粗米糠、燕麦、海带、芹菜、韭菜、菠菜等，每日膳食纤维素应增加到30g，减少刺激性食物。多喝水，每天1 500～2 000ml，晨起喝一杯温水，以确保肠道有足够的润滑。可适当取蜂蜜20～30ml温开水溶化，早上空腹饮用，营养丰富，有助通便。

（3）保持运动：鼓励老年人积极参加活动，如散步、慢跑、太极、气功、园艺、绘画等。应协助卧床患者进行体力活动；定期翻身和腹部按摩，可以改善消化和促进排便。

（4）调整心态：调整老年人的生活方式，保持乐观的心态，消除精神紧张，改善消化功能。

（5）避免用力排便。用力排便可导致冠状动脉、脑血管血流改变，引起心绞痛、急性心肌梗死、心律失常、动脉瘤或室壁瘤破裂、高血压、急性脑血管疾病，甚至猝死。因此，建议有心血管疾病的老年人排便时，身旁备硝酸甘油等，以防发生意外。

Section 2　Care of the Elderly with Urinary Incontinence

Urinary incontinence refers to the bladder can not control the flow of urine, urinary incontinence can occur in patients of all age groups, but more common in elderly patients, and lower urinary tract aging and changes in the way of urination. The incidence of urinary incontinence was higher in women than in men (1.5:1), which was related to the factors such as pregnancy and childbirth, estrogen deficiency and shortening of urethra. Due to the fact that older people have more urinary incontinence, people mistakenly believe that urinary incontinence is an inevitable natural consequence of aging. In fact, there are many causes of urinary incontinence in the elderly, many of which can be controlled or avoided. Urinary incontinence is not a direct impact on the lives of most elderly people, but can cause skin erosion, body odor, recurrent urinary tract infection, etc., is one of the causes of elderly people with autism, depression. Urinary incontinence is not the normal performance of aging, it is not irreversible, so we should look for a variety of reasons, to take reasonable treatment.

I. Etiology

i. Temporary Urinary Incontinence

If risk factors are eliminated, temporary incontinence could stop.

1. Acute urinary tract infection.

2. Atrophic vaginitis and urethritis. There is 80% of older women have atrophic vaginitis; atrophic vaginitis easily associates with urethritis and trig one of bladder inflammation, so that reduce urethral pressure occurring incontinence.

3. Medication, such as sleeping pills, diuretics like furosemide, methylxanthine like theophylline, smooth muscle relaxants, calcium channel blockers, α-adrenergic receptor antagonists, vincristine, E_1 class of prostate medication and angiotensin converting enzyme inhibitors, those medications can cause incontinence.

4. Excessive urine. There are many factors, such as taking more diuretics or metabolic abnormalities like hyperglycemia and hypocalcaemia.

5. Limitation of activities. Incontinence closely

第二节　尿失禁老年人的护理

尿失禁是指膀胱不能控制排尿而自行流出，尿失禁可发生于所有年龄段的患者，但以老年人更为常见，与下尿道老化及排尿方式的改变有关。尿失禁的发病率女性高于男性（1.5:1），这与女性的妊娠及分娩、绝经期雌激素缺乏、尿道长度缩短等因素有关。由于老年人尿失禁较多见，致使人们误以为尿失禁是衰老过程中不可避免的自然后果。事实上，老年人尿失禁的原因很多，其中有许多原因是可控制或避免的。尿失禁对大多数老年人的生活无直接影响，但可造成皮肤糜烂、身体异味、反复尿路感染等，是引起老年人孤僻、抑郁的原因之一。尿失禁不是衰老的正常表现，也不是不可逆的，应寻找各种原因，采取合理的治疗方法。

一、病因与发病机制

（一）暂时性尿失禁

暂时性的尿失禁是指消除引起尿失禁的因素，暂时性尿失禁可能会停止。

1. 急性尿道感染。

2. 萎缩性阴道炎和尿道炎。80% 老年妇女有萎缩性阴道炎，萎缩性阴道炎容易伴尿道炎和膀胱三角炎，使尿道的关闭压力降低而发生尿失禁。

3. 药物，如安眠药，利尿剂如呋塞米、甲基黄嘌呤剂如茶碱，平滑肌松弛剂，钙通道阻滞剂，α－肾上腺素受体拮抗剂，长春新碱，前列腺 E_1 类药物和血管紧张素转换酶抑制剂等都可引起尿失禁。

4. 尿量过多的原因有摄入过多、利尿药、代谢异常（如高血糖症和低钙血症）等。

5. 活动受限。尿失禁与活动受限有密切

relates with paralysis, many age-related diseases often enable the elderly to mobility limitation, such as arthritis, hip deformity, asthenia, orthostatic hypotension, intermittent claudicating, spinal stenosis, heart failure, poor vision, fearing fell, stroke, confusion and others. If elders delay urination, stand difficultly, stand up slowly and tension, so that can increase pressure of abdomen and bladder causing incontinence.

6. When feces blockade, there are mechanical dysfunction of the bladder or urethra, so that elders cause overflowing incontinence. According to statistics, more than 10% of hospitalized elderly patients with incontinence caused by feces blockade.

7. Delirium.

8. Psychological factor.

ii. Long-term Incontinence

There is still incontinence excluding temporary incontinence, then should consider the following reasons.

1. Excessive detrusor activities　It is the most common cause of urinary tract diseases, commonly referred to the uninhibited bladder contraction. It may incidentally occur in the normal elderly, acute cerebrovascular diseases, prostatic outlet obstruction or stress incontinence.

2. Urethra regurgitation　It is the second common cause of incontinence by older women. Coughing, sneezing, laughing, stoop, and weightlifting, those activities can increase intra-abdominal pressure occurring incontinence. They mainly relate with multiple birth or birth trauma that cause muscle relaxation of bladder or pelvic. May also be related to the injuries after surgery.

3. Urethra obstruction　Benign prostatic hyperplasia, prostate cancer and urethral stricture can lead to obstruction; it is the second common cause of incontinence in elderly men. When spinal cord lesions, the signals which reach the pontine urination central nervous are obstructed, there is dyssynergia between the bladder contraction and urethral dilation, so that can cause severe urethra obstruction.

4. Detrusor inability　If detrusor movements are too weak, that could cause urinary retention and overflowing incontinence, which accounting for 5% to 10% of the elderly with incontinence. Degenerative intervertebral disk diseases or tumor can harm the nerves of urinary bladder. Diabetes, multiple sclerosis, pernicious anemia, spinal tuberculosis or alcoholism

关系，多种老年性疾病包括关节炎、髋部畸形、体力不支、直立性低血压、间歇性跛行、椎管狭窄、心力衰竭、视力障碍、害怕跌倒、卒中、意识障碍等常使老年人运动受限。老年人一旦膀胱充盈，排尿动作稍许推迟、站立困难、起立缓慢、紧张等，使腹部和膀胱内压力增加，导致尿液溢出。

6. 粪便嵌塞时，膀胱或尿道的机械性功能紊乱，使老年人发生充溢性尿失禁。据统计在住院的老年尿失禁患者中10%以上患者是由于粪便嵌顿所致。

7. 谵妄。

8. 心理因素。

（二）长期性尿失禁

老年人在排除暂时性尿失禁的可能原因后仍有尿失禁，应考虑以下原因：

1. **逼尿肌活动过度**　是老年性尿失禁最常见的尿路原因，通常指不稳定膀胱。它可偶发于正常老年人及急性脑血管疾病、前列腺出口梗阻或压力性尿失禁。

2. **压力性尿失禁**　是老年妇女尿失禁的第二位最常见原因。在咳嗽、喷嚏、大笑、弯腰、举重等腹内压增加的动作时，可发生压力性尿失禁。大多与多次分娩或产伤所致的膀胱支持组织和盆底松弛有关；也可能与手术后损伤等有关。

3. **尿道梗阻**　良性前列腺增生、前列腺癌和尿道狭窄可导致尿道梗阻，是老年男性尿失禁的第二个最常见原因。脊髓病变时，到达脑桥排尿中枢的通道发生阻断，膀胱收缩和尿道内口松弛之间协同失调，可造成严重的尿道梗阻。

4. **逼尿肌活动过弱**　逼尿肌活动过弱可引起尿潴留和充溢性尿失禁，占老年尿失禁的5%～10%。椎间盘退行性病变或肿瘤可累及支配膀胱的神经，糖尿病、多发性硬化、恶性贫血、脊髓结核或酒精中毒等疾病可引起后神经根或后角细胞破坏，均可使逼尿肌

and other diseases of the urinary bladder can damage nerve roots or the posterior horn cells, to weaken detrusor movements.

5. Functional incontinence Environmental factors, intelligence, activity, dexterity and medical factors also can cause incontinence, such as hip fractures.

II. Nursing Assessment

i. Health History

1. Assess the elderly state of incontinence incidence Including the starting time, occasional or regular, frequency of urination, urine output, whether urgency, dysuria, and barrier or not, at night or heaven in the day.

2. Possible factors Including living environment, activities and energy, fluid intake, history of medication use, disease and so on.

ii. Clinical Manifestation

Incontinence is mainly that patients cannot control urination flowing unconsciously. The elderly with long-term incontinence are easy to suffer from perinea eczema, pressure sores, urinary tract infections, sepsis, falls, fractures and other complications.

iii. Experimental and Other Test

1. Rectal examination by fingers Asses the anal sphincter, bulbocavernosus reflex, size and texture of prostate, stool incarcerated or not.

2. Female genitalia examination Make sure whether the vaginal bulging, uterine prolapsed, atrophic vaginitis and so on.

3. Urethral pressure test Determine the diagnosis of stress urinary incontinence. When the bladder of the elderly full of urine, when he or she has cough or lift heavy objects in the standing position, he or she will experience a leakage of urine.

4. Pad test The elderly do exercises with pads, then weight the increased weight of pad to know the volume of leakage of urine.

5. Others Urinalysis and urine culture whether there is urinary tract infection. Liver and kidney's function tests. If the elderly have polyuria, should show check blood glucose, serum calcium and albumin to identify the causes.

活动过弱。

5. **功能性尿失禁** 环境因素、患者智力、活动能力、操作灵巧性及医疗因素也可引起尿失禁，如髋部骨折。

二、护理评估

（一）健康史

1. **评估老年人尿失禁发病的情况** 包括起始时间，偶发还是经常，排尿次数、尿量，是否有尿急、排尿困难、尿液点滴等情况，是否夜间或白天加重等。

2. **了解可能引起老年人尿失禁的因素** 包括居住环境、活动和体力、液体摄入、服药物史、疾病等。

（二）临床表现

尿失禁主要表现为排尿不能控制而自行流出。老年人因长期尿失禁而容易发生会阴湿疹、压疮、尿路感染、败血症、跌倒、骨折等并发症。

（三）实验室及其他检查

1. **直肠指检** 了解肛门括约肌张力、球海绵体肌反射、前列腺的大小和质地、有无粪便嵌顿。

2. **女性外生殖器检查** 了解有无阴道前后壁膨出、子宫下垂、萎缩性阴道炎等。

3. **尿道压力测试** 确定压力性尿失禁的诊断方法。当老年人膀胱内充满尿液时，于站立位时咳嗽或举起重物，以观察在膀胱加压时是否出现漏尿情况。

4. **尿垫试验** 在老年人内裤里放置一块已称重的卫生垫后让其运动，运动后再次称卫生垫的重量，以评估漏尿的程度。

5. **其他** 尿常规、尿细菌培养，了解有无泌尿系感染。检测肝肾功能，有多尿现象时应检测血糖、血钙和清蛋白等，以协助查清原因。

iv. Psychosocial Aspect

Assess whether the elderly have some mental illness, such as limited activity, less communication due to smelly urine, alone, loneliness, shame, depression and withdrawal and others. Asses self-care ability, family support, source of care costs, difficulties and so on.

III. Nursing Management

i. Psychological Support

1. Fully understand and respect the elderly, protect their privacy, help the elderly to establish the confidence of the treatment, and communicate with their families to get family's support and help, then maintain patients' self-esteem as much as possible and to provide convenience. No talking and no blaming the elderly with incontinence. Don't bother and urge the elderly during urination. Taking urination on the bed at night.

2. Guide urination regularly, and develop a schedule of urination, such as early morning, before meals, before sleep, outside treatment, before checking, so as to urinate in advance.

3. Train bladder's function, and try to hold back urine in non-regular time, until urine at the scheduled time, makes the interval of urination from short to long.

ii. Convenient Living Environment

In the elderly living environment, there are seats with suitable height, non-slip ground, bathroom with easy access and close to bedroom, toilet with handrails and next to the aisle, and light enough. Clothes should be loose and easy to take off. It necessary that helps elders find the toilet location to avoid incontinence before moving to a new house.

iii. Intermittent Catheterization and Indwelling Catheter

For the temporary incontinence, nurses can offer pseudo-catheterization. For long-term incontinence, nurses may provide indwelling catheter, and take care according to the nursing principle of indwelling catheter, set up a regular urination to avoid wet skin and skin ulceration.

iv. Keep the Skin Clean

If the elder patients are conscious, nurses can use

（四）心理社会状况

评估尿失禁患者有无因活动能力受限、尿臭等不愿与他人交往，有无孤独、寂寞、羞耻、抑郁和退缩等心理障碍。了解尿失禁患者自我护理能力、家人支持状况、护理费用来源及困难等。

三、护理措施

（一）给予心理支持

1. 充分理解和尊重老年人，注意保护其隐私。帮助老年人树立治疗的信心，并与家属进行沟通，取得家庭的支持和帮助，尽可能维护老年人的自尊。不谈论、不责难老年人尿失禁，尽可能提供方便和照顾。排尿时，尽可能让无关人员避开，不打扰、不催促，夜间床边放置便器。

2. 指导老年人建立定时排尿习惯，帮助制订如厕时间表，如晨起、饭前、睡前排尿。户外治疗、检查或活动前，事先排尿。

3. 训练膀胱功能，在非规定排尿时间内尽量憋住尿液，直到预定的时刻将尿液排尽，排尿间隔时间由短逐渐延长。

（二）创造便利的生活环境

在老年人生活区域内，设置座椅高矮适宜，保持地面平整、防滑，卫生间布局应方便出入且靠近卧室，马桶旁和走道应有扶手，光线良好。衣裤宜宽松，方便松解。如乔迁新居，应帮助老年人提前熟悉厕所的位置，有助于减少尿失禁的发生。

（三）给予导尿和留置导尿管

暂时性尿失禁老年人可采用假性导尿，长期尿失禁的老年人采用导尿术留置导尿管，按留置导尿管护理，定时放尿，避免浸湿皮肤，发生皮肤破溃。

（四）保持皮肤清洁卫生

对神志清醒的男性老年人可用便壶接尿，

urinal which connects with skin pad with soft paper or cloth to prevent the local skin discomfort because of long-term contact, and clear in time. If the elderly men are unconscious or restless, nurses can use available condom to fix on the penis, connect with the drainage tube, and keep the pipeline open to prevent poor drainage for folding, soaking penis and causing erosion. When turning body, the care providers should prevent skin damaging. The female can use pads or bedpan for urination. For the elder patients with intractable incontinence, they should be used the indwelling catheter. Keep strict aseptic technique to prevent urinary tract infection. Keep the bed clean and dry, replace the wet in time, and clean the perineum and anus with warm water and soft towel after urination or wet body by urine.

v. Treat Related Diseases as Possible

Many diseases can cause incontinence; urinary incontinence may disappear after treatment of these diseases. Therefore, according to the factors of the diseases, use of antimicrobial agents control infection, low-dose estrogen control atrophic urethritis and vaginitis, heart failure, and improve nutrition. Stress incontinence caused by the weakened internal sphincter, generally require surgery.

vi. Health Education

1. Guide the elderly and their families reduce the induced factors as much as possible that cause or worsen incontinence.

2. Avoid increasing intra-abdominal pressure for elder patients with stress incontinence, instruct them avoid laughing, coughing, sneezing, and constipation, stop to increase abdominal pressure. Don't hold back urine if there is feeling of urination, it is timely urination.

3. Drink properly amount of water tell the elderly in general every day to drink water 2 000-2 500ml in order to ensure adequate urine. Control drinking after dinner; avoid drinking caffeinated beverages, in order to avoid too much urination at night or incontinence caused by the stimulated bladder.

4. Avoid the use of inappropriate medication. Some medication which can cause incontinence should be used with caution or forbidden, in order to avoid the occurrence of medication-induced urinary incontinence. There are some medications, such as analgesics, ethanol preparations which can reduce the sensitivity of the sphincter of the urination reflex, and so it should be useless. Those elder

便壶口与皮肤接触处垫以软纸或软布，以防壶口长期刺激局部皮肤引起不适；每次排尿后及时倾倒，冲洗便壶。对神志不清、躁动不安的男性老年人，可用阴茎套固定于阴茎上，顶端剪一开口与引流管连接，保持管道通畅，防止管道折叠引流不畅，尿液浸泡龟头，引起糜烂，翻身时应防止损伤皮肤。女性老年人可垫尿布或用、便盆接尿。对老年人顽固的尿失禁，应给予留置导尿管。导尿操作及留置尿管的处置应严格无菌操作，防止泌尿系感染。保持被褥整洁、干燥，潮湿及时更换，并用温热水及软毛巾擦洗会阴、肛门周围，必要时涂油保护。

（五）遵医嘱积极治疗相关疾病

多种疾病可引起尿失禁，当这些疾病得到治疗后，尿失禁可能消失。因此根据患者的病因不同，采用抗生素控制感染、小剂量雌激素治疗萎缩性尿道炎和阴道炎、控制心衰、改善营养不良等。对内括约肌功能减弱发生的压力性尿失禁，一般需要手术治疗。

（六）健康教育

1. 指导老年人及家属尽可能减少引起或加重尿失禁的因素。

2. 防止腹内压增加。对于压力性尿失禁的患者，指导患者避免大笑、咳嗽、打喷嚏及便秘等导致腹压增高；不要憋尿，如有尿意，应及时排尿。

3. 适量饮水。告诉老年人一般每天宜饮水 2 000～2 500ml，以保证足够的尿量。晚餐后宜控制饮水量，避免饮含咖啡因的饮料，以免夜尿过多或引起膀胱刺激发生尿失禁。

4. 避免使用不当的药物。老年人应慎用或禁用能够引起尿失禁的药物，以免引起药源性尿失禁的发生，如镇痛剂、乙醇制剂等可降低括约肌对排尿反射的敏感性，应尽量少用。心、肾疾病需要用利尿剂时，尽可能采用早晨顿服，以减少夜间尿失禁的发生。

patients with heart and kidney diseases need to use diuretics, used in the morning as far as possible in order to reduce the occurrence of nighttime incontinence.

5. Guide patients to the exercise of pelvic floor muscle and bladder's function; enhance the ability to control urination, such as sit-ups, the training of the levator muscles, and intermittent urination. The training of the levator muscle, which is the elder patient with standing position, sitting position or a combination, deeply breath and slowly relax combined with breathing exercises, in continuous 5 to 10 times accumulated 10 to 20 minutes a day. Intermittent urination which is that patients consciously interrupt urination for several times, so that imitate holding back urine and urination, 3 to 4 times a day, every 5 to 10 minutes. Every time is 3 to 5 seconds, which can relieve stress urinary incontinence.

5. 指导患者进行盆底肌和膀胱功能锻炼，增强控制排尿的能力，如仰卧起坐、肛提肌训练、间隙排尿法等。肛提肌训练：患者取立位、坐位或侧卧位，与呼吸运动相结合，深吸气慢慢放松，连续 5~10 次，日累计 10~20 分钟。间隙排尿法：排尿时患者有意识地中断尿流数次，即模拟憋尿和排尿活动，每天进行 3~4 次，每次 5~10 分钟。每次 3~5 秒钟，可缓解压迫性尿失禁。

Section 3　Care of the Elderly with Fecal Incontinence

第三节　大便失禁老年人的护理

Fecal incontinence is status of involuntary defecation not controlling anal sphincter. Due to the weakening of the anal sphincter and sensation of anal canal and rectum, the elderly with fecal incontinence are so common. As reported, incidence of home elderly fecal incontinence is approximately 10%, ever up to 60% in nursing homes in the United States. Incidence of fecal incontinence in the female is higher than in the male, it caused by injury of pubic nerve and the pelvic tissue during childbirth.

大便失禁是指肛门括约肌不受意志控制而不自主地排便。老年人由于肛门括约肌张力减弱，肛管、直肠感觉功能减退，大便失禁发生较为常见。据报道，大便失禁在居家老年人中发生率约 10%，在美国的一些疗养院高达 60%。女性因为分娩时所致耻骨神经及盆底组织损伤，大便失禁的发生率高于男性。

I.Etiology

一、病因与发病机制

There are basically three risk factors of fecal incontinence: fecal impaction, symptomatic fecal incontinence, and neurogenic fecal incontinence.

大便失禁的原因大致有三大类：粪便嵌塞、症状性大便失禁及神经源性大便失禁。

i. Stool Impaction

Stool impaction or fecal impaction is the most common factor in the elderly with fecal incontinence, which is one of the complications of chronic constipation. Because of fecal impaction in the colon or the rectum, then the dry defecation stimulates the colon and glands to form large amounts of mucus, water flow to the rectum next to the space of dry defecation, if rectum is sensitive with that water, which would flow from the anus to form

（一）粪便嵌塞

粪便嵌塞是老年大便失禁的最常见原因，它是慢性便秘的并发症之一。因粪便嵌塞在结肠下部和直肠，形成硬粪刺激结肠和腺体产生大量黏液，粪水经粪块旁间隙流到直肠，如直肠对流出的粪水敏感，就会从肛门流出，形成大便失禁。10%~20% 的老年便秘患者有此并发症，生活不能自理或长期卧床的老年

fecal incontinence. There are 10%-20% of elderly patients with constipation are suffering complications of fecal incontinence, and are more common of self-caring invalid or bedridden.

ii. Symptomatic Fecal Incontinence

It is caused by dysfunction of anal sphincter. Because of liquid stool deregulation anal sphincter, sensory nerves of the anal canal weaken the ability to distinguish the liquid stool in the rectum and the expansion of gases, so diarrhea by any factors are easy to cause symptomatic fecal incontinence. A common factors include digestive diseases: gastroenteritis, ulcerative colitis, ischemic colitis, colonic diverticulitis, colon cancer, rectal prolapsed and so on. The metabolic disorders and endocrine diseases: Diabetes, hyperthyroidism psychosis and so on. Latrogenic factors: Excessive laxatives, imbalance of intestinal flora by anti-bacterial medication, the stimulation of iron on the intestinal mucosa, postoperative complications (such as anal sphincter slitting), and so on.

iii. Neurogenic Fecal Incontinence

In normal, the gastroscopic reflex promotes colon contents into the rectum, then rectal distension forms sense of defecation, under the control of the senior center nervous, form the rectal contraction and anal sphincter relaxation then defecation. Otherwise, postpone defecation. The elderly disorder of delayed defecation may also cause fecal incontinence. Such as central nervous system lesions or sacral nerve damage, that cannot control defecation known as neurogenic fecal incontinence. The frequency of that fecal incontinence is one or two times a day, and stools have shape. Common factors including: acute cerebrovascular disease, dementia, disturbance of consciousness, spinal cord diseases and so on.

II.Nursing Assessment

i. Health History

1. Assess something related to the elderly defecation, including habits, time, frequency, character, amount, with or without constipation, diarrhea and so on. If the elderly with fecal incontinence all day long, it may relate with stool impaction; if the frequency is one or two times a day, it may relate with diet, and this may be neurogenic fecal incontinence.

2. Know the elderly diet, if the elderly take a long-term low-residue diet, their fecal incontinence may be

人更为多见。

（二）症状性大便失禁

症状性大便失禁是因肛门括约肌功能失常所致。老年人肛门括约肌对液体粪便的调节失调，具有感觉神经的肛管对直肠内液体粪便和气体膨胀的分辨能力减弱，所以，任何原因引起的腹泻都容易引起大便失禁。这类大便失禁的常见原因包括：①消化系统疾病包括胃肠炎、溃疡性结肠炎、缺血性肠炎、结肠憩室、大肠肿瘤、直肠脱垂等；②代谢内分泌疾病包括糖尿病、甲状腺功能亢进症等；③医源性原因包括泻剂过量、抗生素引起的肠道菌群失调、铁剂对肠黏膜的刺激、术后并发症（如肛门括约肌撕裂）等。

（三）神经源性大便失禁

正常情况下，胃结肠反射促进结肠内容物进入直肠，直肠扩张产生便意，在高级中枢控制下，直肠收缩、肛门括约肌松弛进行排便。反之，则暂缓排便。老年人的这种延缓排便的动作出现障碍，也可发生大便失禁。如中枢神经系统病变或骶神经损伤，不能随意控制排便称神经源性大便失禁。这种大便失禁每天1~2次，粪便成形。老年人这类大便失禁的常见原因有急性脑血管疾病、痴呆、意识障碍、脊髓疾病等。

二、护理评估

（一）健康史

1. 评估老年人排便情况包括排便习惯、排便时间、次数、性状、量、有无便秘、有无腹泻等。如果全天大便失禁，可能与粪便嵌塞有关；若一天只出现1~2次，且与进食有关，很可能是神经源性大便失禁。

2. 了解老年人最近进食情况，如果长期低渣饮食，则大便失禁可能与便秘有关；近

associated with constipation; if there are recent changes in diet or eating contaminated food, fecal incontinence may relate with diarrhea.

ii. Clinical Manifestation

1. Defecation Abnormal. Defecation is frequent, or shape stool in one or two times a day. There is no feeling of defecation, so that the elderly usually defecate in bed or pants.

2. Skin Lesions. Skins are always dipped by stool incontinence, and suffer from skin erosion, eczematous changes. Skin lesions are easy to cause local or systemic infection.

iii. Experimental and Other Tests

1. Rectal microscopy. Observe the color of the rectal mucosa, with or without ulceration, inflammation, hemorrhage, tumor, and stricture and so on.

2. Fecal bacteriological examination, abdominal plain film, barium enema may find some help for fecal incontinence.

iv. Psychosocial Aspects

Because fecal incontinence causes inconvenience of the elderly participate activities and communication with psychological burden, the elderly are unwilling to go to public places, unwilling to communicate with others, worried about the family abandon, so that they often take away from the community, feel lonely, shame and depression. In addition, due to fecal incontinence polluting clothes and bedding, those may increase the burden of family and self-care, may cause families' complains much.

III. Nursing Management

1. Treat the primary disease or deal with the symptoms. If fecal incontinence is caused by feces incarcerated, it is mainly to treat constipation. Symptomatic fecal incontinence should treat the primary diseases; neurogenic fecal incontinence should re-establish a conditioned reflex through diet or medication, allow patients to get up and sit on the commode drinking water until defecation. In addition, use opioids or neostigmine to reconstruct defecation conditioned reflex as prescribed.

2. Adjust diet and lifestyle. Intake food which is nutrient-rich, digestible and less residue oil, avoid eating coarse and strong irritant food, in order to reduce the burden of the gastrointestinal tract. Drink plenty of

期饮食变化或进食不洁食物，可能与腹泻有关。

（二）临床表现

1. **排便异常** 排便频繁不止，或每天有1～2次成形粪便，无排便感觉，排在床上或裤子内。

2. **皮肤损害** 因肛周受失禁粪便的浸渍，出现皮肤糜烂、湿疹样改变，容易引起局部或全身感染。

（三）实验室及其他检查

1. 直肠镜检。观察直肠黏膜的颜色，有无溃疡、炎症、出血、肿瘤、狭窄。

2. 粪便细菌学检查、腹部平片、钡剂灌肠对大便失禁的原因查找有一定的帮助。

（四）心理社会状况

老年人因大便失禁给其活动和社交造成不便，产生心理负担，不愿进出公共场合、不愿和他人交往，担心家人嫌弃，常常远离社会，内心感到孤独、耻辱、抑郁。另外，因大便失禁污染衣裤和被褥，加重家庭和自我照顾的负担，长时间可能引起家人抱怨。

三、护理措施

1. 积极治疗原发病，必要时对症处理，如大便失禁由粪便嵌塞引起，则主要治疗便秘；如为症状性大便失禁，以治疗原发病为主；如神经源性大便失禁，可通过饮食或药物重新建立条件反射，可让患者起床后坐在马桶上饮水，直到粪便排出后再起身。另外，可遵医嘱使用阿片制剂或新斯的明等药物重建排便条件反射。

2. 调整饮食和生活习惯。宜摄取营养丰富、容易消化吸收、少渣少油的食物，避免进食粗糙和刺激性强的食物，以减轻胃肠道的负担。便秘时，多饮水，补充体液；若无

water to add body fluids when constipation, if there are no taboos, the elderly should intake 3 000ml of liquid a day. Treating severe diarrhea, may use short-term fasting, or eat dedicate and liquid food or semi-liquid in recovering. After the diarrhea stopped, eat soft food, such as custard, pureed vegetables, lean meat particles and soft rice.

3. Develop regular defecation. If Circumstance allowing, encourage elderly people to take activities or exercise which will help establish a normal defecation reflex; try to take the sitting defecation in same time every day, if necessary, provide bedside commode and assistive devices such as wheelchairs, crutches, or helping the patient into the toilet, so that patients can be timely defecation.

4. Keep dry skin of perineum and anus, and defecate after bath to prevent rupture. The skin around the anus is stimulated to become red due to frequent defecation which can use zinc oxide ointment. In severe cases, use local bake lights twice a day, each one lasts 20 to 30 minutes in order to keep the skin dry. As those patients of continuous loose stools, may select the appropriate fecal incontinence appliances, such as incontinence pads, ostomy bag.

5. Health education.

(1) Guide to develop good defecation habit; do not arbitrarily suppress the sense of defecation which would affect the defecation and patterns of life.

(2) Encourage the elderly to adhere whatever activities such as walking, jogging, Tai Chi, Qi Gong, gardening, painting and so on. As bedridden patients, should do physical activities, and regularly turn body and massage; intentionally exercise the function of the abdominal muscles, diaphragm, levator muscle, so that to promote defecation.

(3) Encourage the elderly to maintain a positive mental state, participate in appropriate communication, and eliminate the psychological tension, which would help to improve digestive function.

(HUANG Jin)

Key Points

1. Elimination disorders cannot be avoided in aging process, and have a tremendous influence on the physical and mental health of the elderly.

2. Urinary incontinence is not a part of normal aging. It is a symptom, not a disease, caused by drugs or by environmental, psychologic, or physiologic disturbances.

禁忌，老年人每天摄入 3 000ml 液体；腹泻严重时，可短期禁食；恢复期进食流食或半流食；腹泻停止后，进食软食，如蛋羹、菜泥、瘦肉末、软饭等。

3. 建立规律的排便习惯。在病情允许的情况下，鼓励老年人活动或锻炼，有助于建立正常的排便反射；排便时尽量采取坐姿；必要时，提供床旁便器和辅助器具如轮椅、拐杖，或帮助患者如厕，使患者能及时排便。

4. 保持会阴部及肛门周围皮肤干燥，便后坐浴，以防破溃。

肛门周围的皮肤因频繁的稀便刺激发红，可涂抹氧化锌软膏。严重者使用烤灯每日两次局部皮肤烘烤，每次 20～30 分钟，以保持皮肤干燥；稀便常流不止者，选择合适的大便失禁器具，如失禁垫、造口袋等。

5. 健康教育。

（1）指导老年人养成良好的排便习惯，不要随意抑制便意而影响排便和生活规律。

（2）鼓励老年人坚持力所能及的活动，如散步、慢跑、打太极拳、练气功、养花、绘画等；卧床不起的老年患者可做肢体活动，并定时翻身和进行腹部按摩，有意锻炼腹肌、膈肌、肛提肌功能，促进排便。

（3）鼓励老年人保持积极乐观的精神状态，参与适当的社交活动以消除紧张心理，且有助于改善消化道的功能。

（黄　金）

本章要点

1. 排泄障碍是机体老化过程中无法避免的，对老年人的身心健康产生了极大影响。
2. 尿失禁不是正常老化的表现。尿失禁是一种症状，而不是疾病，常由药物、环境、心理或生理紊乱引起。

3. Elderly constipation is the most common complication of fecal impaction, leading to intestinal obstruction, colonic ulceration, overflowed fecal incontinence or contradiction diarrhea.

4. There are basically three risk factors of fecal incontinence: fecal impaction, symptomatic fecal incontinence and neurogenic fecal incontinence.

Critical Thinking Exercise

1. How does the fecal impaction affect urinary incontinence?

2. Maria, aged 60, mother of 4 children: "I know I must smell of urine and others don't want to be around me. It has gotten to the point where I don't want to go anywhere. I know my husband Harry gets irritated with me when I need to stop so often to find a bathroom. But, even so, I can't always hold the urine no matter how I try. My friends Beth told me about an incontinence clinic in the city. I guess I really need to find out if they can help me."

Question:
What do you think of the following lived experience?

批判性思维练习

1. 老年人粪便嵌塞是如何引起尿失禁的？

2. 玛丽亚，60 岁，是 4 个孩子的母亲。患者如下自述："我知道我身上总能闻到尿味，别人会嫌弃我身上的这种味道，不想待在我身边，因此我只想待在家，不想外出。因为外出时我时常要上厕所，我丈夫 Harry 很讨厌我这一点。我想尽一切办法憋尿，但是还是憋不住。朋友 Beth 告诉我有一个治疗尿失禁的诊所，我特别想知道治疗是否有用。"
问题：
你如何看待患者的这种表述并如何作答。

Chapter 15 Sleep Management for Elderly

第十五章 老年人睡眠障碍的护理

Learning Objectives

Upon completion of this chapter, the reader will be able to:

- Explain differences between younger and older adults in sleep stages and cycles;

- Identify age-related changes in sleep;

- Describe factors that may disturb sleep in older adults;

- Discuss three sleep disorders in older adults;

- List the components of a sleep history;

- Describe sleep hygiene measures;

- Describe pharmacologic and non-pharmacologic means to promote sleep.

学习目标

学完本章节，应完成以下目标：

- 解释年轻人和老年人在睡眠结构和周期中的差异；

- 识别年龄相关的睡眠变化；

- 描述可能影响老年人睡眠的因素；

- 讨论老年人的三种睡眠障碍；

- 列出睡眠史的主要内容；

- 描述睡眠卫生措施；

- 描述促进睡眠的药物和非药物疗法。

Sleep is a vital physiologic process with important restorative functions for the body and mind; sleep is a state of inactivity or repose that is required to remain active. Notable qualitative and quantitative changes in sleep occur with age. Moreover, many sleep-related disorders occur with increasing frequency among elderly people, more than 50% of older adults complain of difficulty sleeping. These conditions affect health and well-being, as inadequate quality or quantity of sleep is associated with risks to physical and mental health. This chapter discusses age-related changes and sleeping disorders in the elderly with highlights on methods of sleep management and the role of nurse in assisting older individuals to adapt to sleep changes.

睡眠是重要的生理现象，对人的体力、精力恢复和机体的生长发育具有重要作用。由于生理和病理的原因，老年人睡眠质量普遍偏低。严重威胁了老年人的身心健康，造成注意力不集中、记忆力减退和生活质量下降。因此，本章节将讨论与年龄有关的睡眠障碍，并探讨管理睡眠的方法以及护士在促进老年人睡眠过程中的角色。

Section 1　Sleep Architecture

第一节　睡眠结构

Sleep can be divided into two distinct states, namely, non-rapid eye movement (non-REM) and rapid eye movement (REM) sleep. Non-REM sleep is further subdivided into light sleep, stages 1 and 2, and deep sleep, formerly stages 3 and 4. Non-REM sleep accounts for 75%-80% of sleep cycle, REM sleep accounts for the remaining 20%-25%. A normal sleep cycles ranges from 70 to 120 minutes in length and transits through stages 1 to 4 and REM sleep. There are usually four to six cycles occurring in a night.

正常睡眠结构包括快速眼动（rapid eye movement，REM）睡眠和非快速眼动（non rapid eye movement，NREM）睡眠两个睡眠时相，且两个睡眠时相在整个睡眠过程中交替出现。非快速眼动睡眠包括4个阶段：Ⅰ、Ⅱ阶段睡眠较浅，易被唤醒；Ⅲ、Ⅳ阶段睡眠又称深睡眠期。非快速动眼时期占据整个睡眠周期的75%～80%，快速眼动睡眠占据剩下的20%～25%。一个正常的睡眠周期持续70～120分钟，包括快速动眼睡眠和非快速动眼睡眠的交替。一晚上大约有4～6次的循环周期。

Stage 1 and 2 constitute light sleep; stage 3 and 4 comprise deep sleep. Deep sleep generally is more refreshing. To achieve revival, a person experiences series of sleep stages, each stage with different characteristics (table 15-1). Stage 1 is the lightest level of sleep, which can be easily awakened. Sleep progressively deepens from stage 1 to stage 4, so stage 4 is the deepest level. During non-REM sleep, eye movements are relatively infrequent, muscle tone, pulse, blood pressure, and respiratory is moderately reduced as compared with waking levels. The electroencephalogram shows a gradual slowing of frequency and an increase in amplitude through the four stages of non-REM sleep; stages 3 and 4 are often called slow wave sleep (SWS) or delta sleeps. During REM sleep, muscle tone, pulse, blood pressure, and respiratory

第一阶段和第二阶段构成轻度睡眠；第三和第四阶段组成深度睡眠。深度睡眠通常更提神。要想恢复活力，一个人需要经历一系列睡眠阶段，每个阶段都有不同的特点（表15-1）。第一阶段睡眠最浅，很容易被唤醒。睡眠从第一阶段到第四阶段逐渐加。在非快速动眼睡眠中，眼球运动相对较少，肌肉张力、脉搏、血压和呼吸相比于清醒时稍低。在非快速眼动睡眠的四个阶段，脑电图的频率逐渐降低，振幅增加；阶段3和阶段4通常称为慢波睡眠（SWS）。在快速眼动睡眠中，肌肉张力、脉搏、血压和呼吸明显增加，

increase markedly, bursts of conjugate gaze occur, and the electroencephalogram shows low-amplitude, fast-frequency activity similar to that seen during wakefulness. REM sleep is associated with dreaming.

脑电图显示低振幅、快频率的活动图像，与清醒时相似，并与做梦有关。

Table 15-1　Normal Stages of Sleep

Stage	Type of Sleep	Characteristics
	Non-rapid eye movement	
Stage1	Light sleep	Easily awakened
Stage2	Medium deep sleep	More relaxed than in stage 1 Slow eye movements Fragmentary dreams Easily awakened
Stage3	Medium deep sleep	Relaxed muscles Slow pulse Decreased body temperature Awakened with moderate stimuli
Stage4	Deep sleep	Restorative sleep Body movement rare Awakened with vigorous stimuli
	Rapid eye movement sleep	
	Active sleep	Rapid eye movement Increased or fluctuating P/BP/R Dreaming occurs

表 15-1　正常睡眠阶段

阶段	睡眠类型	特点
	非快速动眼期	
阶段 1	浅睡眠	易被唤醒
阶段 2	中等睡眠	深度较阶段 1 更为放松 慢速眼动 断续的梦境 易被唤醒
阶段 3	中等睡眠	深度肌肉放松 脉搏缓慢 体温下降 中等强度刺激可唤醒
阶段 4	深睡眠	养精蓄锐 身体活动减少 强刺激才可被唤醒
	快速动眼睡眠	
	主动睡眠	快速眼动 脉搏、血压、呼吸增加或波动 进入梦境

Changes in sleep architecture do occur with aging, the total amount of REM sleep is reduced, the amount of stage 1 sleep is increased, and stage 3 and 4 sleep are less deep. A large meta-analysis of 65 overnight studies representing 3 577 subjects across the entire age spectrum reported that, with age, the percentage time of rapid eye movement (REM) sleep decreased while the percentages of light sleep (stage 1 and stage 2 sleep) increased.

Circadian rhythms, such as core body temperature, hormone secretion and the sleep-wake cycle, oscillate approximately every 24-hour. The sleep-wake cycle is regulated by an endogenous pacemaker and exogenous stimuli. The hypothalamic suprachiasmatic nucleus controls many circadian rhythms, considered the endogenous clock of the brain and the mediator of circadian rhythms. Circadian rhythms are naturally entrained by exogenous stimuli, or zeitgebers (time cues), including the perception of time, travel across time zones, light exposure, seasonal changes, living habits, stress, illness, and medication.

For older adults, factors associated with aging are identified as contributors to the desynchronization of rhythms. The circadian pacemaker itself degenerates with age and results in less robust rhythms. With age there is also a gradual decrease in rhythm amplitude which likely contributes to less consistent periods of sleep–wake across a 24-hour day. The endogenous secretion of melatonin at night is also reduced with age, which results in a weaker circadian rhythm. The most common clinical consequence of changes in circadian network is an advance of the circadian rhythm, namely phase advance. Older adults feel sleepy in the early evening and awaken in the very early morning hours. Adjusting schedules to accommodate the altered biorhythms and increasing natural light are useful.

Section 2 Age-Related Changes in Sleep

With aging, important changes in sleep structure occur (box 15-1). Nevertheless, some older adults do not consider them as sources of distress, but more than 50% of older adults do complain about their sleep. With the aging process, the total amount of time asleep shortens: infants and young children sleep an average of 16-20

随着年龄的增长，睡眠结构会发生变化，快速眼动睡眠的总时长会减少，第一阶段睡眠时长增加，第三和第四阶段睡眠深度会减少。一项针对 65 项夜间研究，包括 3 577 名受试对象的 meta 分析报告显示随着年龄的增长，快速眼动（REM）睡眠时间的百分比有所下降，而浅度睡眠（第一阶段和第二阶段睡眠）的百分比有所上升。

昼夜节律，如核心体温、激素分泌和睡眠－觉醒周期，大约每 24 小时波动一次。睡眠－觉醒周期受内源性和外源性刺激的影响。下丘脑视交叉上核是昼夜节律的中枢。昼夜节律受到外部刺激或时间的影响，包括对时间的感知、跨时区旅行、光照、季节变化、生活习惯、压力、疾病和药物治疗。

对老年人而言，与衰老相关的因素是导致节律失同步的主要因素。随着年龄的增长，生理节律会退化，幅度也在逐渐减小，这可能导致 24 小时内的睡眠－觉醒周期不太一致。此外，夜间褪黑素的分泌也随着年龄的增长而减少，导致昼夜节律较弱。昼夜节律变化最常见的临床后果是昼夜节律的提前。老年人表现为傍晚感到困倦，早晨醒的早。调整作息时间和这种生物节律相适应或者增加阳光的照射时间可能有效。

第二节　与年龄相关的睡眠改变

随着年龄的增长，睡眠结构发生变化（box 15-1）。超过 50% 的老年人抱怨他们的睡眠质量。然而正常情况下，随着年龄的增长，人的总睡眠时间会缩短：如婴幼儿平均每天睡眠 16～20 小时；成年人则为 7～8 小时；

hours per day, adults 7-8 hours, and people over 60 years of age 6.5 hours daily. Deep sleep (stages 3 and 4), the deepest and most refreshing form of sleep, diminishes with age. While the need for sleep may not change with age, the ability to get the needed sleep does decrease with age. The sleep changes experienced by many older adults include increased sleep latency, reduced sleep efficiency, more awakening in the night, increased early morning awakenings, and increased daytime sleepiness. A survey revealed that 10% of that aged 55-64 years old with daytime sleepiness, reported by 25% of that aged 75-84 years old. Poor sleep puts the older adult at greater risk for decreased physical functioning, problems with memory, increased risk of falls and mortality.

Box 15-1 Typical Sleep Changes with Aging

1. Decreased total nocturnal sleep time.

2. Delayed onset of sleep.

3. Advanced circadian phase: early to bed, early to rise.

4. Reduced slow-wave sleep.

5. Reduced rapid-eye-movement (REM) sleep.

6. Reduced threshold for arousal from sleep.

7. Fragmented sleep with multiple arousals.

8. Daytime napping.

I. Factors Contributing to Sleep Problems

Proper sleep is essential for a person's sense of well-being and health. Feeling tired and less alert after a poor night's sleep lead to a less active and productive day. Normal age-related changes in sleep and rhythms alone do not result in a pathological sleep problem. It is more often the comorbidities that precipitate or perpetuate sleep problems. Multiple causes could be responsible for reduced capability to achieve sufficient sleep with age, including medical or psychiatric illnesses, life changes (e. g. retirement, bereavement, decreased social interactions), environmental changes (e. g. placement in a nursing home), pain, dietary influences, and polypharmacy. Nocturia is common in elderly, 80% of individuals aged 80 and older with nocturia.

II. Consequences of Poor Sleep in Elderly

Sleep complaints in older adults are often considered a normal part of aging. However, poor sleep in older adults

60 岁以上则为每天 6.5 小时。深度睡眠（阶段 3 和阶段 4）随着年龄的增长而减少。许多老年人经历的睡眠变化包括睡眠潜伏期增加、睡眠效率降低、夜间醒来次数增多、清晨醒来次数增多以及白天嗜睡。一项调查显示，在 55～64 岁的人群中，有 10% 的人白天嗜睡，而在 75～84 岁的人群中，这一比例为 25%。睡眠不足会增加老年人身体功能下降、记忆力减退、跌倒和死亡的风险。

Box 15-1 老年人典型睡眠特征改变

1. 夜间总睡眠时间减少。

2. 入睡时间推迟。

3. 老年生理阶段：早睡早起。

4. 慢波睡眠减少。

5. REM 睡眠减少。

6. 睡眠中更易被唤醒。

7. 碎片化睡眠，多觉醒。

8. 白天打盹。

一、导致睡眠障碍的因素

适当的睡眠对一个人的健康至关重要。夜间睡眠不足会导致白天活动和效率降低。正常情况下，与年龄有关的睡眠变化本身并不会导致病态的睡眠问题。更多的睡眠障碍是由其他病引起的。随着年龄的增长，睡眠不足是多种原因造成的，包括身体或精神疾病、生活变化（如退休、丧亲之痛、社会交往减少）、环境变化（如住进养老院）、疼痛、饮食影响和多种药物治疗。老年人的夜尿症状是引起睡眠不足的主要原因，大约 80% 的 80 岁及以上老人都有夜尿症。

二、老年人睡眠不足的危害

老年人的睡眠问题通常是衰老的正常现象。然而，老年人睡眠不足与健康状况不佳、

is substantially associated with poor health, decreased physical function, falls, cognitive impairment, and mortality, etc. In a study conducted among older patients in 11 primary care practice settings, symptoms of poor sleep, including daytime sleepiness, feeling un-refreshed in the morning, and difficulty sleeping, were all found to be markers of poor physical and mental health ($P <$ 0.001). Several studies have examined the relationship between poor sleep and physical function and falls. Polysomnography and wrist actigraphy measurements in 2 862 elderly elderly indicated that poor sleep at night, spending more than 90 min awake at night and sleep efficiency $<$ 80% were all associated with lower grip strength, slower walking speed, inability to stand from a chair without assistance, and inability to complete a narrow walk course. The authors concluded that disrupted sleep at night resulted in reduced physical performance. Older adults with sleep problems report high incidences of balance, ambulatory and visual difficulties, even after adjustment for medication use, all of these difficulties result in an increased risk of falling. Older adults with sleep difficulties have slower reaction times and suffer from more cognitive dysfunction such as impaired memory. The slowed response and decreased attention may increase the likelihood of falls, fractures, and automobile accidents. Poor sleep is associated with significant mortality and morbidity in older adults. Patients with sleep difficulties report decreased quality of life as well as higher rates of depression and anxiety. Poor sleep is an important clinical entity with a potentially significant impact on older adults and society, which requires awareness from the health professionals and family caregivers.

身体功能下降、跌倒、认知障碍和死亡率等因素密切相关。在一项对 11 个初级保健机构的老年患者进行的研究中，睡眠不足的症状，包括白天嗜睡、早晨精神萎靡和睡眠困难，都与老年人身心健康不良有关（$P <$0.001）。有研究证实了睡眠不足与身体功能以及跌倒之间的关系。研究者用多导睡眠图和手腕活动检测仪对 2 862 位老年人测试结果显示夜间有 90 分钟不在睡眠状态或者睡眠效率＜80% 的老人都会有比较明显的握力低下、行走速度慢等问题。此外，有睡眠障碍的老年人，他们的平衡能力、行走能力低下，视觉障碍的发生率很高，反应速度较慢，认知功能障碍发生率高，如记忆力受损。而反应迟缓和注意力下降可能会增加跌倒、骨折和车祸的可能性。睡眠不足还与抑郁和焦虑情绪以及老人的死亡率相关。

Section 3　Sleep Disorders in the Elderly

第三节　老年人常见的睡眠障碍

Approximately half of the adult population complains of sleep disorders, with the major complaint being insomnia. In addition to insomnia, sleep disordered breathing (SDB), restless legs syndrome (RLS)/periodic limb movements in sleep (PLMS), and REM sleep behavior disorder (RBD) can disturb sleep in older adults.

老年人群中半数以上存在睡眠障碍，常见的有失眠（老年人中的慢性失眠障碍）、睡眠呼吸暂停综合征、不宁腿综合征和周期性腿动、REM 期睡眠行为障碍等。

I. Insomnia

Insomnia is the most common sleep disorder reported by older people. Epidemiologic data have shown a higher prevalence of insomnia in older persons than in younger individuals. In the US, an estimated 30%-50% of the elderly are affected by insomnia, a prospective study revealed 49% of the elderly aged 80 years and older with insomnia. Insomnia is defined as the complaint (or perception) of inadequate or poor-quality sleep because of one or more of the following: difficulty falling asleep; waking up frequently during the night with difficulty returning to sleep; waking up too early in the morning; or unrefreshing sleep. Insomnia is not defined by the number of hours of sleep a person gets or how long it takes to fall asleep. Individuals vary normally in their need, and their satisfaction with sleep. Insomnia may cause problems during the day, such as tiredness, lack of energy, difficulty concentrating, and irritability.

Insomnia affects all age groups, among adults, insomnia affects women more often than men, and the incidence tends to increase with age. In a survey among 1 820 individuals aged 65 and older in China, 32.9% reported frequent insomnia symptoms, and 8.9% had insomnia symptoms with daytime consequences, multivariate analysis indicated that individuals aged 75 years and older (odds ratio = 2.0) were associated with elevated risks for insomnia. Geriatric insomnia has multifactorial causes, it is often comorbid with chronic medical and psychiatric conditions in the older adult (figure 15-1).

The insomnia of old people can be primary, but more secondary to other body diseases, mental disorder or medication. According to the length of the course, insomnia can be divided into acute insomnia, subacute insomnia and chronic insomnia. Acute insomnia, also known as transient insomnia, lasts less than 1 week and may be related to stress experience, illness and changes in sleep patterns, once the cause of insomnia is removed, the symptoms can disappear. Subacute insomnia, also known as short-term insomnia, lasts for 1 week to 1 month, and there is a clear correlation between this insomnia and stress, such as major physical illness or surgery, death of relatives and friends, serious family, work or interpersonal

一、失眠

失眠是老年人最常见的一种睡眠障碍，美国数据显示老年人有失眠主诉者可达 30%~50%，一项前瞻性的研究显示 80 岁以上的老人有失眠症状者占 49%。失眠是指入睡困难和/或睡眠的维持发生障碍，导致睡眠时间或睡眠质量不能满足个体生理需要，并且影响日间功能。失眠的定义不是一个人睡了多少小时或需要多长时间才能入睡。每个人对睡眠的需求和满意度都是不同的。失眠可能会导致白天的问题，如疲劳、缺乏能量、难以集中注意力和易怒。

失眠症影响所有年龄段，在成年人中，女性受失眠症的影响多于男性，且发病率随年龄增长而增加。流行病学调查资料显示：随着年龄增长，失眠发生率增加，且老年女性较男性更容易出现失眠症状（可能与女性绝经期后雌激素缺乏有关）。一项针对 65 岁以上老年人的睡眠情况调查，共纳入我国 5 个城市共 1 820 例老年人，结果显示：老年人平均每日睡眠 7.1 小时，32.9% 的老年人主诉有失眠症状，8.9% 的老年人的失眠症状影响到白天的活动。多因素分析结果显示 75 岁以上高龄老人的失眠风险增加（OR=2.0）。老年失眠具有多方面的原因，常与老年人的慢性疾病和精神疾病并存（图 15-1）。

老年人的失眠可原发，但多继发于躯体疾病、精神障碍或药源性。根据病程长短，失眠可分为急性失眠、亚急性失眠和慢性失眠。急性失眠也称为短暂性失眠，持续时间小于 1 周，可能与压力体验、生病及睡眠规律改变有关，一般不需药物治疗，一旦导致失眠的原因解除，症状可消失。亚急性失眠也称为短期性失眠，时间持续 1 周~1 个月，这种失眠与压力明显存在相关性，如重大躯体疾病或手术、亲朋好友过世、发生严重的

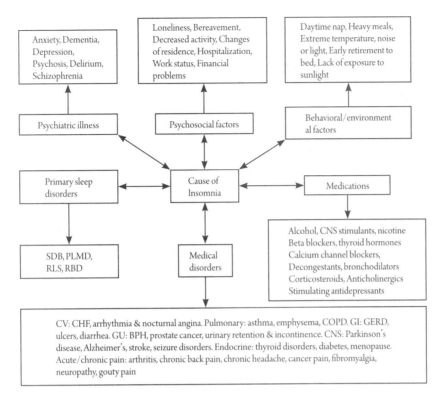

Figure 15-1　Cause of insomnia

problems. Chronic insomnia lasts for more than 1 month, and its causes are complex and difficult to find. Many chronic insomnia is the result of the combination of multiple factors, which requires special neuropsychological and spiritual tests.

For the treatment of insomnia in the elderly, it is firstly preferred to use non-drug treatment methods such as treatment and healthy sleep habits, and drug therapy should follow the principles of minimum effective dose and short-term treatment (3-5 days), and it is not recommended to increase the dose gradually. Meanwhile, close observation should be paid.

II. Sleep-Disordered Breathing / Sleep Apnea

Sleep-disordered breathing (SDB) describes a range of respiratory events that occur periodically during sleep. Individuals with sleep apnea experience at least 5 episodes of cessation of breathing for each hour of sleep, The number of apnea and hypopnea (partial reduction in airflow) per hour of sleep is called the Apnea-Hypopnea Index (AHI). SDB diagnosis is made when a patient has an AHI > 5-10. The incidence increases with age, and it's two times greater in men than in women.

家庭、工作或人际关系问题等。慢性失眠，持续时间大于 1 个月，其原因复杂且较难发现，许多慢性失眠是多种因素联合作用的结果，需要经过专门的神经心理和精神等的测试。

治疗老年人失眠，首选对因治疗和培养健康的睡眠习惯等非药物治疗手段，必要时采取药物治疗。药物治疗应遵循最小有效剂量、短期治疗（3～5 天）的原则，不主张逐渐加大剂量，同时要注意密切观察。

二、睡眠呼吸暂停综合征

睡眠呼吸暂停综合征（SDB）是指睡眠过程中由多种原因导致的反复发作的呼吸暂停，可引起低氧血症、高碳酸血症的临床综合征。睡眠呼吸暂停低通气指数（AHI）是指每小时睡眠时间内呼吸暂停和低通气的次数，当患者的 AHI > 5～10，即可诊断为 SDB。睡眠呼吸暂停综合征患病率随年龄增长逐渐增加，男性患病率是女性的 2 倍。

Risk factors associated with SDB include older age, gender, obesity, and symptomatic status. In addition, other risk factors include use of sedating medications, alcohol consumption, family history, race, smoking, and upper airway configuration. The symptoms are snoring and excessive daytime sleepiness. Older adults with SDB report insomnia, awakening with headache and confused, and daytime cognitive impairment including difficulty with concentration, attention, and short-term memory loss.

Sleep apnea can be caused by a defect in central nervous system (central sleep apnea), a blockage in the upper airway (obstructive sleep apnea), or mixed. It may exacerbate these cognitive deficits for the older adult, it's a risk factor for other health problems, including hypertension and cardiac and pulmonary problems, which can then lead to increased risk of mortality.

Several treatments exist for SDB, which consist of loss weight, continuous positive airway pressure (CPAP), or surgery to remove obstructive. People with SDB should avoid the supine position when sleep, for it allows the tongue to fallback and block the airway. They should also quit alcohol and smoke. If daytime drowsiness is present, they should be careful with driving and using machines.

III. Periodic Limb Movements in Sleep / Restless Legs Syndrome

Periodic limb movements in sleep (PLMS) is characterized by clusters of repeated leg jerks, each jerk may last 0.5-5 seconds and occur every 20-40 seconds, causing a brief awakening. It's a condition characterized by at least five kicks per hour of sleep, each causing an arousal. The prevalence of PLMS in older adults is estimated at 45%, versus 5%-6% in younger adults.

Restless leg syndrome (RLS) is a condition characterized by leg dysesthesia, used to be described as "creepy-crawly, electric current, crazy legs, worms moving, ants crawling or pain". The etiology of RLS and PLMS is unknown, they always associate with each other, approximately 80% of the elderly who have RLS have PLMS, and 30% of PLMS affected older adults have RLS.

The most common complaints of patients with

SDB 的危险因素有高龄、性别、肥胖、家族史、上呼吸道结构改变等，疲劳、安眠药、酒精、吸烟等因素也可加重睡眠呼吸暂停。随年龄增长，参与呼吸的肌肉协调能力下降，上呼吸道更易塌陷，特别是老年人，其对睡眠中气道塌陷更为敏感。患有 SDB 的老年人经常会有失眠，醒来时头痛、疲倦，白天难以集中注意力，注意力和短期记忆丧失等表现。

睡眠呼吸暂停可由中枢神经系统缺陷（中枢睡眠呼吸暂停）、上呼吸道阻塞（阻塞性睡眠呼吸暂停）或二者共同引起。它会加剧老年人的认知缺陷，也是其他健康问题的风险因素，如高血压、心肺功能下降。

睡眠呼吸暂停综合征的处理措施包括避免饮酒、吸烟，采取侧卧位，减肥，适当运动等。对于老年患者，外科治疗有一定的风险，有条件的患者需采取持续气道正压通气治疗（CPAP），这是目前最可靠的治疗方法。

三、周期性肢体运动障碍、不宁腿综合征

周期性肢体运动障碍（PLM）和不宁腿综合征（RLS）均为睡眠相关的神经–肌肉功能失调。周期性肢体运动障碍（PLM）是在睡眠中重复出现下肢肌肉收缩，又称夜间肌阵挛，每次持续时间为 0.5～5 秒，大约每隔 20～40 秒出现 1 次，可引起睡眠觉醒。特点是每小时睡眠至少踢五次，每次都会引起觉醒。据估计，老年人 PLMS 的患病率为 45%，而年轻人为 5%～6%。

不宁腿综合征（RLS）是一种内源性的睡眠紊乱，其特点是腿部感觉异常，患者主诉深部疼痛、虫咬、烧灼或爬行感觉，这些症状多发生在入睡时，从而导致患者入睡困难、睡眠中觉醒次数增多。RLS 和 PLMS 的病因尚不清楚，它们相互关联，大约 80% 的老年 RLS 患者有 PLMS，30% 的老年 PLMS 患者有 RLS。

PLMS 和 RLS 患者最常见的症状是难以

PLMS and RLS are difficulty insomnia and excessive daytime sleepiness. Patients may or may not be aware of their leg jerks, only report simply having difficulty falling asleep or staying asleep. For PLM and RLS patients, the first thing to avoid is the use of caffeinated foods, drinks, and medications that can aggravate symptoms, including calcium channel blockers, metoclopramide, antihistamines, phenytoin, etc. Dopamine receptor agonists such as ropinirol are effective in both diseases, reducing symptoms and the number of attacks.

IV. REM Sleep-behavior Disorder

Dreaming always occurs during rapid eye movement (REM) sleep. Fortunately, the voluntary muscles are actively inhibited in this phase of sleep, which makes us incapable of "acting out" our dreams. Rapid eye movement (REM) sleep behavior disorder (RBD) is a sleep disorder in which patients appear to physically act out dreams during REM sleep, characterized by the loss of this normal muscle atonia. The behaviors may be simple or complex, including talking, singing, yelling, walking, kicking, and jumping from the bed, etc. The patient's uncontrolled movements are sometimes aggressive and violent, so the potential for serious self-harm or bed-partner harm is high. RBD is more common in the elderly, with a significantly higher prevalence in older men. It is frequently associated with neurodegenerative disorders such as Parkinson's disease, multiple sclerosis or Alzheimer's dementia.

For patient with Parkinson's disease or multiple system atrophy, ensuring nocturnal safety of the patient and bed-partner is important by removal of potentially dangerous objects from the bedroom. Both patient and bed partner should be educated in all aspects of the disorder, especially the potential for inadvertent self-harm at night. When drug treatment is thought to be available, Clonazepam is the first-line therapy, appearing to have some benefit in the majority of cases. If clonazepam is non-effective or contraindicated, levodopa, dopamine agonist, and melatonin can then be considered.

入睡和白天嗜睡。患者可能意识不到自己的腿在抽搐，但是同床共枕的人往往能意识到腿部的运动。对 PLM 和 RLS 患者，首先要避免使用可加剧症状的含咖啡因的食物、饮料，以及药物，包括钙通道阻滞剂、甲氧氯普胺、抗组胺类、苯妥英钠等。罗匹尼罗等多巴胺受体激动剂对这 2 种疾病有效，可减轻症状和减少发作次数。

四、REM 睡眠行为障碍

REM 睡眠与做梦相关，但正常情况下，REM 睡眠期肌张力几乎消失，因此梦境中的动作不会表现在现实中。REM 睡眠行为障碍（RBD）是以 REM 睡眠期肌肉弛缓状态消失为特点，并出现与梦的内容有关的复杂运动行为，包括讲话、大笑、喊叫、哭泣、咒骂、伸手、抓握、拍击、踢腿、坐起、跃下床、爬行和奔跑等，并可能对自身和同伴造成伤害。RBD 在老年人中更为常见，尤其是老年男性患病率明显较高。通常与神经退行性疾病有关，如帕金森病、多发性硬化和阿尔茨海默病。

对于帕金森症或多系统萎缩的患者来说，保证安全的睡眠环境是非常重要的；对患者和同伴进行教育，预防夜间对自身和同伴的伤害；避免使用诱发和加重 RBD 的药物，如 SSRI 类抗抑郁药物。药物治疗方面，氯硝西泮一般常规用于该病的治疗，如果该药物无效或者有禁忌证，可以使用左旋多巴、多巴胺激动剂和褪黑素。

Section 4　Promoting Sleep in Elderly

I. Evaluation

The first step in developing interventions to improve the amount and quality of sleep is collecting sleep history. A sleep history should include information from both the patient and family members.

1. This includes information about sleep patterns, habits, and identified triggering/promoting factors, etc. (box 15-2). Relevant personal and societal factors (isolation, loneliness, loss of spouse, change in residence, security, or financial concerns) that may indicate a temporary situational insomnia are key historical factors. Medical and psychiatric conditions that can impair sleep, including drug and alcohol history, also should be carefully investigated.

BOX 15-2　Sleep History Components

- Sleep quality

—The self-report of the older adult, described as poor, fair, good, or excellent.

- Sleep quantity

—The number of hours asleep per 24hours, including daytime naps.

- Bedtime routines
- Place of sleep
- Characteristics of the bed, bedding, and bedroom environment

- Food and fluid intake in the evening and at bedtime
- Use of alcohol and caffeine-containing beverages
- Medications (prescription and nonprescription)
- Characteristics of the sleep disturbance

—Difficulty falling asleep.

—Difficulty staying asleep.

—Frequent nocturnal awakening.

—Daytime sleepiness.

- The older adult's account of the reasons for the disturbed sleep

第四节　促进老年人睡眠的措施

一、及时评估老年人睡眠

为改善睡眠质量而制订干预措施的第一步就是收集睡眠相关的病史。睡眠状况的评估有助于了解病情变化和对疗效做出评价。

1. **对睡眠状况的评估**　包括睡眠结构、习惯和影响因素等信息（box 15-2）。相关的个人和社会因素（如孤立、孤独感、丧偶、住所的改变、安全或经济问题）可能会造成短暂性情境性失眠。此外，还应仔细调查可能损害睡眠的身体和精神疾病，包括药物和酒精史。

Box 15-2　睡眠史的内容

- 睡眠质量

——睡眠差、中等、好或非常好。

- 睡眠数量

——每 24 小时内睡眠时间，包含日间睡眠。

- 常规就寝时间
- 睡眠地点
- 床铺的特征以及卧室睡眠环境

- 夜间所摄入的食物以及饮品
- 服用酒水或含咖啡因饮料
- 药物（处方或非处方）
- 睡眠障碍的表现特征

——入睡困难。

——睡眠维持困难。

——夜间频繁觉醒。

——日间困倦。

- 老年患者睡眠障碍的原因分析

2. A sleep diary (box 15-3) keep by the older adults can provide details initially unrecognized, helpful in recalling the amount of sleep, bedtime routines, and possible symptoms of disturbed sleep over a 24-hour period. It is one of the most practical, economical and widely used sleep assessment methods.

Box 15-3　Simple Sleep Diary

● Daytime activities and pre-sleep ritual (completed before bedtime) .

● Naps (how many/how long).

● Exercise (what type/how long).

● Alcohol and caffeine (amount/how many).

● Food and drink (heavy or light; eat/drink timing).

● Feelings (1, very tired; 2, somewhat tired; 3, fairly alert; 4, wide awake).

● Stress/irritability level before bedtime (1, none; 2, some; 3, moderate; 4, high).

● Medications or sleep aids (types/dose/timing).

● Activities the last hour before bedtime.

● Bedtime routine (meditation/relaxation/how long).

● Bed time, time of "light out".

● Sleeping and getting back to sleep (completed on awakening).

● Wake-up time, time of "lights on".

● Time to fall asleep (minutes).

● Sleep breaks (number of awakening and total time awake).

● Quality of sleep (0-10; 0 worst to 10 best ever).

● Total sleep time (in hours).

Date must be documented daily for a minimum sample time of 2 weeks.

3. Laboratory examination includes polysomnography, electroencephalogram, electrocardiogram, electroencephalogram, electromyography and respiratory apparatus and other modern means can provide objective basis for the diagnosis, classification and differential diagnosis of sleep disorders, as well as important reference information for the selection of treatment methods and evaluation of treatment effects. It is the gold standard for the diagnosis of various sleep disorders.

4. The questionnaire survey is mainly used to comprehensively evaluate sleep quality, sleep

2. **老年人记录的睡眠日记**　睡眠日记（box 15-3）可以提供很多没被发现的细节，有助于回忆睡眠时间、就寝时间以及 24 小时内可能出现的睡眠紊乱症状。它是最实用、经济和应用最广泛的睡眠评估方法之一。

Box 15-3　简单睡眠日记

● 日间活动以及睡觉前进行的活动（在睡觉前完成）。

● 小睡（几次、多长时间）。

● 锻炼（什么类型、多长时间）。

● 酒精和咖啡因（数量、多少）。

● 食品和饮料（重量、食用时间）。

● 感觉（1，很累；2，有点累；3，相当警觉；4，清醒）。

● 压力/睡前易怒水平（1，没有；2，一些；3，温和；4，高）

● 促进睡眠的药物或其他辅助措施（类型/剂量/时间）。

● 睡前最后一小时的活动。

● 睡前常规（冥想/休闲/多长时间）。

● 就寝时间，熄灯时间。

● 入睡及觉醒时间。

● 起床时间，开灯时间。

● 入睡时间（分钟）。

● 睡眠休息（觉醒数量和总时间清醒）。

● 睡眠质量（0~10，0 为最差，10 为最好）。

● 总睡眠时间（小时）。

以上日常必须记录，至少 2 周以上。

3. **实验室检查**　包括多导睡眠图、脑电图、心电图、眼电图、肌电图和呼吸描记器等现代手段，为睡眠障碍的诊断、分类和鉴别诊断提供客观依据，也为选择治疗方法及评价治疗效果提供重要的参考信息，是诊断多种睡眠障碍的金标准。

4. **睡眠问卷**　主要用于全面评估睡眠质量、睡眠特征和行为，以及与睡眠相关的症状

characteristics and behaviors, as well as sleep-related symptoms and attitudes. The Stanford sleepiness scale (SSS) measures feelings of sleepiness or tiredness at specific times. The Epworth sleepiness scale (ESS) is a brief instrument to screen for severity of daytime sleepiness in the community setting. The Pittsburgh sleep quality index (PSQI) is useful to screen for sleep problems in the home environment and to monitor changes in sleep quality, including additional questions for the bed partner (appendix 1-3).

II. Sleep Hygiene Education

Through sleep health education, it can help the elderly establish health awareness, develop good behavior habits, such as avoiding alcohol, coffee and other stimulants before bed ; creating a good sleep environment; relieving stress and keeping calm; strengthening the management of sleep duration, avoiding daytime naps, daily routine and adjusting sleep rhythm are conducive to improving sleep quality.

Box 15-4　Sleep Hygiene Education— Instruction for Patients

- Behavioral Patterns

—Keep a regular sleep/wake schedule (including weekends and holidays).

—Do not go to bed unless sleepy.

—Decrease or eliminate daytime naps (≤ 30 min, no later than the early afternoon).

—Exercise regularly (but not within 3-5 h of bedtime).

—Increase exposure to natural light and bright light during day and early evening; avoid exposure to bright light close to bedtime or when awakening during night.

—Avoid heavy meals and liquids within 3 h of bedtime.

—Limit or eliminate alcohol, caffeine, and nicotine, especially before bedtime.

—Keep relaxing routine (windows down before bedtime, maintain a routine period of preparation for bed, use warm bath/socks).

—Wear comfortable bed clothing.

—Avoid distressing "pillow talk" with bed partner.

—Do not use bed for reading or watching television.

—Get out of bed once awake.

和态度。目前较常使用的有斯坦福睡眠量表（SSS）、匹茨堡睡眠质量指数量表及 Epworth 嗜睡量表等。斯坦福睡眠量表用于测量特定时间的困倦感或疲劳感；Epworth 嗜睡量表（ESS）用于在社区环境中筛选白天嗜睡的严重程度；匹兹堡睡眠质量指数（PSQI）有助于筛查家庭环境中的睡眠问题，并监测睡眠质量的变化，包括对床伴提出的其他问题（附件 1~3 ）。

二、积极开展睡眠卫生教育

通过睡眠卫生教育帮助老年人树立健康意识，养成良好的行为习惯，如睡前避免饮酒、喝咖啡等兴奋剂；创造良好的睡眠环境；缓解压力，保持心情平静；加强睡眠时限管理，避免白天小睡，起居规律，调整睡眠节律，有利于提高睡眠质量。

Box 15-4　患者睡眠卫生教育

- 行为模式

——保持正常的作息时间（包括周末以及假期）。

——若不困倦就不睡觉。

——减少日间睡眠时间（≤30分钟）。

——常规锻炼（入睡前 3~5 小时尽量避免）。

——增加自然光照时间，入睡前或醒来时避免接受强光照射刺激。

——睡前 3 小时避免过量饮食。

——限制或减少酒精、咖啡因以及尼古丁的摄入，尤其是睡觉之前。

——日常保持放松（睡觉前放下窗帘、做好入睡准备、洗个热水澡）。

——穿着舒适的睡衣。

——避免与他人夜间谈话。

——不在床上阅读或看电视。

——醒来后立即起床。

—If unable to fall asleep within 30 min, get out of bed and relax (by listening to soft music or light reading).

● Sleep Environment

—Identify snoring or disruptive bed partners.

—Keep bedroom cool and dark.

—Eliminate as much noise from sleeping quarters as possible.

—Place clocks out of sight.

—Address pets that interfere with sleep.

III. Non-drug Therapy to Promote Sleep

The primary focus of non-pharmacologic strategies in the treatment is aimed at correcting behaviors that are not conducive to healthy sleeping. Evidence suggests that non-pharmacologic therapies, especially behavioral therapies, are as effective as pharmacotherapy, especially in older adults who are at high risk for adverse drug reactions.

The most effective behavioral therapy is cognitive behavioral therapy (CBT). Cognitive behavior therapy can produce significant, lasting improvement in all measures of sleep disorder and may be an effective alternative to drugs in chronic users. Cognitive behavioral therapy helps patients build confidence, reduce fear, and rebuild sleep beliefs. Behavioral therapy often includes sleep restriction, stimulus-control therapy, and relaxation training. Stimulus-control therapy aims to restore the bed's function as a sleep signal, weaken the connection between the bed and sleep unrelated activities, and establish a regular sleep-wake rhythm. Patients are instructed to use the bed strictly for sleeping and not for any other activities. Therefore, patients are instructed to get out of bed if they fail to fall asleep 15- 20 min and stay out of bed until they feel sufficiently sleepy. If unable to fall asleep 15-20 min, they are asked to repeat the process. This therapy attempts to break the association between the bed and wakefulness, to increase sleep efficiency by limiting the amount of time the patient is allowed to stay in bed. Sleep restriction therapy demands that patients can stay in bed for 15 minutes longer than the time of actual sleep they report each night. This results in daytime sleepiness that allows for an increased sleep drive in the following night. As sleep improves each week, the amount of time allowed in bed in gradually increased. Relaxation therapy reduces physical and mental stress just before bedtime through progressive muscle relaxation. Relaxation therapy includes

——若上床 30 分钟内无法入睡，起床进行放松（通过听轻音乐或阅读）。

● 睡眠环境

——识别打呼噜的室友。

——保持卧室清凉黑暗。

——尽量消除噪声干扰。

——将钟表至于视线之外。

——安置好干扰睡眠的宠物。

三、适时提供非药物治疗

非药物治疗的主要目的是纠正不利于健康睡眠的行为。有证据表明，非药物疗法，尤其是行为疗法，与药物疗法一样有效，尤其是对那些药物不良反应风险较高的老年人。

最有效的行为疗法是认知行为疗法（CBT）。认知行为疗法综合了认知疗法、行为疗法以及睡眠健康教育，可有效治疗失眠，被认为是药物疗法的有效替代。认知行为疗法帮助患者树立信心，减少恐惧，重建睡眠信念。行为疗法通常包括刺激控制疗法、睡眠限制法以及放松训练等。刺激控制疗法的目的在于恢复床作为睡眠信号的功能，减弱床和睡眠不相关活动的联系，建立规律性睡眠－觉醒节律。该方案要求当患者只在有睡意时才上床，而如果 15～20 分钟内无法入睡，则起床离开卧室，做些轻松的活动，直到产生睡意才回卧室睡觉；有必要时重复以上活动；这种疗法试图打破床和清醒之间的联系，通过限制患者在床上停留的时间来提高睡眠效率。睡眠限制疗法要求患者每天晚上在床上的时间比他们报告的实际睡眠时间长 15 分钟。这会导致白天嗜睡，从而导致第二天晚上的睡眠驱动力增加，随着每周睡眠的改善，允许在床上的时间逐渐增加。放松疗法通过渐进式肌肉放松来减轻睡前的身心压力。放松疗法有肌肉放松训练、冥想放松及自我暗示法等，通过放松训练减少精神和躯体的紧

muscle relaxation training, meditation relaxation, and self-suggestion. Relaxation training reduces mental and physical tension to treat insomnia. . The disadvantages include noncompliance with adherence, taking a long time (at least 2 weeks) for effectiveness. Considering the safety profile and less expensive nature, the behavioral therapies should be given high priority and implemented as first line in the treatment and be continued even when pharmacotherapy is needed.

In addition, phototherapy also has certain therapeutic effect on the elderly patients who have insomnia with the change of sleep-wake rhythm. Phototherapy might modulate melatonin release. Timed exposure to bright lights has improved sleep efficiency and increased total sleep time, rapid-eye-movement (REM) sleep and slow-wave sleep in older people. Although the mechanism by which light exposure improves sleep is not fully understood, the effects are significant, so all long-term living places should be in a well-lit environment with access to natural light.

IV. Pharmacotherapy to Promote Sleep

Pharmacological treatments should only be considered for chronic insomnia, when the older adult cannot or will not comply with non-pharmacological interventions or when treatment of the primary cause is insufficient to alleviate insomnia. Several different medications are used to treat insomnia such as sedative-hypnotics, antihistamines, antidepressants, antipsychotics, and anticonvulsants. However, the National Institutes of Health State-of-the-Science Conference on Insomnia concluded that there is no systematic evidence that these medications are effective for insomnia and that the risks outweigh the benefits. These treatments therefore are not recommended for the elderly. Research suggests that selective short-acting non-benzodiazepines (e. g. , eszopiclone, zaleplon, zolpidem) and melatonin receptor agonists (e. g. , ramelteon) are safe and effective for older adults. Sedatives must be used with the utmost care. As with all medications prescribed to older patients, lowest doses and shortest durations of administration are preferable, and gradual dose tapering is safer and less likely to lead to rebound or withdrawal symptoms compared with abrupt discontinuation when treatment is complete. Monitoring for dependency and abuse (including patient resistance to tapering or requests for higher doses) is always required. Hypnotics are best avoided in patients with a substance abuse history, myasthenia, moderate-

张来治疗失眠。

此外，光疗对睡眠 - 觉醒节律改变的老年失眠患者也有一定的治疗效果。光疗可以调节褪黑素的释放，在老年人中，定时暴露在强光下可以提高睡眠效率，增加总睡眠时间、快速眼动（REM）睡眠和慢波睡眠。尽管光线照射改善睡眠的机制尚不完全清楚，但其影响非常显著，因此，所有长期居住场所都应该是一个光线充足的环境，并能接触到自然光线。

四、必要时提供药物治疗

只有当老年人不能或不愿接受非药物干预或者非药物干预措施效果不理想，才应考虑用药物治疗他们的慢性失眠。常用的药物有镇静催眠药、抗组胺药、抗抑郁药、抗精神病药和抗惊厥药。但是，美国国立卫生研究院失眠研究所称没有系统性的证据表明这些药物对失眠有效，而且风险可能大于益处。因此，药物治疗失眠不应该是老年人的常规治疗。研究表明，选择性短作用的非苯二氮䓬类药物（如埃索匹克隆、扎勒普隆、唑吡坦）和褪黑素受体激动剂（如雷麦酮）对老年人是安全有效的。使用镇静剂必须谨慎。与所有老年用药一样，采用低剂量、短疗程给药，减量时应循序渐进，才可能不会导致严重的戒断症状。用药期间要持续监测老年人的反应（包括老年人对于药物剂量的依从性）。有药物滥用史、肌无力、中度至重度呼吸系统疾病和近期中风的患者最好避免使用安眠药。在治疗的第一周内对老年人进行随访以评估药物的有效性和不良反应。药物更换时，应鼓励老年人每两周复查一次，鼓励他们写睡

severe respiratory disease, and recent stroke. Follow-up with the older adult within the first week of treatment is essential to assess the effectiveness as well as adverse effects of medications. Older adults should be seen approximately every 2 weeks while changes are being made. Encourage them to keep sleep diaries and report the results of therapy in every visit. If insomnia persists despite the treatments, reevaluate for secondary causes, such as severe depression, anxiety, or sleep-related disorders.

The advantages of using a combination of pharmacologic and behavior therapies are that the pharmacologic therapy offers short-term respite during the period before benefits of behavior therapies appear but combined with the durability of the CBT.

(LIANG Tao, GUO Hong)

眠日记。如果治疗后仍然失眠，重新评估失眠的原因，如严重的抑郁、焦虑或睡眠相关障碍。

药物治疗和非药物治疗结合的优点就是药物治疗作用更快，而非药物治疗效果个更加持久。

（梁　涛　郭　宏）

Key Points

1. Age-related sleep changes include increased sleep latency, reduced sleep efficiency, more awakening in the night, increased early morning awakenings, and increased daytime sleepiness. Multiple factors influence sleep, including medical or psychiatric illnesses, life changes (e. g. retirement, bereavement), environmental changes, pain, diet, and medication use.

2. The first step in developing interventions to improve sleep is a thorough sleep history.

3. Sleep history includes questions about sleep patterns, habits, and identified triggering/promoting factors (e. g. sleep environment, activities, diet, and medications).

4. Sleep hygiene measures emphasize regular schedules, friendly sleep environment, eliminating stimuli that interfere with sleep, stress reduction.

5. The most effective behavioral therapy for insomnia is cognitive behavioral therapy. The cognitive portion of CBT deals with misconceptions about sleep, the behavioral component involves a combination of stimulus control and/or sleep restriction plus cognitive restructuring, relaxation, and good sleep hygiene.

6. With all medications prescribed to older patients, lowest doses and shortest durations of administration are preferable, and gradual dose tapering is safer.

本章要点

1. 老年相关的睡眠变化包括增加的睡眠潜伏期，睡眠效率降低，夜间觉醒次数增加，清晨早醒，白天嗜睡。睡眠受很多因素影响，包括身体或者精神疾病、生活变化（例如，退休、丧亲）、环境变化、疼痛、饮食和药物使用。

2. 睡眠病史的评估是实施干预措施的首要步骤。

3. 睡眠史包括睡眠的模式、习惯以及阻碍或促进因素（例如，睡眠环境，活动，饮食和药物）。

4. 睡眠卫生措施强调作息规律，良好的睡眠环境，减少干扰睡眠的刺激，以及减轻压力。

5. 失眠的最有效的行为治疗是认知行为治疗。CBT 的认知部分涉及关于对睡眠的误解，行为部分是刺激控制和 / 或睡眠限制、认知重构，放松、良好的睡眠卫生习惯的组合。

6. 老年患者使用药物时，应优选服用最低剂量以及选择最短的疗程，并且剂量逐渐递减，这样才最安全。

Critical Thinking Exercise

1. In nursing facility, an old woman tells you she hasn't slept well, how do you assess the sleep condition, what

批判性思维练习

1. 在护理机构时，一位老妇人告诉你她睡得不是很好，你该如何评估睡眠状况，你会问

questions do you ask to assess her sleep quality and quantity?

2. What non-pharmacologic measures can be incorporated into an older adults' lifestyle to facilitate sleep?

3. In a clinic, you meet with an older man accompanied by his wife. She reports that he is snoring loudly every night and always falling asleep during the day. Which type of sleep disorder do you suspect? What recommendations should be informed to the client?

什么问题来评估她的睡眠质量和数量？

2. 促进老年人睡眠的非药物疗法有哪些？

3. 在诊所里，你遇到一位老人，由他的妻子陪伴着。他妻子说，丈夫每晚大声打鼾，而且总是白天想睡觉。你怀疑是哪种类型的睡眠障碍？应提供哪些建议？

Chapter 16 Pain Management for Elderly

第十六章　老年人的疼痛管理

Learning Objectives

On completion of this chapter, the reader will be able to:

- Define the concept and classification of pain;

- Understand the pathology of pain in the elderly;

- Describe the main characteristics of pain in elderly;

- Use a pain assessment tool to rate client's pain intensity;

- Apply pain management strategy for the elderly.

学习目标

学完本章节，应完成以下目标：

- 定义疼痛的概念并能阐述疼痛的级别；

- 理解老年人疼痛的病理机制；

- 描述老年人疼痛的主要特点；

- 使用疼痛评估工具评估被照顾者疼痛程度的等级；

- 采取针对老年人的疼痛管理策略。

Pain is an unpleasant sensory and emotional experience, which is usually associated with injury or a pathophysiologic process that causes an uncomfortable experience and is usually described in such terms. There are not always objective biologic markers of pain, an individual's description and self-report usually provides accurate, reliable, and sufficient evidence for the presence and intensity of pain.

The incidence of pain is more than doubles after the age of 60 years old. In an emergency room or in hospitals, it is quite common to encounter older people who are in pain. The special characteristics of the elderly make pain assessment and management quite different from other age group, for example, the presence of dementia and communication difficulties can interfere with assessment.

疼痛是一种不愉快的感觉和情绪体验，往往与外伤或病理生理改变有关。疼痛有时并不存在客观的生物学指标，但患者的主诉常可准确、有效地提示疼痛存在与否以及疼痛的强度。

疼痛在老年人群中非常普遍，老年人罹患致痛疾病的风险增大，60岁以后疼痛的发生率增加1倍以上。老年人由于其年龄特点，疼痛的评估和管理有别于其他年龄群，如痴呆和沟通困难可妨碍对疼痛的评估。疼痛可严重影响老年人的健康、功能和生活质量，若未能缓解，常可导致抑郁、焦虑，社交减少、睡眠障碍、活动下降，医疗资源利用增加，医疗负担加重等。医务人员应该提高对老年人疼痛问题的认识，保证老年人的疼痛得到最佳的评估与治疗。

Section 1　Introduction

Older adults are at higher risk for pain-inducing situations during their life span. Pain has major implications for older adults' health, functioning, and quality of life. If unrelieved, pain is associated with depression, anxiety, decreased socialization, sleep disturbance, impaired ambulation, and increased healthcare utilization and costs. Although less thoroughly described, many other conditions are known to be worsened potentially by the presence of pain, including gait disturbances, slow rehabilitation, and adverse effects from multiple drug prescriptions. Health professionals should be aware of the serious issues related to pain and the fundamental right to have pain assessed and treated to the greatest extent possible.

I. Definition of Pain

Pain is an unpleasant sensory and emotional experience, which is usually associated with injury

第一节　疼痛的定义与分类

老年人更容易引起疼痛。疼痛对老年人的健康，功能和生活质量具有重大影响。如果无法缓解，则疼痛会与抑郁、焦虑、社交活动减少、睡眠障碍、移动障碍以及医疗保健利用率和成本增加有关。尽管描述得不够详尽，但已知许多其他情况可能会因疼痛的存在而恶化，包括步态障碍，缓慢的康复以及多种药物处方带来的不良影响。卫生专业人员应意识到与疼痛有关的严重问题，以及最大程度地评估和治疗疼痛。

一、疼痛的定义

疼痛是与实际或潜在的组织损伤有关的一种不愉快的感觉和情感体验，或是对这种

or a pathophysiologic process. American Geriatrics Society Panel on the Pharmacological Management of Persistent Pain in Older Persons defines pain as pain is a complex phenomenon caused by noxious sensory stimuli or neuropathological mechanisms. An individual's memories, expectations, and emotions modify the experience of pain. It is worthy noticing that pain is always subjective. Each individual learns the application of the word through experiences related to injury in early life. Biologists recognize that those stimuli which cause pain are liable to damage tissue. It is undoubtedly a sensation in a part or parts of the body, but it is also always unpleasant and therefore also an emotional experience. Experiences which resemble pain but are not unpleasant, e. g., pricking, should not be called pain. Unpleasant abnormal experiences (dysaesthesia) may also be pain but are not necessarily so because, subjectively, they may not have the usual sensory qualities of pain.

II. Classification of Pain in Elderly

Pain may be considered acute or persistent. Acute pain is defined by rapid onset and relatively short duration and a sign of a new health problem requiring diagnosis and analgesia. It is normally suffered as a result of trauma, such as from a fall or from a surgical procedure. In contrast, persistent pain is defined as a painful experience that continues for a prolonged period of time that may or may not be associated with a recognizable disease process. The terms persistent and chronic are often used interchangeably in the medical literature.

Persistent pain in the elderly is more common than acute pain and often disabling, which has become a label associated with negative images and stereotypes often associated with longstanding or drug-seeking behavior. A Louis Harris telephone survey found that one in five older Americans (18%) are taking analgesic medications regularly (several times a week or more), and 63% of those had taken prescription pain medications for more than 6 months. Older people are more likely to suffer from arthritis, bone and joint disorders, back problems, and other chronic conditions. Studies of both the community-dwelling and nursing home populations have found that older people commonly have several sources of pain, which is not surprising, as older patients commonly have multiple medical problems.

损伤的描述。许多学者认为：①疼痛由伤害性刺激或神经损伤引起，受到个体的记忆、期望值、情感等的影响；②疼痛常与令人不快的组织损伤或神经病理改变有关。疼痛是一种复杂的生理心理活动，包括痛感觉和痛反应两部分。痛感觉具有经验属性，是种复合感觉，其产生往往和其他躯体感觉混杂在一起，并常伴有强烈的情绪色彩，构成相当复杂的心理活动，如害怕、恐怖、焦虑、厌恶等。痛反应是在伤害性刺激作用下，在意识领域内产生疼痛感觉的同时出现各种躯体和内脏活动改变，有时可伴随情绪和行为变化，包括躯体－运动性反应、植物－内脏性反应和神经－精神性反应三大方面。因此疼痛包含多个方面，如感觉／鉴别（如痛阈）、情感／动机（如疼痛忍耐度）、认知／评价（如疼痛记忆）和自主／神经内分泌反应等。

二、老年人疼痛的分类

老年人的疼痛可分为急性疼痛和慢性疼痛。急性疼痛发作快、持续时间较短（<6个月），多由急性疾病或损伤引起，如跌倒、手术等，常需及时处理。而慢性疼痛，也称为持续性疼痛，是指急性疾病或损伤治愈后持续存在的疼痛，或与慢性疾病有关的疼痛，持续或反复发作时间较长（>6个月）。

慢性疼痛在老年人中比急性疼痛更为常见，致残率高，老年人常因慢性疼痛而用药。一项调查发现，18%的美国老年人经常服用镇痛剂（一周几次或更多），63%的老年人服用处方止痛药超过6个月。引起老年人慢性疼痛的常见疾病有关节炎、骨关节疾病、背部问题和其他慢性疾病。

The clinical manifestations of persistent pain are commonly multifactorial. Because of the complex interplay among these factors across several domains (physiologic, psychological, and social), discriminating which factors are most important for the purpose of treatment can be very challenging. Further complicating this task is the fact that pain expression and hence the importance of specific factors commonly varies, not only across individuals but also over time in one individual.

Persistent pain is common in older people. A survey found that 45% of patients who take pain medications regularly had seen three or more doctors for pain. Previous studies have suggested that 25% to 50% of community-dwelling older people suffer important pain problems.

To describe the pathophysiology of individual pain syndromes in classifying persistent pain, there are four basic categories that encompass most syndromes:

1. Nociceptive pain may be visceral or somatic and is most often derived from the stimulation of pain receptors. Nociceptive pain may arise from tissue inflammation, mechanical deformation, ongoing injury, or destruction. Examples include inflammatory or traumatic arthritis, myofascial pain syndromes, and ischemic disorders. Nociceptive mechanisms usually respond well to traditional approaches to pain management, including common analgesic medications and non-drug strategies.

2. Neuropathic pain results from a pathophysiologic process that involves the peripheral or central nervous system. Examples include diabetic neuropathy, trigeminal neuralgia, post-herpetic neuralgia, post stroke central or thalamic pain, and post amputation phantom limb pain. These pain syndromes do not respond as predictably as do nociceptive pain problems to conventional analgesic therapy. However, they have been noted to respond to unconventional analgesic drugs, such as tricyclic antidepressants, anticonvulsants, or antiarrhythmic drugs.

3. Mixed or unspecified pain is usually regarded as having mixed or unknown mechanisms. Examples include recurrent headaches and some vasculitic pain syndromes. Treatment of these syndromes is more unpredictable and may require trials of different or combined approaches.

4. There may be rare conditions (e. g. , conversion reaction) where psychological disorders are responsible

慢性疼痛有多方面的临床表现。疼痛常受生理、心理和社会因素的影响，且这些因素之间还会互相作用。疼痛还存在个体差异，患者表述复杂多变。尽管正确评估疼痛的主要影响因素非常棘手，但是对于治疗非常重要。

慢性疼痛在老年人中很常见。患有慢性疼痛的老年人中 45% 的患者常去看医生。初级保健医生是管理慢性疼痛的主要卫生人员。有研究显示，25% 到 50% 的社区老年人有严重的疼痛问题，但是多数情况下慢性疼痛没有得到充分治疗。

根据疼痛的原因，可将慢性疼痛分为4 类：

1. **损伤性疼痛**　指由痛觉感受器受到损伤性刺激引起的疼痛，可表现为内脏痛和躯体痛。组织炎症、结构破坏，如炎性或外伤性关节炎，可引起损伤性疼痛。传统的疼痛治疗方法，包括常见的药物或非药物治疗，可有效治疗损伤性疼痛。

2. **神经性疼痛**　指由周围或中枢神经系统的病理生理改变引起的疼痛，如糖尿病性神经病变、三叉神经痛、带状疱疹后神经痛、脑卒中后的中枢性疼痛、截肢后的幻肢痛等。传统的疼痛治疗方法治疗神经性疼痛的效果较差，但一些非传统的止痛药，如抗抑郁药、抗惊厥药等药物，却表现出一定的治疗效果。

3. **混合性疼痛**　指兼由以上两种致痛机制，或由其他机制产生的疼痛。混合性疼痛采用单一的治疗方法难以奏效，常需尝试一种以上的治疗方法。

4. **精神性疼痛**　指疼痛的发作、强度、迁延、恶化与心理障碍直接相关的疼痛。一

for the onset, severity, exacerbation, or persistence of pain. Patients with these disorders may benefit from specific psychiatric treatments, but traditional medical interventions for analgesia are not indicated.

般不太提倡对该类疼痛使用传统的药物进行治疗，而是采用相应的精神 – 心理疗法，其治疗效果明显。

Section 2 Characteristics and Assessment of Pain in Elderly

I. Pathophysiology of Pain in the Elderly

The physiological, psychological, and environmental changes that accompany aging and restrict homeostasis may further exacerbate the consequences of persistent pain. Homeostasis (i. e., 'maintaining stability through change') is the response of the body to stress by activation of physiological reserves. These reserves include cognitive and emotional resilience to stress and activation of the neuroendocrine system, the autonomic nervous system, and the immune system. In contrast to the homeostasis of maintained internal equilibrium through the adjustment of physiological processes, homeostenosis is the constraint of an ageing organism's ability to effectively respond to stress because of diminished biological, psychological, and social reserves. When the inherent reserve capacity is exceeded, this may result in disability or death.

A key distinction between the elderly and younger individuals with persistent pain is the normal and pathological ageing-associated brain changes that may contribute to pain homeostenosis. That is, the older adult's experience of pain may be altered because of dysfunctional brain changes that cause impaired descending inhibition. Intact descending inhibition is a key component of modulation of the barrage of sensory input from the periphery that ascends to the brain, as described in the gate control theory of pain (GCT). Impaired descending inhibition caused by fear, dysfunctional coping, depression, and anxiety has been found to play a major role in driving disability in younger patients with persistent pain.

The effects of age on pain threshold are contradictory. It has been reported that somatosensory thresholds for non-noxious stimuli increase with age, whereas pressure pain thresholds have been reported increase or decrease;

第二节　老年人疼痛的特点及评估

一、老年人疼痛的病理生理特点

老化带来的生理、心理变化，可能进一步加剧疼痛的影响。应激反应时机体稳态（即动态中的平衡）是通过激活生理代偿功能而维持的。这些代偿功能包括认知和情绪调节，还有自主神经系统、神经内分泌系统、免疫系统的调节。老年人由于生理、心理、社会各方面的老化，导致了机体调节能力的减退。如果超出了生理代偿功能，会造成机体障碍甚至死亡。

老年人患慢性疼痛与年轻人最主要的区别在于大脑生理和病理的改变，导致了机体对疼痛的调节能力下降。由于大脑对疼痛的控制作用减退，因此老年人对疼痛的感觉可能会与年轻人不同。疼痛的全过程始终处于机体自身的调控之中，这在"闸门控制学说"中有所论述。研究发现恐惧、应对障碍、抑郁和焦虑引起的疼痛控制障碍也是年轻人发生慢性疼痛的主要原因。

年龄与疼痛阈值的关系不一致。生理疼痛阈值随年龄而升高，压力痛觉可能既有升高也有降低，热痛阈值与年龄无关。老年人

heat pain thresholds may show no age-related changes. Threshold and tolerance of experimentally induced ischemic pain is significantly less in older than in younger adults. Apart from an enhanced temporal summation of heat pain, pain summation may not be critically affected by age. However, recent work has suggested that the nociceptive system of older subjects may indeed have a reduced capacity to down-regulate subsequent to sensitization. The relationship between these physiological changes observed in the laboratory and clinical pain states is unknown, although data suggest that older adults with persistent pain may function at a higher psychological and physical level than their younger counterparts.

The pathophysiology of both mild age-related changes and more severe changes associated with dementia is neuronal death and gliosis. Areas of the brain involved with pain perception and analgesia are susceptible to these pathological changes. Functionally, neuronal death and gliosis may directly interrupt neuronal tracts involved in descending inhibition, especially those involved with the periaqueductal gray, locus coeruleus, and nucleus raphe magnus, areas rich in opioid and monoamine receptors.

In addition to functional changes, another result of aging and disease is changes in behavior. Many older adults have excellent coping skills and live with persistent pain that is not disabling. Some individuals such as those who suffer from comorbid dementia and/or depression; however, may experience behavioral changes including decreased ability to cope with pain, impaired ability to effectively express needs and distress, and difficulty with adhering to an analgesic or other somatic regimen.

II. Main Characteristics of Pain in the Elderly

The elderly segment of our population is a demographic group that bears a significant burden of pain. The elderly continue to be an under recognized and under-treated population with respect to pain. The elderly have been defined as those age 65 years or older. However, patients who are the greatest challenge in geriatric medicine are those older than age 75 years. These patients are frequently the frail with multiple medical problems, little social support, and multiple medication use. This age group is the fastest growing segment of our society. The prevalence of pain in people older than age 60 years is twice that in those younger than 60 years of age. Studies suggest that 25% to 50% of community-dwelling

对实验诱发的缺血性疼痛的耐受力和痛阈值明显低于年轻人。热痛觉敏感性与年龄无关，除非延长热痛的时间。但是，最近的研究表明老年受试者的痛觉敏感度的确有下降。尽管患有慢性疼痛的老年人可能比年轻人具有更好的生理和心理状态，但是这些生理变化是否与疼痛的临床表现相关尚不清楚。

大脑老化和更严重的痴呆病理生理改变均是神经元死亡和神经胶质增生。与疼痛感知有关的大脑区域易受这些病理生理变化的影响。功能上，神经元死亡和神经胶质增生可能直接影响疼痛抑制的神经传导，特别是病变发生在灰质、蓝斑核、中缝大核、富含阿片和单胺受体的区域。

除了功能改变外，衰老和疾病也会导致行为改变。生活中许多老年人对一般的慢性疼痛有很好的应对技巧。然而，一些患有痴呆或抑郁症的老年人，可能会发生行为改变，包括疼痛应对能力下降、需求表达能力受损、无法坚持服止痛药和应用物理疗法。

二、老年人疼痛的主要特征

虽然疼痛不是人体老化的必然现象，但疼痛仍是老年人的常见问题。老年人由于组织器官衰退，机体防御能力和对疾病的反应性均有不同程度的下降，老年人疼痛性疾病较为常见。60 岁以上人群的疼痛患病率是 60 岁以下人群的两倍。

older people suffer pain. Pain is quite common among nursing home residents. It is estimated that pain in 45% to 80% of nursing home patients contributes to functional impairment and a decreased quality of life. Functional impairment is most concerning in that it fosters learned helplessness, social isolation, and greater health care costs because of increased dependency in activities of daily living and therefore greater nursing care needs.

More than 80% of older adults have chronic medical conditions that are typically associated with pain, such as osteoarthritis and peripheral vascular disease. The majority of hospitalized older patients suffers from both acute and persistent pain due to multiple medical conditions, both chronic and/or acute, and may suffer from multiple types and sources of pain. In addition, older adults with cognitive impairment experience pain but are often unable to verbalize it.

III. Epidemiology and Scope of Pain

Although acute pain probably occurs at much the same rate across all age groups, self-report of chronic pain seems to increase among the elder people. Chronic pain in older people is more often experienced in major joints, the back, legs and feet. Pain prevalence among residents of nursing homes varied from 3.7% to 79.5%. The prevalence of pain appeared to be influenced by the research methods and data sources used to detect the resident's pain, such as self-reporting by the residents or staff records.

Pain is mostly due to the increasing prevalence of age-related disorders among older people, such as arthritis, osteoporosis, and peripheral vascular diseases. Pain often leads individuals to seek medical treatment. In older adults, pain often results in a decrease in the activities of daily living (ADL) and quality of life, which in turn leads to higher health care costs due to greater nursing care needs. Pain is a common symptom among older residents of nursing homes and can lead to adverse effects such as a decrease in the activities of daily living and quality of life. From the existing literature it was clear that older residents commonly suffer from pain and other serious problems related to pain. It was also reported that higher pain

研究显示，80% 以上的老年人存在与疼痛相关的慢性疾病，如骨关节炎、骨质疏松、周围血管疾病；大部分住院的老年人也因各种疾病而经历急、慢性疼痛。老年人的疼痛不仅普遍，而且发病因素复杂，患病率高，常导致日常生活功能障碍和生活质量下降。疼痛影响老年人的身体健康、日常功能和生活质量。研究显示，如果疼痛不能及时消除，可导致抑郁、焦虑、食欲缺乏、睡眠障碍、社交减少或孤立、活动减少或受限，并能延缓疾病康复进程、增加病死率和对医疗资源的使用，从而导致医疗费用的增加。

三、流行病学与疼痛范围

老年人的慢性疼痛更常见于关节，背部，腿部和脚部。老年人疼痛发生率从 3.7% 到 79.5% 不等。由于检测方法或记录方法不同，疼痛的发生率会有较大差异，例如住院患者的疼痛主要来源于患者的自我报告或医务人员的病历记录。

疼痛主要由老年慢性病引发（例如，关节炎，骨质疏松症和周围血管疾病）。疼痛常导致日常生活活动（ADL）和生活质量下降，进而增加医疗、护理费用。由于老年人群的特殊性，医务人员在诊断和治疗老年人的疼痛问题时面临着巨大的挑战。护理人员需要了解老年疼痛患者的特殊护理需求，持续、准确的疼痛评估对有效管理疼痛非常重要。老年人疼痛管理的目标为：①缓解疼痛；②控制引起疼痛的疾病；③保持活动能力和日常生活功能；④提高疾病自我管理的能

intensity led to greater limitations in the activities of daily living. Insufficient use of analgesics for treating residents with pain was often reported, particularly in residents with a low cognitive status. Adequate pain management is important, particularly for nursing home residents, because these are mostly vulnerable residents who require long-term care, constant assistance in ADL, and/or medical attention.

IV. Pain Assessment

Assessment is crucial to identify pain in the elderly. Assessment should include a functional observation of the individual. However, assessment can be fraught with other issues particular to underlying psychiatric problems, cognitive impairment, and sensory impairments. There may be multiple medical and pain problems.

Assessment of pain in the elderly presents unique challenges. Older patients themselves may make accurate pain assessment difficult. They may be reluctant to report pain despite substantial physical or psychological impairment. Many older people expect pain with aging and do not believe that their pain can be alleviated. They may fear the need for diagnostic tests or medications that have side effects, or fear addiction to and dependence on strong analgesics. Some patients accept pain and suffering as atonement for past actions. While denying the presence of pain, many older adults will acknowledge discomfort, hurting, or aching. Sensory and cognitive impairment, common among frail older people, make communication more difficult; fortunately, pain can be assessed accurately in most patients by the use of techniques adapted for the individual's handicaps.

i. General Principles of Pain Assessment

Pain management is most successful when the underlying cause of pain is identified and treated definitively. A thorough initial assessment and an appropriate work-up are necessary to determine whether disease-modifying interventions could address the cause of a patient's persistent pain. Assessment should include evaluation of acute pain that might indicate new concurrent illness rather than exacerbation of persistent pain.

力；⑤提高生活质量。通过对患者及家属进行健康教育和优质护理可实现这些目标。

四、老年人疼痛的评估

疼痛评估对识别老年人疼痛的原因、程度和影响，指导疼痛治疗和监测治疗效果非常重要。疼痛评估需注意评估的内容和方法。

疼痛是一种复杂的生理心理活动，疼痛的表现和表达受到躯体疾病、疼痛经历以及患者对疼痛的认知、态度和信念等多种因素的影响，同时疼痛反过来也会影响患者的生理、心理和社会等功能。因此疼痛评估要全面系统：不仅要评估疼痛的强度、部位、性质、发作频率、持续时间、加重和缓解的因素，还要详细了解病史，进行全面的体格检查，重视老年人的年龄、性别、个性和文化背景，评估患者有无躯体功能（如日常生活功能、睡眠、食欲）、心理社会功能（如情绪、人际交往、应对方式）、认知功能（如意识、感觉、记忆思维）等的障碍。明确疼痛的病因，对疼痛进行对因治疗往往是最有效的；与年轻人相比，躯体功能对老年人更为重要，可用来指导设计治疗方案，制订治疗目标，以及评价治疗效果。

（一）疼痛评估的一般原则

根据病因管理疼痛最为有效。因此，必须全面检查和评估，明确疼痛的病因才能确定干预措施。比如，急性疼痛往往提示新的病变，而不是慢性疼痛的加重反应。

In the evaluation process, interdisciplinary assessment may help identify all the potentially treatable contributors to the pain. For those in whom the underlying cause is not remediable or is only partially treatable, an interdisciplinary assessment and treatment strategy is often indicated. Patients who need specialized services or skilled procedures should be referred to a specialist with appropriate expertise. Such patients include those with debilitating psychiatric complications, substance abusers, and those with life-altering intractable pain.

The most accurate and reliable evidence of the existence of pain and its intensity is the patient's report. Clinicians as well as family and caregivers must believe patients and take their reports of pain seriously.

A variety of pain scales have been accepted for use among older adults, even among those with mild to moderate cognitive impairment. A verbally administered 0–10 scale is a good first choice for measuring pain intensity in most of the older persons. The Joint Commission on Accreditation of Healthcare Organizations has often accepted and many institutions have adopted this method for routine assessment or "pain-the 5th vital sign" monitoring programs. In this case, the clinician simply asks the patient "On a scale of zero to ten, with zero meaning no pain and ten meaning the worst pain possible, how much pain do you have now?" However, a substantial portion of older adults (with and without cognitive impairment) may have difficulty responding to this scale. Other verbal descriptor scales, pain thermometers, and faces pain scales also have accepted validity in this population and may be more reliable in those who have difficulty with the verbally administered 0–10 scale. Thus it is important to utilize a scale that is appropriate for the individual and document and use the same tool with each assessment.

Health status and functional status must be assessed. An underlying reason for pain usually must be identified and treated. An assessment should include an evaluation of the presence of acute pain superimposed over persistent pain. Observations from using a pain scale must be evaluated along with the report of pain from the patient himself or herself. Standard pain assessment tools can be used. The same scale should be used with the patient on every assessment and the observation appropriately documented as the 5th vital sign.

另外，由于老年人疼痛和疾病的复杂性，多学科协同合作有助于老年人疼痛的全面评估。更加复杂的情况，如精神衰弱者，存在药物滥用以及顽固性疼痛的患者需要专业人员进行评估和治疗。

目前，在没有客观、稳定的生物学指标的情况下，患者的疼痛主诉是公认的诊断疼痛的"金标准"。应当重视老年人的疼痛主诉，患者的任何疼痛主诉均需认真对待。

目前可使用一些疼痛评估量表对老年人的疼痛进行评估与监测。轻度至中度认知障碍者也可以使用疼痛量表来进行评估。这些评估量表一般可分为自评和观察性评估量表两大类。前者主要有视觉模拟量表、数字评定量表、词语描述量表、面部表情量表、McGill 疼痛问卷，及简洁疼痛问卷，通过直接询问患者，由患者主诉疼痛的情况；后者如语言沟通障碍老年人疼痛评估表，由他人（包括医生、护士、家属等）通过观察言语、表情、行为和体征等来反映老年人的疼痛情况，主要用于认知、语言功能有障碍、疼痛主诉能力下降或主诉结果不可靠的老年人，如痴呆患者。

健康状况和功能状况的评估也很重要，可以借此确定疼痛的根本原因继而采取治疗。慢性疼痛急性加重时也应及时评估。使用疼痛量表进行评估时必须结合患者主诉。在每次评估中，都应使用相同的量表。疼痛被当作第五生命体征备案记录。

Patients' mood and ability to cope with their own pain may also affect the perception of pain. Establishing a rapport with patients allows them to tell their own pain story. Patients should be identified for suffering from pain, treated, and followed for success of treatment. All observations and interventions should be documented. The elderly should be routinely assessed at every encounter for pain along with the other vital signs.

The elderly may not acknowledge pain but instead describe a discomfort or an aching. The cognitively impaired can be assessed for pain by observation of body language. The clinician may observe grimacing, sighing, moaning, guarding, increased pacing or rocking, aggressive behavior, changes in appetite or sleep patterns, crying, increased confusion, or irritability in the cognitively impaired elder as signs of pain.

Other unique characteristics of the elderly should be taken into consideration when assessing for pain. The elderly may be reluctant to report pain. Many elderly expect pain with aging, fear diagnostic tests, do not believe their pain can be alleviated, or fear addiction from analgesics. Other impairments considered in the pain assessment process besides cognitive impairments are impairments of hearing and vision, as well as difficulty in speaking or selecting and comprehending certain terms. Pain assessment should take into consideration patients' ethnicity and cultural beliefs. Assessment and treatment strategies need to be sensitive to culture and ethnicity, as well as the values and beliefs of individual patients and families. Information from family and other caregivers should also be included in the assessment.

情绪和耐受力也会影响对疼痛的感知。良好的护患关系可以促进患者向医务人员描述疼痛。确定疼痛后要给予及时治疗，并跟踪治疗效果。每次评估和干预均应记录在案。疼痛和其他生命体征需要定期评估。

老年人可能否认疼痛，或把疼痛描述为不适。当患者主诉有困难时，医护人员可以通过观察肢体语言来评估认知障碍者的疼痛程度，如患者表情、叹气、呻吟、警惕、攻击行为、睡眠方式变化、哭泣、精神错乱或易怒等都可提示疼痛症状。

评估疼痛时，应考虑老年人的其他独特特征。老年人可能害怕进行诊断检查，或者害怕止痛药成瘾。在疼痛评估过程中，除了认知障碍外，还应考虑其他障碍，包括听觉和视觉障碍，以及言语障碍。向老年人询问时要避免专业术语。疼痛评估还应考虑患者的种族和文化信仰。

Box 16-1 Core Principles of Pain Assessment for Providers

● Every older adult has the right to appropriate assessment and management of pain. Pain should be assessed in all individuals living in nursing homes.

● Pain is always subjective. Therefore, the individual's self-report of pain[1] is the single most reliable indicator of pain. The clinician needs to accept and respect this self-report.

● Physiological and behavioral (objective) signs of pain (e. g. , tachycardia, grimacing) are neither sensitive nor specific for pain. Such observations should not replace individual self-report unless the individual is unable to communicate.

Box 16-1 疼痛评估的核心原则

● 每位老年人的疼痛都应该得到合理的评估和恰当的管理，这是他们的权利之一。所有在老人院的老年人都应该得到疼痛的评估服务。

● 疼痛是一种主观感受，所以个体对疼痛的自我汇报是最可靠的依据，医务人员需要接受并尊重来自个体的自我疼痛汇报。

● 生命体征（如心率加快等）和个体的行为对疼痛来说既不是敏感的信号也不是特殊性的标志。除非遇到不能交流的服务对象，此类观察不可代替个体对疼痛的自我汇报。

- Assessment approaches, including tools, must be appropriate for the individual. Special considerations are needed for those with difficulty communicating. Family members should be included in the assessment process, when possible.
- Pain can exist even when no physical cause can be found. Thus, pain without an identifiable cause should not be routinely attributed to psychological causes or discounted.

- Different levels of pain in response to the same stimulus may be experienced by individuals; that is, a uniform pain threshold does not exist.

- Pain tolerance varies among and within individuals depending on factors including heredity, energy level, coping skills, and prior experiences with pain.

- Individuals with chronic pain may be more sensitive to pain and other stimuli.

- Unrelieved pain has adverse physical and psychological consequences. Therefore, clinicians should encourage the reporting of pain by individuals who are reluctant to discuss pain, deny pain when it is likely present, or fail to follow through on prescribed treatments.

- Pain is an unpleasant sensory and emotional experience, so assessment should address both physical and psychological aspects of pain.

ii. Comprehensive Assessment of Pain in Older Adults

The assessment of all people who are having pain, especially persistent pain, should involve consideration of medical, psychosocial, cognitive, neuropsychological, and behavioral factors. The assessment of pain in older adults can be extremely challenging given the multiple co-morbidities that often are present and the variety of issues that impact pain presentation.

A comprehensive assessment of pain must include the identification of relevant underlying physical pathologies and other conditions that may influence pain perception, report, and management. Assessment of functional limitations (e. g. , impairment in performance of basic, instrumental, and advanced activities of daily living (ADL), mobility, sleep, and appetite), psychosocial

- 疼痛评估手段必须适合要每个不同个体。对于沟通困难者应该给予特殊的考虑。可能的情况下在疼痛评估的过程中应该考虑邀请家庭成员的加入。
- 即使没有身体疾病的原因疼痛也是可以存在的，所以找不到原因的疼痛绝不应该被常规的认为是心理原因或者不被重视。

- 每个不同的个体对相同的刺激导致的疼痛的程度可以是不同的，所以说根本不存在标准的痛阈值。
- 每个不同的个体对疼痛的容忍度是不同的甚至同一个个体不同的时候对疼痛的容忍度也是不同的，起决定性的因素包括遗传，个体能量水平，应对能力和既往疼痛的经历。
- 患有慢性疼痛的个体可能会对疼痛和其他刺激原更敏感。
- 没有得到缓解的疼痛对个体的身体和心理健康都有负性的影响。所以对于那些有可能正在承受疼痛但否认疼痛的人或者不愿意讨论疼痛的人，还有那些不遵照疼痛的处方进行治疗疼痛的人，医务人员要鼓励他们汇报疼痛。
- 疼痛是一种不愉快的感觉和情感经历，所以对疼痛的评估一定要把疼痛的生理和心理两方面都要强调到。

（二）老年人疼痛综合评估

对所有疼痛尤其是持续性疼痛的人进行评估时，应考虑医学、心理、认知、神经心理学和行为因素。鉴于经常出现的多种合并症以及影响疼痛表现的各种问题，对老年人的疼痛评估可能极具挑战性。

对疼痛的全面评估必须包括识别潜在的生理病理和其他可能影响疼痛感知，主诉和管理的状况。评估功能限制（例如，日常基本生活能力，工具和高级活动能力，活动能力，睡眠和食欲的表现受损），社会心理功能（例如，情绪，人际互动，对疼痛的信念，对

function (e. g. , mood, interpersonal interactions, beliefs about pain, fear of pain-related activity), and cognitive function (e. g. , dementia or delirium) is necessary. As with younger adults, information on functional limitations is extremely important for older persons because this information is used to guide therapy, establish reasonable and attainable goals, and to track outcomes. Interdisciplinary evaluation and collaboration are often necessary to address the full range of the older person's health-related circumstances.

Pain assessment is situation and context-dependent (i. e. , patient care or clinical research, acute or persistent, new symptom or ongoing, crisis or routine, outpatient or inpatient, etc.). The core outcome domains and measures recommended by the initiative on methods, measurement, and pain assessment in clinical trials (IMMPACT) for evaluating chronic pain treatments provide a valuable foundation for guiding a comprehensive pain assessment in older adults. Specifically, the IMMPACT initiative recommends that the following domains be routinely considered in pain clinical trials: pain intensity, physical functioning, emotional functioning, patient report of global improvement or satisfaction, and symptoms and adverse events. The comprehensive approach of pain assessment is shown in Figure 16-1.

疼痛的恐惧）和认知功能（例如痴呆或谵妄）是必要的。与年轻人一样，有关功能限制的信息对老年人也极为重要，因为该信息用于指导治疗，建立合理和可实现的目标以及追踪结果。跨学科评估和协作通常是解决老年人健康相关状况的必要条件。

疼痛评估取决于具体情况和情境（即患者护理或临床研究，急性或持续性，新症状或持续，危机或常规，门诊或住院等）。临床试验方法，测量和疼痛评估倡议（IMMPACT）推荐的用于评估慢性疼痛治疗的核心结果领域和措施，为指导老年人进行全面的疼痛评估提供了宝贵的基础。具体而言，IMMPACT倡议建议在疼痛临床试验中常规考虑以下领域：疼痛强度、身体功能、情绪功能、患者总体改善或满意度的报告以及症状和不良事件。疼痛评估的综合方法见图 16-1。

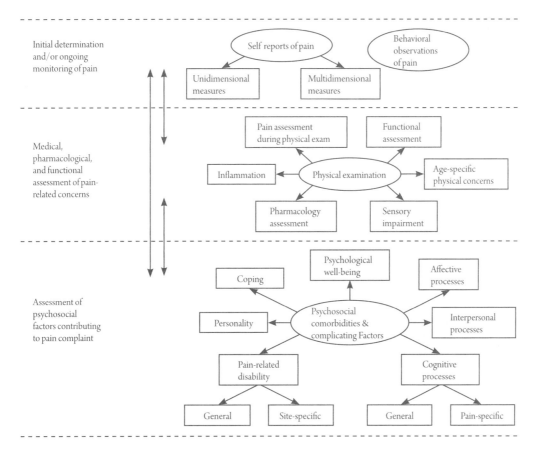

Figure16-1 Graphically depicts the comprehensive approach of pain assessment

iii. Brief Summary of Assessment Parameters

1. Assumptions

(1) The majority of hospitalized older patients suffer from both acute and persistent pain.

(2) Older adults with cognitive impairment experience pain but are often unable to verbalize it.

(3) Both patients and health care providers have personal beliefs, prior experiences, insufficient knowledge, and mistaken beliefs about pain and pain management that (a) influence the pain management process, and (b) must be acknowledged before optimal pain relief can be achieved.

(4) Pain assessment must be regular, systematic, and documented to accurately evaluate treatment effectiveness.

(5) Self-report is the gold standard for pain assessment.

2. Strategies for pain assessment

(1) Reviewing medical history, physical exam, and laboratory and diagnostic tests to understand sequence of events contributing to pain.

(2) Assessing present pain, including intensity, character, frequency, pattern, location, duration, and precipitating and relieving factors.

(3) Reviewing medications, including current and previously used prescription drugs, over-the-counter drugs, and home remedies. Determine which pain control methods have previously been effective for the patient. Assess patient's attitudes and beliefs about use of analgesics, adjuvant drugs, and non-drug treatments.

(4) Using a standardized tool to assess self-reported pain. Choose from published measurement tools and recall that older adults may have difficulty using 10-point visual analog scales. Vertical verbal descriptor scales or faces scales may be more useful with older adults.

(5) Assessing pain regularly and frequently but at least every 4 hours. Monitor pain intensity after giving medications to evaluate effectiveness.

(6) Observing for nonverbal and behavioral signs of pain, such as facial grimacing, withdrawal, guarding, rubbing, limping, shifting of position, aggression, agitation, depression, vocalizations, and crying. Also watch for changes in behavior from the patient's usual patterns.

(7) Gathering information from family members about the patient's pain experiences. Ask about the

（三）评价参数小结

1. 假设

（1）大多数住院的老年患者都患有急性和持续性疼痛。

（2）有认知障碍的老年人会感到疼痛，但通常无法将其表达出来。

（3）患者和医疗保健提供者都对疼痛和疼痛管理有个人信念，先前的经验，知识不足和错误的信念，这些信念影响疼痛管理过程，并且必须认识后认，才能实现最佳的疼痛缓解。

（4）疼痛评估必须定期，系统且有文件记录，以准确评估治疗效果。

（5）自我报告是评估疼痛的金标准。

2. 疼痛评估策略

（1）了解病史、体格检查、辅助检查、心理社会等情况，找出疼痛的可能原因。

（2）评估疼痛的临床表现，包括强度、性质、频率、部位、持续时间、加重和缓解的影响因素。

（3）了解用药史及治疗过程，识别曾对该患者疗效显著的止痛方法；评估患者对止痛药、辅助药和非药物治疗的态度、信念。

（4）采用合适的疼痛评估工具进行疼痛自评。

（5）每4小时至少评估一次疼痛；每次给药后评估疼痛强度以评价疗效；记录评估结果。

（6）观察疼痛的行为表现，如有无痛苦表情、退缩、防卫、按摩、跛行、体位改变、攻击、激惹、抑郁、哼声和哭泣等；注意与患者平日的表现进行比较。

（7）向家属了解患者的疼痛相关信息，询问患者有无疼痛的语言和行为表现。

patient's verbal and nonverbal/behavioral expressions of pain, particularly in older adults with dementia.

(8) When pain is suspected but assessment instruments or observation is ambiguous, institute a clinical trial of pain treatment (i. e. , in persons with dementia). If symptoms persist, assume pain is unrelieved and treat accordingly.

3. Assessing pain in older adults and in persons with dementia In nursing homes, assessment and management of pain is often problematic. Older residents in nursing homes often have several chronic problems, such as cerebrovascular accidents, arthritis, and/or dementia. Physical and cognitive impairments often make it difficult for such residents to report pain to the staff. Furthermore, older residents often do not actively report pain, because of the stigma associated with it or because of their own forbearance/stoicism. The heavy workloads of nursing home staff may compound the problem, making it difficult to identify pain among residents. In addition, nurses tended to estimate severe pain and pain tolerance significantly lower than patients. Therefore, nursing home staffs need to be aware of these problems and efforts should be directed toward improving pain assessment and management.

（8）当怀疑存在疼痛、而疼痛工具或观察结果显示阴性时，应进行试验性治疗；如果症状缓解，则说明存在疼痛。

3. 评估老年人和痴呆老年人的疼痛　在养老院，疼痛的评估和管理难以开展。因为养老院的老年居民常患有各种慢性病。疾病和认知障碍常使老年人难以向工作人员表述疼痛。此外，养老院工作人员工作繁重可能会忽视对老年人疼痛的识别，同时护理人员对严重疼痛和疼痛耐受性的评估明显低于患者感受。因此，需要意识到这些问题，并努力改善疼痛评估和管理。

Section 3　Pain Management for the Elderly

第三节　老年人的疼痛管理

In 2004, the International Association for the Study of Pain and the World Health Organization promoted the concept of pain relief as a human right. Health professionals may need to be more aware of serious problems related to pain among elders and their fundamental right to be treated for their pain to the greatest extent possible.

2004 年，国际疼痛研究协会和世界卫生组织提出了缓解疼痛是人的权利的概念。卫生专业人员可能需要更多地了解与老年人疼痛相关的严重问题，以及他们应获得最大程度的疼痛治疗的基本权利。

I. Clinical Guidelines

一、疼痛管理临床指南

Recommendations for the treatment of pain in the elderly, particularly for persistent pain, have been published. However, the recommendations are not supported by strong published scientific evidence because there are few randomized trials studying patients in the age range of 75 to 85 years. In 2002, the American Geriatrics Society published guidelines on the management of chronic or persistent pain in the frail elderly, taking into consideration limited social and financial resources of

关于老年人疼痛，特别是持续疼痛的建议已经公布。然而，这些建议没有得到强有力的科学证据的支持，因为很少有随机试验研究 75 ~ 85 岁的患者。2002 年，美国老年医学会公布了关于管理体弱老人慢性或持续疼痛的指南，同时考虑到这一人口有限的社会和财政资源。该指南的一些临床影响是提高

this population. Some of the clinical implications of the guidelines were an enhanced awareness on the part of clinicians to assess patients at every encounter for pain and the changing attitude to a more favorable view of the use of opioids in the treatment of persistent pain. Increasing age is associated with the pain of osteoarthritis. The American Pain Society published guidelines in 2002 on the management of osteoarthritis with emphasis on the pain experienced by older adults. Recommendations for the treatment of cancer pain have been recently updated from the 1994 Agency for Healthcare Policy and Research Guidelines. These guidelines have been published by the American Pain Society.

II. Co-morbidities Associated with Pain

Co-morbidities in the aged with complaints of pain must be recognized and treated. Associated problems include psychiatric co-morbidities such as depression or anxiety. The patient may experience sleep disturbances, decreased socialization leading to isolation, and impaired functioning in activities of daily living. Medical co-morbidities must also be identified and treated to ensure optimal pharmacotherapeutic outcome for pain. To manage all aspects of pain and associated co-morbidities, an interdisciplinary approach to patient care is suggested. Specialized services can be provided by the mental health professional, physical or occupational therapist, pharmacist, and social worker. Non-pharmacological treatment strategies are important in the complex treatment of the elderly. Cognitive and behavioral coping strategies, along with regular participation in physical activities to restore function and reduce pain, will enhance quality of life.

III. Pain Treatment for the Elderly

Pharmacotherapy must be adjusted in the elderly with consideration for age and organ function. The pharmacokinetics of drug therapy may be altered in the elderly with respect to absorption, distribution, metabolism, and excretion.

Absorption of sublingual tablets can be reduced in the elderly when there is decreased saliva formation. This may be exacerbated by the concomitant administration of anticholinergic drugs. Stomach acid production in the elderly is reduced and may be further reduced by administration of commonly used histamine 2

临床医生的意识来评估患者每次遇到疼痛和态度改变，以更有利的观点使用阿片类药物治疗持续疼痛。年龄的增长与骨关节炎的疼痛有关。美国疼痛协会于 2002 年发布了关于骨关节炎管理的指南，重点是老年人所经历的痛苦。关于治疗癌症疼痛的建议最近更新了 1994 年颁发的保健政策和研究指南。这些指南已经由美国疼痛协会发布。

二、疼痛的合并症

必须识别并治疗老年人中因疼痛而引起的合并症。相关问题包括精神疾病合并症，例如抑郁症或焦虑症。患者可能会出现睡眠障碍，社交能力下降，导致孤独感以及日常生活活动功能受损的情况。还必须确定医学上的合并症，以确保获得最佳的疼痛药物治疗结果。为了处理疼痛和相关合并症的所有方面，建议采用跨学科的患者护理方法。精神卫生专业人员，物理或职业治疗师，药剂师和社会工作者可以提供专业服务。在老年人的综合治疗中，非药物治疗策略很重要。认知和行为应对策略以及定期参加体育活动以恢复功能并减轻痛苦，将改善生活质量。

三、疼痛的治疗

老年药物治疗中的药物动力学问题必须根据年龄和器官功能在老年人中进行调整。药物治疗的药理动力学在老年人的吸收、分布、新陈代谢和排泄方面可能会发生变化。

当唾液形成减少时，老年人对舌下片剂的吸收可以减少。抗胆碱药物的施用可能会加剧这种情况。老年人的胃酸生成减少，而常用组胺 2 拮抗剂或质子泵抑制剂可能进一步减少胃酸。腹膜减少增加便秘、恶心和呕吐

antagonists or proton pump inhibitors. Peristalsis is reduced, increasing the risk of constipation, nausea, and vomiting, especially from opioids. Aging is associated with increased body fat, which allows for an increased volume of distribution of lipophilic medications and delays elimination and the onset of effect. Conversely, many elderly are frail, lean, and under-nourished, which also influences the volume of distribution depending on the pharmacokinetic characteristics of each medication. In general, hepatic metabolism of drugs in the elderly will be reduced as compared to the younger patient. The elderly are at increased risk of side effects and adverse reactions due to these age-related hepatic differences in metabolism.

Elimination of active drugs and metabolites is similarly compromised in the elderly. In general, it is not uncommon for a patient older than age 65 years to have at least a 50% reduction in creatinine clearance. Medications really cleared have an associated toxicity in patients who are experiencing age-related renal insufficiency and/or dehydration. In circumstances such as this, as well as with severe hepatic insufficiency, the medication dosing interval should be lengthened and/or the dose reduced to avoid poor outcomes associated with medication use. The scheduled administration of pain medications should be avoided in patients who are oliguric or anuric. Instead, pain medications should be administered strictly on an as-needed regimen.

Because opioids offer an important pain treatment option, their pharmacokinetics is of particular interest. All opioids and their metabolites, with the exception of methadone, are 90% to 95% renally excreted. Methadone is approximately 50% excreted renally and 50% excreted hepatically. The metabolites of morphine are morphine-3-glucuronide and morphine-6-glucuronide. Morphine-6-glucaronide is the active analgesic metabolite with a longer half-life than morphine itself and is many times more potent than the parent drug. In older patients, morphine utilization may be compromised because of the accumulation of the metabolites secondary to renal and hepatic insufficiency. All of the phenanthreneopioids—codeine, hydrocodone, hydromorphone, morphine, and oxycodone—follow first-order kinetics and exhibit similar pharmacological behavior. Peak plasma concentration (C_{max}) is reached approximately 60 to 90 minutes after oral (including enteral feeding tube) or rectal administration, 30 minutes after subcutaneous or intramuscular injection, or 6 minutes after intravenous injection. Elimination is direct and predictable, irrespective of the dose. After

的风险，特别是服用阿片类药物的时候。衰老与身体脂肪增加有关，这让亲脂药物的分配量增加，同时药物代谢延迟，使得药物的作用时间逐渐延长。相反，许多老年人体弱、瘦弱、营养不足，这也影响了各种药物的药理动力学特性，影响分布量。一般来说，与年轻患者相比，老年人的药物肝代谢会减少。这些与年龄相关的肝代谢差异使老年人患副作用和不良反应的风险增加。

活性药物和代谢物的清除在老年人群体中相当缓慢。一般来说，65 岁以上的患者肌酸清除量至少减少了 50% 的情况并不少见。对于年龄相关的肾功能不全和 / 或脱水的患者来说，真正清除的药物对他们具有一定的毒性。在这种情况下，以及严重的肝功能不全，药物剂量间隔应延长和 / 或减少剂量，以避免与药物使用相关的不良结果。在少尿或无尿患者中应避免按计划施用止痛药，止痛药应严格按照需要的治疗方案进行。

由于阿片类药物成为疼痛治疗的主要选择，因此它们的药代动力学特别受关注。除美沙酮外，所有阿片类药物及其代谢物 90%～95% 经肾脏排泄。美沙酮大约 50% 通过肾脏排泄，而另外 50% 通过肝脏排泄。吗啡的代谢产物是吗啡 –3– 葡糖醛酸和吗啡 –6– 葡糖醛酸。吗啡 –6– 葡糖醛酸是一种活性止痛药代谢物，其半衰期比吗啡本身更长，而且功效比母体药物高出许多倍。在老年患者中，由于肾脏和肝功能不全而导致的代谢产物积累，可能会影响吗啡的使用。所有的菲类阿片类药物（可待因，氢可酮，氢吗啡酮，吗啡和羟考酮）都遵循一级动力学，并且表现出相似的药理行为。口服（包括体内饲管）或直肠给药后约 60～90 分钟，皮下注射或肌内注射后 30 分钟，或静脉内注射后 6 分钟达到血浆峰值浓度（C_{max}）。药物清除是直接且可

hepatic conjugation, the kidney then excretes 90% to 95% of the metabolites. The rate of renal clearance influences the half-life ($t_{1/2}$) of the opioid metabolite. The effective half-life ($t_{1/2}$) of the phenanthrenesis approximately 3 to 4 hours if the renal clearance is normal. After 4 to 5 half-lives, the plasma concentration of these drugs approaches steady state when dosed repeatedly. Thus, steady-state plasma concentrations are usually attained within a day.

Methadone is structurally classified as a diphenylheptane. Methadone has a long and variable half-life estimated to be between 18 to 120 hours. The half-life on average, however, is approximately 24 hours. The effective dosing interval for analgesia varies. Methadone is hepatically metabolized, resulting in several metabolites. About half of the parent drug and its metabolites are excreted by the intestines, as well as the kidney. In general, methadone is longer acting than immediate-release morphine. With chronic administration, the immediate analgesic effect of methadone lasts from 6 to 12 hours. Depending on the patient's unique pharmacokinetic profile regarding hepatic and renal clearance, the methadone effective dosing interval maybe every 12, 8, 6, or sometimes 4 hours. The uncertainty of the methadone dosing interval, as well as the fact that methadone exhibits incomplete cross tolerance when converting from other opioids, contributes to the phobia for using methadone in pain management. Only practitioners knowledgeable on the unique characteristics of methadone can ensure its safe and effective use. We ensure the safe and effective use of methadone in our own clinical practice by supporting daily follow-up for 7 to 10 days after the initiation of methadone.

IV. General Principles of Alternative Therapies in Pain Management

Alternative therapies, such as physical, cognitive and behavioral therapies, have been given attentions by geriatric practitioners, the elders and their caregivers. Clinical experience suggests that most non-drug therapies work well with mild pain, or in combined use of pharmacological therapies in older people.

1. Physical therapies Physical therapies include application of heat and cold, therapeutic touch, massage, acupuncture, nerve stimulations and exercise.

2. Heat and cold Application of heat can decrease pain by increasing blood flow, oxygen and

预测的，与剂量无关。肝结合后，肾脏会排泄90%~95%的代谢产物。肾脏清除率会影响阿片类药物代谢的半衰期（$t_{1/2}$）。如果肾脏清除率正常，则菲的有效半衰期（$t_{1/2}$）大约为3~4小时。在4~5个半衰期后，这些药物的血浆浓度在重复给药时会达到稳定状态。因此，通常在1天之内就可以达到稳态血浆浓度。

美沙酮在结构上被分类为二苯基庚烷。美沙酮的半衰期长且可变，估计在18~120小时之间。其平均半衰期约为24小时。用于镇痛时，有效剂量的间隔时间有所不同。美沙酮通过肝脏代谢，产生几种代谢物。大约一半的母体药物及其代谢物通过肠和肾脏排泄。通常，美沙酮比速释吗啡的作用时间更长。长期服用后美沙酮的立即镇痛作用持续6~12个小时。根据患者在肝脏和肾脏清除方面的独特药代动力学特征，美沙酮有效给药间隔时间可能每12小时、8小时、6小时或有时4小时一次。美沙酮服药间隔的不确定性以及美沙酮从其他阿片类药物转化时表现出不完全的交叉耐受性这一事实，让美沙酮在疼痛控制中无法成为优先考虑的药物。只有熟悉美沙酮特殊性的医生才能确保其安全有效地使用。我们需要在开始使用美沙酮治疗后的7~10天内进行每日随访，确保在我们自己的临床实践中安全有效地使用美沙酮。

四、疼痛的非药物替代治疗

疼痛的替代疗法，例如物理疗法，认知疗法和行为疗法，已经被老年科医生及其老年人照护者所关注。临床经验表明，大多数非药物疗法或联合使用药物疗法对老年人轻度疼痛效果很好。

1. **物理疗法** 物理疗法包括冷热敷、治疗接触、按摩、针灸、神经刺激和锻炼。

2. **热疗和冷疗** 热疗可以通过促进血液流动、氧气和向患处输送营养物质来减轻疼

nutrition delivery to the affected areas; application of cold can decrease pain by reducing inflammation and edema after injury. Nurses and caregivers can use methods of heat and cold application as introduced in fundamental nursing skills. Due to the reduced skin sensitivity among elders, it is important to follow the protocol of heat and cold applications to prevent injuries and complications such thermal burn and cold sores.

3. Exercise   For older adults, stretching and other low intensive balancing exercise can help older adults decrease pain by maintaining function, relieving muscle spasms and preventing stiffness. Before starting exercise, it is important to assess older adults' physical condition and obtain medical consultation to ensure safety. In some cases, analgesic medication can be given shortly before exercise.

4. Cognitive and behavior therapies   The elders' conception and perception of pain greatly influence their pain behavior and coping strategy. Some strategies such as music therapy, meditation, therapeutic and healing touch, and education may have effects on elder's pain perception, emotion and sense of control. For example, studies have shown that therapeutic touch had comfort effects on the elders. It not only provides pain relief through relaxation of muscle spasms, it can decrease the anxiety level as well. However, for elders with cognitive impairments, these therapies may be not efficient.

V. Nurses' Contribution in Pain Management

It is important to manage pain for nursing home residents by providing individually tailored care for each resident. To promote individually tailored care, it is essential to obtain all necessary information about the pain, such as its causes, intensity, and other related factors. Pain assessment and management should also be based on the best available evidence from studies and tailored for the residents' circumstances and needs. There is an increase in the number of such studies worldwide that examine pain prevalence among nursing home residents and explore the factors related to pain.

The most common strategy to manage pain is to use analgesic drugs. Unfortunately, older patients have been systematically excluded from clinical trials of such drugs. In one report of 83 randomized trials of non-steroidal anti-inflammatory drugs (NSAIDs) including nearly 10 000 subjects, only 2.3% were aged 65 or over and none were aged 85 or over. Despite the fact that older people are more likely to experience the side effects of analgesic

痛；冷疗可以减轻受伤后的炎症和水肿，从而减轻疼痛。护理人员可以使用基础护理学中介绍的热疗和冷疗方法。由于老年人的皮肤敏感性降低，因此要严格遵循热疗和冷疗的原则，以防止受伤和并发症，例如热灼伤和冻疮。

3. 锻炼　伸展运动和其他低强度的平衡锻炼可通过维持功能，缓解肌肉痉挛和防止僵硬来帮助老年人减轻疼痛。在开始运动之前，要评估老年人的身体状况并制订运动处方，以确保安全。必要时，可以在运动前服用止痛药。

4. 认知和行为疗法　老年人对疼痛的观念和认知很大程度地影响了他们的疼痛行为和应对策略。音乐疗法，冥想，治疗和康复接触以及教育等策略可能会对老年人的疼痛感，情感和控制感产生影响。例如，研究表明，治疗性接触对老年人有安慰作用。它不仅可以通过放松肌肉痉挛来缓解疼痛，还可以降低焦虑水平。但是，对于有认知障碍的老年人，这些疗法可能无效。

五、护士在疼痛管理中的作用

通过为每位居民提供个体化的护理来管理疗养院居民的疼痛，这一点很重要。为了促进个体化的护理，获取有关疼痛的完整信息（例如其原因，强度和其他相关因素）至关重要。疼痛评估和管理还应基于循证研究中获得的最佳证据，针对老年人的情况和需求个体化定制。在全世界范围内，调查疗养院居民中的疼痛患病率并探讨与疼痛相关因素的研究数量正在增加。

解决疼痛的最常见策略是使用止痛药。然而，老年患者已被系统地排除在此类药物的临床试验之外。在一项包括近 10 000 名受试者的 83 项非甾体抗炎药（NSAID）随机试验的报告中，只有 2.3% 的受试者年龄在 65 岁或以上，而没有一个受试者的年龄在 85 岁或

medications, they appear to be more sensitive to analgesic properties, especially those of opioid analgesics. For example, single-dose studies comparing younger and older patients with postoperative and cancer pain have observed higher pain relief and longer duration of action among older patients for morphine and other opioid drugs.

The use of opioid analgesic drugs for persistent non–cancer-related pain remains controversial, although consensus statements from major professional pain organizations endorse their use in appropriate situations (e. g. , American Academy of Pain Management and American Pain Society). Reluctance to prescribe these drugs has probably been over-influenced by political and social pressures to control illicit drug use. In fact, the incidence of addictive behavior among patients taking opioid drugs for medical indications appears to be very low. Moreover, the exercise of careful professional responsibility reduces the risk of abuse. This does not imply that opioid drugs should be used indiscriminately, but only that fear of addiction and other side effects does not justify failure to treat severe pain.

i. Nursing Care Strategies

1. Prevention of pain

(1) Assess pain regularly and frequently to facilitate appropriate treatment.

(2) Anticipate and aggressively treat for pain before, during, and after painful diagnostic and/or therapeutic treatments.

(3) Educate patients, families, and other clinicians to use analgesic medications prophylactically prior to and after painful procedures.

(4) Educate patients and families about pain medications and their side effects; adverse effects; and issues of addiction, dependence, and tolerance.

(5) Educate patients to take medications for pain on a regular basis and to avoid allowing pain to escalate.

(6) Educate patients, families, and other clinicians to use non-drug strategies to manage pain, such as relaxation, massage, and heat/cold.

2. Treatment guidelines

(1) Pharmacologic

以上。尽管事实上老年人更可能会遇到止痛药的副作用,但他们似乎对止痛药的特性更加敏感,尤其是阿片类止痛药的特性。例如,单剂量研究比较了年轻患者和老年患者术后疼痛和癌症疼痛,观察到老年患者对吗啡和其他阿片类药物的镇痛效果更强,作用时间更长。

尽管主要专业疼痛管理机构一致声明他们支持适当地使用阿片类镇痛药治疗非癌症相关的持续性疼痛(例如,美国疼痛管理学会和美国疼痛学会),但仍存在争议。处方中不愿开这些药的原因可能受到控制非法药物使用的政治和社会压力的影响。实际上,服用阿片类药物进行治疗的老年患者中,成瘾行为的发生率很低。此外,审慎的医疗态度降低了滥用的风险。但这并不意味着可以不加选择地使用阿片类药物,而是不能因为对成瘾和其他副作用的恐惧而不去治疗严重的疼痛。

(一)护理措施

1. **疼痛预防**
(1)常规评估疼痛。

(2)若某项诊断或治疗可能产生疼痛,需给予预防性的止痛措施。

(3)在手术前后,教育患者,家庭和其他临床医生预防性使用止痛药。

(4)教给患者和家属有关止痛药的使用、不良反应、耐受、依赖、成瘾等知识。

(5)向患者强调遵医嘱服药的重要性,并避免疼痛加剧。

(6)教给患者和家属非药物的止痛方法,如放松训练、按摩和冷热疗法等。

2. **疼痛治疗**
(1)药物治疗

1) Older adults are at increased risk for adverse drug reactions.

2) Monitor medications closely to avoid over-or under-medication.

3) Administer pain drugs on a regular basis to maintain therapeutic levels; avoid PRN drugs.

4) Document treatment plan to maintain consistency across shifts and with other care providers.

5) Use equianalgesic dosing and the WHO three-step ladder to obtain optimal pain relief with fewer side effects.

(2) Nonpharmacologic

1) Investigate older patients' attitudes and beliefs about, preference for, and experience with nonpharmacological pain-treatment strategies.

2) Tailor nonpharmacologic techniques to the individual.

3) Cognitive-behavioral strategies focus on changing the person's perception of pain (e. g. , relaxation therapy, education, and distraction) and may not be appropriate for cognitively impaired persons.

4) Physical pain relief strategies focus on promoting comfort and altering physiologic responses to pain (e. g. , heat, cold, TENS units) and are generally safe and effective.

(3) Combination approaches that include both pharmacological and nonpharmacological pain treatments are often the most effective.

3. Follow-up assessment

(1) Monitor treatment effects within 1 hour of administration and at least every 4 hours.

(2) Evaluate patient for pain relief and side effects of treatment.

(3) Document patient's response to treatment effects.

(4) Document treatment regimen in patient care plan to facilitate consistent implementation.

ii. Expected outcomes

1. Patient

(1) Will be either pain free or pain will be at a level that the patient judges as acceptable.

1）老年人发生药物不良反应的风险增加。

2）严密监测用药情况，防止药物滥用或用药不足。

3）按时给药以维持治疗水平的药物浓度，尽量避免临时用药。

4）记录治疗方案，以保证各班次人员疼痛护理的一致性。

5）按 WHO 三阶梯疗法用药，以最小剂量达到最佳止痛效果，减少不良反应。

（2）非药物治疗

1）评估患者有关非药物止痛方法的态度、信念、偏好和体验。

2）制订个体化的非药物治疗方案。

3）认知－行为疗法重于改变人们对疼痛的感知（如放松疗法，教育和分心），不适用于认知功能障碍的患者。

4）应用冷热疗法、体育锻炼等方法时，注意保证患者的安全和治疗效果。

（3）包括药物和非药物疼痛治疗的组合方法通常是最有效的。

3. 效果监测

（1）给药后 1 小时内需评估疼痛，常规每 4 小时至少评估疼痛一次。

（2）评估患者疼痛缓解情况和治疗的不良反应。

（3）了解患者对治疗效果的评价。

（4）记录治疗效果，以保证疼痛管理的连续性。

（二）预期目标

1. 患者

（1）疼痛消除或减轻至患者可忍受的水平。

(2) Maintains highest level of selfcare, functional ability, and activity level possible.

(3) Experiences no iatrogenic complications, such as falls, GI upset/bleeding, or altered cognitive status.

2. Nurse

(1) Will demonstrate evidence of ongoing and comprehensive pain assessment.

(2) Will document evidence of prompt and effective pain management interventions.

(3) Will document systematic evaluation of treatment effectiveness.

(4) Will demonstrate knowledge of pain management in older patients, including assessment strategies, pain medications, nonpharmacological interventions, and patient and family education.

3. Institution

(1) Facilities and institutions will provide evidence of documentation of pain assessment, intervention, and evaluation of treatment effectiveness.

(2) Facilities and institutions will provide evidence of referral to specialists for specific therapies (e. g. , psychiatry, psychology, bio-feedback, physical therapy, or pain treatment centers).

(3) Facilities and institutions will provide evidence of pain management resources for staff (e. g. , care-planning and pain management references, pain management consultants).

(WU Lihua)

Key Points

1. A comprehensive understanding of pain in the elderly is crucial in geriatric care, which request all the health care professionals have the knowledge and skills to conduct ongoing assessment and management as needed among this population.

2. Pain assessment should be compulsory in nursing care plan in hospitals. It must be an ongoing process, from admission to discharge. For home-based residents and nursing homes, staff should have sufficient training in terms of pain recognition and assessment and management.

（2）自我管理能力、日常生活功能和活动能力保持在最佳水平。

（3）避免医源性的并发症，如跌倒、胃肠道出血、意识改变等。

2. 护士

（1）能对疼痛进行持续、全面的评估。

（2）能及时记录疼痛管理措施的效果。

（3）能对治疗方案进行系统评价。

（4）掌握老年人疼痛管理的知识，能有效开展对患者及家属的健康教育，包括评估方法、药物和非药物止痛方法等。

3. 机构

（1）提供有关疼痛评估，干预和治疗效果评估的文件证明。

（2）转诊时向专家提供特殊治疗（例如，精神病学，心理学，生物反馈，物理疗法或疼痛治疗中心）的证据。

（3）为员工提供疼痛管理的培训或学习资料（例如，护理计划和疼痛管理参考资料，疼痛管理指南）。

（吴丽华）

本章要点

1. 全面了解老年人的疼痛对于老年护理至关重要。老年护理要求所有医疗保健专业人员具备相关知识和技能，根据护理需求对老年人进行持续的评估和管理。

2. 疼痛评估是护理计划中必须实施的项目。它是连续进行的，应包含入院到出院的整个过程。对于居家者和疗养院，工作人员应该在疼痛的识别、评估和管理方面有足够的培训。

3. For pain management, pharmacological pain management is widely used in hospitals with analgesics, opioid analgesics, and other additional medications. Non-, pharmacological therapies include physical methods using cold, heat and massage; relaxation and distraction etc.

4. Nurses have an important role in pain management, it is necessary to assess pain continuously and evaluate the effect of employing any of these methods.

5. Barriers of effective pain management in the elderly include the misconception that intolerance to pain is age related, underreporting of pain, lack of access to diagnostic services, cognitive and functional impairment, the inability to communicate etc.

Critical Thinking Exercise

An 86 years old gentleman was brought to the Emergency and accident department after a fall at home. He did not only suffer from the fall itself, there is a long list of diseases in his medical history: chronic heart failure, pace-maker insertion (he is on warfarin), renal impairment and dementia.

Question:

Please discuss how you would like to assess his pain and what is nursing plan in pain management for this patient.

3. 对于疼痛管理，药物治疗被广泛用于医院，包括镇痛药，阿片类镇痛药和其他。非药物治疗包括使用冷，热和按摩等物理方法、放松训练和转移注意力等。

4. 护士在疼痛管理中具有重要作用，必须对疼痛连续评估并评价各种处理的效果。

5. 老年人疼痛管理的难点在于其对疼痛不耐受，疼痛评估不充分，缺乏诊断路径，认知和功能障碍，沟通困难等。

批判性思维练习

一名 86 岁的男性患者在家中跌倒后被送到急诊。他不仅有跌倒造成的外伤，同时还患有多种慢性病，包括慢性心力衰竭，起搏器插入（正在服用华法林），肾功能不全和痴呆。

问题：
请讨论你如何对他进行疼痛评估和疼痛管理，并实施护理计划。

Chapter 17 Skin Care for Elderly
第十七章　老年人皮肤的护理

Learning Objectives

On completion of this chapter, the reader will be able to:

- Describe the differences in skin structure between normal and aged skin;

- List the common problems of aged skin;

- Define the pruritus;

- Identify factors that precipitate itching;

- Discuss the general principles in the management of pruritus;

- Describe the etiology of pressure ulcers;

- Identify risk factors for pressure ulcer development;

- Implement pressure ulcer preventive strategies;

- Discuss the basic principles of pressure ulcer management.

学习目标

学完本章节，应完成以下目标：

- 描述正常和老年人的皮肤结构之间的差异；

- 列举老年人皮肤的常见问题；

- 瘙痒的定义；

- 明确促进瘙痒的因素；

- 讨论瘙痒管理的一般原则；

- 描述压疮的病因；

- 明确压疮发展的危险因素；

- 实施压疮的预防策略；

- 讨论压疮管理的基本原则。

The skin is the protective outer covering of the body. Concerning its area and weight, it is the largest organ of the body. Serving as a barrier between the internal environment and the world outside, the skin has many functions including preventing fluid loss or dehydration, protecting the body from ultraviolet (UV) rays and other external environmental hazards, and protecting underlying organs from injury. As life expectancy increases, skin aging becomes a complex, multifactorial process accelerated by environmental, mechanical, or socioeconomic factors. Together these factors lead to cumulative alterations of skin structure, function and appearance. This chapter has three sections. First section reviews characteristics of aged skin; second and third sections discuss nursing care of elders with pruritus and pressure ulcers.

Box 17-1　Case Study

Mrs. Yang is 80 years old suffered a stroke two years ago. She is cared for by her daughter at home. Mrs. Yang is dependent for position changes and is unable to communicate her needs. She is unable to feed herself. She has a stage Ⅱ pressure ulcer on her sacrum.

Questions:

1. How to take care of Mrs. Yang's pressure ulcer on her sacrum?

2. What contents should be included in the teaching plan for her daughter?

Section 1　Characteristics of Aged Skin

The intrinsic structural changes of aged skin increase skin fragility, decrease the ability of the skin to heal, and produce aesthetically undesirable effects like wrinkling and uneven pigmentation. As aged patients represent a larger segment of the population, the skin aging problems deserve our attention.

皮肤是身体的保护外壳。就它的面积和重量而言，它是人体最大的器官。作为内部环境和外部世界之间的屏障，皮肤具有许多功能，包括防止水分流失或脱水，保护身体免受紫外线光的辐射和其他外部环境的危害，保护内在器官免受损伤。随着预期寿命的增加，皮肤的老化变成一个复杂的和多方面的过程，而且环境、机械或社会经济因素能加速这一过程。这些因素一起导致皮肤结构、功能和外观的累积改变。这一章包括三节内容：第一节回顾老年人皮肤的特点；第二和第三节讨论伴有瘙痒和压疮的老年人的护理。

Box 17-1　案例

杨女士，80岁，两年前卒中，在家由她的女儿照顾。杨女士不能独立变换体位，而且无法表达自己的需要，不能自行进食。在她的骶骨部位有一个Ⅱ期压疮。

问题：

1. 如何照料杨女士骶骨部位的压疮？

2. 在对她女儿的教学计划中，应包括什么内容？

第一节　老年人皮肤特点

老年人皮肤内在结构的变化可增加皮肤脆性、降低皮肤愈合的能力，并产生审美上的不良影响，如起皱和不均匀的色素沉着。随着年龄的增长，受环境、社会心理学等因素的影响，老年人皮肤的触觉、痛觉、温觉减弱，表面的反应性衰减、失调，对不良刺激的防御功能降低。老年人的皮肤老化问题值得我们关注。

I. Structure and Function of Normal Skin

The skin is commonly divided into three layers: epidermis, dermis, and hypodermis.

1. Epidermis The epidermis is the outermost layer of the skin. It is a dynamic system whose metabolic activity is largely regulated by the integrity of the permeability barrier, which is responsible for maintaining the fine balance between clinically normal and dry skin. This layer contains primarily keratinocytes which are completely replaced about every 30 days. The stratum corneum is a dynamic and metabolically interactive tissue comprised of about 60% structural proteins, 20% water, and 20% lipids. Skin is considered clinically dry when the moisture content falls below 10%, at which point the stratum corneum becomes less flexible and begins to crack or fissure. The primary function of the epidermis is to be a protective barrier.

2. Dermis The dermis is the most important part of the skin and is sometimes referred to as "true skin". It is a layer composed of strong connective tissues that contain the sweat glands, blood vessels, and nerve endings. The primary function of the dermis is to provide strength, support, moisture, blood, and oxygen to the skin. The dermis also protects the muscles, bones, and organs.

3. Hypodermis Below the dermis is the hypodermis, an innermost skin layer which binds the skin to internal organs. It is composed of adipose and connective tissue, which provides a cushion between skin layers, muscles, and bones. It is also in charge of thermoregulation and skin stability by connecting dermis to internal organs.

一、正常皮肤的结构和功能

皮肤由表皮、真皮、皮下组织三层组成，并含有附属器官（汗腺、皮脂腺、指甲、趾甲）以及血管、淋巴管、神经和肌肉等。

1. **表皮** 表皮是皮肤最外面的一层，平均厚度为 0.2mm，根据细胞的不同发展阶段和形态特点，由外向内可分为 5 层：角质层、透明层、颗粒层、棘细胞层和基底层。角质层由数层角化细胞组成，含有角蛋白。它能抵抗摩擦，防止体液外渗和化学物质内侵。角蛋白吸水力较强，一般含水量不低于 10%，以维持皮肤的柔润，如果低于此值，皮肤则干燥，出现鳞屑或皲裂。基底层由一层排列成栅状的圆柱细胞组成，此层细胞不断分裂，逐渐向上推移、角化、变形，形成表皮其他各层，最后角化脱落。基底细胞分裂后至脱落的时间，一般认为是 30 天，称为更替时间。基底细胞间夹杂着黑色素细胞，能产生黑色素，决定着皮肤颜色的深浅。表皮的主要功能是起保护屏障作用。

2. **真皮** 真皮位于表皮和皮下组织之间，由中胚层分化而来。真皮的主要成分为纤维、基质和细胞。纤维有胶原纤维、网状纤维和弹力纤维 3 种。其中胶原纤维是真皮结缔组织的主要成分。基质是水、电解质、营养物质和代谢产物进行交换的场所。真皮内还有血管、淋巴管、神经及皮肤附属器，如毛发、皮脂腺、大小汗腺及肌肉等。真皮是皮肤最重要的一部分，有时被称为"真正的皮肤"。真皮的主要功能是为皮肤提供力量、支持、水分、血液和氧气。真皮也保护肌肉、骨骼和器官。

3. **皮下组织** 位于真皮下方，由疏松结缔组织及脂肪小叶构成，其下紧邻肌膜。皮下组织中含有汗腺、毛根、血管、淋巴管及神经等。皮下组织的厚薄依年龄、性别、部位及营养状态而异，有防止散热、储备能量和抵御外来机械性冲击的功能。

II. Structural Changes in Aged Skin

Although skin is incredibly durable, it is affected, like all other organ systems, by aging. As the skin ages, changes are seen in skin thickness and quality of the epidermis and dermis as discussed later (box 17-2).

Box 17-2 Age-related Skin Changes

● Loss of thickness, elasticity, vascularity, which can delay the healing process and increase the skin tears and bruising.

● Decline of replacement rate of the stratum corneum which can slower the healing process and reduce barrier protection.

● Structure of sweat glands becomes distorted, numbers of functional sweat glands decreases.

● Decrease in number of blood vessels.

● Change in distribution of subcutaneous fat.

1. Skin thickness changes The skin thins progressively over adult life at a rate which accelerates with age. This change is most pronounced in exposed areas, including the face, neck, upper part of the chest, and the extensor surface of the hands and forearms. Epidermal thickness decreases about 6.4% per decade, and decreases even faster in females. Dermal thickness also decreases, but at the same rate in both genders.

2. Epidermal changes With the aging process, the replacement rate of the stratum corneum, the first layer of epidermis, declined by 50%. This decline results in slower healing and reduces barrier protection. A thinner epidermis allows more moisture to escape and may compound previously existing skin problems. The number of melanocytes decreases with age, providing older adults less protection from UV rays, paler skin, and graying hair. Melanocytes also produce uneven pigmentation, causing the development of lentigines, also known as "age spots" or "liver spots".

3. Dermal changes The decrease in dermal cells results in a reduced number of blood vessels, nerve endings, and collagen. These changes lead to diminished thermoregulatory function and inflammatory responses, decreased tactile sensation, reduced pain perception, and development of wrinkles.

二、老年人皮肤结构的变化

虽然皮肤非常持久耐用，但和所有的其他器官系统一样受衰老影响。随着皮肤的老化，老年人皮肤厚度以及表皮和真皮质量的发生变化，见 box 17–2。

Box 17-2 年龄相关的皮肤变化

● 厚度、弹性、血管分布的损失，可延迟愈合过程，增加皮肤的撕裂和擦伤。

● 角质层更新率的下降可以减慢愈合过程，减弱屏障的保护。

● 汗腺结构变得扭曲，功能性汗腺的数量减少。

● 血管数量减少。

● 皮下脂肪的分布改变。

1. 皮肤厚度的改变 皮肤厚度随着成年生活逐渐变薄，而且会随着年龄的增长加速。这种变化在裸露的部位最为明显，包括面部、颈部、上胸部以及手和前臂伸肌表面。表皮厚度每十年下降约 6.4%，并且在女性中下降更快。真皮厚度也下降，但男女下降速度相同。

2. 表皮的改变 随年龄的增长，表皮角质层的更新率减慢，导致愈合较慢和屏障保护功能减弱。表皮变薄可使水分流失更多，并可能加重之前存在的皮肤问题。随着年龄的增长，黑色素细胞数量减少，导致老年人紫外线抵抗力减弱，皮肤暗淡。黑色素细胞也产生不均匀的色素沉着，导致"雀斑"发展，也被称为"老年斑"或"肝斑"。

3. 真皮的改变 随着年龄增长，真皮乳头减少、变薄、萎缩。结缔组织减少，弹性纤维的弹性蛋白变性致使弹性纤维失去弹性，胶原纤维变得更坚实，导致皮肤松弛、弹性降低。此外，老年人皮肤毛细血管减少，皮

4. Hypodermal changes The overall volume of subcutaneous fat typically diminishes with age. Fat distribution changes as well. The fat in the face, hands, and feet decreases whereas a relative increase is observed in the thighs, waist, and abdomen. These changes decrease the cushioning function in the extremities.

III. Common Problems of Aged Skin

Because of these age-related changes in the skin structure, many problems occur among old adults, like pervasive dryness and itching, skin infection and pressure ulcer. In fact, most people over 65 have at least one skin disorder, and many have two or more.

Section 2　Care of Elderly with Pruritus

Pruritus (extremely itching skin) is a common skin problem in persons over the age of 65 years. Pruritus can have a profound impact on the quality of life in the elderly, especially through sleep deprivation. Nurses should take measures to identify the source of the pruritus, to relieve the symptom, and to prevent the secondary complications.

I. Etiology of Pruritus

Pruritus in elderly may result from a variety of etiologies. Xerosis (dry skin) is the most common cause of pruritus. As skin ages, the integumentary and vascular systems undergo atrophy, leading to suboptimal moisture retention. Other skin changes in elderly that may contribute to itch include decreased skin surface lipids, reduced sweat and sebum production, and diminished barrier repair.

A decline of normal immune function with aging also produces a higher incidence of autoimmune skin disorders

肤的体温调节功能下降；神经末梢的密度显著减少，故老年人皮肤感觉迟钝。

4. **皮下组织改变**　随年龄增长，皮下脂肪的含量逐渐减少，脂肪的分布也相应发生改变。面部、双手及双足的脂肪含量下降，然而大腿、腰部以及腹部的脂肪含量相对上升。这些改变降低了四肢末端皮下脂肪的缓冲作用。

三、老年人常见的皮肤问题

随着年龄增长，老年人的皮肤结构发生了很大变化。许多皮肤问题随之而来，如老年人皮肤干燥、瘙痒、皮肤感染以及压疮的发生。事实上，在 65 岁及以上的老年人中，大多患有一种皮肤病，有的甚至患有两种甚至更多。

第二节　老年人皮肤瘙痒的护理

皮肤瘙痒是 65 岁以上老年人常见的皮肤问题，皮肤瘙痒会产生睡眠剥夺，严重影响老年人的生活质量。护士应采取措施明确瘙痒的来源以缓解症状和防止继发性并发症。

一、皮肤瘙痒的病因

皮肤瘙痒可以由各种各样的原因导致，而皮肤干燥病是最常见的原因。随着皮肤的老化，表皮和血管系统开始萎缩，导致皮肤湿度下降。另外，皮肤老化导致的皮下脂肪含量减少、汗液分泌下降和屏障修复功能减弱也易引起瘙痒。

随着年龄增长，人体免疫功能下降，瘙痒性自体免疫性皮肤疾病（如大疱性类天疱

(e. g. , bullous pemphigoid and postherpeticneuralgia) that can induce pruritus. Certain cutaneous disorders such as atopicdermatitis and seborrheic dermatitis, and systemic disorders such as chronic kidney disease, hepatic dysfunction, hematologic disease, and endocrine disorders that are associated with pruritus are also more prevalent in elderly. Infectious etiologies of pruritus, including scabies and lice, may be more common in elderly, especially within institutionalized care settings. In addition, medications frequently used in this age group increase the possibility of drug-induced pruritus (e. g. , aspirin, opioids, and angiotensin converting enzyme inhibitors).

The mechanism of itching is not fully understood. Histamine is considered as a mediator of pruritus. Heat, sweating, sudden temperature changes, cleaning products, fatigue, and emotional stress can precipitate the itching, and itching can be more severe in winter.

II. Management of Pruritus

Physical and cognitive limitations, multiple diseases, and multiple medications affect the management of pruritus in the elderly. The management of pruritus in the elderly must be managed with a proven individualized management plan.

1. Assessment A full skin assessment is needed when an older adult complains of pruritus. The location, intensity, and onset of itching should be obtained by interviewing the older adult. The nurse should inquire about any patterns of behavior that induce itching such as anxiety, environmental exposures, and friction. Information about bathing practices and kinds of soaps, detergents, and skin products used should be obtained. The nurse should also check for the signs that suggest a skin disorder such as rashes, vesicles, scaling, and erythema.

2. Intervention There are a number of general measures in the management of pruritus in the elderly, irrespective of the underlying cause. Education is central to the management of pruritus. The older adult and family members should be taught about etiologic factors, the need to prevent skin trauma from scratching, and treatment measures to increase compliance and involvement in care. Identifying and removing aggravating factors are often the initial steps. Breaking the "itch-scratch" cycle is critical and simple measures, such as keeping finger nails short, may help to interrupt this cycle. Warmth can heighten the sensation of pruritus, thus, measures such

疮和带状疱疹后遗神经痛)的发生率增加。一些老年人常见的皮肤病变，如过敏性皮炎和脂溢性皮炎，或者机体器官功能失调，如慢性肾脏疾病、肝功能失调、血液系统疾病和内分泌失调等疾病都和皮肤瘙痒有着紧密的联系。在老年照顾机构常见的一些传染性皮肤病，如疥疮等也会引起皮肤瘙痒。另外某些药物也导致皮肤瘙痒(如阿司匹林、阿片类药物和血管紧张素转换酶抑制剂)。

目前，瘙痒的机制还不清楚，但认为组胺是中介物质。高热、出汗、突然的温度改变、清洁物品、疲劳、压力等都会诱发其产生，并且瘙痒在冬天会更严重。

二、皮肤瘙痒的管理

老年人身体和认知功能的受限、多种疾病、多种用药等影响着其皮肤瘙痒管理。老年人皮肤瘙痒的管理必须采取行之有效的个体化管理方案。

1. **评估** 对主诉有皮肤瘙痒症状的老年人进行评估非常必要。应询问老年人瘙痒的部位、强度、发生的时间，以及诱导瘙痒产生的原因，如焦虑、环境改变、摩擦等。还要收集老年人沐浴的方式、沐浴时使用的清洁产品等。护士还要检查皮肤是否有出疹、水疱、伤疤和红斑等。

2. **干预** 一般的皮肤瘙痒管理措施有很多，健康教育是重中之重。老人和家庭成员都应该了解皮肤瘙痒的病因、诱发因素、防止抓伤的必要性和治疗方法。明确和去除加重瘙痒的因素是干预的第一步，打破瘙痒-抓伤循环是关键，剪短指甲是防止抓伤最简单有效的方法。温暖会增强皮肤瘙痒的感觉，可以采用温水洗澡、穿轻便单薄的衣服、使用空调等保持皮肤凉爽。

as tepid showering, wearing light clothing, and the use of air conditioning should be undertaken to keep the skin cool. In order to maximize compliance and limit potential adverse drug reactions, simple topical regimens are preferable.

Moisturizers, emollients, and barrier repair creams are recommended to use, if dry skin is present with no lesions or erythema. These nonpharmacologic compounds help to prevent transepidermal water loss and possibly prevent the entry of irritants and other itch-causing agents, thus reduce pruritus through improving barrier function. Emollients should be applied at least twice daily and applied to moist skin immediately after bathing.

Topical antipruritic (e. g. , topical corticosteroids, menthol, and topical calcineurin inhibitors) and systemic antipruritic agent (e. g. , antihistamines and antidepressants) are also used to relieve itching. These treatments should be administered under a specialist setting and be used with caution to avoid the significant side-effects associated with these medications.

If pruritus is persistent, a diagnostic workup may be conducted to identify any systemic cause. If anxiety or stress is the source of itching, the nurse should assess the older adult's self-esteem and coping strategies and identify factors that may lead to anxiety or stress. The nurse should also discuss stress management strategies and assist to determine effective ones. A referral to a professional such as psychologist, or psychiatrist may be needed for continued guidance and support.

3. Prevention and care of dry skin Dry skin is the most common cause of itching in the elderly. Preventing dry skin is possible one of the effective strategies for managing pruritus. Meiner and Miller provide the following information about preventing and care of dry skin (box 17-3).

Box 17-3 Preventing and Care of Dry Skin

1. Include adequate amounts of fluid in the daily diet. Drink at least 1 500 to 2 500 ml of water a day if not contraindicated by other medical conditions.

2. Use humidifiers to maintain environmental humidity levels of 40% to 60%.

3. Bathing or showering with warm water should not exceed a frequency of every other day. Pat skin dry and avoid brisk drying with a towel. Bath oil can be used in a

如果皮肤干燥，在没有皮肤破损和红斑的情况下，可以使用保湿剂、润肤油、面霜等保持皮肤湿润。这些非药物的混合物有助于防止皮肤的水分丢失，可能防止刺激物和其他引起瘙痒的物质进入，从而通过改善屏障功能减少瘙痒。每天至少两次涂抹润滑油，并且洗澡后立刻使用。

必要时可使用局部止痒剂（如糖皮质激素、薄荷醇、局部钙调磷酸酶抑制剂）或系统止痒剂（如抗组胺药和抗抑郁药）来止痒，但应在专业人员的指导下应用以防止药物的副作用。

如果瘙痒很顽固，应进行系统的全身检查。如果焦虑和压力是导致瘙痒的原因，护士应该评估老年人对于焦虑和压力的自我概念和应对策略以及明确可能导致焦虑或压力的因素。护士应帮助老年人选择有效的压力应对策略。

3. 干燥皮肤的护理和预防 皮肤干燥是老年人发生皮肤瘙痒最常见的原因，预防皮肤干燥是皮肤瘙痒管理的必要措施。Meiner 和 Miller 总结了预防和护理干燥皮肤的方法（box 17–3）。

Box 17–3 干燥皮肤的预防和护理

1. 适当的液体摄入，在没有禁忌的情况下每天至少喝 1 500～2 500ml 的水。

2. 使用加湿器使环境湿度达到 40%～60%。

3. 最多每隔一天用温水洗澡一次，轻轻拍干皮肤而不要用浴巾擦干，洗澡后用护肤油。

basin when sponge bathing but not in the tub or shower. Apply oil after bathing.

4. Avoid the use of harsh soaps; instead use a superfatted soap in limited quantities with only one lathering.

5. Apply moisturizing lotions twice daily or as needed. Use heavy emollient lotions or creams containing urea or lactic acid after bathing when skin is moist.

6. Never use alcohol, perfumes or other drying rubs on skin.

7. Avoid tight-fitting clothes that rub against the skin.

The management of pruritus in the elderly poses a particular challenge because of the multitude of variables that come with advanced age. Physical and cognitive limitations, multiple comorbid conditions, and polypharmacy are factors that influence the management in this age group. Management must take an individualistically tailored approach with consideration of the older adults' general health, the severity of symptoms, and the adverse effects of treatment.

Section 3　Care of the Elderly with Pressure Ulcers

National Pressure Ulcer Advisory Panel defined apressure ulcer as a "localized injury to the skin and/or underlying tissue, usually over a bony prominence, as a result of pressure or pressure in combination with shear and/or friction". Elders who have mobility or activity limitations increase the risk of development of pressure ulcers and this risk is a major problem with far-reaching negative functional consequences. As the incidence of pressure ulcer increases, the serious consequences of pressure ulcers have been increasing attention in recent years. Preventing pressure ulcers in acute settings has been a major focus of quality improvement programs and identifying pressure ulcers has been a quality indicator for long-term care facilities. Many clinical practice guidelines on prevention and treatment pressure ulcers were published. Most recently published guidelines were the evidenced-based guidelines developed by the NPUAP in collaboration with the European Pressure Ulcer Advisory Panel (EPUAP) in 2009. These guidelines continue to be the recommended guides for pressure ulcers.

4. 避免使用刺激性的肥皂，使用含油脂多的清洁用品。

5. 每天两次使用保湿乳液或按需使用，在洗澡后使用强效的润肤乳或含尿素和乳酸的润肤用品。

6. 不要使用酒精或香水等导致皮肤干燥的物品。

7. 避免穿紧身衣或摩擦力强的衣服。

由于年老伴随大量变化，对老年人瘙痒的管理提出了特别的挑战。老年人身体和认知功能的受限、多种疾病、多种用药等影响着其皮肤瘙痒管理。老年人皮肤瘙痒的管理必须采取考虑到老年人的健康状况、症状的严重程度和治疗副作用的个体化的管理方案。

第三节　老年人压疮的护理

美国压疮咨询委员会将压疮（又称压力性溃疡）定义为：由压力或压力联合剪切力和摩擦力造成的皮肤和／或深层组织的局部损伤，以骨隆突处多见。活动受限的老年人发生压疮的危险增加，对躯体功能的影响严重。压疮所耗费的资源巨大，逐渐引起人们的重视，预防压疮成为照护机构的重要质量指标。由美国国家压疮控制小组与欧洲压疮控制小组在 2009 年联合制订的预防和治疗压疮的临床实践指南是目前广为接受和应用的指南。

I. Epidemiology of Pressure Ulcers

Lyder and Ayello reported an almost 80% increase in pressure ulcers in hospitalized patients between 1993 and 2006. In hospitals, the incidence of pressure ulcers ranges from 2.7% to 60% and the prevalence rate ranges from 3.5% to 29.5%, while in long-term care facilities, the prevalence rate of pressure ulcers ranges from 2.4% to 23%. Because of the heterogeneous case-mix and staffing patterns, the incidence rates vary among nursing facilities.

II. Etiology of Pressure Ulcers

The development of pressure ulcers is a complex process involving many variables. The intensity of pressure leading to capillary closure, combined with the duration of pressure and tissue tolerance, results in tissue anoxia, ischemia, edema, and eventually tissue necrosis. Risk factors for unrelieved pressure include immobility, decreased activity, and decreased sensory perception. Factors influencing tissue tolerance include extrinsic factor (e. g. , friction, shearing, and moisture) and intrinsic factors (e. g. , advanced age, nutrition, hypotension, skin temperature, emotional stress, and smoking).

Pressure ulcers usually begin at the point of contact between soft tissue and a bony prominence or other hard surface. As a result, an upside-down cone-shaped wound with the largest area of breakdown being near the bone develops. The sacrum (in a supine position), ischial tuberosity (in an upright sitting position), lateral malleolus and trochanter (in a lateral position), and heels (in a supine position) are the common bony prominences susceptible to pressure ulcers development.

The incidence of pressure ulcers is increased in elderly, particularly in those over 70 years old. Tangalos reported seventy percent of pressure ulcers occur in persons older than 70 years. With aging, thickness of the epidermis and dermis decreases, elasticity decreases, dermal–epidermal junction flattens, and vessels degenerate. These age-related changes increase the susceptibility of older skin to injury and the effects of mechanical stress, impair the early warning sign of erythema, delay early immunologic responses, and hinder the healing process. Thus the elders are at risk for the development of pressure ulcers.

一、压疮的流行病学特点

Lyder 和 Ayello 报道在 1993 至 2006 年间，住院患者中压疮增长了近 80%。压疮在医院的发生率在 2.7%～60% 之间，流行率在 3.5%～29.5% 之间，在长期照护机构，流行率在 2.4%～23% 之间。由于护理机构间的病例组合和人员配置模式存在差异，其发病率各不相同。

二、压疮的病因学特点

压疮的发展是一个复杂的过程。压力、施压时间和组织耐受力是形成压疮的基本原因。超常的压力使毛细血管收缩，组织缺氧，局部水肿，最终导致组织坏死形成溃疡。压力的风险因素包括长期卧床、缺乏运动、感觉减退。影响组织耐受力的因素包括外在因素（如摩擦力、剪切力和湿度）和内在因素（如高龄、营养、低血压、皮肤温度、压力和吸烟）。

压疮通常发生在软组织和骨隆突出的连接处或其他坚硬的表面。因此，在骨附近形成了具有最大损伤面积的倒置的锥形伤口。骶骨（仰卧位），坐骨结节（直立坐位），外踝和转子（侧卧位）和脚跟（仰卧位）是常见的容易发生压疮的骨隆突出部位。

老年人压疮的发生率在增加，特别是 70 岁以上的老年人。Tangalos 报道 70% 的压疮发生在 70 岁以上的老年人。随着年龄增加，表皮和真皮的厚度减少，弹性降低，真皮和表皮的连接趋于平缓，血管退化。这些和年龄相关的变化可增加老年皮肤对损伤和机械压力影响的易感性，损害早期警告信号、延迟早期免疫反应和阻碍康复过程。因此老年人压疮发生的风险增高。

III. Risk Assessment Tools

In order to successfully prevent pressure ulcers, early identification of at-risk elders is essential. It has been well recognized that a risk assessment should be conducted on all persons who are bed-bound, chair-bound, frail, disabled, incontinent, nutritionally compromised, or having altered mental status. Identified high-risk persons should be reassessed at regular intervals if mobility or activity is impaired.

Numerous instruments have been developed to identify at-risk individuals for pressure ulcer formation. The Braden and Norton tools are used frequently in the clinical setting in predicting individuals at risk for pressure ulcers. The two assessment tools have been subjected to vigorous evaluation of reliability and validity testing.

The Norton scale was developed in the late 1950s and was disseminated in 1962. It was the first pressure ulcers risk assessment tool designed for use in a geriatric nursing study. The Norton scale has five assessment categories: physical condition, mental condition, activity, mobility, and incontinence. In a later study, Norton suggested that nutritional status as an important parameter would have to include in the risk assessment. Individuals with a total score of 16 or lower are considered to be at risk for pressure ulcer development.

The Braden scale for predicting pressure sore risk is commonly used risk assessment tool and extensive testing supports its validity and reliability. This tool is recommended by the Hartford Institute for Geriatric Nursing as the best practice for identifying elders who are at risk for the development of pressure ulcers. The Braden scale includes six subscales of sensory perception, skin moisture, activity, mobility, nutrition, and friction and shear. Individuals scoring 15-18 on the Braden scale are considered to be at risk; scoring 13-14 at moderate risk; scoring 10-12 at high risk, and scoring less than 9 at severe risk.

IV. Pressure Ulcer Prevention

Pressure ulcers are costly health problems that adversely affect elders' quality of life. The geriatric nurse has responsibility to identify elders at risk for pressure ulcers and to implement evidence-based preventive strategies to against pressure ulcers. Pressure ulcer prevention includes the following aspects:

三、压疮的危险评估工具

早期发现高危人群是成功预防压疮的关键。对于长期卧床、长期使用轮椅、身体虚弱、残疾、尿失禁、营养缺乏者或精神障碍者都要进行危险评估。被识别的高危人员应定期重新评估移动或活动是否受损。

许多工具已被开发用于评估压疮发生的高危人群。Braden 和 Norton 量表是经过信效度检验，目前临床上应用最为广泛的危险评估工具。

Norton 量表发展于 1950 年代末期，于 1962 年广泛使用。这是首个在老年护理研究中使用的压疮风险评估工具。该量表包含 5 个维度：一般状况、精神状况、活动能力、运动能力和大小便失禁。在以后的研究中，Norton 认为营养状况作为一个重要的参数必须包含在风险评估中。总分在 16 分及以下提示有发生压疮的危险。

Braden 量表是一个广泛使用，且信效度得到大量试验检验的风险评估工具，被 Hartford 老年护理研究院推荐为评估老年人压疮危险的最佳量表。Braden 量表包含 6 个维度：感知觉能力、皮肤潮湿度、活动能力、运动能力、营养状况及摩擦力和剪切力。总分在 15～18 分提示有危险，13～14 分为中度危险，10～12 分为高度危险，9 分及以下为极度危险。

四、压疮的预防

压疮这一健康问题花费较大，严重影响老年人的生活质量。老年科护士有责任明确老年人的压疮风险，并实施以证据为基础的预防性策略来防止压疮发生。压疮的预防包括以下几个方面：

1. Risk assessment   Nurses should assess all elders who are bed-bound or chair-bound, incontinent, nutritional compromised, or whose ability to reposition is impaired, or mental status decreased at the time of admission to health care facilities using Norton scale or Braden scale. When elders are identified as being at risk, reassessment should be conducted at regular intervals and a prevention plan should be developed and implemented. The care plan should be modified according to the individual factors.

2. Skin care   All elders identified as being at risk should have a daily skin inspection with close attention to bony prominences. Signs other than redness (e. g., localized heat, edema, and induration) should be assessed for darkly pigmented skin. The skin of an incontinent elder should be cleansed with a mild and nonirritating cleanser using warm water at the time of soiling. Topical barriers (e. g., zinc oxide) can be applied after cleansing and gently drying the skin. Absorbent underpads or diapers can be used to maintain a dryer skin surface. For dry skin, moisturizers should be used to keep the skin from drying and cracking. Skin should not be rubbed or massaged over bony prominences. Proper turning, transferring, and positioning should be used to minimize skin injury from friction or shearing forces.

3. Nutrition monitoring   Nutritional status should be closely monitored by assessing caloric intake, weight, hemoglobin, hematocrit, levels of serum albumin and cholesterol, and total lymphocyte count (TLC). Diets high in protein, carbohydrates, and vitamins are necessary to maintain and promote tissue growth. Nutritional supplementation or support is considered for nutritionally compromised elders. Low levels of serum protein, cholesterol, and TLC are associated with malnutrition and pressure ulcer development. Therefore a serum albumin level below 30 g/L, cholesterol level below 1.5 g/L, and a TLC below 1 200/mm^3 warrant aggressive nutritional support. Hydration status should also be monitored because dehydration can contribute to pressure ulcer development. An elder requires a minimum of 2 000 to 2 500 ml of water daily unless contraindicated.

4. Mechanical loading and support surfaces The AHCPR clinical guidelines suggest reposition bedbound persons at least every 2 hours and chair-bound persons every hour. However, capillary closing pressure varies with each individual, the turning schedule should be determined based on development of erythema. Elders should be turned only at a 30-degree obliqueangle to decrease pressure intensity over the trochanter and lateral

1. 危险评估　护士应该在老年人进入卫生保健机构时，使用 Norton 量表或 Braden 量表评估所有卧床不起或坐轮椅的、大小便失禁、营养受损、体位改变能力受损或精神状态下降的老年人。当老年人被评估为有风险时，应定期重新评估，并制订和实施预防计划。根据个体情况调整护理方案。

2. 皮肤护理　对高危老年患者，应每天评估皮肤情况，特别是骨隆突处。除了发红处，应评估皮肤颜色较深的迹象（如局部发热、水肿和硬结）。有大小便失禁的患者应采用中性的、无刺激性的清洁剂和温水进行污物清洗。在清洗后可使用皮肤保护剂（如氧化锌软膏），并轻轻地擦干皮肤。也可使用吸水性敷料或尿布来保持皮肤干燥。对于干性皮肤，应该使用保湿霜防止皮肤干燥和皲裂。避免按摩骨隆突上脆弱的皮肤。在给患者翻身和更换体位时，采用合适的技术减少皮肤的摩擦力和剪切力。

3. 营养监测　应该通过评估摄入的卡路里量、体重、血红蛋白、血细胞比容、血清白蛋白和胆固醇水平和总淋巴细胞计数（TLC）密切监测营养状况。富含蛋白质、碳水化合物、维生素的饮食是维持和促进组织生长所必需的。营养不良的老年患者，可食用营养补充剂。低水平的血清蛋白、胆固醇和 TLC 与营养不良和压疮的发展相关。因此，血清白蛋白水平低于 30g/L，胆固醇水平低 1.5g/L，TLC 低于 1 200/mm^3 时需要积极的营养支持。因为脱水会导致压疮发展，所以应监测水合状态。除非有禁忌证，老年人每天至少需要 2 000 ～ 2 500ml 水。

4. 避免局部组织长期受压　美国卫生保健政策研究所临床指南建议卧床不起的人至少每隔 2 小时改变一次体位，坐轮椅的人每 1 小时改变一次体位。然而，每个人毛细血管关闭的压力不同，应依据红斑的发展确定翻身的频率。老年人应在倾斜 30° 的角度上翻身，以减少大转子和外侧踝部骨隆突处的压

malleolus prominences. Pillows should be placed under the calves to lift the feet and heels off the bed to decrease pressure intensity on the heels. Other devices can also be used to suspend the heel, maintain or correct foot-ankle position, and protect the elder from neurosensory damage. The nurse should use lifting devices (e. g. bed linen or trapeze) to move rather than drag persons during transfers and position changes. To minimize shearing forces, the nurse should not elevate the head of the bed greater than 30 degrees and should last for as short a time as possible.

At-risk elders should be placed on a pressure-reducing device such as mattress overlays, chair cushions or overlays, and specialized beds to prevent pressure ulcer development by decreasing pressure intensity. When using these pressure reducing devices, their negative effects should be considered. For example, the mattress overlays may increase the height of the bed, making it more difficult to get in and out of bed; may decrease the protective height of bed side rails; may trap moisture and heat, which can be uncomfortable. Furthermore, these devices do not eliminate the need for meticulous nursing care; therefore elders must still be repositioned, assessed, and kept clean and dry.

5. Education　Structured, organized, and comprehensive educational programs for the prevention of pressure ulcers should be developed for all levels of health care providers, elders, family, and caregivers. Information on etiology of and risk factors for pressure ulcers, risk assessment tools, skin assessment, and preventive strategies should be included in the educational programs.

V. Pressure Ulcer Management

The management of pressure ulcers requires interdisciplinary collaboration. Nurses play a key role and as an expert in pressure ulcer management. Meiner indicates three basic principles guiding successful pressure ulcer management: a. minimize or eliminate precipitating factors such as pressure, friction, and shearing; b. monitor nutritional status and provide nutritional support; and c. create and maintain a clean, moist wound environment with adequate oxygenation and circulation. Information related to the first two principals have discussed in pressure ulcer prevention and those preventive measures also apply to treatment. The following discussion focuses on pressure ulcer wound care.

力强度。枕头应该置于小腿下，从床上抬起足部和脚跟，以减少脚跟的压力强度。其他设备也可以用于悬空脚跟，保持或纠正脚踝位置，防止老年人感觉神经的损伤。在转移位置和变换体位时，护士应该使用提升装置（如床单或吊带）移动，而不是拖拽患者。为了减少剪切力，护士在提升床头时，不应该使床的倾斜度超过30°，而且应尽可能减少提升的时间。

应该将高危老年人置于一个减压设备上，如床垫、椅垫或覆盖物，以及专门通过减少压力强度防止压疮发展的床。当使用这些减压设备时，应考虑它们的负面影响。例如，床垫可能增加床的高度，增加了上床和下床的困难；可能减少了床栏杆的防护高度；可能不利于水分与热量的散发，使患者感到不舒服。此外，这些设备并不能排除细致的护理，因此老年人仍需要改变体位、评估、保持清洁和干燥。

5. 健康教育　对老年患者和照顾者进行综合的健康教育，教育内容应包括压疮的发生、发展和预防的一般知识，评估工具、皮肤自身评估的方法等。指导患者和照顾者学会预防压疮的方法，鼓励他们经常进行皮肤检查，如发现异常，及时告知医护人员。

五、压疮的管理

压疮的管理要求各学科间的协作，护士作为该领域的专家扮演着重要的角色，Meiner提出了压疮管理的三大基本原则：①减小或消除压力、摩擦力、剪切力等危险因素；②监控营养状况并提供营养支持；③创造和维持一个干净的、湿润的、有利于愈合的伤口环境。前两项原则已在预防措施中进行了讨论，下面重点讨论压疮伤口的护理。

1. Assessment　Assessment of an established pressure ulcer involves a complete medical evaluation including the onset and duration of ulcers, risk factors, previous wound care, health problems and medications, psychological health, behavioral and cognitive status, social and financial resources, and access to caregivers. The nurse should examine the ulcers, noting the number, location, size (length, width, and depth) and color of ulcers; any discharge, bleeding, or odor; presence of sinus tracts; necrosis or eschar formation, tunneling, or undermining; pain or tenderness; amount of erythema surrounding the wound edges, healing (granulation and epithelialization), and wound margins. Most importantly, the nurse should determine the stage of each ulcer.

The internationally used staging system for pressure ulcers includes four stages. In 2007, the NPUAP added the term category to each stage Ⅰ-Ⅳ and two additional stages to the system. Following describes and illustrates the six pressure ulcer stages:

(1)Suspected deep tissue injury: Purple or maroon localized area of discolored intact skin or blood-filled blister resulting from damage to underlying soft tissue from pressure or shear. The area may be preceded by tissue that is painful, firm, mushy, boggy, warmer or cooler when compared to adjacent tissue. Deep tissue injury may be difficult to detect in persons with dark skin tones.

(2) Stage/category Ⅰ-non-blanchable erythema: Intact skin with non-blanchable redness of a localized area, usually occurs over a bony prominence. Darkly pigmented skin may not have visible blanching, and its color may differ from the surrounding area. The affected tissue may be painful, firm, soft, or warmer or cooler compared to adjacent tissue.

(3) Stage/category Ⅱ-partial thickness: Partial thickness loss of dermis appears as a shallow open ulcer with a red pink wound bed, without slough. It may also appear as an intact or open/ruptured serum-filled blister. This category should not be used to describe skin tears, tape burns, perineal dermatitis, maceration or excoriation.

(4) Stage/category Ⅲ-fullthickness tissue: Loss subcutaneous fat may be visible but bone, tendon or muscle is not exposed. Slough may be present but does not obscure the depth of tissue loss. It may include undermining and tunneling. The depth of a stage Ⅲ pressure ulcer varies by location from shallow (e. g. , on

1. 压疮的评估　完整的评估包括溃疡的发生和持续时间、危险因素、先前的伤口护理、目前的健康问题和用药、心理健康、行为、认知状况、社会和经济状况以及照顾者等。护士应该检查和记录溃疡的数目、位置、大小（长度、宽度、深度）和溃疡的颜色；有无分泌物、出血和气味；是否存在静脉窦、坏疽或焦痂、瘘管或窦道；疼痛或压痛；伤口边界红斑的范围、愈合情况（肉芽和上皮形成）和伤口的边界。另外，还应判断伤口的分期阶段。

国际上将压疮分为 4 期。2007 年，美国压疮咨询委员会扩展了四期分类法，并新添加了 2 个期。以下描述和阐明了压疮的 6 个阶段：

（1）疑似深部组织损伤期：由于压力和剪切力造成皮下软组织受损，在完整的皮肤上出现紫色或者褐红色的局部变色区域，或形成充血性水疱。与邻近组织相比，该区域的组织可能会先出现疼痛、硬肿、糊状、潮湿、皮温较冷或较热等表象。

（2）阶段 / 分类Ⅰ——不可变色的红斑：局部区域的皮肤完整，发红，但按压不变白，通常在骨隆突出处发生。肤色较深的皮肤可能不易看见皮肤变白，并且它的颜色可能不同于周围部分。相比邻近组织，受影响的组织可能会感到疼痛、僵硬、柔软、皮温升高或降低。

（3）阶段 / 分类Ⅱ——部分厚度：部分真皮层缺失，出现带有粉红色创面的表浅的开放型溃疡，底部无坏死组织；也可以表现为完整的皮肤或已破损的充满血清的水疱。此期不能被用来描述皮肤撕裂、烫伤、会阴部皮炎、浸渍、抓痕等。

（4）阶段 / 分类Ⅲ——全层组织丢失：皮下脂肪层可见，但是骨、肌腱或肌肉尚未暴露，可有坏死组织但组织缺失的深度未知，此期也可包括瘘管和隧道。Ⅲ期压力性溃疡的深度随解剖部位的表浅（如鼻子、耳朵、

nose, ear, occiput, malleolus) to very deep where there is significant adiposity.

(5) Stage/category IV-full thickness tissue loss with exposed bone, tendon or muscle: Slough or eschar may be present on some parts of the wound bed. It often includes undermining and tunneling. Depth of a stage IV pressure ulcer varies by location from shallow to deep, and may extend into muscle and/or supporting structures (e. g., fascia, tendon or joint capsule), making osteomyelitis possible. Exposed bone/tendon is visible or directly palpable.

(6) Unstageable/unclassified: Full thickness tissue loss in which the base of the ulcer is covered by slough (yellow, tan, gray, green or brown) or eschar (tan, brown or black) in the wound bed. The true depth cannot be determined until enough slough and/or eschar is removed to expose the base of the wound. Stable (i. e., dry, adherent, intact without erythema or fluctuance) eschar on the heels should not be removed because it is protective.

In individuals with dark skin pigmentation, a stage I ulcer may appear as a persistent red, blue, or purple discoloration. If an ulcer is covered with eschar, a stage/category cannot be determined until the eschar is removed to expose the base of the wound. Ulcers do not progress through stages in formation or healing.

Assessment of the wound should be on an ongoing basis and supported with documentation. The NPUAP recommends the use of the pressure ulcer scale for Healing (PUSH) tool for assessing changes in pressure ulcers. The PUSH tool scores pressure ulcers according to size, exudates, and tissue type and changes in the PUSH score over time indicates the progression or regression of the pressure ulcer. All new pressure ulcers wounds should be described (i. e., location, color, discharge, tenderness, and stage) and measured. The measurements should include length, width, and depth. The nurse should measure undermining using a cotton-tipped applicator, marking depth on the applicator, and placing it next to a tape measure to obtain dimension. The position of undermining should also be noted (e. g., 3cm at 2 o'clock).

2. Management of infections A wound infection exists if the pressure ulcer has a pale wound bed, pus, increased tenderness, persistent exudate. The nurse should obtain a culture first. The EPUAP-NPUAP treatment guidelines recommend obtaining a tissue biopsy or quantitative swab technique for pressure ulcer

枕部、脚踝部）和脂肪肥厚的深部区域而异。

（5）阶段/分类IV——全层组织丢失伴随骨骼、肌腱或肌肉暴露：创面可出现坏死组织和焦痂，通常存在瘘管和隧道。IV期压疮的深度随解剖部位的表浅和深度而异，可能延伸至肌肉或支持结构（如筋膜、肌腱或关节囊）而并发骨髓炎。暴露的骨头或肌腱明显可见。

（6）不可分的/无类别的组织——全层缺损：溃疡的创面床上完全被坏死组织（黄色、褐色、灰色、绿色或棕褐色）或焦痂（褐色、棕褐色、黑色）所覆盖。除非彻底清除坏死组织和焦痂以暴露出创面基底部，否则无法确定溃疡的深度。不应该清除足跟部稳固的焦痂（如干燥的、附着紧密的、完整无红肿或波动感），因为它相当于机体的保护屏障。

在肤色较深的人中，I期压疮可能出现持续的红色、蓝色或紫色变色。如果溃疡覆盖着焦痂，除非彻底清除焦痂以暴露出创面基底部，否则无法确定溃疡的阶段或分期。溃疡在形成或愈合阶段不会进展。

溃疡伤口的评估是一个持续的过程并且要进行记录。美国压疮咨询委员会建议使用压疮愈合量表（PUSH）评估压疮的变化。该工具根据压疮的大小、渗出液和组织类型给压疮计分，得分随时间的变化可表明压疮的进展和好转。所有新发的压疮伤口都应该进行描述（如位置、颜色、液体、软度和阶段）和测量。测量应包括长度、宽度和深度。护士应该使用棉签测量瘘管，标记棉签的深度，并在旁边放置一个卷尺来获取尺寸。瘘管的位置也应该记录（如2点钟方向3cm）。

2. 感染的管理 如果压疮创面苍白，有脓液，压痛增加，渗出物增多，则存在伤口感染。护士应该了解欧洲压疮咨询委员会和美国压疮咨询委员会的治疗指南推荐获得组织活检或定量拭子技术鉴定感染。然后局部

cultures. Then the infected wound is managed topically with antiseptics or systemically depending on the severity and risk of osteomyelitis. Regarding the use of antiseptic solutions (e. g. providone-iodine or acetic acid), there is great controversy because of their cytotoxic effects. The keys to successful use of antiseptic solutions are using only when the wound is obviously infected, dilution, short-term use (e. g. , 3-5 days) and never using on a healthy, granulating wound bed.

3. Debridement　Debridement is the removal of necrotic tissue, exudate, and metabolic waste from a wound. Necrotic tissue promotes bacterial growth and impairs wound healing, and it should be debrided as soon as possible. Measures such as wet-to-dry dressings or topical antimicrobials should be taken to resolve bacterial insults until purulent discharge has dissipated. Dry and hard eschar which slows the migration of epithelial cells and delays healing should be considered to remove, however, heel ulcers that have stable, dry eschar without edema, erythema, fluctuance, or drainage should be left intact. If the elder has diabetes with a dry and hard intact eschar, the eschar may be left in place prudently and must be monitored.

Debridement methods include mechanical, autolytic, chemical, and surgical. Mechanical debridement is effective for removing slimy or stringy exudates. It includes wet-to-dry dressings, hydrotherapy, wound irrigation, and whirlpool bath debridement. Wet-to-dry dressings adhere to devitalized tissue, which is removed with dressing changes. The nurse should protect wound borders from maceration with zinc oxide or stoma adhesive when using wet-to-dry dressings because viable tissue may also be removed. Hydrotherapy via whirlpool bath debridement or irrigation may loosen debris and should be reserved for large, exuding wounds. Mechanical debridement may be painful and may destroy fragile epithelial cells; therefore, a more efficient method should be sought first.

Autolytic debridement uses the body's own enzymes and moisture to re-hydrate, soften, and liquefy hard eschar and slough. It is useful for removing stringy slough when less than half of the wound bed is involved and the wound is not infected. Autolytic debridement can be achieved with the use of hydrocolloid, hydrogel, and transparent film dressings. Autolytic debridement is selective and only necrotic tissue is liquefied; however, it takes longer to be effective.

Chemical debridement involves the topical use of enzymatic gels and solutions to dissolve necrotic tissue

使用消毒剂管理感染的伤口，根据骨髓炎的风险和严重程度进行系统治疗。关于使用消毒液（如聚维酮碘或醋酸）有很大的争议，因为其具有细胞毒作用。只有当伤口有明显的感染时才可以使用消毒液，并且需要稀释和短期应用（如3~5天），避免在正常的、有肉芽生长的疮面使用。

3. 清创术　清创术是为了去除坏死组织、分泌物和伤口代谢产生的废物。坏死组织促进细菌的生长并阻碍伤口的愈合，应尽快清除。应采取干燥敷料或局部抗菌剂的措施解决细菌的侵害，直到脓性分泌物消散。干的和硬的焦痂减缓了上皮细胞的迁移，延误愈合，应该考虑去除；但是，如果足跟溃疡有稳定的、干的焦痂，没有水肿、红斑、波动或渗出液，应保持其完整性。如果老年糖尿病患者有干的、硬的、完整的焦痂，焦痂可谨慎保留在原处，并且必须严密观察。

清创术的方法有机械式、自溶式、化学式和外科手术式清创。机械式清创适用于除去黏性分泌物。它包括干燥敷料，水疗，伤口灌洗和漩涡浴清创术。干燥敷料依附于衰亡组织，可随敷料的变化而移除。护士在使用干燥敷料时应该保护伤口边界避免氧化锌或气孔黏合剂的浸渍，因为可再生的组织也可能被移除。通过漩涡浴的水疗清创或灌溉可能松开碎片组织，应该用于较大的、有渗液的伤口。因机械式清创可能会有疼痛感，会破坏脆弱的上皮细胞，应首先考虑其他更为有效的清创方法。

自溶式清创术使用人体自身的酶和水分重新水合，软化和溶解焦痂和蜕皮，此法对于没有感染的伤口清除分泌物十分有效。自溶式清创术可以使用水胶体，水凝胶和透明膜敷料实现。自溶式清创术选择性强，只作用于坏死组织，但起效时间较长。

化学式清创术采用局部使用酶凝胶和溶液的方法来溶解坏死组织。它主要是家中或

from the wound. It is primarily used in the home setting or long-term-care facility where surgery is not an option. Chemical debridement is effective for removing yellow, tender eschar that is difficult to remove surgically. When used, the chemical enzyme should be limited to the area of necrosis or slough because the enzyme may destroy granulation tissue and epithelial cells.

Surgical debridement is needed if infection occurs or to remove thick and extensive eschar. Surgical debridement using a sterile scalpel or scissors may be performed at bedside or in the operating room if more extensive debridement needed. Surgical debridement is very selective and fast, but painful. After surgical debridement, the nurse should apply wet-to-dry dressings moistened with an antiseptic every shift for 1 to 3 days to prevent infection.

4. Woundcleansing Wound cleansing helps optimize the healing environment and decreases the potential for infection by loosening and washing away debris such as bacteria, exudate, purulent material and residual topical agents from previous dressings. Pressure ulcer wounds should be cleansed initially and with each dressing change. Devices such as a catheter-tip syringe, butterfly tubing with the needle cut off and connected to a Luer-Lok syringe, or a syringe with a 19-gauge needle are recommended to use to irrigate the wounds gently. Use of normal saline (20-50 ml per time) is preferred. Wound cleansing with antiseptic agents (e. g. , povidone-iodine, hydrogen peroxide, acetic acid, and sodium hypochlorite) should be avoided because they are cytotoxic and destroy granulation tissue.

5. Wound dressings Dressings that maintain a moist wound environment facilitate wound healing and can be used for pressure ulcers treatment. There are numerous dressing options; therefore the nurse should understand the healing trajectory and select the best treatment option based on clinical judgments and wound characteristics. Synthetic dressings are often used because they reduce caregiver time, cause less discomfort, and provide more consistent moisture. Synthetic dressings include transparent films, hydrogels, hydrocolloids, alginates, and foams. Transparent films effectively retain moisture, and are used for stage Ⅰ or Ⅱ pressure ulcers. They are also used to secure dressings, protect vulnerable areas from friction, and facilitate autolysis. Transparent films are semipermeable allowing exchange of air, thus do not use to cover enzymatic debriding agents, gels, or ointments. Transparent films can be left on for 3 to 7 days with checking at least once a day.

长期照护机构中的非手术选择。对于外科手术难以移除的黄色、柔软的焦痂很有效。在应用时，应注意将酶仅限于坏死组织，因为酶会破坏肉芽组织和上皮细胞。

如果有感染或要移除大面积的焦痂时应采用外科手术式清创。手术清创需使用无菌手术刀或剪刀，可以在床边进行，如果需要更广泛的清创术，则在手术室中进行。外科清创术具有快速、选择性强的优点，但是患者的疼痛比较明显。手术清创后，护士应每隔1～3天使用一次用消毒剂润湿的干燥敷料，以防止感染。

4. 伤口清洁 伤口清洁有助于促进愈合环境，并通过松开和洗去碎片物质，如细菌、渗出物、脓性物质和以前的敷料中残留的局部药剂，减少感染的可能性。压疮的伤口应在最初和每次换药时进行清洁。推荐使用导管尖端注射器，具有切断的针头并连接到Luer-Lok注射器的蝶形管或19号针的注射器等装置轻轻地冲洗伤口。优选使用生理盐水（每次20～50ml）。应避免使用消毒剂（例如聚维酮碘，过氧化氢，乙酸和次氯酸钠）清洁伤口，因为它们具有细胞毒性，并能破坏肉芽组织。

5. 伤口敷料 敷料可以维持伤口的湿润并促进伤口愈合，可以用于压疮的治疗。有很多敷料可以备选，因此护士应该针对临床诊断和伤口情况做出最优的选择。合成敷料因其减少照护时间、降低不舒适感，并能提供持续的湿润环境而常被选用。合成敷料包括透明膜、水凝胶、水解胶体、海藻酸盐和泡沫。透明膜能有效地保持水分，适用于Ⅰ或Ⅱ期压疮。它们还用于固定敷料，保护脆弱部位免受摩擦，并促进自溶。透明膜是半透性的，允许空气交换，因此不用于覆盖酶清除剂，凝胶或软膏。透明膜可以放置3～7天，每天至少应检查一次。

Hydrogels consist primarily of water and can be used for deep wounds with light exudate. Hydrogel dressings should not be used on infected wounds because they retain humidity. Hydrogels must use another dressing to keep in place and secure with tape or film. The cover dressing (e. g. , gauze, foam, and transparent films) should be selected based on the health of the surrounding skin and the degree of wound exudates.

Hydrocolloids are sticky, non-permeable wafers that retain moisture and facilitate granulation. They are used on noninfected, shallow stage Ⅲ pressure ulcers and to protect body areas at risk for friction injuries or injury from tape. Hydrocolloid dressings should never be used for ulcers that are infected, have purulent discharge, or have a suspected infection. Hydrocolloid wafers can be left in place for 3 to 7 days.

Alginates are manufactured from seaweed and are useful for wounds with moderate to heavy exudate. In most cases they are safe to use on infected wound. As alginate dressings have excellent exudates handling properties, they are useful in wounds and around drainage tubes when the wound fluid causes periwound skin maceration.

Foam dressings are nonadherent and absorbent dressings that protect an ulcer and assist in minimizing maceration of ulcer edges. They are used for stage Ⅱ and shallow stage Ⅲ pressure ulcers, exudating cavity ulcers, painful ulcers, and ulcers at risk for shear injury.

Gauze dressings are primarily used for debriding and cleaning up a wound bed since moisture was identified as a facilitator of healing. When a wound has tunneling or undermining, loosely packed, saline-moistened gauze can be used with caution not having the moistened gauze touching the healing surface surrounding the ulcer.

6. Biophysical agents Acoustic (ultrasound), mechanical, and kinetic energy, and energy from the electromagnetic spectrum (EMS) are also used in the management of pressure ulcers. Infrared (thermal) radiation, ultraviolet light, and laser are used as electrical/electromagnetic stimulation. Negative pressure wound therapy is an early adjuvant for deep stage Ⅲ and Ⅳ pressure ulcers and hydrotherapy is used as an adjunct for wound cleaning.

Pressure ulcers are common in elderly and are a costly health care problem. It takes only hours for an ulcer to develop; however, complete healing can take

水凝胶主要由水组成，可用于具有轻度渗出物的深层伤口。由于水凝胶敷料有一定湿度，不应该用于感染的伤口。水凝胶必须使用另一种敷料保持在适当位置，并用胶带或薄膜固定。应根据周围皮肤的健康和伤口渗出物的程度来选择覆盖敷料（如纱布，泡沫和透明膜）。

水胶体是黏性的，水分不可渗透，能保持水分并促进肉芽组织生长。它们适用于非感染性的、浅层的Ⅲ期压疮，并保护身体部位免受摩擦损伤或约束带损伤。水胶体敷料绝不能用于感染、有脓性排泄物或怀疑感染的溃疡。水胶体晶片可以保留3至7天。

海藻酸盐由海藻制成，并且适用于具有中度至重度渗出物的伤口。在大多数情况下，他们可以安全地用于感染的伤口。由于藻酸盐敷料处理渗出物的功能较好，当伤口渗出液引起伤口周围皮肤浸渍时，它们可用于伤口和引流管周围。

泡沫敷料是非黏附的和可吸收的敷料，能保护溃疡并且有助于溃疡边缘的浸渍达到最小化。它们可用于Ⅱ期和Ⅲ期浅层压疮，渗出性溃疡，疼痛性溃疡和具有剪切损伤风险的溃疡。

由于水分被认为可以促进愈合，纱布敷料主要用于清创和清洁伤口床。当伤口具有窦道或瘘管，包扎松散时，可以使用盐水润湿的纱布，注意避免湿润的纱布接触溃疡周围正在愈合的疮面。

6. 物理疗法 声学的（超声），机械的和动能，以及来自电磁谱（EMS）的能量也用于压疮的管理。红外（热）辐射，紫外光和激光被用作电刺激或电磁刺激。负压伤口治疗是Ⅲ期深部和Ⅳ期压疮的早期辅助治疗，水疗辅助伤口清洁。

压疮在老年人中很常见，并且是花费较大的健康问题。溃疡的发展只需要几个小时，然而完全愈合可能需要几个月。预防是防止

months. Prevention is the first line of defense against the development of pressure ulcers. Nurses have the responsibility to conduct pressure ulcer risk assessment and implement preventive measures. Successful pressure ulcer management requires a multidisciplinary approach. Nurses play a key role in pressure ulcer management and in developing collaborative relationship with other professionals.

(LIU Hongxia)

Key Points

1. Pruritus is the most common skin complaint in the elderly.

2. Xerosis (very dry skin) is the most common cause of generalized pruritus.

3. Pruritus can occur with certain cutaneous disorders and systemic disorders such as renal, liver, hematologic, and thyroid conditions.

4. Management of pruritus in the elderly requires an individualistically tailored approach with consideration of the elder's general health, the severity of symptoms, and the adverse effects of available treatments.

5. Elders are at greater risk for development of pressure ulcers.

6. Pressure ulcers are costly health care problems that adversely affect elderly clients' quality of life.

7. Braden and Norton scales are valid and reliable tools to identify risk factors for pressure ulcer development.

8. Prevention is the first-line strategy for care of pressure ulcers.

9. Preventing strategies for at-risk elders including preventing moisture, avoiding friction and shearing, changing position frequently, and ensuring optimum nutritional status.

10. The key to successful pressure ulcer management is to create and maintain a clean, moist wound environment that supports healing.

压疮发展的第一道防线。护士有责任进行压疮风险评估和实施预防措施。成功的压疮管理需要多个学科方法。护士在压疮管理和与其他专业人员发展合作关系中发挥关键作用。

（刘红霞）

本章要点

1. 老年人最常见的皮肤问题是皮肤瘙痒。

2. 干燥症（非常干燥的皮肤）是皮肤瘙痒最常见的病因。

3. 皮肤瘙痒能引起皮肤功能紊乱，还能使全身系统紊乱，如肾脏、肝脏、血液系统以及甲状腺疾病。

4. 老年人皮肤瘙痒的管理需要根据老年人自身的健康状况、瘙痒的严重程度以及治疗的不良影响采取个体化的方案。

5. 老年人是发生压疮的高危人群。

6. 压疮在卫生保健中的花费较多，它严重影响了老年患者的生活质量。

7. Braden 和 Norton 量表是信效度较好的评估压疮风险的工具。

8. 预防是护理压疮的首选方式。

9. 对于有压疮风险的老年人，预防压疮的措施有保持皮肤干燥、避免摩擦力和剪切力、频繁地更换体位和保持良好的营养状态。

10. 成功管理压疮的关键是保持创面清洁、潮湿，这样有助于创面的愈合。

Critical Thinking Exercise

1. Mrs. Hao is 75-year-old who has a history of chronic pruritus. The symptom of itching is more severe in the winter and she often cannot sleep well at night. She has some scratching lesions on her arms. Please develop a nursing care plan for Mrs. Hao.

2. Discuss the psychosocial implications of pressure ulcers on the elders.

批判性思维练习

1. 郝女士，75 岁，有慢性皮肤瘙痒史。其皮肤瘙痒的特征是冬天瘙痒加重，严重影响夜间睡眠。在她的胳膊上有一些抓痕。请为高女士制订一份护理计划。

2. 讨论压疮对老年人社会心理方面的影响。

Chapter 18 Care of Elderly with Delirium

第十八章 老年人谵妄的护理

Learning Objectives

On completion of this chapter, the reader will be able to:

- Define the concept of delirium;

- Describe the symptoms and diagnostic tests of delirium;

- Identify risk factors of delirium;

- Describe the major components of assessing the elderly with delirium;

- Identify and implement appropriate nursing interventions to care for the elderly with delirium.

学习目标

学完本章节，应完成以下目标：

- 定义谵妄的概念；

- 描述谵妄的症状和评定；

- 识别谵妄的危险因素；

- 描述评估老年人谵妄症状的主要特点；

- 对谵妄的老年人制订并实施适当的护理干预措施。

Delirium, also known as acute confusional state, is a common, serious, and potentially preventable source of morbidity and mortality among hospitalized older patients. Delirium has particular importance because patients over 65 years of age account for more than 50 percent of all days of hospital care. Moreover, the incidence of delirium will probably increase with the aging of the population. It contributes to increased morbidity and mortality, longer hospital stays, functional impairment, and more permanent forms of cognitive impairment if it is not recognized and treated in a timely fashion. Substantial additional costs accrue after discharge from the hospital, because of the increased need for institutionalization, rehabilitation, and home care. It is very important for clinicians and nurses to understand that delirium is reversible if it is recognized as an acute change and causes are removed in a timely fashion. Assisting with the prevention, diagnosis, and treatment of these cognitive impairments is an important responsibility of the gerontological nurse.

谵妄，也称为急性脑病综合征，是老年住院患者常见的严重问题，会加重病情，增加死亡率，但是可预防。谵妄的发生率与年龄相关，65 岁以上老年住院患者谵妄发生率高达 50%。随着人口老龄化，谵妄的发生率可能会增加。如果不及时识别和治疗，它会影响疾病预后，延长住院日，导致功能受损甚至增加死亡率。谵妄发生后对住院，康复和家庭护理的需求增加，增加医疗费用。临床医生和护士如果能及时判别谵妄并且消除诱因，谵妄是可预防的。协助预防，诊断和治疗谵妄也是老年护士的重要责任。

Box 18-1　Case Study

Mr. A is a 91-year-old man who was admitted from his home after falling in the garden. He had cataracts, diabetes and osteoarthritis, but was not on any regular medication. He underwent successful surgery for a fractured neck of femur. A few days later, he becomes confused, disorientated and agitated. He tried to pull his intravenous cannula out and was found wandering outside the ward. He became paranoid, anxious and believed that the hospital staff wanted to harvest his organs.

Questions:

1. What has happened?

2. What will be the consequences?

Box 18-1　案例

A 先生，91 岁，男性。他在家中花园摔倒后受伤入院。患有白内障，糖尿病和关节炎，但没接受任何正规药物治疗。他成功接受股骨颈骨折手术。术后几天，他变得思维混乱，定向力障碍和情绪不安。他试图去拔静脉插管出来。护士还曾发现他在病房外徘徊。他变得偏执，焦虑，认为医院的工作人员想获取他的器官。

讨论：

1. 患者出现了什么症状？

2. 可能会造成什么后果？

Section 1　Introduction of Delirium

I. Definition

The word delirium comes from the Latin "delirare". In its Latin form, the word means to become "crazy or to rave". According to the *Diagnostic and Statistical Manual*

第一节　概述

一、谵妄的概念

谵妄这个词来自拉丁语 delirare，意味着变得"疯狂"。根据《精神疾病诊断和统计手册》（DSM-IV-TR，APA，2000），谵妄被定

of Mental Disorders (DSM-IV-TR, APA, 2 000), delirium is defined as a transient, organic mental syndrome characterized by reduced level of consciousness, reduced ability to maintain attention, perceptual disturbances, and memory impairment. Delirium affects 10%-20% of all hospitalized adults, and 30%-40% of elderly hospitalized patients and up to 80% of ICU patients. In ICU patients or in other patients requiring critical care, delirium is not simply an acute brain disorder but in fact is a sign of much greater likelihood of death within the 12 months which follow the ICU patient's hospital discharge.

II. Pathophysiology

The underlying pathophysiology of delirium is not well understood and there may be many different pathogenic mechanisms that contribute to the development of delirium. These include acute stress response, drug toxicity, and inflammation. All of these can contribute to the disruption of neurotransmission. Recently, there is a growing evidence to support a role for cholinergic deficiency in delirium. Anticholinergic drugs are known to precipitate delirium and certain metabolic abnormalities may decrease acetylcholine synthesis in the central nervous system and contribute to the development of delirium.

More than 50% of hospitalized adults 65 years and older experience cognitive impairment during their hospital stay. It occurs with higher frequency in those with pre-existing cognitive impairment. Compared with other patients, these patients are more prone to falls, injuries, pressure ulcers, restraints, use of urinary catheters, and inadvertent exposure to agents with anticholinergic properties, all of which can lead to delirium, especially in the intensive care unit (ICU). Delirium in the ICU is an independent predictor of longer stays in the hospital and ICU, increased health care costs, and higher mortality rates.

III. Clinical Importance

The problem of delirium is far from an academic one. Not only does the presence of delirium often complicate and render more difficult the treatment of a serious illness, but also it carries the serious possibility of permanent irreversible brain damage. The clinical importance of delirium is that it is associated with increased mortality,

义为一过性的、波动性的、以兴奋性增高为主的高级神经中枢急性活动失调状态，又称为急性脑病综合征。其特征是表现为意识清晰水平改变，定向力差，注意力障碍，思维混乱。谵妄在成人住院患者中发生率为10%～20%，老年住院患者为30%～40%，ICU患者发生率可高达80%。在ICU患者中，谵妄不仅仅是一种急性脑部问题，更有可能造成患者出院后12个月内死亡。

二、谵妄的病因

目前谵妄的发病机制不明确，可能有许多不同的机制导致谵妄的发生，如急性应激反应、药物毒性、炎症等。所有这些都可以干扰大脑神经递质的传递。最近，越来越多的证据支持胆碱缺乏与谵妄密切相关。如抗胆碱能药物会促发谵妄，某些代谢异常可能会降低中枢神经系统中乙酰胆碱的合成，从而导致谵妄的发生。

65岁及以上的住院患者更容易发生认知障碍。在已有认知障碍的人群中，它的发生频率更高。与其他患者相比，这些患者更容易发生跌倒损伤、压疮、身体约束、使用导尿管等，并使用抗胆碱能药物，所有这些都可以导致谵妄，特别是在重症监护病房（ICU）。谵妄是ICU住院时间、医疗费用增加、高死亡率的独立预测因子。

三、谵妄临床管理的重要性

谵妄的问题不仅仅是一个学术问题。谵妄会使疾病的治疗复杂化，而且还会造成永久性不可逆的脑损伤。谵妄对临床而言非常重要，因为能增加死亡率，延长重症监护病房（ICU）的住院时间，造成意外拔管或移除

prolonged duration of intensive care unit (ICU) and hospital length of stay, greater risk of unplanned extubation and device removal, and long-term cognitive sequelae. Delirium is frequently seen in older patients in the emergency department and ICU. Patients with delirium diagnosed have a 12-month mortality rate of 10%-26%, comparable to patients with sepsis or acute myocardial infarction.

Despite its seriousness, delirium is missed by physicians in 57%-83% of cases. As many as 25% patients with unrecognized delirium are discharged from the emergency department. Historically, patients discharged with undetected delirium are nearly three times more likely to die within three months than those in whom delirium is recognized in the ED. The Society for Academic Emergency Medicine Task Force has recommended delirium screening as a key quality indicator for emergency geriatric care, and researchers have identified delirium as a crucial aspect of geriatric emergency medicine requiring additional research.

Section 2 Nursing assessment of Elderly with Delirium

I. Identify the Risk Factors

Rarely is delirium caused by a single factor; rather, it is a multifactorial syndrome, resulting from the interaction of vulnerability on the part of the patient (i. e., the presence of predisposing conditions, such as cognitive impairment, severe illness, or visual impairment) and hospital-related insults (i. e., medications and procedures). Individual, physiological, environmental, and pharmacological factors have been identified as common risk factors associated with delirium. They are identified in table 18-1. We recommend routine monitoring of delirium in older ICU patients.

Research has revealed that the risk of delirium increases as the number of risk factors increase. Between two and six factors may be contributing in any one case of delirium. It is important for nurses not to assume that there is just one single factor and stop in the search for any and all potentially contributing factors when assessing a patient's risk of delirium. In most situations most risk factors may not be modified, but nurses may be alerted to patients at highest risk and early surveillance and

设备的风险以及带来长期认知后遗症。谵妄常见于急诊科和 ICU 的老年患者。谵妄的患者 12 个月内死亡率高达 10%~26%，堪比脓毒症或急性心肌梗死这类危重症的死亡率。

尽管谵妄后果严重，但在 57%~83% 的病例中，医生都漏诊了谵妄。多达 25% 的漏诊谵妄患者从急诊部出院。（由于谵妄漏诊未收到正确护理）这类漏诊的患者在三个月内死亡的概率比确诊的患者高出近三倍。急诊医学工作组建议将谵妄筛查作为老年护理的关键质量指标，研究人员将谵妄视为老年急诊医学的关键方面，建议学者对其进行重点研究。

第二节　谵妄的护理评估

一、危险因素评估

谵妄很少由单一因素引起，相反，它是多种原因共同作用的结果，如来自患者的因素（疾病、认知障碍或视力障碍），或医院相关的因素（即药物和治疗）。个体，生理，环境和药理学因素已被确定为与谵妄相关的常见危险因素。护理人员应该常规地监测谵妄的危险因素（表 18-1）。

研究表明，随着危险因素数量的增加，谵妄的风险也会增加。发生谵妄的病例中，往往有两到六个危险因素。医护人员在评估导致谵妄发生的原因时，不要只发现一个导致谵妄的原因就停止对其他谵妄原因的继续追寻，否则会影响谵妄原因的去除和谵妄的治疗。尽管大多数危险因素难以避免，但护

monitoring may allow for more timely interventions. In addition, pharmacological factors can contribute to delirium with anticholinergics, benzodiazepines, and narcotics being the major offenders. Over-the-counter medications must also be considered.

士可以对高危患者进行早期监测和干预。此外，抗胆碱能药，苯二氮䓬类药物和麻醉药是导致谵妄的药理学因素，同时非处方药也必须谨慎使用。

Table 18-1　Risk Factors for Delirium

Individual Factors	Physiological Factors	Pharmacological Factors	Environmental Factors
Advanced age	Postoperative state	Polypharmacy	Stress
Visual impairment	Infection	Withdrawal from alcohol or drugs	New or change in environment
Hearing impairment	Dehydration		Excessive or lack of sensory input, isolation
Preexisting cognitive impairment	Hypoxia		Use of bladder catheters
Preexisting brain disorders (stroke, Parkinson's disease)	Anemia		Absence of clock, watch, reading glasses
Previous delirium episodes	Malnutrition		
Severe chronic illnesses	Vitamin B_{12}, folate deficiencies		
Immobility (including restraint use)	Hypovolemia		
Disordered sleep	Hyponatremia, hypernatremia		
Depression	Low perfusion states		

表 18-1　谵妄的危险因素

机体因素	生理因素	药物因素	环境因素
高龄	术后	多种药物治疗	压力
视力下降	感染	药物或酒精戒断	环境改变（新环境）
听力下降	脱水		感觉剥夺或超负荷隔离
预先存在的认知损害	缺氧		应用导尿管
预先存在的脑损害（脑卒中，帕金森病）	贫血		没有钟表、手表、阅读用的眼镜
谵妄发作史	营养不良		
严重的躯体疾病	维生素 B_{12}、叶酸缺乏		
应用限制措施（如约束带）	低血容量		
睡眠紊乱	高血钠，低血钠		
抑郁	低灌注状态		

II. Clinical Manifestations

Typically, the onset of delirium is rapid—over a few hours or days, and the symptoms can be highly variable and intermittent. Variability in attention, arousal or both can occur unpredictably and irregularly, often worsening at night. This may be witnessed as different behaviors occurring within a relatively short time, due to the fluctuation. For example, drowsiness, hypervigilance, normal wakefulness, and agitation, may occur within minutes to hours of each other. There are three subtypes of delirium which are hyperactive, hypoactive, and mixed variants. They are different on clinical manifestations.

The hyperactive subtype is the classic picture of the patient who is agitated, combative, restless, and hyperalert. Patients may have fast or loud speech, be distractible, and have quick motor responses. These patients always try to pull out intravenous lines and catheters, climb over bedrails, and are at greatest risk for complications due to injury and physical or chemical restraints. They also require increased nursing surveillance and care, often straining already depleted staffing resources. These cases account for less than 25% of all cases but have the worst outcomes, including nursing home placement or death in short time.

The hypoactive subtype includes patients who have decreased alertness, slow speech, lethargy, slowed movements, and apathy. These patients may not be identified as delirious timely because they are quiet and do not present nursing staff with increased demands for care or surveillance.

The mixed variant subtype includes symptoms of both hyperactive and hypoactive subtypes with patients cycling between the two and accounts for more than 50% of cases. These patients often are not identified as being delirious until they become agitated and confused with more symptoms of the hyperactive state. For example, some patients may present with an alternation between falling asleep during a conversation and trying to get out of bed to go home.

Overall, symptoms of delirium fluctuate and may include difficulty maintaining concentration or attention to external stimuli and a language disturbance, including slurred, forced, or rambling speech. Disorganized thinking demonstrated by tangential reasoning and conversation is often the presenting symptom. Other common symptoms of delirium include:

二、谵妄的临床表现

谵妄常在几小时或几天内迅速发作，并且症状多变，呈间歇性发作。注意力不集中、易激惹是临床常见表现，且常在夜间发作。这是急性高级神经系统功能活动失调的状态。根据临床表现，谵妄可分为3型。

活动亢进型：表现为高度警觉状态，不安，对刺激过度敏感，可有幻觉或妄想。这类患者常因试图拔出静脉输液针管、导管等，或翻爬床栏而受伤。他们需要加强监护，耗费紧张的人力资源。尽管此类发生率不到25%，但患者结局最差，需要医疗救治甚至短期死亡。

活动抑制型：表现为警觉性降低、言语迟缓、嗜睡、活动减少及冷漠，此型在老年人中较常见，因症状不易被察觉，常被漏诊。

混合型谵妄：混合型兼有亢进型和抑制的症状，发生率在50%以上。混合型谵妄症状常在不断变化，患者精神状态也随时在改变，患者可能在一段时间内情感淡漠，短时间又变得不安宁、焦虑或易激惹。例如，患者一会儿出现嗜睡，一会又吵着回家。

总体而言，谵妄的症状波动，包括注意力不集中、易激惹和语言障碍。沟通时思维混乱往往是谵妄的征兆。谵妄的其他常见症状包括：

- Clouding of consciousness or fluctuation of awareness.

  - Misperceptions, illusions, or hallucinations.
  - Disorientation to persons, place, and time.
  - Memory problems.
  - Increased or decreased physical activity.
  - Impaired judgment.

III. Identify the Presence of Delirium

A variety of conditions can impair cerebral circulation and cause disturbances in cognitive function. Sometimes the history, physical examination, or laboratory tests will indicate the presence of an organic factor that has caused the disturbance; however, without such evidence, the diagnosis of delirium can be established by the symptoms and lack of any non-organic mental disorder that could cause them.

The American Psychiatric Association's Diagnostic and Statistical Manual, 5th edition (DSM-V), provides five key components of delirium (Association AP 2013): a disturbance in attention and awareness; the disturbance is acute and develops over a short period of time while fluctuating during the course of the day; a disturbance in cognition occurs; these disturbances are not explained by another neurocognitive disorder and do not occur during a state of reduced level of arousal including coma; and there is evidence to suggest that the disturbance is caused by a medical condition, substance intoxication or withdrawal, or side effect of a medication.

There are several tools can be used for nurses to identify delirium. The most commonly used is the confusion assessment method (CAM, table 18-2) developed by Inouye and colleagues in 1990. The CAM is a simple tool that can be used quickly and accurately at the bedside by all clinicians to diagnose delirium. It has a sensitivity of 94%-100% and a specificity of 90%-95%. The diagnosis of delirium requires the presence of features 1 and 2 and either 3 and 4. It can also help differentiate between delirium and dementia. The CAM-ICU is a version developed specifically for use in critical care settings and can be used with ventilated patients.

- 意识模糊或意识障碍。

  - 理解困难，出现幻觉。
  - 对人、地点和时间障碍。
  - 记忆障碍。
  - 亢奋或活动减少。
  - 判断力受损。

三、谵妄的分级评定

多种病症可损害脑功能并引起认知功能紊乱。通常，病史、体检或实验室检查可帮助提供谵妄的原因或危险因素分析。但是，因为谵妄没有类似于血液成分检查或影像检查等客观的检查手段来进行诊断，医护人员常使用神经心理学诊断量表进行谵妄的识别。

根据美国《精神疾病诊断与统计手册第5版》（DSM-V）诊断标准，谵妄有五个特点：①意识障碍（注意力障碍和环境识别力下降）；②认知功能改变（记忆力缺陷、定向力障碍及言语混乱）或知觉异常（如视错觉、幻觉）；③快速起病（数小时至数天），病情在一天内起伏变化；④有引起谵妄的生理情况证据（躯体疾病、治疗及全身情况）；⑤不能以其他精神认知障碍来解释，通常不会在觉醒水平降低时发生，如昏迷。

在识别谵妄的量表中，Inouye 及其同事在1990 年开发的谵妄评定表（confusion assessment method，CAM）是使用最为广泛的标准化诊断谵妄的工具，可以协助临床医生床边快速准确地诊断谵妄。它有 4 项评定内容，评定时间只需要 5 分钟即可完成（表 18-2）。该方法简洁、有效，诊断敏感性为 94%～100%，特异性为 90%～95%。当评定发现第 1 和第 2 项存在时，再加上第 3 或第 4 项中的任一项（因为 3、4 项都在提示意识障碍的问题），可诊断为谵妄。它还可以帮助区分谵妄和痴呆。CAM-ICU 是专为ICU 开发的版本，适合医护人员床边使用，对不能很好交流的 ICU 患者进行谵妄发生的鉴别。

Table 18-2   Description about the Confusion Assessment Method (CAM)

Items	Descriptions
1. Acute onset and fluctuating course	Usually obtained from a family member or nurse and shown by positive responses to the following questions: "Is there evidence of an acute change in mental status from the baseline?" "Did the abnormal behavior fluctuate during the day which tends to come and go, or increase and decrease in severity?"
2. Inattention	Shown by a positive response to the following: "Did the patient have difficulty focusing attention, for example, being easily distractible or having difficulty keeping track of what was being said?"
3. Disorganized thinking	Shown by a positive response to the following: "Was the patient's thinking disoriented or incoherent, such as rambling or irrelevant conversation, unclear or illogical flow of ideas, or unpredictable switching from subject to subject?"
4. Altered level of consciousness	Shown by any answer other than "alert" to the following: "Overall, how would you rate this patient's level of consciousness?" Normal=alert Hyperalert=vigilant Drowsy, easily aroused=lethargic Difficult to arouse=stupor Unarousable=coma

表 18-2   谵妄评定表（CAM）

条目	描述
1. 急性发作和波动病程	通常询问家庭成员或护士："精神状态是否有急性变化？""过去一天内行为是否有波动（症状出现或消失，加重或减弱）？"
2. 注意力不集中	患者注意力是否难以集中，例如容易注意涣散或难以交流
3. 思维混乱	患者的思维是否凌乱或不连贯，例如，谈话主题散漫，思维不清晰，或从一个话题突然转到另一个话题
4. 意识改变	总体上看，患者的意识水平如何？是否存在不正常的改变，如： 警醒：正常 警觉：过度敏感 嗜睡：瞌睡，易于唤醒 昏睡：难以唤醒 昏迷：不能唤醒

Box 18-2   Several Tools can Be Used for Nurses to Identify Delirium

The diagnosis of delirium is based on clinical assessment and is guided by standard criteria. *The Delirium Diagnostic Criteria of the International Classification of Diseases*, tenth edition (ICD-10) and the recently published *Diagnostic Statistical Manual of Mental Disorders*, fifth edition (DSM-V) represent definitive standards in terms of diagnosis, based on the best available evidence and maximal expert consensus at the time of their publication.

To date, most studies have used earlier DSM versions, as they have been easier to operationalize and standard user-friendly tools have been developed to meet this need,

Box 18-2   谵妄评定工具

谵妄的诊断基于临床表现，并有统一的诊断标准。《国际疾病分类谵妄诊断》第 10 版（ICD-10）和最近公布的《精神障碍诊断统计手册》第五版（DSM-V）的谵妄诊断是国际通用标准。

但目前，大多数研究还使用早期的 DSM 版本，因为它们更易于临床操作如谵妄评定表（CAM），这是临床实践和研究中最广泛使用谵妄评定工具。诊断谵妄的金标准

such as the confusion assessment method (CAM), the most widely used tool to diagnostically screen for delirium in both clinical practice and research studies. The gold standard for diagnosis of delirium is the DSM-V criteria applied by a trained psychiatrist, but this method is often not feasible in the hospital setting as psychiatric services are not available around the clock. As a result, multiple delirium detection tools have been developed and validated against DSM-V criteria for use in the ICU. The confusion assessment method for the intensive care unit (CAM-ICU) and the intensive care delirium screening checklist (ICD-SC) are the most commonly used tools.

Because features of delirium, dementia, and depression may coexist in an individual, it is very important for nurses to be able to differentiate features of delirium from other two in older patients. Nurses should always investigate a change in cognitive or behavioral signs and symptoms in elderly patients, and never assume they are "normal". The family or other caregivers should be asked if the patient had ever experienced previous episodes of delirium and under what circumstances. The table 18-3 listed the differences among delirium, dementia, and depression.

是 DSM-V，但仅限于专业的精神科医生应用，因此在临床使用有限。此外，重症监护室（CAM-ICU）和重症监护谵妄筛查检查表（ICD-SC）也是最常用的工具。

因为谵妄、痴呆和抑郁症的表现有共同点，所以对于护士来说，能够在老年患者中区分三者是非常重要的。护士应该随时了解老年患者的认知水平或体征和症状的变化，并且意识到这些变化是非"正常的"。应向家属或其他护理人员询问老年患者以前是否有过谵妄发作史以及在什么情况下发作的。表 18-3 列出了谵妄、痴呆和抑郁症之间的差异。

Table 18-3　Clinical Features of Delirium, Dementia, and Depression

Clinical Feature	Delirium	Depression	Dementia
Mini-Mental State Examination	Acute fluctuations	Performance fluctuates over time	Moderately stable with decreasing scores over time
Onset	Sudden onset	Can be abrupt or associated with life events	Months to years
Duration	Hours to days	Weeks to months	Long term or lifetime
Mood	Labile; suspicious, mood swings	Consistent; sadness, anxiety, irritability	Fluctuating; depressed, apathetic, uninterested
Behavior	Variable; hypokinetic or hyperkinetic	Variable; may have psychomotor retardation or agitation	Variable with psychomotor retardation or agitation
Orientation	Impaired with variable severity	Selected disorientation	Slow decline over time
Alertness	Lethargic or hypervigilant	Normal	Generally normal
Memory	Impairment of recent memory and attentiveness	Selective impairment	Early recent and later remote memory impairment

continued

Clinical Feature	Delirium	Depression	Dementia
Thought processes	Difficulty maintaining concentration; disorganized; fragmented	Intact with themes of hopelessness, helplessness, and self-depreciation	Impoverished; impaired abstract thinking; word-finding difficulties; impaired judgment
Perception	Possible visual, auditory, and tactile hallucinations or delusions	Normal	Misperceptions not generally present
Speech and language	Slurred, forced, or rambling	Normal to slowed	Disordered; word-finding difficulties

表 18-3　谵妄、痴呆和抑郁症的差异

临床特点	谵妄	抑郁症	痴呆
简易精神状态检查（MMSE）	急性波动	随着时间波动	随病程分数逐渐下降且较稳定
开始	突然发作	突发或与生活事件相关联	缓慢起病
持续时间	数小时至数天	数星期至数月	余生
情绪	无规则波动；疑虑、时起时落	持续性；悲伤、焦虑，易怒	波动；沮丧，冷漠，不感兴趣
行为	异常；减弱或过度	异常；可能会有智力障碍或混乱	逐渐失去智力，头脑日益混乱
定向力	障碍	部分障碍	逐渐障碍
警觉	昏迷或过度警觉	正常	较正常
记忆	近期记忆损害	部分损害	近期和远期记忆均损害
思维过程	注意力难以集中；思维混乱；不连贯	绝望、无助、自卑	思维贫困、抽象思维受损、描述困难、判断力受损
知觉	幻听、幻视、幻觉，妄想症	正常	一般正常
言语和语言	模糊、强迫或漫游	正常或语速减慢	混乱、找词困难

Section 3　Nursing Management of Elderly with Delirium

Many cases of delirium are potentially preventable, and primary and secondary care services should be taking active steps in order to do prevent this condition. Primary prevention is probably the most effective strategy. Once delirium has occurred, nursing intervention strategy will be less effective and less efficient.

第三节　谵妄的护理措施

谵妄多数是可以预防的，应积极采取护理措施，预防谵妄发生。一级预防可能是最有效的策略。一旦发生谵妄，护理措施效果不佳。

I. Identify and Treat Underlying Medical Conditions

It is critical for nurses to remember that delirium is rarely caused by only one factor. It is important to review and treat all possible contributing factors. The mnemonic DELIRIUM which is outlined below is helpful to nurses to identify reversible causes of delirium.

1. Drugs Nurses should review the record for the list of medications. Particularly, they should note of anything newly added or omitted that may lend a clue as to the cause of the change in mental status. Even if a person has been on a medication for years, this does not mean that it is not the cause for a delirium. Nurses should ask themselves if the patient is undergoing withdrawal, taking any over-the-counter medications, or the drug levels are changed which might induce toxic effects.

2. Electrolyte abnormalities & dehydration Since a urine-specific gravity and color can indicate hydration status, nurses should carefully check the patient's usual blood work to identify imbalances in sodium, potassium, blood urea nitrogen, creatinine, calcium, and glucose.

3. Low oxygen states An oxygenation saturation level should be checked quickly especial in patients with myocardial infarction or stroke to rule out a low oxygen state as a contributing factor.

4. Infection A urinary tract infection is a common cause of mental status changes. It can be verified by a urinalysis and culture. Pneumonia is another common cause of delirium, but it often presents without classic signs of fever and cough in an older adults. A change in mental status may be the only indication of an underlying pulmonary process. Auscultation of the patient's lungs and an elevated white blood count can also indicate an acute infection.

5. Reduced sensory input Nurses need to ask themselves if the patient is without his or her glasses or hearing aids, the patient is in an understimulating or overstimulating environment, the patient has access to orienting devices (e. g. , watch, calendar), the patient has recently undergone multiple transfers across settings (home to ED, to ICU, to general unit)?

6. Intracranial (cerebrovascular accident, transient ischemic attack, seizure) Does the patient have a history of a recent fall, which might indicate a slowly accumulating subdural hematoma? A screening neurological examination might reveal deficits that

一、识别和处理谵妄潜在的风险

谵妄很少由独立因素引起。护理重要的是审查和处理所有可能造成谵妄的因素。字符串 DELIRIUM 有助于识记谵妄的原因。

1. **药品** 护士应该查看用药记录。尤其是护士应该注意到任何新增或缩减的可能造成精神状态改变的线索。即使患者已经服药多年，也并不意味它不会造成谵妄。护士应该评估患者是否正在经历戒断（如酒精），或服用非处方药物，或药物剂量有所改变，因为这些会增加药物的毒性反应。

2. **电解质异常和脱水** 尿比重和颜色可以提示机体缺水，护士应仔细检查患者的血常规，如血钠、血钾、血尿素氮、肌酐、钙和葡萄糖的水平。

3. **低氧** 在心肌梗死或脑卒中患者中要快速检查氧饱和水平，要排除低氧造成谵妄的因素。

4. **感染** 尿道感染是精神状态变化的常见原因。可以通过尿常规和尿细菌培养来检查。肺炎是谵妄的另一个常见原因，但肺炎在老年患者中通常没有典型的发热和咳嗽症状。精神状态改变可能是肺炎的唯一症状。对患者肺部听诊和白细胞计数升高也可提示肺部急性感染。

5. **感觉输入减少** 护士应评估患者有无眼镜或助听器、患者是否处于感觉剥夺或过度的环境中、患者是否能够使用增进定向力的设备（如手表，日历）、患者是否最近经历了多次转移（家庭到急诊，到 ICU，或转到病房）？

6. **脑损害** 如患者发生脑血管意外、短暂性脑缺血发作、癫痫发作等。评估患者是否最近有跌倒史，这可能提示缓慢积累的硬膜下血肿。神经学检查可能提示脑血管损害

indicate vascular compromise. Determine if the patient has a history of seizures or other neurological conditions or impairments. Patients may undergo brain imaging, either CT or MRI, to rule out structural abnormalities.

7. Urinary or fecal retention An abdominal and rectal examination and review of the intake and output sheet gives a clue as to whether retention of urine or stool is a cause.

8. Myocardial (congestive heart failure, MI, arrhythmia) In the older adult, an MI may present with only a change in mental status instead of the classic signs of substernal chest pain. Nurses should ask themselves, "Does the patient have a history of heart disease, including MI or arrhythmia?" A thorough cardiovascular assessment including an electrocardiogram can help determine cardiac abnormalities.

II. Supporting Safety and Recovery

When the underlying causes of delirium are identified and treated, nurses should provide care to support and protect the patient. Appropriate nursing care of patients with delirium generally includes psychosocial, behavioral, and environmental support. Interventions work best when they are tailored to the patient's degree of confusion. For example, reorienting, cueing, and explaining hospital routines were useful strategies when a patient was less confused or agitated. The same cognitive strategies were not useful in patients who were highly confused because they were found to agitate patients further. For these patients, environmental strategies of minimizing stimulation, dimming lights, and minimizing physical presence (i. e., limiting the number of unnecessary interactions) were useful. The following are the caring strategies that nurses may use for patients with delirium:

1. Foster orientation Frequently reassure and reorient patient (unless patient becomes agitated); utilize easily visible calendars, clocks, caregiver identification; carefully explain all activities; communicate clearly.

带来的问题。确定患者是否有癫痫或其他神经系统疾病的病史。患者可以进行 CT 或 MRI 检查，以排除脑形态方面异常。

7. 尿潴留或便秘 腹部和直肠指检以及对出入液量的检查可判断是否尿潴留或便秘。

8. 心脏疾病 如充血性心力衰竭，心肌梗死，心律失常等。在老年患者中，心肌梗死可能只出现精神状态的变化，而不出现典型的胸痛。护士应该评估"患者是否有心脏病史，包括心肌梗死或心律失常？"心电图在内的全面心血管评估检查可以帮助确定心脏方面的异常。

二、谵妄老年人的安全和康复护理

谵妄发生时，护士应当根据谵妄发生的原因实施护理。谵妄患者的护理包括心理，行为和环境支持。针对患者的谵妄程度量实施干预措施效果最佳。例如，当患者意识障碍或情绪亢奋症状较轻时，护士帮助患者重新定位，提示和解释住院规定往往有效。但是，相同的护理措施对于思维混乱较重的患者没有用，反而会刺激患者。对待这些患者，减少刺激，调暗灯光和减少约束才有用。护士应该明确一点：谵妄要着重于一级预防，因为一旦发生，护理措施往往效果不佳。以下是护士可能对谵妄患者使用的护理策略：

1. 加强患者的定向能力 住院患者在医院中容易失去方向感。在病房内使用易见的时钟和日历，在病房内白板上写明今天的日期和星期几，护士的名字，当天要做的检查和治疗等会有所帮助。另外，鼓励亲友探视，但探视时间应该分散开，避免探视者的人数过多和探视时间过长，以免患者疲劳。

2. Provide appropriate sensory stimulation　Quiet room; adequate light; one task at a time; noise-reduction strategies.

3. Facilitate sleep　Back massage, warm milk or herbal tea at bedtime; relaxation music/tapes; noise-reduction measures; avoid awakening patient.

4. Foster familiarity　Encourage family/friends to stay at bedside; bring familiar objects from home; maintain consistency of caregivers; minimize relocations.

5. Maximize mobility　Avoid restraints and urinary catheters; ambulate or active range of motion three times daily.

6. Communication　Communicate clearly, provide explanations.

7. Reassure and educate family.

8. Minimize invasive interventions.

9. Consider psychotropic medication as a last resort.

III. Documentation

Because the nature of delirium is that symptoms wax and wane, and because there are many components of delirium, documentation is essential as it is helpful

2. **提供感官输入**　缺乏感知觉的输入可能会导致老年患者发生谵妄。一方面要避免感觉剥夺，包括给老人佩戴度数合适的眼镜，用放大镜，看适合的电视节目，戴助听器，听喜欢的音乐和广播、新闻节目等；另一方面要避免感觉超负荷，如将光线控制到柔和状态，减少工作人员的噪声。

3. **确保充足睡眠**　应鼓励可以下床活动的患者白天下床活动，在活动期间注意安全。白天尽量减少患者的睡眠时间，鼓励患者夜晚入睡，以帮助患者形成合适的睡眠－觉醒节律。夜间灯光应柔和暗淡，防止黑暗给患者带来恐惧，同时注意不能用灯光直接照射患者；尽量在 11p.m.～5a.m. 期间协调和限制各种护理操作，减少对谵妄患者的夜间叫醒次数；减少噪声，最大限度地降低各种监护仪报警声和电话铃声等。使用这些措施以确保患者充足睡眠，促进大脑功能恢复。

4. **增强熟悉感**　安排患者家属或朋友在病床边照料，或使用家中常用物品，提供固定的护理人员，减少生活环境变动。可以鼓励患者讨论时事，追忆往事，或者指导家属带一些患者日常熟悉的物品如家庭照片、日报等，与患者共同回忆这些照片或者过去的情景。

5. **提高活动度**　避免身体约束和导尿管。每日三次步行或主动活动。

6. **交流**　与患者交流时要语言清楚，并提供解释。

7. 安抚和教育患者家属。

8. 减少侵入性操作。

9. 必要时才使用药物治疗。

三、及时准确的评估和记录谵妄的变化

因为谵妄主要分为亢进型和衰退型，并且有许多症状，所以详细的护理记录很必要，因为它有助于做出准确的诊断。谵妄的记录

in making an accurate diagnosis. However, nurses consistently underdocument cognitive symptoms. Documentation of delirium should include onset and course of the syndrome and disturbances in consciousness, attention, and cognition. Sometimes, nurses tend to focus on orientation, which is just one marker of cognitive functioning. A good example of documentations is "Patients asked me if he was in a salon room. He spoke slowly and halting, repetitive, awake most of the night, restless and attempting to get out of bed. " This gives information about orientation, speech, sleep, and psychomotor activity. On the following day, the nurse wrote "he was falling asleep while I was talking to him" or "trouble following directions, appears not to be able to focus".

It is also important that nurses accurately describe and document patients' cognitive status during times of transition (i. e. , from community to hospital, from nursing home to hospital, from unit to unit). One example of this kind description is "patients with a long history of dementia who had been cared at home by her husband became acutely confused during hospital stay but has slowly returned to prehospitalization baseline. She is oriented to place only, is now calm and cooperative. "

(JIN Rongchen)

Key Points

1. Delirium is a medical emergency and should not be considered a normal part of aging, or a normal occurrence associated with hospitalization, even though more prevalent in the elderly.

2. Delirium is associated with increased mortality, increased hospital costs, and long-term cognitive and functional impairment.

3. Delirium can be prevented with recognition of high-risk patients and the implementation of a standardized protocol.

4. Delirium may be under-recognized by physicians and nurses when it develops.

5. Routine screening for delirium should be part of comprehensive nursing care of older adults.

应包括各个发作过程以及意识、注意力和认知的波动情况。有时，护士倾向于专注于定向力，但这只是认知功能的一个标志。一例较好的记录如"患者问我是否在沙龙室。他语速缓慢，时有停顿、重复，夜不能寐并试图离床活动。"这条记录提供了关于定向力、言语、睡眠和精神运动活动的信息。第二天，护士记录到"我正和患者说话时他睡着了"或"患者不能按照指领做事，注意力无法集中"。

护士在环境转换期间（从社区到医院，从养老院到医院，从病区到另一病区）也应该准确地描述和记录患者的认知状态。

（晋溶辰）

本章要点

1. 谵妄是急性症，不应被视为老年人的正常表现，或与住院相关的正常情况，即便这种问题在老年人中更普遍。

2. 谵妄会增加死亡率，提高医疗成本，并造成长期认知功能障碍。

3. 护士可以通过识别高危患者和实施标准化方案来防止谵妄。

4. 医生和护士可能会忽视谵妄的发作。

5. 谵妄评定应该成为老年护理的组成部分。

Critical Thinking Exercise

1. Mrs. Li is an 80-year-old woman who has been admitted to the hospital for 2 days. She fell in a park and suffered a fractured at right hip and had an open reduction with internal fixation yesterday afternoon. However she did not get a good sleep last night due to the pain. When Mrs. Li first arrived, she was quiet and pleasant but now she is agitated, attempting to pull out intravenous lines and get out of bed, yelling, and throwing her pillows on the floor. The nurse attempts to reason with her and reassure her, but she is not responding. What have happened on her? Mrs. Li's daughter requests that she be restrained to prevent falls. She has seen patients with waist restraints and feels the use of this device will keep her mother safe from injury. Will restraining Mrs. Li be a good way to protect her in this situation?

2. The manager of a nursing home referred Mrs. B, an 80-year-old woman with a moderate degree of dementia, who suffered a sudden change in her level of confusion and orientation. Although responsive, she appeared lethargic, apathetic and was incoherent. She refused medication and food, and had disturbed sleep, being awake and alert during the night, but drowsy at times during the day. She was subsequently admitted to a general hospital, and was found to have suffered a stroke.

Sometimes, the carers might recognize that the elderly patient is confused but fail to appreciate the significance of this change in condition and, consequently, the problem may not be addressed until further deterioration ensues. Analyzing how early to avoid misdiagnosis of delirium. What can we do to avoid this?

批判性思维练习

1. 李女士是一名 80 岁的女性，已住院 2 天。昨日下午她在公园里跌倒，造成了右髋骨折并行内部固定减压术。昨晚由于疼痛，她睡眠不太好。当李女士入院时情绪平和，但此刻她很激动，试图拔出静脉输液管，并离床大喊大叫，她把枕头扔在地板上。护士试图向她解释并安慰她，但她没有应答。她发生了什么问题？

李女士的女儿看到有使用腰部约束的患者，她认为使用这种装置能保护她母亲安全，因此她建议护士把母亲束缚以防止坠床。在这种情况下，约束李女士是否是保护她的好方法？

2. 一所养老院的护士接诊了 B 女士，她是一名 80 岁的中度痴呆症患者。她的意识水平和定向力突然发生了改变。患者虽然对外界刺激有反应，但嗜睡、表情淡漠、不合作。她拒绝服药和进食，睡眠紊乱，昼夜颠倒。她后来被送进一所综合医院，诊断患有脑卒中。

有时，护理人员会观察到老年患者认知能力有所改变，但缺乏分析症状变化的临床意义，从而影响了疾病的预后。为避免早期谵妄误诊，我们该提供哪些护理措施呢？

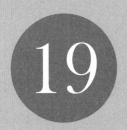

Chapter 19　Care of Elderly with Depression

第十九章　老年人抑郁的护理

Learning Objectives

On completion of this chapter, the reader will be able to:

- Define depression;

- Identify factors associated with depression in older adults;

- Describe differences between younger and older adults in clinical manifestations of depression;

- List the main screening process and assessment tools of depression in the elderly;

- Describe pharmacologic and non-pharmacologic approaches to manage depression.

学习目标

学完本章节，应完成以下目标：

- 了解抑郁症定义；

- 识别老年人抑郁症的相关因素；

- 能描述抑郁症在老年人与成年人之间的差异；

- 熟悉老年抑郁症评估内容和主要筛选工具；

- 描述抑郁症管理药物和非药物的方法。

Depression in the elderly is not a normal consequence of aging. It is a persistent or recurrent psychological disease and it complicates the treatment of other physiological diseases, negatively affecting patient's social function of patients, and bringing great suffering and burden to patients and their families. However, it is often under-recognized and usually under-treated so far.

Box 19-1　Case Study

An 86-year-old female complained sore muscle, dizziness, constipation, poor sleep and a loss of appetite. She repeatedly visited doctors with vague symptoms. Her daughter reported she was noncompliance with a wave of anger. Her husband died 1.5 years ago, so she lived alone. She missed her husband very much and felt that her husband had died recently.

Questions:

1. What's the main nursing problem for this patient?

2. What needs to be assessed?

3. What kind of actions the clinical nurse might suggest to the daughter to support her mother?

4. How to care for the patient?

Section 1　Basic Information

I. Definition and Prevalence

Depression is one of the mental illnesses, which results in the sufferer continuously being in a prolonged state of sadness and withdrawal from his/her personal, and social and occupational activities. Depression in the elderly refers to the depression existing in the aged (≥ 60 years), including primary depression (young or adult onset, senile relapse) and secondary depression in old age. It appears most frequently among older adults in abroad, affecting up to 15%-25% of community-based older persons, 30%-45% of geriatric inpatients and 20%-50% of residents in long-term care facilities. The study of small sample size in different regions of China showed that the prevalence of depression among the elderly was 10.2%-45.3% in the community, 31.6%-36.3% in the institution, while in the patients with chronic diseases; it was estimated to be 50.4%-66.7%. Depression in the elderly

老年抑郁症是一种持续性或反复发作性心理疾病。它使其他生理疾病的治疗变得复杂。其极大地影响患者的社会功能，给患者及其家人带来极大的痛苦和负担。目前抑郁症诊断和治疗常常不足。

Box 19-1　案例

一位 86 岁女性患者，主诉肌肉酸痛、头晕、便秘、睡眠差、食欲下降。她反复看医生，述说的症状不确切。她的女儿诉说她不合作，偶有愤怒。她目前独居，丈夫 1 年半前去世。患者说非常思念她的丈夫，感觉丈夫才离开她不久。

问题：

1. 患者的主要护理问题是什么？

2. 需要继续评估哪些内容？

3. 护士可以建议患者的女儿对其母亲进行哪些家庭支持？

4. 如何对该患者进行照护？

第一节　概述

一、老年人抑郁症的定义和发病情况

抑郁症是一种精神疾病，患者长期处于抑郁心境，并且其个体、社会和职业活动退缩。老年抑郁症（depression in the elderly）泛指存在于老年期（≥60 岁）这一特定人群的抑郁症，包括原发性抑郁（含青年或成年期发病，老年期复发）和老年期的各种继发性抑郁。严格而狭义的老年期抑郁症是指首次发病于 60 岁以后，以持久的抑郁心境为主要临床特征的一种精神障碍。抑郁症是老年人最常见的精神疾病之一。国外 65 岁以上老年人抑郁症患病率在社区为 15%～25%，住院老年人为 30%～45%，老年护理机构约为 20%～50%。我国不同地区样本量偏小的研究提示，老年

can lead to disability, cognitive impairment, exacerbation of medical problems, increased use of health-care services and family care burden, increased suicide and risk of falls. This chapter discusses factors associated with depression and differences in clinical manifestations of depression in the elderly with highlights on nursing management of depression.

II. Etiology

Depression is a complex disorder which can manifest itself under a variety of circumstances and may be caused by multiplicity of factors, including biological, physical and psychosocial factors.

1. Biological factor　Genetic and prior episode of depression, as well as aging changes and disease in neurotransmission disorders play a role in contributing to depression.

(1) Genetic factor: It has been consistently observed that depression tends to cluster and run in families. Early-onset depression is influenced by genes for depression, whereas late onset may represent a biological or psychological response to the events that are more common in late life.

(2) Prior episode of depression: The one with prior episode of depression tends to develop depression more easily in his/her old stage.

(3) Neurobiology factor: This is a lot of evidence demonstrates altered brain structure and function in depression patients. Depression involves many neurotransmitters dysfunction, including monoamines (serotonin, norepinephrine, and dopamine), gamma-aminobutyric acid, glutamate. The early theoretical models tend to believe that depression is due to decrease neurotransmission of monoamines, particularly serotonin and norepinephrine. It now seems that the onset of depression appears to involve more complex dynamics. It is still a matter of debate whether the abnormalities in brain structure and function and various neurochemical systems in the brain cause depression, or are themselves the result of depression.

人抑郁症患病率在社区老年人为 10.2%～45.3%，机构老年人为 31.6%～36.3%，而在慢性病患者中高达 50.4%～66.7%。老年期抑郁症会导致老年人失能、认知障碍、疾病加重，增加其门诊或住院治疗的概率和家庭照护负担，增加自杀以及跌倒风险。本章讨论与抑郁症相关的因素以及老年人抑郁症临床表现的差异，重点介绍抑郁症的护理管理。

二、病因

老年期抑郁症病因复杂，多因生理、心理和社会因素交互作用引起。

1. **生物因素**　遗传、既往发生过抑郁症以及老化和疾病导致神经传递障碍影响抑郁症的发生。

（1）遗传因素：早年发病的抑郁症患者，具有明显的遗传倾向。

（2）早期抑郁症：青年或成年期发病的抑郁症患者到老年阶段更容易发生抑郁。

（3）神经生物学：许多证据表明抑郁症患者脑部结构及功能出现改变。抑郁症包括单胺类（5- 羟色胺、去甲肾上腺素和多巴胺）、γ - 氨基丁酸和谷氨酸等神经递质的功能异常。早期理论模型认为由于 5- 羟色胺和去甲肾上腺素等单胺类神经传递减少导致抑郁症。但现在看来抑郁症的发生似乎涉及更复杂的动力学。大脑机构及功能、神经化学系统的异常对抑郁症发病的影响，目前尚需要进一步研究。

2. Physical factor

(1) Specific disease: A number of chronic diseases or medical disorders are associated with the development of depression in the elderly, including cardiovascular disorders (such as congestive heart failure, myocardial infarction), endocrine disorders (such as hypothyroidism, hyperthyroidism and diabetes mellitus), neurologic disorders (such as dementia, stroke, and Parkinson disease), metabolic and nutritional disorders (such as vitamin B_{12} deficiency), infectious diseases, advanced macular degeneration, sleep disorders, etc.

(2) Chronic medical conditions and loss of physical function: Some chronic medical conditions, especially with pain or loss of function, may contribute to depression in the elderly. Impaired vision or hearing and cognitive impairment are similarly associated with depression. Loss of independence occurring with the acute declines in function may result in further cause depression.

(3) Exposure to drug: Some medications used by older adults can lead to a significant risk for depression (box 19-2).

Box 19-2 Medications that can Cause or Worsen Depression

- Blood pressure medication.
- Beta-blockers.
- Sleeping pills.
- Tranquilizers.
- Calcium-channel blockers.
- Medication for Parkinson's disease.
- Ulcer medication.
- Heart drugs containing reserpine.
- Steroids.
- High-cholesterol drugs.
- Painkillers and arthritis drugs.
- Estrogens.

3. Psychosocial factor A number of important psychosocial factors may lead to the development of depression. These factors include unresolved conflicts (e. g. anger, guilt, negative thought patterns) cognitive dysfunction (memory loss and dementia), personality disorders, being unmarried, separated and divorced, living alone, lack of social support, recent loss and prolonged

2. 躯体因素

（1）特殊躯体疾病：一些慢性疾病与老年抑郁症的发展有关。其中包括癌症，心血管疾病，内分泌疾病（如甲状腺疾病和糖尿病），神经系统疾病（如老年痴呆、脑卒中和帕金森病），代谢和营养障碍（如维生素 B_{12} 缺乏），传染病，晚期黄斑变性，睡眠障碍等。

（2）慢性疾病及躯体功能障碍：某些慢性疾病尤其是疼痛或功能丧失，都是导致老年人抑郁症的主要问题之一。视觉或听力受损和认知障碍同样与抑郁症有关。急性功能丧失，可能会进一步导致抑郁症的发生。

（3）药物因素：老年人使用一些处方药物的会造成抑郁症（box 19-2）。

Box 19-2 导致或加重抑郁的药物

- 降压药。
- β受体阻滞剂。
- 安眠药。
- 镇静剂。
- 钙通道阻滞剂。
- 治疗帕金森病药物。
- 溃疡的药物。
- 含有利血平的心脏药物。
- 类固醇。
- 治疗高胆固醇的药物。
- 止痛药和关节炎药物。
- 雌激素。

3. 心理社会因素 许多重要的心理因素可能导致抑郁症的发展。这包括解决冲突（如愤怒、内疚、消极的思维模式），认知功能障碍（记忆丧失和痴呆）、人格障碍，未婚、分居和离婚，独居，缺乏社会支持，长

bereavement (especially the death of family members and friends) and stressful life events, isolation, being a caregiver for family member, loss of job and income and lower socioeconomic status, etc.

时间的丧亲之痛（特别是家庭成员和朋友的死亡）和应激性生活事件，隔离；还包括作为一个家庭成员的照顾者，工作、收入损失和社会经济地位低等。

Section 2　Nursing Assessment

I. Health History

Ask the elderly about the past /current substance abuse, nearest major life events, family history of depression, history of depression or suicide attempt, history of diseases and medication.

II. Clinical Manifestations

The typical symptoms of the depression include: ①depression experience, depression, sadness, etc; ②depression cognition, helplessness, no value, etc; ③the external manifestations of depression, decline or lack of interest, restlessness, etc. Without typical symptoms of depression presented in the young, depression in elderly is characterized by greater clinical heterogeneity, disability, severe somatic symptoms and more chief complaints.

1. Insidious manner　Somatic complaints often predominate in the clinical manifestation rather than psychological symptoms. As the physical condition covers up the depression symptoms, patients' repeated visits, referring to as "masked depression". Older adults are less likely to endorse cognitive-affective symptoms of depression, including dysthymia and worthlessness/guilt, than younger adults. Sleep disturbance, fatigue, loss of appetite, pain, weight loss, restlessness, loss of interest in living, and hopelessness about the future may be more prevalent in late-life depression. And many above symptoms of depression in the elderly are common to a number of physical ailments, often resulting in misdiagnosis. Negative results of thorough medical examination and effective outcome of polite study by taking antidepressants are presumptive evidence of depression.

2. Hypochondriasis　Hypochondriasis is preoccupation with the idea or fear that the elderly patient

第二节　护理评估

一、健康史

询问老年人过去／目前药物情况，最近主要生活事件，有无抑郁症的家族史，个人是否有抑郁病史或自杀未遂，疾病及用药史。

二、临床表现

抑郁症的典型表现包括：①抑郁症的经历，包括抑郁、沮丧和悲伤等；②抑郁认知，如患者丧失希望、无助，认为自己无用等；③抑郁的外在表现，如兴趣降低或缺乏、焦躁不安等。与年轻人抑郁症相比，老年人抑郁症常常不典型，具有更大的临床异质性，失能，严重躯体症状和更多主诉不适。

1. 隐匿性　抑郁症的核心症状是心境低落，但老年抑郁症患者大多数以躯体症状作为主要表现形式，常见的躯体症状有睡眠障碍、头疼、疲乏无力、胃肠道不适、食欲下降、体重减轻、便秘、颈背部疼痛、心血管症状等，情绪低落不太明显，因此极易造成误诊。隐匿性抑郁症常见于老年人，以上症状往往查不出相应的阳性体征，服用抗抑郁药可缓解、消失。

2. 疑病性　患者常从一种不太严重的身

has a serious disease. These patients may actually have some medical disorders but will not explain the patient's concerns or the nature and severity of the symptoms reported. The elderly tend to express depression through somatic symptoms unexplained by demonstrable physical illness, go to see doctors frequently for the same complaints. The chief complaints are usually of various physical discomforts such as constipation, loss of appetite, pain, insomnia, fatigue, weight loss, and restlessness. A competent and thorough medical examination is really necessary; after that, depression should rise to the top of the list of suspicions.

3. Suicide　A particularly tragic potential outcome of depression in late life is suicide. Suicidal behavior is more likely to be fatal for the elderly with a higher level of intent and more planning but less verbalization of suicidal thoughts than at any other age. Older adults are particularly likely to visit a physician shortly before the death, so it is very important that screening and assessment of depression for the elderly patients when they visit a physician.

4. Agitation　Severe depression patients aged at least 45 years are usually identified by anxiety, fear, and worry about themselves and their families suffering misfortune all day, appearing agonizing, insomnia every night, repeated unpleasant memories. Such patients lose interest in life, and even take suicidal behavior. Older individuals often deny having a dysphoric mood.

5. Inability to concentrate　It is common that older patient inability to concentrate with resultant impairment of memory and other cognitive functions. Depression is also sometimes associated, particularly in the elderly, with a reversible decline in intellectual functioning known as pseudodementia. After antidepressant treatment, it can be improved.

6. Other　Apathy and withdrawal, loss of self-esteem are common in the older individuals, but feelings of guilt are less prominent.

III. Screening and Assessment

Depression in the elderly can be assessed with standardized rating scales or a comprehensive nursing assessment including several key clinical manifestations of depression.

Older adults may be more likely to report physical or somatic symptoms than emotional symptoms when talking to their primary care doctor or specialist. Primary

体疾病开始，继而出现焦虑、不安、抑郁等情绪，由此反复去医院就诊，要求医生给以保证，如要求得不到满足则抑郁症状更加严重。疑病性抑郁症患者疑病内容常涉及消化系统症状，便秘、胃肠不适是此类患者最常见也是较早出现的症状之一。

3. 自杀倾向　自杀是抑郁症最危险的症状。老年人自杀常常致命。因为与其他年龄段相比，老年人有较强烈的自杀意图，并且做较多准备工作而较少语言表达自杀的想法。老年人特别可能在自杀前不久去看医生，因此老年患者就诊时的抑郁筛查和评估非常重要。

4. 易激惹　45 岁后发病的严重抑郁症患者常表现为焦虑、恐惧，终日担心自己和家庭遭遇不幸，出现坐卧不安，夜间失眠，反复的回忆不愉快的记忆。患者失去生命的乐趣，甚至产生自杀的想法。但老年患者往往否认有烦躁不安的情绪。

5. 注意力不集中　老年患者常常无法集中注意力，伴有记忆力下降和其他认知功能障碍。抑郁症性假性痴呆常见于老年人，为可逆性认知功能障碍，经过抗抑郁治疗可以改善。

6. 其他　老年患者冷漠和退缩，自尊的丧失表现较突出，但内疚感不常见。

三、筛查评估

可以用标准化的评定量表或护理综合评估进行老年抑郁症评估，后者包括评估抑郁症的几个主要表现。

与初级保健医生或专家交谈时，老年人更可能诉说的躯体症状，而不是情感症状，

care physicians frequently accept the patients' attribution of their symptoms, consequently missing the underlying depression. Thus, it is important to ask older individuals directly about depression using brief screening tools or even by just asking whether they feel depressed.

There are a number of instruments developed to screen adults for adult depression. But in the elderly commonly used ones are the two-question screen (TQS), geriatric depression scale (GDS), etc. (table 19-1). The severity of depression can be assessed by using a standardized rating scale, such as the GDS-15, and center for epidemiologic studies depression scale (CESD). Among them, GDS exists in both short and long forms. The short, 15-item version of the GDS (GDS-15) and 5-item version of the GDS (GDS-5) are validated for screening elderly patients in community-dwelling, hospitalized, and institutionalized settings. 5-item version of the GDS (GDS-5) has good receiver operating characteristics all elderly populations (appendix 4). The patient health questionnaire (PHQ), nine-item and two-item scale, have increasingly been used to evaluate depression for the elderly. The two-item measure can be used for preliminary screening followed with a longer measure if the individual's answer suggests that the patient may be depressed.

Some depression tools have been used with specific diseases, for example, the Cornell depression scale is used to screen for depression in older patients with dementia. The stroke aphasic depression questionnaire is for depression in older patients with stroke and aphasic. The screening instruments for late-life depression are shown in primary care shown in table 19-1.

初级保健医生经常重视患者的躯体症状，忽略对潜在的抑郁症。因此，使用简短的筛选工具直接询问老年人关于抑郁症的情况，甚至通过直接询问他们是否感到沮丧非常重要。

已有许多评估量表被开发用来筛查成人抑郁症，但在老年人中常用的有两个问题筛查表（TQS）、老年抑郁量表（GDS）等（表19-1）。抑郁的严重程度可以通过标准化的评定量表来评估，对抑郁的严重程度可采用标准化评定量表进行评估，如老年抑郁量表（GDS-15）、流调中心用抑郁量表（CES-D）等。其中，GDS以长、短两种形式存在。简短的15项GDS（GDS-15）和5项GDS（GDS-5）用于筛查社区、医院和机构中的老年患者。5项GDS（GDS-5）具有良好的接收器操作特性（见附录4）。其中GDS包括长、短两种形式量表，简短GDS-15条目（GDS-15），GDS-5条目（GDS-5）常用于筛查社区，医院和养老机构老年人（见附录4）。患者健康问卷（PHQ），9条目和2条目，已越来越多地被用于评估老年人抑郁症。如果患者的回答表明患者可能有抑郁，用2条目初步筛查，如果老年人的答案提示其可能有抑郁，再用较长量表评估。

一些抑郁症评估工具已被使用于特定疾病的抑郁评估，如康奈尔抑郁量表筛查老年痴呆患者的抑郁。脑卒中后失语患者抑郁问卷，筛选脑卒中失语老年患者的抑郁。初级保健常用老年抑郁筛查工具见表19-1。

Table 19-1　Screening Instruments for Late-life Depression in Primary Care

	Sensitivity percent	Specificity percent	Inpatient	Outpatient	Physically ill	Cognitively impaired
Two-question screen (TQS)	97	67	Unknown	Yes	Unknown	No
Geriatric depression scale (GDS) (5-item)	94	81	Yes	Yes	Yes	Unknown

	Sensitivity percent	Specificity percent	Inpatient	Outpatient	Physically ill	Cognitively impaired
PHQ-9 depression questionnaire (9-item)	88	88	Unknown	Yes	Yes	Unknown
Cornell depression scale (CDS 19-item)	90	75	Yes	Yes	Unknown	Yes
Center for epidemiologic studies- depression scale (EPDS) (20-item)	93	73	No	Yes	Unknown	No

表 19-1　临床实践老年抑郁筛查工具

	敏感性	特异性	住院患者	院外患者	身体疾病	认知障碍
2 个问题的筛查表（TQS）	97	67	不确定	是	不确定	否
老年抑郁量表（GDS-5）	94	81	是	是	是	不确定
9 条目患者健康问卷（PHQ-9）	88	88	不确定	是	是	不确定
康奈尔痴呆患者抑郁量表（CDS 19）	90	75	是	是	不确定	是
流行病学研究中心 – 抑郁量表（20 项）	93	73	否	是	不确定	否

IV. Other

The other comprehensive nursing assessment consists of physical examination, mental status examination, nutritional situation, family assessment, and performance of ADLs. Diagnostic tests, such as certain laboratory tests, the function test of renal, liver and thyroid, electrocardiogram (ECG), magnetic resonance imaging (MRI) and computed tomography scans may be useful in ascertaining the presence of depression instead of other illness.

四、其他

其他护理综合评估包括体格检查，精神状态，营养状况，家庭功能和日常生活能力、性能功能等评估。诊断试验，如某些实验室检查，肾、肝、甲状腺功能，心电图（ECG），核磁共振成像（MRI）和计算机断层扫描，有利于鉴别抑郁和其他疾病。

Section 3　Nursing Management

I. Nursing Problem and Management Goal

i. Main Questions of Mangement

The following is a list of main samples of nursing diagnoses commonly identified in the elderly experiencing

第三节　护理管理

一、护理问题和管理目标

（一）主要护理问题

以下列出的是对发生过郁症的老年人进行全面评估后，其常见的护理诊断：

depression after a comprehensive assessment of depression.

1. Ineffective response Ineffective individual coping related to numerous recent losses.

2. Decreased self-care ability Self-care deficit related to depressed mood, lack of motivation, fatigue, medications.

3. Social isolation High risk for suicide related to depressed mood.

4. Risk of suicide Social isolation related to depression mood, cognitive impairment.

5. Nutritioningestion lower than the body needs Impaired nutrition-more or less than body requirements related to depression, cognitive impairment, inactivity, suicidal attempt.

6. Sleep pattern disturbance Sleep problems caused by underlying physiological or psychological problems such as pain, anxiety, depression, shortness of breath, gastritis, or unrealistic sleep expectations.

ii. Goals of Management

The goals of management for depression include decreasing symptoms, reducing risk of relapse and recurrence, increasing quality of life, improving medical health status, and decreasing health care cost and mortality.

II. Management Measure

Management is individual and based on medical history, concurrent illness, and severity of illness. Treat the disease that may lead to depression first, and stop taking any medications that may cause or aggravate depressive symptoms are needed. If these steps do not work, further treatment and care measures can be used for manage depression in the elderly. The evidence-based treatment modalities are shown in table 19-2.

1. **应对无效** 与不能满足角色期望、无力解决问题、认为自己丧失工作能力成为废人、社会参与改变、对将来丧失信心、使用心理防卫机制不恰当有关。

2. **自理能力下降** 与抑郁、缺乏积极性、疲劳、治疗用药相关。

3. **社会孤立** 与抑郁，认知功能障碍相关。

4. **有自杀的危险** 与严重抑郁悲观情绪、自责自罪观念、有消极观念和自杀企图和无价值感有关。

5. **营养低于机体需要** 与抑郁、焦虑、认知障碍和自杀企图相关。

6. **睡眠型态紊乱** 与潜在的生理或心理问题有关，如疼痛、焦虑、抑郁、呼吸急促、胃炎或不切实际的期望有关。

（二）管理的总体目标

管理的总体目标是老年抑郁症患者能减轻抑郁症状，减少复发的危险，提高生活质量，促进身心健康状况，减少医疗费用和降低死亡率。

二、护理措施

护理措施个体化，其效果与病史、以往治疗效果、并发疾病和疾病的严重程度相关。首先治疗可能导致抑郁症的疾病，停止服用任何可能使抑郁症恶化的药物。如果以上措施无效，需要早期进一步治疗和护理。抑郁症的循证治疗措施见表 19-2。

Table 19-2　Evidence-based Treatment Modalities for Depression

Treatment	Evidence	Level description of the management
Medication	A	Tricyclic antidepressants, selective serotonin reuptake inhibitors, monoamine oxidase inhibitors can all effectively treat depression
Hormone therapy	C	Estrogen use in women given as a patch, cream, injection implant, or suppository was effective only in women post hysterectomy Use of testosterone in men orally, by injection, as skin patches, or as a gel, single group study showed decrease in depression among a small group of older men
Cognitive behavior therapy	A	Active time-limited therapy that aims to change the thinking and behavior of individuals that influences their depression. Effective when compared to no treatment
Exercise	B	Aerobic activity such as running or brisk walking was found to be more effective than education in lowering depression scores Resistance exercise focused on muscle strengthening activity alone has been less effective
Electroconvulsive therapy (ECT)	A	Involves delivering a brief electric current to the brain to produce a cerebral seizure ECT is better than placebo (sham ECT)

NOTES: A, supported by one or more high quality randomized trials; B, supported by one or more high-quality nonrandomized cohort studies or low-quality RCTs; C, supported by one or more case series and/or poor quality cohort and/or case-control studies.

表 19-2　抑郁症循证治疗模式

治疗	证据级别	措施描述
药物治疗	A	三环类抗抑郁药，选择性 5- 羟色胺再摄取抑制剂，单胺氧化酶抑制剂均能有效地治疗抑郁症
激素治疗	C	女性的雌激素的使用，包括贴剂，乳、霜，注射植入物，栓剂，对女性子宫切除后患者有效 使用男性的睾丸激素的口服，注射，皮肤贴剂，或作为凝胶在单组一小样本老年男性研究表明减少抑郁症
认知行为疗法	A	活动时间有限的疗法，旨在改变这种状况影响了他们的抑郁症的思想和个人的行为。与没有治疗相比有效
运动	B	有氧运动如跑步或快走，被认为是比教育更有效地降低抑郁分数 抗阻力训练的重点在于加强肌肉活动，单独运用效果不明显
电刺激（ETC）	A	涉及向大脑传递一个短暂的电流，以引起大脑癫痫发作，疗效优于安慰剂

注意：A，一项或多项高质量的随机试验支持；B，一项或多项高质量的非随机队列研究或低质量的 RCT 支持；C，由一个或多个病例序列和 / 或质量较差的队列和 / 或病例对照研究支持。

1. Management of pharmacotherapy　For patients who are treated with antidepressants and hormones, they should be administered correctly according to medical order.

（1）Observing effect and side effect: Early treatment of depression with pharmacologic agents is highly recommended in the elderly. The broad classes of available medications for antidepressants include tricyclic antidepressants (TCAs), selective serotonin reuptake inhibitors (SSRIs), monoamine oxidase inhibitors (MAOIs), and others. TCAs have been responsible for increased cardiac disorders and deaths in people with ischemic heart disease. The required dietary restrictions to

1. 用药管理　对于运用抗抑郁药和激素治疗的患者按照医嘱正确用药。

（1）密切观察作用及副作用：老年抑郁症患者应早期应用药物治疗。抗抑郁药种类较多，包括三环类抗抑郁药（TCAs）、选择性 5- 羟色胺再摄取抑制剂（SSRIs）、单胺氧化酶抑制剂（MAOIs）等。TCAs 增加了缺血性心脏病患者的心脏疾病和死亡风险。使用 MAOIs 使老年人需要饮食限制，以防止高血压危象和

prevent hypertensive crises and orthostatic hypotension from MAOIs can make the elderly problematic. TCAs and MAOIs have important side effects and thus poorly selected for the elderly patient, unless other therapies have failed. SSRIs are considered to be the first choice of antidepressant for most elders with depression and especially for those with conduction defects, ischemic heart disease, glaucoma, and prostate disease. Nurses need to monitor carefully and tell the elderly and the caregivers about the side effects, including xerostomia, diaphoresis, urinary retention, indigestion, constipation, hypotension, blurred vision, drowsiness, increased appetite, weight gain, photosensitivity, and fluctuating blood glucose levels. Sedation usually occurs during the initial few days of therapy, so precautions should be taken to reduce the risk of falls. Hormone related side effects also should pay attention to when hormone therapy is used.

(2) Adherence to medication: Because the patients' motivation may be very low, it is important to observe side effects of the medication closely and encourage patients' participation in the treatment plan and compliance with antidepressant dosage. Therapeutic effects will be displayed for at least 1 month of therapy; patients should be supported during this period. In addition, the importance of adherence to long-term medication should be emphasized because of relapse of depression in older people. For most patients, medications should be continue to take for 2 years, and for a number of recurrent patients, the period of meditation should be lengthened.

2. Cognitive-behavioral therapy Cognitive-behavioral therapy focuses on negating cognitive errors that are common to mildly depressed elderly. It includes milieu, individual, family, and group therapy. Group therapy is particularly effective with older adults because it allows them to express feelings and receive support. Reminiscence therapy, as a specific type of group therapy, can encourage older adults to discuss past events to identify problem-solving skills that have worked for them in the past. Most reminiscing is about happy or pleasant events from the past, the goal is to stimulate older adults to take control and make decisions, and explain what they want and what they enjoy or appreciate.

3. Exercise Two main types of exercise: aerobic activity and resistance training. Evidence from a

直立性低血压。TCAs 和 MAOIs 有严重副作用，因此除非其他治疗方法无效，老年患者一般不选择使用。SSRIs 常作为大多数老年期抑郁症患者药物治疗的首选，尤其是那些有心脏传导问题、缺血性心脏病、青光眼和前列腺疾病的患者。护士需要仔细监测并告知老年人和照护者药物相关副作用，包括口干、多汗、尿潴留、消化不良、便秘、低血压、视物模糊、嗜睡、食欲增加、体重增加、光敏性和血糖波动。镇静副作用通常发生在最初几天的药物治疗中，应采取预防措施以减少跌倒的风险。激素治疗应注意观察患者与激素相关的副作用。

（2）坚持服药：因抑郁症治疗用药时间长，有些药物有不良反应，患者往往对治疗信心不足或不愿治疗，可表现为拒药、藏药或随意增减药物。要耐心说服患者严格遵医嘱服药，不可随意增减药物，更不可因药物不良反应而中途停服。药物治疗至少 1 个月后治疗效果才会显示出来，在此期间应该支持患者。另外，由于老年抑郁症容易复发，所以要强调长期服药。对于大多数患者应持续服药 2 年，而对于有数次复发的患者，服药时间应该更长。

2. 认知行为疗法 认知行为疗法侧重于否定认知错误，是老年人轻度抑郁常用干预方法。它包括环境、个人、家庭和团体治疗。老年人小组治疗效果较好，因为其允许老年人表达和接受支持。怀旧治疗，作为一种特定类型的团体治疗，可以鼓励老年人讨论过去的事件，鉴别其解决问题的能力。怀旧治疗是通过引导老年人回顾以往的生活，重新体验过去的生活片段，并给予新的诠释，协助老年人了解自我，减轻失落感，增加自尊及增进社会化的治疗过程。多数回忆过去的最愉快的事件，其目的是激发老年人采取控制和作出决定，表达其需求，有喜欢的事物。

3. 运动干预 运动主要包括有氧运动和耐力训练。一个系统评价提示运动干预和持

systematic review implied that exercise interventions and ongoing physical activity can improve depression in older adults.

4. Electroconvulsive therapy (ECT) It is a safe and effective treatment for severe depression when patients refused to other treatment. Informed consent should be agreed by patients or their agents before treatment. More attention should be paid to pre-ECT evaluation, especially for patients with cardiopulmonary disease and prior surgeries (prior surgeries anesthesia type, any complications, history of skull fracture).

Hypertension patients should control blood pressure and patients with pulmonary disease should optimize pulmonary function. Medication to prevent detrimental tachycardia and hypertension should be taken before and during treatment. About 2 hours before ECT treatment, patients should take antihypertensive and anti-reflux medications with a small sip of water (except diuretics, to avoid increasing the amount of urine in the bladder during ECT). Adverse side effects need be observed such as the aspiration pneumonia, fracture, dental and tongue injuries, headache, and nausea. Antidepressants may continue to be used during treatment, but the benzodiazepine drugs need to be reduced and withdrawal.

5. Suicide prevention Suicidal ideation and behavior are the most serious and dangerous symptoms in the depression patients. The elderly (≥60 years) have the highest suicide rate among all age groups. The ratio of attempts to completed suicides is 4 to 1 in the elderly, much higher than the younger person.

(1) Identification of suicide attempt: Higher risk of suicide should be focused on male, old age, widowed or divorced, in poor health, retired, alcoholic, with a family history of unsatisfactory relationships and mental illness. In addition to recognizing obvious suicide attempts, nurses need to recognize symptoms that are more subtle but equally destructive desire to die, such as self-starvation, opposing a therapeutic need (e. g. , ignoring dietary restrictions or refusing a particular therapy).

(2) Psychological support: It is important to take interventions to prevent suicide. Approaches, for example, establishing lifesaving connections with individuals, especially the family and groups, such as phone call-in counseling could provide ongoing, long-term counseling, emotional support, and reassurance to the suicidal elder. Nurses' willingness to listen and discuss their thoughts and feelings about suicide may prevent patients from taking actions to end their lives.

续的体力活动可以改善老年人的抑郁症。

4. 电刺激治疗 一般临床需要快速达到治疗效果或者患者拒绝治疗时，选择电刺激治疗，这是一种对严重抑郁安全有效的治疗方法。治疗前需要患者或者其代理人知情同意，评估需要特别注意心肺疾病史和既往手术史（麻醉类型和任何并发症，颅骨骨折史等），肺部疾病者优化肺功能状态。治疗前及治疗过程中需要用药物降低可能带来不良后果的过高心率和血压。治疗前约2小时，患者需用一小口水服用其常规服用的抗反流药物、抗高血压药（利尿剂除外，避免增加操作过程中膀胱中的尿量）和抗心绞痛药物。所有肺部疾病患者应在每次治疗前数分钟开始鼻导管吸氧。术后观察患者是否有吸入性肺炎、骨折、牙齿和舌损伤、头痛和恶心等不良反应。治疗期间抗抑郁药继续使用，但苯二氮䓬类需要减量并停药。

5. 预防自杀 自杀观念与行为是抑郁患者最严重而危险的症状。在所有的年龄组中，老年人（60岁及以上）自杀意念和行为发生率最高。老年人企图自杀到完成自杀的比例是在4∶1，远远高于年轻人。

（1）识别自杀动向：对下列有自杀高风险的患者需要更多关注，包括男性、老年人、丧偶或离婚、健康状况不佳、退休、酗酒、与家庭关系不理想、精神疾病史。除了明显的自杀企图，护士必须学会识别那些不明显，但同样可有潜在自杀企图的行为，比如绝食，拒绝需要的治疗（例如，无视饮食限制或拒绝特定的治疗）。

（2）自杀企图患者心理支持：对有自杀企图的患者采取干预是非常必要的。建立与个人（特别是家人）和团体的救助联系，如咨询电话，为有自杀企图的老年提供持续的、长期的心理咨询、情感支持和安慰。护士传达一个愿意倾听和讨论自杀的想法，可能会阻止患者采取行动来结束他们的生命。

(3) Established suicide care: If a suicidal intent has been established, the following immediate managements are necessary: ① To reduce immediate danger by removing hazardous materials to reduce self-injury; safe keeping drug, in order to avoid patients take large doses at once, resulting in acute drug poisoning. ② To evaluate the need for constant attendance, and arrangement for family, friend, or professionals to be present during the period of imminent danger to ensure close observation, careful protection. ③ To evaluate the need for medication and prompt therapy. ④ To mobilize internal and external resources by getting the individual involved with external support and reconnected with internal capacities.

6. General care

(1) Daily life care: Depressed elders may be unable to perform their own ADLs and may have numerous somatic concerns, so meeting their physical needs is also a priority for interventions. Nurses need to meet the physical needs of elderly, and ensure their good activity, sleep, nutrition and regular bowel movements to enhance a healthy physical state, so as to manage depression.

(2) Environment management: Patient accommodation should be bright light, ventilated, clean and comfortable, with murals hung on the brightly colored walls and moderate flowers, in order to facilitate the mobilization of patients with good mood and full of love of life.

(3) Psychological support: The nurses must show unconditional positive regard and empathy in a professional manner so that trust can be developed to build a therapeutic relationship. The nurses help the elderly to block negative thinking, learn new coping skills, and encourage patients to express their thoughts.

7. Health education

Encourage the elderly to avoid isolation, to talk self-feelings with a friend or relative, to exercise regularly, to learn good sleep habits, to take medications correctly, to do funny activities, to learn a new skill. Encourage children and elderly people live together; society should pay more attention to the elderly depression. Community and institutions should create opportunities to allow the elderly to interact and participate in some collective activities for senile depression prevention and mental health promotion seminars, the establishment of the network and telephone hotline for psychological health education and psychological guidance conditional area.

(CHEN Qian)

（3）有明确自杀企图者的照护：如果老年人自杀意图已明确，必须立即采取措施：①通过消除危险物品，以减少自杀危险；安全保管药物，避免患者一次大剂量服用，造成急性药物中毒；②评估每天的需要，并在危险时期安排家人、朋友或专业人员陪伴，密切观察、保护患者；③评价药物的需要，及时治疗；④调动内部和外部资源，通过个人参与的外部支持和重新与内部能力。

6. 常规护理

（1）日常生活护理：护士需要积极帮助老年人满足日常生活需要，保证良好的活动，睡眠，营养和定时排便，增强机体健康状态。

（2）环境布置：患者住处应光线明亮，空气流通，整洁舒适，墙壁以明快色彩为主，并挂上壁画，摆放适量的鲜花，以利于调动患者积极良好的情绪，焕发对生活的热爱。

（3）心理支持：护士必须表现对老年人专业的尊重和同情的态度，使患者信任以建立一个良好的照护关系。护士帮助老年人排除消极思想，学习新的应对技巧，鼓励患者表达自己的想法。

7. 健康教育

健康教育内容包括患者教育及家庭社会支持指导。鼓励老年人多与他人接触，与信任的人交流自己的感受，规律锻炼，保持良好的睡眠习惯，参与社会活动，培养兴趣爱好。鼓励儿女和老年人共同生活。社会应更加关注老年抑郁症，社区和老年护理机构等应创造条件让老年人进行相互交往，参加一些集体活动，有条件的地区可设立网络和电话热线进行心理健康教育和指导。

（陈 茜）

Key Points

1. Depression can manifest itself under a variety of circumstances and relate to a multiplicity of factors.

2. Late-life depression is characterized by greater clinical heterogeneity, disability, and with more serious somatic symptoms and complaints.

3. A brief questionnaire should be used for screening and then followed by a longer screening tool if there is an indication that the patient is depressed.

4. Management should be individual and based on medical history, including pharmacotherapy, individual psychological therapy, cognitive behavioral therapy, exercise interventions, medications, suicide prevention, etc.

Critical Thinking Exercise

A 76-year-old man was admitted on May 10 because of headache, insomnia, loss of appetite for 18 days, and with happening of suicide.

Three years ago, his loved wife passed away, and his only daughter went abroad with her husband and son one year ago. He felt loneliness. On April 22 he perceived moderate to severe headache, could not sleep well, woke up several times during one night and experienced loss of appetite. He had gone to see doctors many times and taken many kinds of drugs, but the manifestations were not improved. He was found lying in bed with taking a lot of Valiums and was sent to the hospital by his neighbor 2 hours ago.

The outcomes of physical examination, ECG, and MIR are normal. The score of the geriatric depression scale (15-item) is 14.

Questions:

1. What's the main medical diagnosis for the patient?

2. Which manifestations and test results support the main diagnosis?

3. Are there any risk factors associated with the diagnosed disease?

本章要点

1. 抑郁症临床表现复杂，与多种因素相关。

2. 老年抑郁症的特点有临床特异性，其失能、躯体症状和主述多并且严重。

3. 抑郁症早期筛查采用简短的问卷调查，如果筛查提示患者有抑郁症可能，再一个较长的工具评估。

4. 管理注重个人化和疾病史，包括药物治疗、个别心理治疗、认知行为治疗、运动干预、药物治疗、预防自杀等。

批判性思维练习

一位男性患者，76岁，于5月10日，因头痛、失眠、食欲减退18天，自杀入院。

3年前，其爱妻去世，他唯一的女儿、女婿、外孙到国外生活。他感到非常孤独。从4月22日起，他感觉到中度到重度头痛，睡眠差，晚上醒来数次，并伴随有食欲下降。他多次就诊，服用多种药物，但症状没有改善。2小时前邻居发现其躺在床上，服用了大量安定片，邻居将其送到医院。

体格检查：ECG、MIR正常。老年抑郁量表（GDS-15）评分为14分。

问题：

1. 患者的主要医疗诊断是什么？

2. 哪些表现和检查结果支持该诊断？

3. 该疾病相关的危险因素有哪些？

Chapter 20 Care of Elderly with Dementia

第二十章 老年痴呆患者的护理

Learning Objectives

On completion of this chapter, the reader will be able to:

- Define the concept of dementia;

- Identify risk factors and possible pathophysiology to dementia;

- Describe the symptoms and diagnostic tests of dementia;

- Identify and implement appropriate nursing interventions to care for the elderly with dementia.

学习目标

学完本章节，应完成以下目标：

- 描述痴呆的定义；

- 确认痴呆发生的危险因素以及相关的病理生理改变；

- 描述痴呆的症状以及诊断方法；

- 为痴呆患者制订适宜的护理计划并实施。

Dementia is the most common disease of the aging brain and represents a growing public health problem as the world population expands and ages. The progressive degeneration of dementia leads to multiple cognitive deficits and results in disability and dependency. As the disease advances, individuals with dementia require more and more care. Nurses play an important role in the screening, diagnosis, and working with families to take care of elderly with dementia.

随着年龄的增长，痴呆已经成为威胁老年人身心健康的重大疾病之一。随着病情的进展，老年人逐渐丧失认知功能和生活自理能力，越来越需要他人的照顾。护士在痴呆患者的筛查、诊断和与患者家庭共同制订照顾计划进而为患者提供良好照顾等方面起到了重要作用。

Box 20-1　Case Study

Mrs. Wang is an 80 year old lady who lives with her elderly husband. She has a history of hypertension (30 years) which needs to be followed up at the community healthcare center. She used to work as a secretary until she retired in her early 60s. She clearly had a good memory. She enjoyed travelling abroad with her husband. However, during the last year, Mrs. Wang got lost for several times around the neighborhood and was picked up by police to be returned at home. Mrs. Wang became disorientated about where she was and be confused about time. She also missed her doctor's appointments for several times.

Questions:

1. What might happen with Mrs. Wang?

2. Which kinds of tests will she need to be diagnosed?

Box 20-1　案例

王夫人今年80岁，她和爱人一起单独居住。她有高血压史30年，需要定期去社区卫生服务中心随诊。王夫人60岁退休前的工作是一名秘书，记忆力很好。她喜欢和先生一起出国旅游。去年开始，王夫人在自己的家附近迷路了几次，都被社区里的警察送回了家里。她的地点定向力和时间定向力出现了问题。她也常常忘记去医院随诊的时间。

问题：

1. 王夫人可能出现了什么问题？

2. 需要对王夫人进行哪些检查以明确诊断？

Section 1　Basic Information on Dementia

I. Definition and Prevalence

Dementia is a syndrome, not a disease. It is characterized by dysfunction or loss of memory, orientation, attention, language, judgment, and reasoning. It also results in changes in the patient's behavior. Ultimately, these problems result in alterations in the individual's ability to work, take care of social and family responsibilities, and maintain activities of daily living.

Dementia occurs most often in older adults. As the number of elderly increases, dementia is becoming a

第一节　概述

一、老年痴呆的定义与发病情况

痴呆是由于脑部疾病引起的获得性智能损害综合征。临床表现为慢性、进行性、持续性的智能损害。其智能损害包括记忆、思维、理解力、判断力、计算力、学习能力、定向力、情感以及人格等各方面。该智能障碍是获得性，而非先天性的，亦不是儿童期精神发育迟滞。它还会导致患者行为的改变。这些问题导致个人工作能力、社会责任、家庭责任以及日常生活活动能力的改变。

随着人们平均年龄的增长，痴呆的患病率将越来越高。痴呆已经成为全世界所面临

challenging public health concern for all countries around the world. Alzheimer's disease international reported an estimated 50 million people worldwide were living with dementia in 2018; this number is predicted to be 150 million in 2050. In the United States, the first national population-based prevalence study of dementia found that nearly 14% of those aged 71 and older suffer from some form of dementia and almost 10% suffer from Alzheimer disease (AD). In China, the prevalence of dementia varies among different cities, generally affecting 2.7% to 7.3% of people aged 60 and over. The incidence of dementia in China is around 5% and, as life expectancy increases, the incidence of dementia will continue to increase.

Despite more than 70 conditions can cause dementia in older adults, Alzheimer's disease (AD) is the most common by far. AD accounts for more than 50% of dementia cases, followed by vascular dementia (VD) (15%-20%). VD and AD often coincide and appear to have additive effects. Between 8% and 30% of cases of dementia have been found to have mixed vascular and Alzheimer's pathologies. Because AD and VD are the two most common causes of dementia, together accounting for nearly two thirds of all dementia cases, this chapter focuses primarily on these two causes.

II. Etiology

The etiology of dementia is still not clear yet. Risk factors and pathophysiology of dementia are listed at the following.

1. Risk factors

(1) Risk factors of AD: Research has focused on genetic, nutritional (i. e. , vitamin B_{12} deficiency), viral, environmental, and other causes of AD. Age is the single most important risk factor for the development of AD, as the number of people with the disease doubles every 5 years beyond age 65.

(2) Risk factors of VD: Risk factors for the development of VD include arteriosclerosis, blood dyscrasias, cardiac decompensation, hypertension, atrial fibrillation, cardiac valve replacements, systemic emboli for other reasons, diabetes mellitus, peripheral vascular disease, obesity, smoking, and transient ischemic attacks.

2. Pathophysiology of dementia

(1) Pathophysiology of AD: The typical pathological changes of AD include the degeneration and loss of nerve cells (neurons), particularly in those regions essential

的公共卫生和社会问题。国际阿尔茨海默病协会报道在 2018 年全球大约有 5 000 万老年痴呆患者；到 2050 年将达到 1.5 亿。在美国，年龄在 71 岁及以上的痴呆症患者中有近 14% 患有某种形式的痴呆症，近 10% 患有阿尔茨海默氏病（AD）。在中国，痴呆的发病率由于没有全国性的调研资料而没有一个统一的数字，60 岁及以上老年人的患病率在 2.7% ～ 7.3% 之间波动，而中国的痴呆发生率大约为 5%。

尽管有 70 多种疾病可导致老年人痴呆，但阿尔茨海默病（AD）是所有痴呆疾病中的最常见的一种类型，约占 50% 以上，其次为血管性痴呆（VD），约占 15% ～ 20%。同时还有 8% ～ 30% 的 AD 和 VD 并患的患者，称为混合性痴呆的患者。

二、老年痴呆的病因学

痴呆的病因学目前并不是很清楚。有关痴呆患病的危险因素以及病理特点介绍如下：

1. 危险因素

（1）AD 的危险因素：研究发现遗传、营养因素（如维生素 B_{12} 缺乏），病毒因素，环境因素以及其他一些因素都可能导致 AD。年龄是 AD 发生中最重要的危险因素，65 岁之后每增长 5 岁，发生 AD 的危险性就增大一倍。

（2）VD 的危险因素：发生 VD 的危险因素包括动脉硬化、血流障碍、心功能不全、高血压、房颤、心脏瓣膜置换后、糖尿病、周围血管疾病，其他原因发生的栓塞、吸烟、肥胖、一过性脑缺血等。

2. 病理特点

（1）AD 的病理特点：阿尔茨海默病（Alzheimer's disease，AD）的病理改变主要为皮

for memory and cognition, and the presence of amyloid plaques and neurofibrillary tangles. Amyloid plaques are accumulations of degenerative nerve endings and other material, with a core of the peptide beta amyloid. Located near synapses, plaques probably interfere with communication between neurons and may also be toxic to healthy cells. Neurofibrillary tangles are twisted strands of protein found within the bodies of nerve cells. Tangles probably interfere with the cells' energy metabolism and the movement of chemicals to cell endings, eventually leading to cell death. This loss of neurons can result in atrophy. Cell loss is most pronounced in the temporolimbic region, particularly the hippocampus, entorhinal cortex, and amygdala, as well as in frontal and temporoparietal areas of the brain. Sensorimotor areas are relatively spared. These patterns of cell loss correspond to typical neuropsychological performance found in AD patients. Accompanying the loss of cells is a decrease of certain neurotransmitters, the chemicals that permit communication across the synapses between neurons. Among the affected neurotransmitters are acetylcholine, serotonin, and norepinephrine.

(2) Pathophysiology of VD: VD is a heterogeneous category of disorders in which the common feature is vascular pathology. The most widely known type of VD, multi-infarct dementia, involves the occurrence of multiple strokes or "infarcts" in the cerebral cortex. Infarcts result in the death of surrounding tissue due to insufficient blood supply. The most common forms, however, are characterized by small-vessel ischemic changes, or lacunas, and extensive white-matter lesions. Lacunar states are caused by occlusion in small vessels in the frontal lobes, basal ganglia, and other areas. White-matter lesions are found among both healthy older people and those with dementia; however, dementia is found when white-matter lesions are more extensive and when they occur in combination with other vascular and nonvascular pathology, including AD and Lewy body dementia.

All these abnormal physiological changes for AD and VD have resulted in impairments of patient cognition and function, and eventually result in loss of self-care ability and become totally dependent on care provided by others.

Box 20-2　Mild Cognitive Impairment (MCI)

Recent studies have confirmed that there are pathological changes in the brain years before symptoms of Alzheimer's disease appear. The transitional stage between normal

质弥漫性萎缩，沟回增宽，脑室扩大，神经元大量减少，并可见淀粉样斑块，神经原纤维结等病变。胆碱乙酰化酶及乙酰胆碱含量显著减少。

（2）血管性痴呆的病理特点：是指由于脑血管病变引起，以痴呆为主要临床表现的疾病，既往称多发性梗死性痴呆，包括高血压性脑血管病。痴呆可发生在多次短暂性脑缺血发作或连续的急性脑血管意外之后，个别人也可发生在一次严重脑卒中后。梗死灶一般较小，但效应可累加。一般在晚年起病，包括多发脑梗死性痴呆。

AD 和 VD 所致的大脑病理改变均导致患者认知功能和日常行为功能的异常，最终导致患者自理能力的丧失，最后完全依赖于他人的照顾。

Box 20-2　轻度认知障碍（MCI）

近年来的研究显示，在 AD 症状出现数年前大脑就已经出现了一定的病理改变。在正常认知和痴呆之间的转换阶段被称为轻度认知

cognitive aging and dementia in which the person has short-term memory impairment and challenges with complex cognitive functions is referred to a mild cognitive impairment. Persons with mild cognitive impairment have a higher risk of developing Alzheimer's disease; research is currently exploring the reason for some persons with this condition progressing on to developing the disease while others does not.

障碍，主要表现为短期记忆力下降、完成复杂任务的能力降低。发生轻度认知障碍的人群发展为 AD 的危险性更高。目前研究也在探讨为什么 MCI 的人群一部分发展为 AD，而一部分不会发展为 AD。

Section 2　Nursing Management

I. Assessment

1. **Health history**　Except the age, other risk factors of dementia are also needed to be assessed which include genetic factors, viral factors, environmental factors, and nutritional factors. Genetic factors especially need to be assessed in cases of presenile dementia, or dementia seen in individuals younger than the age of 65. Viral illness such as herpes zoster, herpes simplex, or viral encephalitis is believed to be a possible risk factor for AD. Environmental factors that are potentially associated with cognitive dysfunction include exposure to toxic substances or chemicals. Vitamin B_{12} deficiency, as one of nutritional factors, has been reported to be related with AD. Hyperhomocysteinemia (plasma homocysteine greater than $14\mu mol/L$) increases the risks for dementia and AD. In addition, detailed history of health problems need to be assessed especially for VD patients. Several medical problems place individuals at risk for the development of VD. These include arteriosclerosis, blood dyscrasias, cardiac valve replacements, systemic emboli for other reasons, diabetes mellitus, peripheral vascular disease, obesity, smoking, and vasospasms in segments of the brain.

2. **Clinical manifestations**　For individuals with dementia, because of the special pathological changes, there are several kinds of symptoms which are abnormal. These symptoms also are the reason why taking care of dementia patients is very challenging. Three broad domains for the impairments in dementia patients have been utilized by many studies. These domains are cognitive function, functional capacity, and behavioral problems. The impairments in these three domains reflect needed care and affect the caregiving process. The care needs are widely considered stressors, which are appraised

第二节　老年痴呆患者的护理

一、护理评估

1. **健康史**　除了年龄之外，还应该评估患者的遗传、病毒、环境以及营养状况等。65岁以前发病者尤其需要评估家族遗传史。疱疹病毒感染史、维生素 B_{12} 缺乏也是危险因素。此外，高同型半胱氨酸血症也增加罹患痴呆和 AD 的危险性。还应仔细询问血管性痴呆患者的既往疾病史，如动脉硬化，血液异常，心脏瓣膜病，糖尿病，周围血管病，肥胖或其他易引发静脉血栓的疾病。

2. **临床表现**　以 AD 为例，痴呆主要有三大综合征，即认知功能障碍，日常生活能力下降，特殊的行为问题。在这三方面的症状中，重度的痴呆患者表现十分突出，早期痴呆患者在认知及行为障碍中可以有些症状，而日常生活自理能力常保持良好，或者症状不明显，所以此三方面的症状并非平衡发展。而且，每一个患者所表现的症状也不完全相同，需要针对个体的具体情况而制订相应的

by caregivers as stressful.

(1) Cognitive function: Cognitive function is critical to an individual's performance in every aspect of life. It is commonly broken down into several domains: attention, memory (calculation/working memory, episodic and semantic memory, implicit and procedural memory), orientation, language, visual-spatial abilities, psychomotor speed, executive/problem solving, and intelligence. Dementia, in contrast to normal age-related cognitive changes, leads to severe, irreversible, and global deterioration of cognitive function.

In early stage of dementia, the pattern of cognitive impairments varies depending on the site of brain damage and the type of dementia. For example, AD is characterized with insidious onset and gradual decline in cognitive function. Memory loss is typically noticed first in AD patients. Initially the patient has difficulty recalling new information such as names or details of conversation (short-term memory), while remote memories are relatively preserved. With progression, the memory loss worsens to include remote memory.

In contrast, for VD patients, impaired memory is not as prominent a symptom as in AD, while frontal executive abilities and language deficits may be prominent at early stage. VD reflects sudden onset and stepwise progression. In all kinds of dementia, as the dementia progresses, global deterioration of cognitive function is revealed.

(2) Functional capacity: Over the years, functional capacity has come to mean a person's ability to perform those activities of daily living deemed necessary to survive adequately in modern society. Functional assessment includes three major domains: activities of daily living (ADLs) (i. e. , dressing, bathing, eating, grooming, toileting, bladder/bowel continence), instrumental activities of daily living (IADLs) (i. e. , cooking, cleaning, shopping, money management, use of transportation, use of telephone, medication administration), and mobility (i. e. , walking, stairs, balance, transferring). During the

治疗护理方案。

（1）认知功能：认知功能是影响一个人生活能力的很重要方面。痴呆老人的认知功能受损常表现为注意力不集中，对事物特别是过去不熟悉的事物丧失了主动的注意，立即发生的事情马上就忘记；记忆力减退，尤以近记忆减退为主要表现，而远记忆下降在中度和重度痴呆时较为明显；定向力受损，包括时间、地点和人物定向力受损，如不知道是白天还是黑夜，不知道具体的季节，不认识自己的住址甚至自己的房间，甚至发生走失，随着痴呆的加重，对周围环境中的人、家人、自己的认识能力下降；语言能力、计算能力、思维障碍，解决问题能力下降等。如外出购物不会算账，不能自己管理财务，语言能力障碍表现为命名困难，找不到合适的词语表达。思维内容障碍表现为产生很多妄想、多疑等。

在痴呆的早期阶段，认知障碍的表现因脑损伤的部位和痴呆的类型而异。例如，AD的特征在于隐匿性发作和认知功能的逐渐下降。AD患者最早常表现为记忆力减退。最初，是近期记忆减退，随着进展，远期记忆将进一步恶化。

相比之下，对于VD患者，记忆障碍的症状并不像AD那样突出，而执行能力和语言障碍可能在早期就很明显。VD常急性发作并进展性加重。

（2）日常生活能力：随着痴呆病情的进展，患者的日常生活能力逐渐下降。早期痴呆患者生活自理活动大致正常，仅仅在灵活度方面显得较为迟钝，需要别人提醒和督促。在中度痴呆时，患者生活自理能力有较明显的下降，学习与工作已经基本无法正常进行。日常生活需要他人协助，如穿衣需要他人提醒，避免内衣外穿或者扣错扣子；如厕也需要定时提醒。不能自己做饭和购物，完全需

normal aging process, even with 50 percent deterioration in many organ systems, an individual can still function adequately because the elder has the ability to compensate for age-related changes. However, for individuals with dementia and the resulting progressive cognitive decline, a gradual loss of the ability to perform everyday tasks occurs. Early on, the ability to carry out complex activities (such as work-related tasks or managing finances) is impaired. Later in the disease, people can no longer perform basic activities of daily living, such as dressing and bathing. Many studies related to dementia care have addressed the importance of determining individual levels of independence in meeting ADLs and IADLs which can aid in understanding the patient's severity of dementia and care needs.

(3) Behavioral problems: In addition to cognitive and functional impairment, behavioral problems are another prominent manifestation of dementia. It is estimated that about 90% of patients with dementia will develop significant behavioral problems at some point in the course of their illness. These problems include, but are not limited to, difficulties with personal hygiene and care, depression, agitation, and aggression. Because of the nature of behavioral problems, they are more burdensome to caregivers than are physical impairments.

Agitation is the term used to describe all behavioral symptoms of dementia. It is defined as inappropriate verbal, vocal, or motor activity that is not explained by needs or confusion per se. Agitated behaviors have been divided into three major syndromes: physically aggressive behavior (hitting, kicking); physically non-aggressive behavior (pacing, disrobing, wandering); and verbally agitated behavior (constant repetitions of words). A more complex taxonomy can be based on a multimethod assessment approach: verbal aggression/vocal agitation (screaming, moaning, complaining), physical aggression (inflicting self-harm or harm to others), affective behavioral disorder (crying, seeking reassurance, rejecting others, coldness), psychotic behavior (delusions, hallucinations, confusion), wandering, and asocial behavior (disrupting others, disrobing, sloppy eating).

AD and VD can increase the likelihood of agitated behavior in several ways. Neurons are lost in key

要他人协助。晚期的患者生活上完全不能自理，吃饭需要他人喂食，穿衣需要他人帮助才能穿上，大小便失禁，有的甚至还会玩弄大小便。有的患者尚能四处走动，但完全没有目的性；有的患者完全卧床、肢体挛缩，无法从语言上表达自己的需要，无法与人进行交流。功能评估包括三个主要领域：日常生活活动（ADLs）（如穿衣、洗澡、饮食，美容，大小便失禁等）、工具性日常生活活动能力（IADLs）（如做饭，购物，资金管理，交通使用，电话使用，药物管理）和出行（即步行，爬楼梯，保持平衡，转移）。在正常的衰老过程中，即使许多器官退化了50%，一个人仍然可以充分发挥功能。与痴呆症护理有关的许多研究都强调了分辨个体化ADLs和IADLs需求的重要性，这有助于分析痴呆的严重程度和护理需求。

（3）行为问题：大约90%的痴呆患者在其病程中会发生某些特殊的行为问题，是导致痴呆患者照顾难度较大的一个原因。如表现为抑郁、情绪不稳定、进行照顾时发生抵抗行为、激越行为等。

激越行为常用来表达痴呆患者的常见行为症状，一般分为三大类：身体激越行为（如打人、踢人）、身体非激越行为（如徘徊、当众脱衣服）和语言激越行为（如重复话语）等。更具体的分类可为语言/声音激越行为（如尖叫、呻吟、抱怨等），身体激越行为（如包括伤害自己和他人的行为），情感行为障碍（如哭闹、反复寻求保证、排斥他人、冷淡）和精神行为障碍（如幻觉、妄想、谵妄等），徘徊，反社会行为（如打搅他人、公众场合脱衣服、不雅的饮食行为等）。

行为障碍的出现以及行为问题的特殊表现与大脑的受损区域相关，导致涉及情绪和

regions of the brain, leading to corresponding deficits in neurotransmitters involved in the regulation of mood and behavior.

Cognitive deficits associated with dementia also make problem behavior more likely. Patients may misunderstand what other people say to them, be unable to communicate effectively, or become frightened by their inability to recognize people, places, or things. They also have more difficulty initiating activities and keeping occupied. These changes create an increased probability of behavior problems.

Individuals with dementia have special pathological changes in the brain compared with others who are aging normally. These pathological changes result in abnormal symptoms of dementia in the cognitive, functional, and behavior domains. The abnormal symptoms result in care demands and make the caring for a family member with dementia especially detrimental. These unique cognitive, functional, and behavioral impairments can contribute substantially to the psychological and physical morbidity of the caregiver as well as caregiver's social function.

3. Experimental and other tests Inorder to differentiate different types of dementia, proper diagnosis will be required. Cognitive testing, laboratory tests, and imaging are usually common diagnosis tests.

(1) Cognitive tests: There are several well used measures to examine cognitive function in dementia patients: mini-mental state examination, global deterioration scale, and clinical dementia rating scale. All these measures can reflect the level of cognitive impairment for dementia patients, and provide information on patients care needs and treatment effects.

a. Mini-mental state examination: The mini-mental state examination (MMSE) is the most widely used screening instrument. It was developed as a short, easy-to-administer measure of mental status and as a screening tool for dementia. It has been used extensively in research involving dementia patients and found to be an acceptable measure of mental status. The MMSE yields a total score of 30, with a score of 24 established as the cutoff point for dementia. It consists of 11 questions or commands, such as "What is the year? " or "Write a sentence", and assesses seven categories of cognitive function including orientation to time and place, registration of three words, attention and calculations, registration of three words, attention and calculations, recall of three words, language, and visual construction. The MMSE takes 5-10 minutes

行为调节的神经递质缺乏。

另外，随着认知功能的下降，患者会误解或者不能理解周围人，加之失去相应的定向力，从而导致某些行为问题的发生。

与正常衰老的人相比，痴呆患者大脑有特殊的病理改变。这些病理变化导致痴呆认知和行为方面的异常症状。异常症状导致特殊护理需求增多，加重了家庭成员和照顾者的负担。

3. 检查和其他诊断方法 为了区分不同类型的痴呆，常常需要对患者进行认知功能检测、实验室检查及影像学检查。

（1）认知功能检测：常使用比较成熟的认知心理学方面的检测量表来完成。较为常用的是简易智力状态检测量表（MMSE）、认知功能全面衰退量表（GDS）、临床痴呆评定量表等。表20-1和表20-2分别列举了GDS和CDR的评分分值所代表的含义。

1）简易智力状态检测量表（MMSE）是使用最广泛的认知障碍筛选工具之一。主要用于痴呆的筛查和评估。MMSE的总分为30，得分24为痴呆症的临界点。它由11个问题组成，例如"今年是哪一年？"或"写一句话"，并评估七种认知功能，包括对包括以下7个方面：时间定向力，地点定向力，即刻记忆，注意力及计算力，延迟记忆，语言，视空间。MMSE需要5～10分钟，并且不需要专业培训即可使用。

and does not require extensive training to administer. Folstein determined that a score of 23 points or less with an individual who had more than 8 years of education can be a diagnostic indication of cognitive impairment.

b. Global deterioration scale: The global deterioration scale (GDS) (table 20-1) is a global rating scale which is used to summarize whether an individual has cognitive impairments consistent with dementia (including Alzheimer's disease). Individuals are rated according to a seven-point scale, as outlined below; a score of 4 or higher is usually considered to be indicative of dementia. A score of 3 on the GDS is considered consistent with mild cognitive impairment (MCI); people with MCI are at heightened risk to develop dementia within the next few years.

2）全面衰退量表（GDS）（表 20-1）是目前全世界最常用的阿尔茨海默症分级体系。把阿尔茨海默症患者从无症状到认知功能严重下降的整个过程分为了 7 个阶段，以提供针对性治疗和护理的参照依据。得分 4 分及以上表示为痴呆症。3 分为轻度认知障碍（MCI）。MCI 患者在未来几年内患痴呆症的风险更高。

Table 20-1　GDS Scale

GDS Rating	Description
1	Patient has no complaints of memory deficit; clinician can detect no memory deficit evident during interview
2	Patient complains of memory deficit (forgetting names, forgetting where one has placed objects), but clinician can detect no objective evidence of a memory deficit during interview
3	Patient shows evidence of mild memory deficit during intensive clinical interview; symptoms include: patient may have gotten lost when traveling to a familiar location, may forget familiar names, may have problems finding the correct word; family and/or co-workers are aware of memory lapses; patient may have lost or misplaced an object of value; patient may show anxiety and/or deficits in concentration
4	Patient shows clear-cut evidence of memory deficit during interview with clinician, including decreased memory of current and recent events, decreased ability to travel or handle finances, inability to perform complex tasks. Patient may also deny there is any problem with his/her memory even though it is evident to friends and family
5	Patient can no longer handle activities of daily life without some assistance; patient is unable to recall a major aspect of current life such as own address or telephone number, and may have trouble choosing proper clothing to wear (e. g. deciding whether a coat is required)
6	Patient is largely unaware of all recent events and experiences; may forget spouse's name, may become incontinent, may show personality changes
7	Patient loses all verbal abilities over the course of this stage; patient is incontinent and requires help with feeding and toileting; patient begins to lose basic motor skills (e. g. ability to walk)

表 20-1　认知功能全面衰退量表（GDS）评分含义

GDS 评分	含义
1	无认知功能减退：无主观叙述记忆不好，临床检查无记忆缺陷的证据
2	非常轻微的认知功能减退：自己抱怨记忆不好（如忘记名字，忘记东西放在哪里），临床检查无记忆缺陷的证据
3	轻度认知功能减退：临床检查期间患者表现出记忆缺陷的证据，症状包括在熟悉的地方发生迷路，可能忘记熟悉的名字，可能找不到合适的词汇，家人或者同事发现其有记忆问题，患者可能遗失贵重物品或者放错地方，患者显示出焦虑或者注意力不能集中

GDS评分	含义
4	中度认知功能减退：临床检查过程中患者表现出明显的认知缺陷，对目前或者最近的时间记忆不清，旅行或管理钱财能力减退，不能执行复杂的任务。患者会否认自己的记忆力有问题即使其家人和朋友确认他存在记忆问题
5	重度认知功能减退：在没有帮助的情况下患者完成日常自理活动出现困难；患者不能回忆与以前生活密切相关的事情，例如自己的家庭住址或者使用多年的电话号码，或者不知道挑选合适的衣服（例如不知道是否需要穿外套）
6	严重认知功能减退：患者对最近的经历和事件大部分忘记；可能忘了配偶的名字，可能出现尿便失禁，可能出现人格改变
7	极严重认知功能减退：丧失语言功能；出现尿便失禁；需要喂食和如厕帮助；丧失基本的精神性运动技能（例如不能走路）

c. Clinical rating scale: The clinical dementia rating (CDR) scale is a 5-point scale used to characterize six domains of cognitive and functional performance applicable to Alzheimer disease and related dementia. The six domains include memory, orientation, judgment & problem solving, community affairs, home & hobbies, and personal care. The necessary information to make each rating is obtained through a semi-structured interview of the patient and a reliable informant or collateral source (e. g. , family member). Appendix 5 provides descriptive anchors that guild the clinician in making appropriate ratings based on interview data and clinical judgment. This numeric scale is used to quantify the severity of symptoms of dementia. Scores in each of the six domains are combined to obtain a composite score ranging from 0 through 3. The overall score is useful to characterize and track a patient's level of impairment with dementia (table 20-2).

3）临床痴呆评定量表（CDR）是一个 5 分制量表，用于评估痴呆认知和行为功能 6 个维度的异常。这六个维度包括记忆、定向、判断和解决问题、社会活动、家务和爱好、个人护理（附录 5）。通过对患者和其家属进行半结构化访谈获得信息。总体得分可用于表征和跟踪患者痴呆症的损伤程度（表 20-2）。

Table 20-2   CDR Scale

Composite rating	Severity
0	Normal
0. 5	Very mild dementia
1	Mild dementia
2	Moderate dementia
3	Severe dementia

表 20-2   临床痴呆评定量表评分含义

综合评分	痴呆严重度
0	认知功能正常
0.5	可疑痴呆
1	轻度痴呆
2	中度痴呆
3	重度痴呆

(2) Laboratory tests: Routine blood tests are also usually performed to rule out treatable causes. These tests include vitamin B$_{12}$, folic acid, thyroid-stimulating hormone (TSH), C-reactive protein, full blood count, electrolytes, calcium, renal function, and liver enzymes. Abnormalities may suggest vitamin deficiency, infection or other problems that commonly cause confusion or disorientation in the elderly. The problem is complicated by the fact that these cause confusion more often in persons who have early dementia, so that "reversal" of such problems may ultimately only be temporary. Testing for alcohol and other known dementia-inducing drugs may be indicated.

(3) Imaging: Currently, there is no validated test available for the diagnosis of AD. Although autopsy remains the gold standard for the diagnosis of AD, clinical diagnosis has become increasingly accurate over the past several years. Magnetic resonance imaging (MRI) and positron emission tomography (PET) scans have been used to identify the hippocampal atrophy associated with the diagnosis AD. Because the costs are prohibitive and the findings similar to those of clinical examination for the diagnosis of AD, these tests are not routinely recommended. For the diagnosis of VD, neuroimaging with either computed tomography (CT) or MRI usually reveals one or more areas of cerebral infarction. VD is most often associated with diffuse or bilateral cortical or subcortical areas of infarction or microinfarction. Other than neuroimaging and clinical examination, no other diagnostic tests or biomarkers exist for the diagnosis of VD.

II. Nursing Intervention

Dementia is a group of symptoms rather than a single disease. Among these symptoms, cognitive impairment is one of the most devastating losses faced by older adults and their caregivers. Although memory loss may be the earliest and most common indication, dementia also causes changes in personality, behavior, sensorimotor function, and language. A goal of care is to promote maximum function, dignity, and quality of life for the person with dementia. The following presents some nursing interventions with a focus on patients, care environments, and their caregivers.

1. Interventions toward the patient

(1) Pharmacological therapies: Currently, there are no pharmacological agents that can cure or stop the progression of dementia. Several agents have been

（2）实验室检查：包括血常规检查，也包括维生素 B$_{12}$、叶酸、促甲状腺激素、C 反应蛋白、电解质、肾功能、肝功能检查等。某些指标的异常可能会引起老年人短暂的认知功能障碍。

（3）影像学检查：包括 MRI 检查和正电子断层扫描检查（PET）等。对于 AD 而言，最具有诊断效力的是大脑的组织病理切片，而 MRI 和 PET 的检测结果只具有一定的参考作用。对于 VD 而言，还没有具诊断意义的特征性的脑 CT 或 MRI 检查结果。如 CT 或 MRI 检查无 CVD 发现，则基本上否定 VD 的诊断，并成为 AD 和 VD 鉴别的有力依据。作为考虑诊断 VD 的依据，脑影像学检查显示的局部解剖结构的损害及严重度至少要达到一定的标准。尽管脑损害的体积与痴呆的关系不肯定，但可能存在累加效应。

二、护理干预

痴呆患者的护理目标是最大限度地保存患者的功能，保证患者的尊严及较好的生活质量。痴呆患者的护理措施可以从患者的角度、照顾环境的角度以及痴呆患者照顾者的角度进行考虑。

1. 对痴呆患者进行护理

（1）药物治疗方法：目前针对痴呆，没有有效的药物可以治愈疾病或者阻止疾病的进程。针对轻度、中度的痴呆患者，一些

developed that may temporarily improve cognitive function or slow its decline for many with mild to moderate AD. Most of these drugs (i. e. , donepezil, rivastigmine, galantamine) act to increase the amount of acetylcholine in the central nervous system, by inhibiting the enzyme cholinesterase. Acetylcholine is a memory and cognition-regulating neurotransmitter. Prolonging the activity of acetylcholine on the cholinergic receptors and in the synapses permits more effective transmission. Although currently approved only for AD, it has been suggested that these drugs may be equally effective for people with VD or Lewy body dementia. Memantine is the first drug shown to be effective in clients with moderate to severe AD. It has been proposed that memantine may reduce neuronal cell destruction.

Other drugs that are being investigated to manage symptoms of dementia include antioxidants (e. g. , ginkgo biloba, vitamin E); nonsteroidal anti-inflammatory drugs; and statins. All the drugs have been shown inconsistent results.

Nurses and caregivers should ensure that dementia patients have had the medicines safely. They should ensure the patients have actually swallowed their medication. In addition, patients and families should be instructed to take medications as prescribed, because higher doses may not increase cognitive benefits, but are likely to increase side effects. To maximize absorption of the drug, galantamine and rivastigmine should be administered with food, whereas donepezil and memantine can be administered without regard to food. The useful information about the medication and side effects are listed in table 20-3.

药物可以暂时性地延缓认知功能下降的程度。由于老年痴呆的一个主要原因是胆碱不足，导致患者记忆减退、定向力丧失、行为和个性改变等。因此，具有增强胆碱能作用的药物在老年痴呆治疗方面发挥了重要作用。目前常用的4种药物是乙酰胆碱酯酶（AChE）抑制剂，包括安理申、艾斯能、加兰他敏。另外还有一种N-甲基-D-天门冬氨酸（NMDA）受体拮抗剂，即盐酸美金刚，其在治疗过程中也具有一定的疗效。

另外，某些改善脑血液循环和脑细胞代谢的药物，如吡拉西坦、都可喜、甲磺酸双氢麦角碱等可以用于老年痴呆患者，改善部分症状。同时，一些研究者利用具有自由基清除作用的银杏叶提取物EGB-761治疗老年痴呆患者，发现有明显的认知功能改善作用。维生素E是重要的抗氧化剂，具有自由基代谢的神经保护作用，还可能通过抑制和清除脑内β-淀粉样蛋白沉积，产生延缓衰老的作用。

护理人员和家庭照顾者一定要确认患者安全地服用了这些药物。同时，护理人员还要保证患者不要服用过量的药物，因为这些药物过量使用会产生一定的副作用。

Table 20-3　Medication and Side Effects

Drug	Total Daily Dose	Adverse Effects
Donepezil	5-10 mg q.d.	Headache, fatigue, insomnia, diarrhea, nausea, anorexia, weight loss, frequent urination
Galantamine	4-12 mg b.i.d.	Fatigue, bradycardia, anorexia, diarrhea, weight loss
Rivastigmine	3-6 mg b.i.d. to a maximum of 12 mg/day, orally or transdermally	Weakness, dizziness, anorexia, nausea, vomiting, weight loss
Memantine	5-10 mg b.i.d.	Dizziness, headache, constipation

表 20-3 常用药物及其副作用

药物	每日剂量	副作用
多奈哌齐	5~10mg q.d.	头疼、疲乏、失眠、腹泻、恶心、食欲缺乏、体重减轻、尿频
加兰他敏	4~12mg b.i.d.	疲乏、心动过缓、食欲缺乏、腹泻、体重减轻
利凡斯的明	3~6mg b.i.d.，最大剂量不超过 12mg/d，口服或者经皮肤给药	虚弱、头晕、厌食、恶性、呕吐、体重减轻
美金刚	5~10mg b.i.d.	头晕、头疼、便秘

(2) Non-pharmacological therapies: As nurses take care of patients with dementia by non-pharmacological therapies, three models might be useful to plan and provide the care. They are the progressively lowered stress threshold (PLST) model, the need-driven dementia-compromised behavioral model (NDB), and the cognitive developmental approach.

The progressively lowered stress threshold model (PLST) developed by Hall and Buckwalter posits that the ability to tolerate stress declines with the progression of the disease. This includes both internal (i. e., pain and fatigue) and external stressors (i. e., overwhelming environmental stimuli). A plan of care directed to patients who be patient-centered. All interventions should support the patient in functioning within the limits of the dementing illness.

The need-driven dementia-compromised behavioral model (NDB) is proposed by Algase. This model reframes disruptive behaviors as an expression of unmet needs of the person with dementia. These unmet needs may be emotional, social, physical, or psychological in nature, but because the person with dementia may have lost language skills necessary to communicate their needs, they do so behaviorally. By assessing and organizing personal and environmental factors, the nurse can identify individuals at risk for dysfunctional behavior and individualized interventions can evolve.

The cognitive developmental approach proposes that cognitive skills and functional abilities are lost in reverse order from which they were originally acquired. The stages of dementia, from diagnosis to death, are equated to the reverse order of Piaget's developmental levels of children for the purpose of individualizing assessment and intervention. This model recommends that interventions should be chosen to match the functional skills of the older adult with dementia to ensure success. Three levels of functional ability direct interventions. For ambulatory individuals, active sports and games and cognitive

（2）非药物治疗方法：护士在使用非药物治疗方法护理患者时，可以使用下面提到的 3 个模式指导护理实践活动：

逐渐递减刺激阈值模型（PLST）：强调护士要明确患者随着病情变化所能忍耐压力的能力。压力包括内部压力（如自身的疼痛、疲乏）和外部压力（如过度的环境压力）。护理计划应该是以患者为中心的，都要以支持患者现有的应对应激的能力为出发点进行具体措施的制订。

以需求为导向的痴呆行为发生模型（NDB）：强调痴呆患者行为问题的发生可能是其需要未被满足的一种表达。这种需要可能是情感的、社会交往的、生理的或者心理方面的。由于痴呆患者可能丧失语言表达能力，不能准确地表达他们的需求，因此他们用这些特殊的行为来进行表达。护士通过仔细评估个体和环境的因素，明确患者的需求，识别可能发生异常行为或者已经发生异常行为的患者，并给予个体化的护理。

认知发展理论：认为痴呆患者的认知功能和日常生活能力的丢失与其获得的顺序恰恰相反。痴呆患者从确诊到死亡的全过程中，患者功能水平的丧失正是按照皮亚杰的发展理论的阶段逆向而行的。这个理论强调护理干预一定要建立在患者现存的功能水平上，与这些功能水平相对应。

stimulation with a motor component are examples of interventions. Activities for the wheelchair-bound individual include exercises and sensory stimulation, and for the nonambulatory individual, range-of-motion exercises, massage, and sensory integration activities are appropriate.

The appendix 6 lists some behavioral management strategies directed to patients with dementia. However, as nurses apply these, they need to revise them as patient-centered which mean to meet the individual special condition and needs. In addition, appendix 7 lists several non-pharmacologic caring techniques to patients with dementia.

Box 20-3 Best Practice Guideline for Accommodating and Managing BPSD in Residential Care

The British Ministry of Health developed *the Best Practice Guideline for Accommodating and Managing BPSD of Dementia in Residential Care* in 2011. The guideline supports physicians, nurses, clinicians and care staff to provide interdisciplinary, evidence-based, person-centered care to those experiencing behavioral and psychological symptoms of dementia (BPSD), with a specific focus on the appropriate use of non-pharmacological interventions and antipsychotic drugs in the residential care setting.

The guideline aims to:

● Improve the quality of care for persons with dementia who live in residential care;

● Improve resident/family/substitute decision maker engagement in consent to care and treatment;

● Identify the appropriate use of antipsychotic drugs in treating BPSD in residential care;

● Increase the capacity of the residential care sector to provide appropriate assessment and care for persons experiencing BPSD.

2. Interventions toward care environment
Whether the person is living at home or in a long-term care facility, it is often necessary to modify the environment to compensate for the person's impaired functional and cognitive status. The primary concern is safety. Potential harmful items (i. e. , sharp objects, toxic fluids) should be removed from the client's environment. Mirrors and photographs which can be confused or frightening

附录 6 列出了针对痴呆患者的一些行为管理策略。附录 7 列出了针对痴呆患者的几种非药物护理技术。护士使用这些工具时需要以患者为中心，满足个人的特殊条件和需求。

Box 20-3 机构痴呆老人 BPSD 的最佳实践指南

英国卫生部于 2011 年发布了《机构痴呆老人精神行为问题症状（BPSD）的最佳实践指南》。以指导医护人员为那些伴有 BPSD 的痴呆人群提供多学科合作的、以患者为中心的照护服务指南。

指南的目的是：

● 促进机构中痴呆患者的照护质量；

● 促进患者、家属、机构决策者能对照护和治疗方式的知情；

● 在机构照护中使用恰当的药物治疗手段；

● 促进机构中的管理部门的能力提升，为伴有 BPSD 的痴呆老人提供合适的评估工具和照护方法。

2. 照顾环境的改善措施 无论痴呆患者是在家居住还是在养老机构居住，其所居住的环境一定要经过相应的改造以适应患者的认知功能和日常生活能力。在环境的改造中，最需要关注的就是环境安全的问题。潜在的可能造成伤害的物品（如锐器、有毒液体）等一定要从患者居住的环境中挪走。房间内

to patients should be covered or removed. Television and radio programming should be monitored for appropriateness. In the living area, clutter, highly polished floors, or scatter rugs can lead to falls in patients who may already suffer from an unsteady gait. To the extent possible, keep belongings, frequently used items, and furniture in the same place, so the person with dementia does not have to relearn their whereabouts and may rely more on habit and routine to negotiate the environment.

Using contrasting colors for the walls and woodwork make it easier for the patients to more clearly distinguish doorways. Patterned wallpaper, curtains, and upholstery can cause confusion and should be replaced with solid colors wherever possible. Furniture should be in a contrasting color to the floor to make it easier to distinguish. Grad bars installed in the bathtub and bedside the toilet provide a measure of safety for all members of the household. A hand-held shower can make bathing less frightening. Replacing the bathroom door and glass shower doors with shower curtains will continue to offer privacy but prevent the person from getting stuck or locked in the bathroom. If the color of the toilet and floor are similar, changing the toilet seat to a contrasting color helps the person distinguish the seat.

In kitchen, removing extra pots, dishes, and utensils help to minimize an overwhelming number of choices. Childproof locks can be installed on cabinet doors and oven doors to restrict access. Control knobs for the stove should be removed to prevent injury.

Cognitive impairment limits the person's ability to differentiate between safe and unsafe acts. Age-related sensory impairments can further contribute to accidents or injury. Modifications made to the living environment are done primarily to maintain the safety of the individual as well as the independence and dignity of the older adults.

3. Interventions toward to family caregivers
It is estimated 70% of persons with dementia are cared for in their own home or a family member's home. Caring for an elderly with dementia triggers significant emotional, physical, and financial stress. These kinds of stress have been linked to some adverse outcomes, including depression, high psychotropic drug use, decline in physical health, and compromised immune response. Nurses are

能引起患者恐惧感的镜子或者某些图片要移除。电视节目和收音机频道也一定要符合患者的功能水平。居住环境中避免有堆积的物品、松动的地毯及过滑的地板等，以免步态不稳的患者发生跌倒。尽可能地将房间内的家具、患者常用的物品等按照患者以往所熟悉的方式摆放，这样痴呆患者就不需要再重新适应新环境，很多患者可以在这个熟悉的环境中根据自己既往的习惯或者常规方式来生活。

在墙壁和家具间可以使用对比色，使得患者容易找寻到房间内的过道。带有图案的墙纸、窗帘和家具装饰用品会引起患者的混乱，应尽可能换为单色的。家具应与地板形成对比色，以便于区分。浴盆和厕所旁都应该装有安全扶手。更换浴室门和浴房门等，换为浴帘，这样做既可以维护患者的隐私，又可以避免患者被锁在浴室或者浴房内。如果厕所的颜色和地面的颜色很接近，要更换厕所座便的颜色使得其与地面有鲜明的对比。

厨房内多余的锅、碗、碟子等都尽量挪走，使得患者对这些物品的选择变得简单。可以使用儿童安全锁对橱柜或者烤箱等锁定，避免患者玩弄。炉灶上的打火按钮也要移除，以避免发生危险。

认知功能障碍使得患者识别危险的能力减弱。而与年龄相关的感官功能衰退又使得患者发生意外伤害的概率增加。照顾环境的改善与调整一方面可以维护患者的安全，另外一方面也可以更好地维持患者的自理能力和自尊水平。

3. 对痴呆患者照顾者进行护理 据统计大约有 70% 的痴呆患者被家人照料。照料痴呆患者使得照顾者产生情感、生理和经济等各方面的压力。这些压力会导致照顾者发生不良结局，如抑郁、精神药物滥用、身体健康状况下降、免疫系统受损等。护士应帮助照顾者具备照顾痴呆患者的相应的知识与技

playing an important role to provide training to empower family members with the knowledge and skills necessary in handling the stressful situation and those problematic behaviors as well, while maintaining their own well-being.

(1) Education and support in caregiving responsibilities: The PLST can be used as the basis for a pyschoeducational intervention for caregivers of dementia. Instruction focused on reducing environmental stressors, compensating for executive dysfunction and communication deficits, providing unconditional positive regard, and planning care based on a lowered stress threshold. An ongoing nursing relationship is pivotal in guiding family caregivers to establish a routine that maximizes abilities and minimizes stress for both the care recipient and the caregiver.

(2) Referral to support groups for care and assistance: Support groups provide an avenue to meet other family caregivers to share feelings and concerns, and provide emotional support and decrease the caregiver burden. Many support groups also provide learning opportunities by formal community experts and the informal expertise of other caregivers.

(3) Nursing home placement: When the family member is no longer able to care for his or her loved one at home, nursing home placement may be warranted. Many caregivers experience decreased depression and burden at 6 and 12 months after placing a family member in the nursing home; however, spouses demonstrate greater burden than adult children caregivers. However, relocation to a nursing home does not necessarily mean an end to the stress experienced by family caregivers. Some family caregivers experience feelings of guilt, betrayal, and inadequacy related to their caregiving role. Nursing home placement necessitates the assumption of a new role for the resident and caregiver. Most families do not know how to make the transition from direct care tasks to a more indirect, supportive, interpersonal role, nor are they likely to receive assistance from nursing home staff in how to go about making changes in their caregiver role. In some cases, families may encounter resistance and resentment from staff who view them as disruptive "outsiders" or "visitors" when they try to carry out decision making and protective care in the facility, resulting in staff-family role conflict.

(LIU Yu)

能，以使得他们更好地应对这个充满压力的照顾任务，并维持自身的健康。

（1）照顾者教育和情感支：PLST 模型可以在这里应用。主要目的是保证家庭照顾者能针对患者的现存功能安排患者的日常活动，使患者发挥其最大功能，且要解决的问题在患者的功能可应付范围内。

（2）向家庭照顾者引荐相应的支持小组和可获取的帮助：支持小组可以帮助多个痴呆患者的家庭照顾者彼此之间互相分享他们各自的情绪体验、面临的问题和关心的焦点。支持小组可以降低照顾者的负担，同时提供照顾者相应的情感支持。在照顾者小组中，还有很多学习如何照顾痴呆患者的讲座，进而扩展照顾者的相关照顾知识和技能。

（3）入住养老机构：当家庭成员不能继续在家中照顾老年人时，往往会将老年人送入养老机构。但是送入之后的一段时间内，家庭照顾者仍然会面临较大的负担。护士一方面应该做好家庭照顾者的内心调节工作，同时应该让家庭照顾者与养老机构的医务人员合作，参与到痴呆老人的计划制订活动中。

（刘　宇）

Key Points

1. Dementia is a syndrome of gradual and progressive cognitive decline. It is not a part of the normal aging process.

2. Management of AD focuses on maintaining cognitive and global function early on in the disease process to postpone the need for institutional care.

3. Individuals who have experienced a CVA have an even greater risk of VD.

4. The effective management of problem behaviors should not focus on trying to change the older person but on modifying factors that may be contributing to these behaviors.

5. The use of physical and chemical restraints has demonstrated no benefit in controlling disruptive behaviors or managing disease.

6. Maintaining social interaction and human contact in a variety of ways is beneficial for older persons with cognitive decline.

7. The nurse's role in dementia care has shifted from caregiver to care coordinator. The nurse teaches and assists the family members with home care, provides supportive care, and serves as a client advocate.

Critical Thinking Exercise

Mrs. Li was a happy lady for over 75 years. She lived in the center of the city and had her daily morning exercise at the community square to chat with her friends. She lost her husband 5 years ago, and her daughter was living in other city. She lived by herself. Her daughter started to notice that something was not right when she visited her mom 3 years ago. During her stay of two weeks, she found that her mom always forgot to take her pills and not went out for exercise and chatting with her friends. She also noticed her mom was sleeping more and not changing her clothes for season and weather. The time from when the daughter first noticed changed in Mrs. Li's cognition to the neurological physician visiting was approximately 3 years. Mrs. Li was found to have difficulty with memory and recall, poor orientation, calculation, and multistep task performance. Her MMSE was recorded as 19/30, and a diagnosis of dementia of the Alzheimer's type was made.

To this day Mrs. Li has not acknowledged any memory

本章要点

1. 痴呆是渐进性的认知功能减退综合征。它不属于正常老化过程。

2. 对 AD 患者的护理应着重从病程的早期开始就关注患者认知功能及整体功能的维持，延缓其入住照护机构的时间。

3. 既往有脑血管意外事件发生的个体，有更大的危险性罹患血管性痴呆。

4. 对痴呆患者行为问题的应对不要去尝试改变患者，而应该去调整引发患者出现行为问题的可能原因。

5. 使用物理约束或者化学约束已经被证明对管理患者的异常行为还是疾病照护都没有益处。

6. 使用多种方法帮助认知功能障碍的老人维持其社交活动和增加社会参与度是非常有益处的。

7. 在痴呆照护中护士的角色已经从照护者转为照护的协调者。护士要教给和帮助家庭照护者提供居家照护，提供支持性的帮助，并作为患者的代言人为患者服务。

批判性思维练习

李夫人在 75 岁之前一直是一位乐观的女士。她住在市中心，每天早晨都到社区中的小广场进行锻炼，同时和老朋友们聊聊天。她的丈夫去世 5 年了，她自己独居，女儿住在另外一个城市里。3 年前她的女儿来看望妈妈时发现有些事情不太正常。在她回家探亲的 2 周里，女儿发现妈妈总是忘记服药，不去锻炼，也不和老朋友聊天了。她发现她妈妈睡觉的时间越来越长，不能随着季节和气候的变化相应地调整衣物。在发现这些异常情况的 3 年后，女儿才带着妈妈第一次去就医。检查发现李夫人的记忆力、回忆力、定向力、计算力以及执行力都非常的差。她的 MMSE 得分为 19 分，被诊断为 AD。

但是李夫人不承认自己的记忆有问题，当被

deficit and when confronted by the family she states "it's part of getting old". It has been difficult for the family to persuade Mrs. Li to attend appointments. The family expressed fear in causing their mother anxiety by insisting on the appointments; thus they delayed the checkup as long as possible.

Family is more often in denial with such statements as "it's her age" or "ever since my father died, she hasn't been quite right". Families tend to generate their own explanatory model for the behavior and symptoms. Many families believe that memory loss is a normal part of aging, and it becomes quite a task to explain otherwise.

Questions:

1. What are some of the possible reasons that prevented the family from seeking a diagnostic workup earlier?

2. What additional information would the nurse need to gather before communicating the diagnosis? How could the nurse assist the family and patient with adjusting to the diagnosis of dementia?

家人提及记忆有问题时，她就解释说这是"老化的一部分"。劝说李夫人及时随诊变得非常困难，家人也害怕在强迫李红就医时导致她过度焦虑，因此随诊的时间被一拖再拖。

家庭成员往往以"她年纪到了，应该这样"，或者"自从我爸爸去世以后，她就有些有不对劲了"这样的借口来否认疾病的发生。家庭成员试图对老人的异常行为和症状寻找解释的借口。很多家庭成员认为记忆缺失是正常老化的一部分，需要多和老人解释和沟通。

问题：

1. 有哪些可能的原因阻止家庭成员尽早带出现异常情况的老人就医和做出诊断？

2. 护士在和家庭成员谈及诊断前还需要收集哪些额外的信息？护士如何帮助家庭成员和患者来适应痴呆这一诊断？

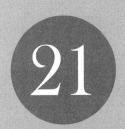

Chapter 21 Hospice Care Issues
第二十一章 老年人的安宁疗护

Learning Objectives

On completion of this chapter, the readers will be able to:

- Describe basic concept of hospice care and the underline philosophy;

- Describe psychological as well as physical care needs of dying individuals;

- Describe common discomforts of the dying individual;

- Describe early development of hospice care;

- List nursing interventions to meet the dying people's need;

- Identify bereavement and grief strategies for survivors and describe ways to support them.

学习目标

学完本章节，应完成以下目标：

- 掌握安宁疗护的基本概念及理念；

- 掌握临终患者的生理、心理需求；

- 掌握临终患者的常见不适症状；

- 了解安宁疗护的发展；

- 应用满足临终患者需求的常用护理措施；

- 掌握沮丧者悲哀的表现和护理措施。

With the growing of aging population and the increasing number of old people suffering from terminal illness and cancer, more and more attention is now on end-of-life care, which is described as hospice care in this chapter. Unfortunately, in the mainland of China, hospice care now stays in the phrase of concept and few special institutions, while most clinical nurses and doctors are not equipped with the essential knowledge and professional skills to deal with the dying elderly. However, the introduction of WHO pain control and hospice care of cancer patients in 1990 to Chinese medical system has remarkably improved the development of hospice care in China.

Box 21-1　Case study

Mr. Luo is a terminally ill nursing facility resident who is suffering from pain secondary to metastasis of his lung cancer to his spine. His pain has been managed with a non-steroid anti-inflammatory drug, because Mr. Luo is seen grimacing with pain periodically throughout the day. A review of his medication administration record reveals that he sometimes asks for his pain medication at 6-8-hour intervals, although he is able to have the drug every 4 hours. The nurses observe that he complains of pain more frequently during the week than on weekends when his family visits.

Question:

What could nurse staffs do to help him to improve pain control for visits?

Section 1　Basic Information and Development of Hospice Care

End of life issues and hospice care are important topics in gerontological nursing. Improving quality of hospice care not only help the elder patients and also their families to cope with difficult situations.

I. Concepts of Hospice Care

Hospice care (or hospice) is a way of caring for the terminally ill with life expectancy of six months or less. Hospice was founded on the philosophy of compassionate, humane nursing care that focuses on patient comfort and quality of life provided by health professionals and volunteers rather than curing the patient's disease. It aids in putting quality and meaning into the remaining

随着社会老龄化及老年人口数量的攀升，肿瘤患者和终末期疾病患者的安宁疗护问题越来越受到关注。然而，在我国，安宁疗护仍处于起步阶段，真正实践安宁疗护（又名临终关怀、舒缓医学、姑息医疗等）的机构相对较少，具备关怀知识和能力的医护人员也相对缺乏。WHO 对于肿瘤和疼痛患者的治疗指南大大促进了我国安宁疗护的发展。

Box 21-1　个案学习

罗先生因肺癌脊柱转移住在安宁疗护机构。患者主诉疼痛，为周期性二级疼痛。非甾体抗炎药作为长期备用医嘱。用药记录中显示患者用药周期为 6 ~ 8 小时（医嘱为每 4 小时可用药）。然而，护士发现，周末家人探望时，老人疼痛会"缓解"。

问题：

护士可以通过哪些措施可以帮助罗先生达到家人探望时疼痛缓解的效果？

第一节　安宁疗护的概念与发展

安宁疗护是老年护理中的重要内容。在实践中提高安宁疗护的护理质量不仅会帮助临终老人还将帮助整个居丧家庭度过危机。

一、基本概念

安宁疗护是医护工作者、社会工作者、志愿者等组织或个人对身患绝症、预期寿命为 6 个月或更短的患者及其家庭成员的多方位、人性化的照顾。安宁疗护是建立在同情和人文关爱的护理理念基础上，医护人员和志愿者更关注患者的舒适度和生活质量，而

period of life. A basic goal of hospice is palliative care and support services, that is, helping the dying live as fully as possible with the highest quality of life on a day-to-day basis, thus to make the dying process in peace, comfort and dignity. Hospice care helps to save medical recourses and prevent hospitals from over-explore of therapeutic checkups and medications with little help to save life. Hospice care employs interdisciplinary efforts to meet physical, emotional, and spiritual needs, which include the following interventions or aspects of nursing care: pain relief, symptom control, emotion support, coordinated home care and institutional care, grief and bereavement counseling.

II. Development of Hospice Care

i. Hospice Care Development

Originally, hospice was a medieval term that meant a place where food, shelter, and care were offered to travelers who were on a long journey. Hospice is concerned with scientific and technological advances of treatment (of a palliative nature) combined with the art of caring and compassion (the spiritual quality that surrounds the patient). "Death is a part of the life cycle and need not be frightening, feared, or violet" has served as a philosophical "backbone" for the twentieth century hospice movement. In 1971, day care and in-home service were added in hospice care in St. Luke's Hospice in Sheffield, England. A North American model of hospice care research and training center was set up by Dr. Balfour Mount in Montreal, Canada in 1973 (table 21-1).

不是治愈疾病。安宁疗护致力于提高临终患者的生命质量，旨在满足临终患者的躯体、情感和精神需求，使患者在平静、舒适的环境下有尊严地离世。安宁疗护关注生命最后阶段的质量和意义，有助于节省医疗资源，防止医院过度实施对挽救生命没有帮助的治疗。安宁疗护综合了医学、社会学、心理学等多学科知识，其具体内容包括缓解疼痛，控制症状，减轻或消除负面情绪，临终患者的生活照护和丧亲者的照护。

二、安宁疗护的发展历程

（一）安宁疗护的起源

Hospice 一词源于中世纪，原意为旅游者提供食物、护理和中途休息的地方。医学上指对临终患者关怀照顾的场所，为养老院。安宁疗护运动促使人们相信死亡是生命周期的一部分，不必害怕或恐惧。1971 年，在英国谢菲尔德 (Sheffield) 的圣卢克收容所 (St. Luke's Hospice) 开展了日托和家庭服务。1973 年，巴尔弗蒙特博士（Dr. Balfour）在加拿大蒙特利尔（Montreal）建立了一个北美模式的安宁疗护研究和培训中心（表 21-1）。

Table 21-1　Brief Review of the History of Hospice in the West

Periods	Name of institution/facility and service offered
Middle Ages	Hospice-offered food, shelter, care to travelers, on their way to the Holy Land
1846	In Dublin the Irish Sisters of Charity opened a hospice that included long-stay patients. Their focus was upon the dying and hospice then became equated with this type of work
1969	In London, Dame Cicely Saunders, M.D. opens St. Christopher's, the first modern hospice (in caring only for the dying). This hospice has served as a model for many western countries
1971	Dr. Eric Welkes opens St. Luke's Hospice in Sheffield, England. Day care and in-home services were added
1973	Dr. Balfour Mount opens the Royal Victoria Hospice in Montreal, Canada. This hospice is associated with a research training hospital and has served as a North American model
1986	Every state in the US is involved in hospice care

表 21-1 西方国家安宁疗护发展史概述

时期	机构名称及所提供的服务
中世纪	Hospice 机构为路人提供食
1846	建立了为病患居住的长期照顾机构，旨在照顾临终患者
1969	Dame Cicely Saunders 医生在伦敦设立第一所现代安宁疗护机构 St. Christopher 医院，成为西方国家安宁疗护的典范
1971	Dr. Eric Welkes 在英国 Sheffield 建立了 St. Luke 安宁疗护机构，加入了日间照护和家庭照护的内容
1973	Dr. Balfour Mount 在加拿大的蒙特利尔建立了 Royal Victoria 安宁疗护机构，同时兼备研究和训练的功能，成为北美洲的典范
1986	全美每个州都成立了安宁疗护机构

2. Early hospice care in China   In China, Beitian Yuan in Tang Dynasty (600 to 900), Futian Yuan in Song Dynasty (900 to 1 200) and Puji Tang in Qing Dynasty (1 600 to 1 900) had the function of taking care of the dying old.

ii. Development of Modern Hospice Care

Chinese Association for Hospice Care and Hospice Care Fund has been established after Tianjin Medical School founded the Hospice Research Center in 1988. After that, different types of hospice agencies developed successively. Nowadays, numerous hospice agencies have been set up all over the country mainly in metropolitans, and extending from medium cities to small remote cities. In April, 2006, the establishment of the Life-care Association indicates that China's hospice care career entered a new development period.

Currently, there are three types of hospice care organizations in China: Specialized Hospice Agencies; The attached hospice wards to comprehensive hospitals, which is the main form in China nowadays. The home hospice care, a community-based service, which takes the family as the unit in hospice care.

iii. Strategy for Further Development

In future, there are a few ways to accelerate the development of hospice care in China. One important strategy is to advocate the concept of quality of life of the dying. Hospice care neither accelerates the process of dying, nor delays it. We should supersede our traditional idea of longevity of life by quality of life. The widespread acceptance of hospice care lies in the extensive understanding of improving quality of life in end-of-life care.

2. 中国早期的安宁疗护   我国唐代（公元 600 至 900 年）的"悲田院"、宋代（公元 900 至 1200 年）的"福田院"以及清代（公元 1600 至 1900 年）的"普济堂"等机构也具有照顾关怀临终老人的功能。

（二）现代安宁疗护的发展

自 1988 年天津医学院创办临终关怀研究中心之后，中国心理卫生协会临终关怀专业委员会和临终关怀基金会成立，目前全国各地建立的安宁疗护机构主要分布于大城市，正向中等城市延伸。2006 年 4 月，中国生命关怀协会成立，标志着我国的安宁疗护事业进入了一个新的发展时期。

当前，我国老年患者安宁疗护组织形式主要有 3 种：①安宁疗护专门机构；②附设的安宁疗护机构，即综合医院内的专科病房或病区，这是目前最主要的形式；③家庭安宁疗护病床，一般以社区为基础、以家庭为单位开展安宁疗护服务。

（三）我国现代安宁疗护的发展策略

国际卫生组织在安宁疗护定义中明确指出安宁疗护既不加速死亡，也不延缓死亡。对生命的重视应从数量上转移到质量上。因此，思想观念的扭转非常重要，应强调教育与宣传并重，让优化生命末端质量的观点深入人心。

Another strategy is systematic hospice care education in professional medical students, which are drawing attention from many medical schools in China.

Another but not the last strategy is to obtain more chances of international cooperation, by attending international hospice care conferences or exchanging scholars who are majored in this field. Those conferences will bring together the latest and updating ideas and knowledge of hospice care, as well as great opportunities of co-operations.

我国安宁疗护起步较晚，教育内容的广度和深度有待发展。在目前的基础上积极开展各种形式的继续教育是一条可行之路。

每年世界各国都会举行安宁疗护的相关会议，国际会议作为国际交流的重要手段，不仅可以拓宽发展思路，把握最新发展动态，借鉴经验，为我国安宁疗护的发展提供参考，同时也提供了很多国际合作的机会。我国应尽可能多地开展国际合作，充分利用已有的研究成果。

Section 2　Supporting the Dying Elderly

I. Basic Needs of the Dying Elderly

Basic needs of the dying person are much similar to the normal adults, but during the end of life, there are some specialties, as for physical, psychological and social aspects respectively. There are three levels of needs, keeping alive, free of pain and die without pain. Therefore, the immediate need of the old people who is dying is peace, stay with the support family members and without disturb. Or some more specific needs such as writing a will, meeting old friends. These psycho-social needs of the dying should not be neglected, and nursing care here aims at helping the client accomplish his journey of life.

i. Physical Aspect

1. Dressing and grooming　Generally speaking, dressing to the dying is not as important as to normal people, so a comfortable warm covering is enough. Attitude to the clothes after death indicates attitude to death and people have different attitudes and perceptions towards death, so caring is supposed to be personalized.

2. Diet and nutrition　Most of the dying people take in few solid food while impending death, and some dying individuals depend on Ⅳ supply or gastric tube to obtain caloric. Nutritional study proves that caloric need of the dying is not as much as one third of the normal adults because of the low caloric burning.

第二节　临终老人的需求与护理

一、临终老人的基本需求

临终老人与正常成人的日常需求状况相似，但也有其特殊性。临终者的基本需求主要包括个人的生理需求、精神心理需求和社会存在的需求几个方面。一般说来，濒死者的需求可分 3 个水平：①保存生命；②解除痛苦；③没有痛苦地死去。当死亡不可避免时，患者主要的需求是安宁，亲属陪伴并给予精神安慰和寄托，或者某些特殊需要，如写遗嘱、与亲友告别等。护士及亲属要尽量给予临终者躯体和精神上的照料和安慰，使他们无痛苦地度过人生最后时刻。

（一）基本生存需求

1. **衣着修饰方面**　一般来说，临终者只求衣着裁剪合身、挡风避寒且透气舒适；有关服装的其他功能对大多数临终者已淡化。要认识到老年人对待死亡的态度和认知是不同的，要依据其喜好和需求提供个体化照护。

2. **饮食营养方面**　老年临终者消化吸收能力大多显减，进食一般量少且稀薄，神志部分人依赖于鼻饲或静脉补液。营养医学证明他们每日所需补充热量最多为正常青壮年的 1/3。进入临终后期，一些老年人几乎不

3. Residence   Dying at home is one of the traditional thoughts in rural areas of China. Family care becomes the main way to offer hospice care.

4. Autonomic activities   Old dying persons could rarely move freely, they spend their last time mostly in bed. Simple movements such as eating, excreting, dressing or meeting a health care worker could bother the dying patients. Every single move has to depend on the help of family members or caregivers. Once the residence place is determined, the living places of the dying would be limited in a special court or room for a long time.

ii. Neurological and Psycho Aspect

The dying process could be just few minutes, such as in a heart attack, or could be years or months, such as in a cerebral stroke or chronic renal failure under medical care. However, whether die naturally or die of illness, the dying person is neurologically active before they lose conscious.

1. Perceptions   Modern neuropsychological studies prove that perception threshold is different at different ages, which means the dying person also has threshold to all kinds of stimuli. The perception of environment stimulus is mainly adjusted by thalamus; therefore it can be maintained to the state of fuzzy. Though the dying persons' perceptions and responds are more and more slow, they can exactly perceive any stimuli around or pain inside until they are in coma (except neurology system diseases).

2. Emotion   There are still certain emotion activities at the end of one's life and such activities are strongly affected by family. Neurophysiologic research suggests that marginal areas of the brain take control of human emotion activities. During the last stage of conscious, the dying person may act out or volatile their mood. The appearance and accompany of relatives and family members is quite important to the dying, to make them feel safe, comfort and happy.

能进食，没有咀嚼和吞咽的动作或意愿，也没有每日几餐的区分，几乎完全依赖静脉补液。弥留之际，老年人需求的可能仅仅是湿润口唇，或是少许能直接提供能量的葡萄糖水。

3. 住所方面   现阶段我国老年人大多选择了在家里度过临终期。因此，我国的安宁疗护服务仍应以居家护理为主，家人和照顾者成为承担安宁疗护的主要人员。

4. 自主活动方面   老年临终者少有行动自如者，多数处于卧床状态，其躯体移动大多数依赖他人及助步工具。譬如穿衣进食、翻身解手、就诊求医等，均要依赖家人或照顾者的帮助。因此，他们的居住处所一旦确定，大部分老年临终者往往长期地限定于一个房间或一个院子之中。

（二）精神心理活动

老年人临终期短则数分钟，如严重突发性脑卒中病例；长则可达数月甚至年余，如现代医学条件下的脏器功能慢性衰竭者。而无论是自然死亡或因病死亡，绝大多数临终老人并非始终陷于昏迷状态；在意识清醒的时候，他们有自己的精神活动。

1. 感知觉   现代神经心理学证明，不同年龄段的人们虽然感知觉阈值不同，但老年临终者在清醒时对超阈值刺激的感知觉还是存在的，且这种能力主要受丘脑调节，可以维持到意识模糊阶段。依此，虽然老年人的感知觉越来越迟钝，但直到昏迷前期还是有感知觉的，此时他们完全可以较确切地感知到身体因受异常刺激所产生的不适和痛苦（神经系统病症患者除外）。

2. 情感   意识弥留之际的临终老人仍然有一定的情感活动能力，这种能力及其心理效果往往带有强烈的亲情色彩。神经生理学研究提示，人类的情感活动调控中枢处于边缘区，这就可解释老年临终者在意识由清醒到模糊时，往往会有至数次波动较大的发作性情绪宣泄。当然，情感活动是有条件的，亲人的守候可以使老年人获得安全、放心、

3. Memory and thinking The instantaneous and short-term memory ability of aged persons recesses obviously, while memory capacity of long-term information also cuts under the situation of stroke or other brain disease. Besides memory decline, the ability of conceive also experience a recession. This is not only affected by the memory recession, but also by the decline of brain function, just as it is said that aged and kids are the same. However it is not so in spiritual aspects, the older dying person is actually in a process of wisdom loosing.

iii. Social Aspect

Old or young, the individual is a molecular of society. Participating in social interactivities reflects the existence and needs of the individual to exchange materials and spirits, to build up one's own confidence and self-esteem. So, as long as the dying person is awake, there are social needs to keep in touch with the outside world. Two forms of communication between the dying individual and the social environment exist: direct and indirect ways. Direct way is supported by the social group or public media while the indirect form is through certain persons such as the family member, caregiver, or health care providers. Generally speaking, though the ability of social interactive is declining with the dying process, it is of great importance to meet the growing needs of the dying to maintain communication with the outside world except the limitation of laivck of direct form of obtaining information. Accordingly, visits or sympathy from social organizations, groups and media agencies during dying period is significantly important for the dying person.

iv. Special Sufferings of the Dying

Sufferings during the dying period would be taken away by the dying person without being repeated and complained. So, it is easy to be ignored. The sufferings of the dying individual could be divided into physical aspect and psychological aspect. On physical aspect, chronic disease can cause tissue damage, organ failure, which is often accompanied by significant somatic symptoms, such as inflammation and pain of tumor. The organ failure or dysfunction in the aged patients is mainly because of the

美满的情感体验，因而对老年临终者极其重要。

3. 记忆和思维 老年人瞬时记忆和短时记忆能力明显衰退，长时记也会消减，若是脑卒中或其他脑病患者情况还会更糟。在记忆能力减退的同时，老年人的思维能力也会发生衰退，这既是受记忆衰退的影响，也是脑神经元易化能力减退致信息传导速度减慢的结果。

（三）社会活动需求

老年人作为社会一分子，参与社会实践既是他们体现自己的存在价值并获取生存物质资料的根本方式，也是他们精神生活中各种外界信息内容的根本来源，还是他们形成各自不同的自信、自尊的心理依据。因此，只要尚未进入昏迷，且不管其社会活动能力保留状态怎样，临终老人都将继续保持一定的沟通社会的内在需求惯性。临终期与社会之间的物质—信息双重交流有直接和间接两种形式，直接的形式是通过社会团体、传媒机构等途径来完成的；间接的形式则是通过家人、监护人或者是亲戚、医护人员等一些特殊"个人"来完成的。一般情况是，临终老人愈是趋近死亡终点，其社会活动能力愈弱，同社会之间的物质—信息双重交流就愈是更多地呈现为间接的形式，结果愈是容易陷入个人禁闭状态，因而愈是具有比过去强烈得多的同外界沟通信息、尽量实现各种类型交往的社会活动需求。相应的，社会性组织、团体的关顾、造访或慰问，对于临终老人便具有十分重要的意义。

（四）临终期痛苦

"临终期痛苦"产生之后往往伴随至死亡，无从复述，因此容易被忽视。老年人的"临终期痛苦"可分为躯体和心理两方面。躯体方面，慢性疾病可致组织损伤、器官衰竭，常伴有显著的躯体症状，如炎症和疼痛等；老年人的器官衰竭一方面是退行性的器官功能改变，另一方面则是慢性疾病导致的

aging process or chronic diseases, especially when the health care provided is much better, it would be a long-term suffering of complications and the discomfort of the disease itself. As to the psychological aspect of the sufferings of the dying person, there are many reasons for it, which could be described as helplessness and hopelessness. Fail to meet the physical needs of the dying person, and fail to avoid those invades from outside, and incapable to deal with the tough situation and to get enough help，all above contribute to such feelings and sufferings. Therefore, the "psychological distress" is not only closely related with the material life conditions, but also with individual spiritual and social factors (table 21-2).

器官功能障碍，如患老年痴呆、老年肺气肿、慢性肾衰竭等。如果接受了良好的医疗照顾，则病程可持续 10 年，甚至是 20 年以上，但往往会伴有并发症，如脑血管意外患者多伴有意识障碍和肢体瘫痪，因卧床时间过久时常发生肺部感染、便秘、压疮等并发症。心理方面，引起老年人临终期"心理痛苦"的原因很多，主要分为两个方面：一是各种基本需求得不到满足，在遭受自然或人为侵害时的无能为力感；二是遭受侵害时得不到有效援助的无助感。因此，老年人临终期"心理痛苦"不仅同物质生活条件密切相关，而且同个体精神生活和社会生活需求能否得到满足密切相关（表 21-2 ）。

Table 21-2　Key Points of the Basic Needs of the Dying

Basic Needs of the Dying	
Physical aspects	Dressing and grooming Diet and nutrition Residence Autonomic activities
Neurological and psycho aspects	Perceptions Emotion Memory and thinking
Social aspects	Advance directives, written instructions regarding the preferred medical care
Special sufferings	Somatic symptoms, such as inflammation and pain of tumor Psychological distress, helplessness and hopelessness

表 21-2　临终患者的主要需求概述

临终患者的需求要点	
生理需求	衣着、饮食、居所、自主活动
神经精神需求	感知、情绪、记忆、思考
社会生活需求	写出自己的医疗需要
其他痛苦	躯体症状，如感染、疼痛、肿瘤；心理症状，如无助、无望等

II. Common Discomforts of the Dying Elderly

Common physical problems and symptoms encountered by terminally ill clients include pain, dyspnea, constipation, delirium, altered urinary elimination patterns, altered skin integrity, loss of appetite, dry mouth, nausea and vomiting, restlessness and sleeplessness, difficulty swallowing, and nutritional problems. Here, we

二、临终前常见症状及护理

老年患者临终的情况各不相同，有的是突然死亡，有的是逐渐衰竭以至死亡。后者可能有较长时间在生和死的边缘挣扎。临终患者常见的生理症状有疼痛、呼吸困难、便秘、谵妄、排泄形态改变、皮肤完整性受损、

share the most typical and common discomforts of the dying elder people.

i. Pain

Concern as to the degree of pain that will be experienced and its management may be a considerable source of distress for dying individuals; nurses are in a position to reassure them with realistic information regarding pain. Legitimate pain killers can improve the quality of life which is not used as "comfort for the dying" and as a "last resort".

Gerontological nurses must be aware that patients will perceive and express pain differently based on their cultural background, medical diagnosis, emotional state, cognitive function, and other factors. Complaints of pain or discomfort, nausea, irritability, restlessness, and anxiety are common indicators of pain; however, the absence of such expressions of pain does not mean pain does not exist. Some patients may not overtly express their pain; in these individuals, signs such as sleep disturbances, reduced activity, diaphoresis, pallor, poor appetite, grimacing, and withdrawal may provide clues to the presence of pain. The presence of pain must be regularly reassessed because it can increase or decrease over time. Pain severity is best assessed by patient self-report and may be aided by visual analogue scales (VASs), numerical rated scales (NRSs) and/or verbal rated scales (VRSs).

For the dying patient, the goal of pain management is to prevent pain from occurring rather than treating it once it does occur. Pain prevention not only helps patients avoid discomfort but ultimately reduces the amount of analgesics used by patients. The WHO guidelines for the management of cancer pain state that analgesic treatment choices should be based on the severity of the pain, not on prognosis. So patients at all stages of cancer could have morphine if their pain is sufficient. Professional competence, correct communication, and a relationship based on trust are the three principle factors taken into consideration by patients when deciding whether or not to start opioid treatment. Alternatives to medications should be included in the pain-control program of dying patients. Such measures could include guided imagery, hypnosis, relaxation exercises, massage, acupressure, acupuncture, and the application of heat or cold.

ii. Respiratory Distress

Respiratory distress is a common problem in dying

食欲缺乏、吞咽困难、营养问题以及恶心、呕吐、烦躁不安和失眠等。但是患者并非同时出现所有的濒死症状,也不是所有的症状都会出现,临终患者最常见的症状和体征如下:

(一)疼痛

疼痛是常见的临终症状,尤其是晚期癌症患者。合理的药物镇痛有利于提高临终患者的生活质量。

老年人的护理人员必须意识到,不同患者认识和表达疼痛的方式不同。患者的文化背景、诊断、情绪、认知功能等因素影响其感知和表达疼痛。常见间接提示疼痛的表述有不舒服、恶心、易怒、烦躁和焦虑。也有患者没有特殊提示,但仍然忍受疼痛。一些患者出现睡眠障碍、活动减少、发汗、脸色苍白、食欲缺乏、面容苍白和畏缩等行为变化也可提示疼痛的存在。疼痛会随着时间的推移而加重或减轻,因此要随时评估。评估最好依据患者主诉,也可通过视觉模拟量表(VAS)、数字评分量表(NRSS)和/或口头评分量表(VRSS)来辅助评估。

对于临终的患者来说,控制疼痛应及时、有效。止痛药应规律、足量应用,而不是必要时才使用,等到疼痛发生时再控制比预防疼痛发生更困难。疼痛预防不仅有助于患者避免不适,而且最终减少了患者使用的止痛药数量。WHO发布的癌症疼痛管理指南指出,镇痛治疗的选择应基于疼痛的严重程度,而不是预后。因此,如果疼痛足够的话,处于癌症各个阶段的患者都可以服用吗啡。临终患者的疼痛控制计划中应包括替代药物。除了药物止痛,还可采用其他方法缓解疼痛,如图像引导、催眠术、放松术、按摩、穴位按压、针灸和热和冷疗法等。

(二)呼吸困难

痰液堵塞、呼吸困难是临终患者的常见

patients. In addition to the physical discomfort resulting from dyspnea, patients can experience tremendous psychological distress associated with the fear, anxiety, and helplessness that results from the thought of suffocating. The causes of respiratory distress can range from pleural effusion to deteriorating blood gas levels. Interventions such as elevating the head of the bed and administering oxygen can prove beneficial. Inhaling therapy may be administered to dilute bronchial secretions; provide oral care to lubricate the dry lips or cover the lips and mouth with moisture gauze dressing if the patient is sleeping with mouth open.

For patients with end-stage lung cancer, noninvasive ventilation (NIV) may be more effective at reducing breathing difficulty than standard oxygen therapy, and has the added advantage of reducing patients' reliance on morphine, thus improving lucidity in their final days. For patients at this stage, even small comforts can be the difference between a peaceful and an agonizing death. Clinical randomized controlled study investigating the relief of respiratory distress in end-stage cancer patients shows that the main advantage over oxygen is that NIV not only improve oxygenation, but also work on breathing.

iii. Hallucinations and Delusions

Cognitively impaired older adults who are dying frequently experience hallucinations and delusions. Hallucinations may occur in any sensory modality – visual, auditory, olfactory, gustatory, tactile, or proprioceptive (sense of balance and position in space). Attempts to confront and reorient the delusional person are usually unsuccessful and may cause additional agitation. A better strategy is to ignore delusional statements and divert the conversation to more neutral topics. The technique of validation, based on empathic understanding of the emotion and messages behind the confusion, is effective in communicating with those experiencing delusions and hallucinations. For instance, if a person, when alone, believes that he or she is talking to his or her mother, asking the client if he or she is feeling lonely or afraid may help the client express underlying emotions and ease some anxiety.

iv. Poor Nutritional Intake

The majority of patients with advanced cancer develop malnutrition. This malnutrition has an important impact on quality of life, performance status and immune status (table 21-3). It can be responsible for increased morbidity, particularly infectious complications and thus mortality. In five to more than 20% of patients with cancer,

症状。除了呼吸困难引起的身体不适外，患者还可能经历恐惧、焦虑和无助等心理痛苦。呼吸困难可源于多种因素，如胸腔积液、血氧分压下降等。可采取抬高床头、吸氧，同时开窗或使用风扇通风，护理人员平静的仪态，用手轻柔地抚摸患者加上和声细语，都有利于帮助患者保持平静。雾化吸入用于稀释支气管分泌物，促使分泌物变稀，易于咳出，床旁备好吸引器。对张口呼吸者，提供口腔护理，用湿巾或棉签湿润口腔，患者睡着时用湿纱布遮盖口部。

对于终末期肺癌患者，无创通气（NIV）比标准氧疗法更能有效地减轻呼吸困难，并具有减少患者对吗啡依赖，从而提高患者终末期的清醒度。对于终末期患者而言，些许的安慰可能意味着平静的离世还是痛苦的离世的差别。随机对照临床研究表明，NIV 的主要优势在于，它不仅可以改善氧合，还可以改善呼吸。

（三）谵妄

认知障碍的老年人濒死时常会出现幻觉和妄想。幻觉可能出现在任何感觉中—视觉、听觉、嗅觉、味觉、触觉或本体感觉（平衡和空间感）。针对妄想的任何纠正往往无效，可能会引起更严重的躁动。更好的策略是忽略妄想的主诉，转移话题。但交流中也要注意理解患者的感受，避免引起患者的不安和不被理解的焦躁情绪。例如，如果患者独处，但认为自己正在和母亲谈话，此时要询问患者会是否感到孤独或害怕，这样的问候有助于帮助其表达潜在的情绪，缓解焦虑。

（四）食物摄入减少

大多数晚期癌症患者会出现营养不良，对患者生活质量、工作状态和免疫状态有大影响，可能导致感染甚至加快死亡（表 21-3）。5% 到 20% 的癌症患者的死亡与晚期恶病质直接相关。许多濒死者都有厌食、恶心和呕吐，

death can be directly related to cachexia in the terminal phase. Many dying patients experience anorexia, nausea, and vomiting that can prevent the ingestion of even the most basic nutrients. Additionally, fatigue and weakness can make the act of eating a monumental task. Serving small-portioned meals that have appealing appearances and smells can stimulate the appetite, as can provide foods that are patient's favorites. Nausea and vomiting can be controlled with the use of anti-emetics and antihistamines.

不能摄入基本营养。此外，疲劳和虚弱也会使进食困难。色香味俱全的食物可以刺激食欲，或者提供患者平时最喜欢的食物。适当使用止吐药和抗组胺药控制恶心呕吐。

　　总之，护理人员要密切观察病情变化，做好预后的估测及抢救的准备；同时让家属做好思想和物质准备，安排善后事宜。

Table 21-3　Key points in common discomforts of the dying individual and nursing strategies

Discomforts	Nursing Care
Pain	**Special concerns in assessing pain:** ● Cancer patients are more likely to experience severe pain ● Pain is under recognized and under treated in dementia patients ● Complaints of pain or discomfort, nausea, irritability, restlessness, and anxiety are common indicators of pain ● Changes in behavior in dementia patients might indicate pain suffering ● Pain severity is best assessed by patient self-report and may be aided by VASs, NRSs and/or VRSs **Relief nursing care strategies:** ● The principle is to prevent pain from occurring rather than treating ● Opioid treatment was the central theme in most cases ● Other therapies include guided imagery, hypnosis, relaxation exercises, massage, acupressure, acupuncture, and the application of heat or cold
Respiratory Distress	**Special concerns in assessing respiratory distress:** ● often accompanied by psychological distress fearing suffocating **Relief nursing care strategies:** ● Elevating the head of the bed ● Administering oxygen ● Inhaling therapy to dilute bronchial secretions ● Oral care to lubricate the dry lips ● Cover the lips and mouth with moisture gauze dressing ● NIV for patients with end-stage lung cancer
Hallucinations and Delusions	**Special concerns in assessing hallucinations & delusions:** ● Occur in any sensory modality: visual, auditory, olfactory, gustatory, tactile, or proprioceptive **Relief nursing care strategies:** ● Ignore delusional statements ● Validate the emotion and messages behind the confusion
Poor Nutritional Intake	**Special concerns in assessing nutritional intake:** ● Anorexia, nausea, and vomiting that can prevent ingestion ● Fatigue and weakness can make the act of eating very difficult **Relief nursing care strategies:** ● Small-portioned meals ● Anti-emetics and antihistamines ● Artificial nutrition and hydration ● Fish oil derivatives ● Mouth washing

表 21-3　临终患者主要症状及护理

症状	护理
疼痛	疼痛评估注意事项 ● 肿瘤患者中严重疼痛常见 ● 认知障碍患者的疼痛往往易被忽视 ● 患者主诉疼痛、恶心、易激惹、烦躁不安以及焦虑等表现提示其可能存在疼痛 ● 认知障碍患者行为改变可提示疼痛 ● 疼痛的最佳评估标准是患者主诉，另外 VASs, NRSs 和 / 或 VRSs 等评估工具可作为辅助 减轻疼痛的护理措施 ● 原则是预防疼痛而不是治疗疼痛 ● 多数患者使用阿片类药物 ● 其他疗法包括想象引导、放松练习、按摩、针灸、冷热疗法等
呼吸窘迫	呼吸窘迫评估注意事项 ● 常常伴随心理压抑，害怕窒息 护理措施 ● 抬高床头 ● 给氧 ● 吸入化痰药物，稀释痰液 ● 口腔护理 ● 湿润口唇 ● 终末期肺癌患者可考虑无创通气
错觉和谵妄	错觉和谵妄评估注意事项 ● 视觉、听觉、嗅觉、味觉、触觉或本体感受均可产生错觉 护理措施 ● 忽略患者对错觉的描述 ● 确认产生错觉的原因
营养摄入不足	评估注意事项 ● 厌食、恶心、呕吐会影响食物摄入 ● 疲倦和虚弱使患者进食困难 护理措施 ● 少量多餐 ● 止吐药物 ● 鼻饲 ● 鱼油或其衍生物 ● 口腔护理

v. Psychological Needs of the Dying Elderly

Social environment influences people's attitude towards death. Different persons with different age and culture background hold different attitude to death. For the dying elderly, their biggest concerned at this time of life would be leaving peacefully and painlessly. However, clinical cases maybe complex. With senility, weakness and pain, it is easy to produce fear instead of accepting the treatment peacefully. Understanding death and its impact on us and expressing fear of death are part of hospice care.

（五）临终老年人的心理特征及护理

社会环境影响人们对死亡的认知和态度。人们对死亡最常见的态度是恐惧。不同年龄段的人对死亡的看法是不一样的。而对于濒死者本人，在治疗不再生效的最后阶段，几乎所有的患者都有面临死亡的恐惧和不安。平静、顺利地度过人生的最后阶段，安详、无痛苦地离开才是临终者此时最为关注的问题。老年患者病情较为复杂，在接受治疗过程中由于年老体弱、疼痛等因素，极易产生恐惧、不配合治疗和护理，从而影响患者的生存质量。理解死亡的客观性及其对我们的影响、表达出来对死亡的恐惧是临终护理的一部分。

1. Psychological stages and nursing measures of the dead elderly   In the terminal stage, besides physical pain, the fear of death is more important for elderly patients. A hospice care expert in the United States believes that "the mental pain before death is greater than the physical pain". So, while controlling the physical pain, the nurses are supposed to perform psychological care at the same time. Kubler-Ross divides psychological react of coming death into five successive stages: denial period, anger period, agreement period, depression period and acceptance period.

The psychological process of the patients at their deathbed varies from person to person and from length to length. Retsinas believes that the following factors should also be considered in the dying stage of the elderly: the elderly think that they are about to die; they may be used to the role of patients and gradually lose their vitality; the role of the dying has been redefined; death is a relief for some elderly people. Figure 21-1 describes the Hierarchy of the dying person's needs.

2. Nursing care strategies   The problems maybe classified into three levels: critical, less critical and non-critical. It is necessary to sort up the problems and make priorities. Nursing plan should be formulated according to the specific physiological and psychological problems at different stages, and adjusted constantly with changing conditions.

1. 临终老年人经历的心理阶段及护理措施   在临终阶段，老年患者除了生理上的痛苦之外，更重要的是面对死亡的恐惧。美国的一位安宁疗护专家就认为"人在临死前精神上的痛苦大于肉体上的痛苦"，因此，一定要在控制和减轻患者机体上的痛苦的同时，做好临终患者的心理关怀。Kubler-Ross 将大多数面临终者的心理分为 5 个连续的阶段，即否认期、愤怒期、协议期、忧郁期和接受期。

患者临终时的心理历程因人而异，长短不一。Retsinas 认为，对老年人的临终阶段还应考虑以下几个因素的影响：①高龄老人认为自己即将面临死亡；②他们可能习惯了患者的角色和逐渐失去生命的活力；③临终者的角色已经被重新定义；④死亡对一些老年人是一种解脱。临终患者的需求结构见图 21-1。

2. 护理措施   将患者需要解决的问题分出等级，即：重点、一般和非重点，分轻、重、缓、急制订出完成时限和采取的对策。护理计划应是根据病程中各个阶段患者的生理、心理上的具体问题制订，并随病情改变而不断加以调整。

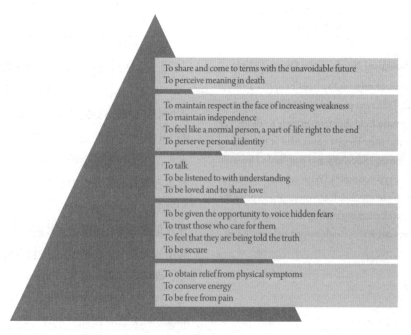

Figure 21-1   Hierarchy of the dying person's needs

(1) Medication: Drug therapy often afflicts the dying elderly, especially patients with advanced cancer. At this time, the focus of nursing is to alleviate pain and symptomatic treatment, so as to alleviate various physical discomfort symptoms. For patients with severe anxiety, depression, fear and restlessness. Sedation and anti-anxiety drugs may be required to alleviate anxiety and negative emotions.

(2) Psychological intervention: Mental care is embodied in every nursing intervention, such as quiet and warm environment, soft and comfortable light, soft words etc. At the same time, nurses can influence or change patients' feelings, perceptions, emotions, attitudes and behaviors through language, expression, posture and behavior. According to different psychological characteristics, different diseases, age, sex, occupation, marriage, belief, cultural level, economic status, family and social environment, and patients' understanding and acceptance ability, it is necessary to choose appropriate communication methods. Death is the last stop of life journey. Nurses should keep abreast of the inner activities of the dying elderly, make full use of the special effect of psychological nursing, so that the dying elderly can pass through the final stage of life calmly and leave peacefully.

(3) Signs that a patient is imminent: As death draws nearer, more obvious changes begin to occur. They may not happen in any particular order – each person is unique. But, there are certain clinical markers that indicate that death is now imminent (can happen anytime). Some of these signs follow: decreased blood pressure; increased pulse rate, weak pulse; dyspnea or apnea; delayed pupil light reflex or no light reflex; pale and cold skin; fecal incontinence; and gradual disappearance of vision and hearing.

Nurses may inform families when there are signs of imminent to allow the families to take the opportunity to spend the last moment with the dying. If the family members cannot be present, medical staff should be around. Hearing is the last sensation that disappears, accordingly, whispering in the ear may help the dying to leave with peace.

（1）药物治疗：临终老人往往深受病痛折磨，尤其是晚期肿瘤患者，此时护理重点是减轻痛苦、对症处理，以减轻各种躯体不适症状。对于严重焦虑、抑郁、恐惧及烦躁不安的患者，可给予安定、多塞平等镇静、抗焦虑药物治疗，以缓解焦虑、摆脱负面情绪。

（2）心理护理：心理护理体现在医疗护理工作的每个细节，如安静温馨的环境，柔和舒适的光线，和蔼可亲的语言，良好的护患关系，熟练的技术操作。同时，护理人员在与患者的接触中，可通过语言、表情、姿态和行为影响或改变患者的感受、认识、情绪、态度和行为，以减轻或消除致病性精神心理因素和由此引起和各种躯体症状。根据患者不同的心理特点，不同的疾病以及年龄、性别、职业、婚姻、信仰、文化水平、经济地位、家庭和社会环境的不同，按照患者的理解、接受能力，选择适当的沟通方法；用通俗易懂的语言、深入浅出的方式帮助患者正视生死。生老病死是人生的自然发展过程，死亡是人生旅程的最后一站，护士应随时了解临终老人的内心活动，充分运用心理护理的特殊功效，使临终老人得以平静地度过人生最后阶段，安详而幸福地离开。

（3）濒死的征兆：随着死亡的临近，会逐渐出现一些更明显的变化。身体功能将会下降，患者临死前的表现有：①血压下降；②脉率增高，脉细而无力；③呼吸困难或呼吸暂停；④瞳孔对光反射迟缓或无对光反射；⑤皮肤苍白、湿冷；⑥大、小便失禁；⑦视觉、听觉逐渐消失。

护理人员了解了濒死的临床表现后就能够在患者濒死前及时通知其家人，使家人有机会陪伴临终者共同度过最后的时光。如果其家人不能及时到场，则要有医务人员在患者身边。临终者去世前最后消失的感官是听觉，因此，家人的陪伴和耳边低语可以帮助临终者放心而没有遗憾地离开。

There are some unpleasant events surrounding death nurses should be prepared for. Sometimes there is a loss of bowel and bladder control at the moment of death. Muscles may twitch and the dying may even try to sit up or stand, but this is most likely a muscle response and not an intentional movement. Sometimes patients yawn or make an audible yell or groan. This isn't a cry or indication of pain; it is just the last big expiration of air passing over her voice box. The eyes can open and the jaw may drop open as well. These are all just normal reflexes as the body dies. After she has been officially pronounced dead by the physician, nurses are supposed to provide postmortem care or by requested by the family members.

另外，有的患者在临终时会出现大小便失禁等情况，护士应做好相应的准备。临终期的患者可能出现肌肉抽搐，或意外的肢体动作，这可能是肌肉的条件反射。有时候患者会大声呻吟，这是气流经过喉头的声音，并不一定是患者痛苦所致。有的临终者睁大眼睛，下巴打开，这些都是临终时身体的正常反应。

Section 3 Challenge to Family

第三节 居丧者面临的主要问题与护理

The society, history and ethic or culture influence individual's attitude to death. Overcome the threatening of death and set up a stable emotional reaction mode to release the fear of death is what the family members could learn from the lost. Mourning occurs when an individual expresses sorrow with outward signs of grief as a result of a loss. The grief process is highly personal, and the person experiencing end-of-life, the family, or the healthcare professional should not try to rush or lengthen it. By understanding the stages of grief, the nurse can play a more effective role as a patient advocate (see figure 21-2).

不同社会、历史、伦理、文化背景的人对于死亡的认识是不一样的。消除对于死亡的恐惧，稳固并重建对生命的认识是人们从失去亲人的悲伤中能够得到的成长。亲人离世，家属和亲友会出现各种各样的情感或心理反应，在为亡人送行的过程包含着惜别、留恋等复杂的情感，悲伤是最为普遍和正常的心理反应。通过了解悲伤的过程，护士可以更有效地扮演患者倡导者的角色（图 21-2）。

I. Normal Grief

一、悲伤过程

Normal grief discusses what happens to people when they lose someone or something important (e.g., health, security, money, material comforts, a home, a job, or a spouse). Westberg is a widely respected pioneer in holistic healthcare and the founder of nursing program, also a Lutheran minister. He states that grief could be divided into healthy or good grief and unhealthy grief and that people should be familiar with the good aspects of grief. He contends that people who handle daily "little grief" in a positive manner prepare themselves for healthy

悲伤产生于人们失去对自己有重要意义的人或事物时，如失去健康、安全、金钱、工作或者配偶时。Westberg 是整体护理领域广受尊敬的先驱。他提出悲伤的表现方式有健康和不健康两种。健康的悲伤是人类情绪的正常表达，对保持心理健康是有益的。当巨大的悲痛来临时，那些能够以积极方式来处理和表达悲伤的人可以做出恰当的反应，反之，便会出现适应不良行为，影响正常的生

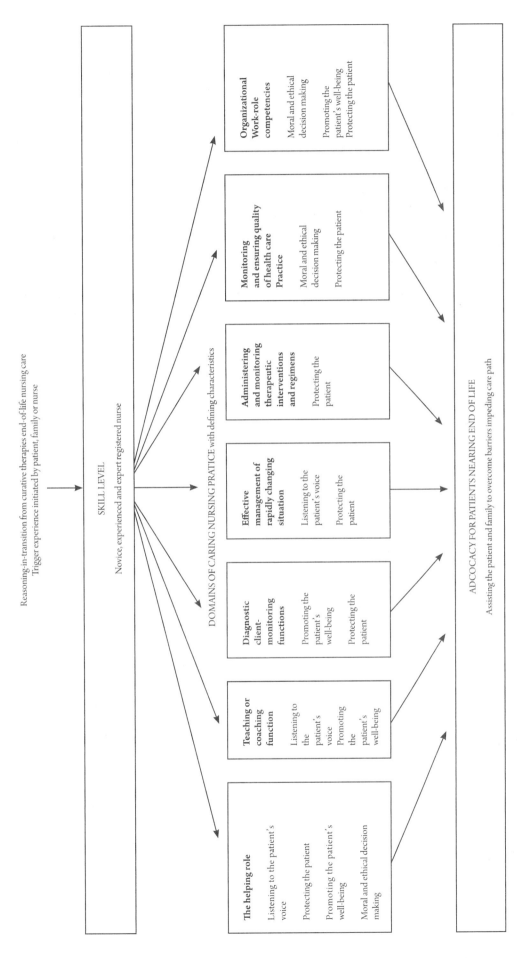

Reasoning-in-transition from curative therapies end-of-life nursing care
Trigger experience initiated by patient, family or nurse

SKILL LEVEL

Novice, experienced and expert registered nurse

DOMAINS OF CARING NURSING PRATICE with defining characteristics

The helping role

Listening to the patient's voice

Protecting the patient

Promoting the patient's well-being

Moral and ethical decision making

Teaching or coaching function

Listening to the patient's voice

Promoting the patient's well-being

Diagnostic client-monitoring functions

Promoting the patient's well-being

Protecting the patient

Effective management of rapidly changing situation

Listening to the patient's voice

Protecting the patient

Administering and monitoring therapeutic interventions and regimens

Protecting the patient

Monitoring and ensuring quality of health care Practice

Moral and ethical decision making

Protecting the patient

Organizational Work-role competencies

Moral and ethical decision making

Promoting the patient's well-being

Protecting the patient

ADCOCACY FOR PATIENT'S NEARING END OF LIFE

Assisting the patient and family to overcome barriers impeding care path

Figure 21-2　Conceptual model of advocacy behaviors in end-of-life nursing care

reactions to larger grief when they occur.

In general, normal or common grief reactions are marked by a gradual movement toward an acceptance of the loss and, although daily functioning can be very difficult, managing to continue with basic daily activities. Normal grief usually includes some common emotional reactions that include emotional numbness, shock, disbelief, and/or denial often occurring immediately after the death, particularly if the death is unexpected. Much emotional distress is focused on the anxiety of separation from the loved one, which often results in yearning, searching, preoccupation with the loved one, and frequent intrusive images of death.

In Westberg's booklet *Good Grief*, he explains that normal grief reactions can be characterized by time: early, middle, and last phases. In the early phase, shock, disbelief, and denial are common. This phase commonly ends as people begin to accept the reality of the loss after the funeral. The middle phase is a time of intense emotional pain and separation and may be accompanied by physical symptoms and labile emotions. Lastly, reintegration and relief occur as the pain gradually subsides and a degree of physical and mental balance returns. The following is a summary of the ten stages of grief as described by Westberg in his book *Good Grief*. Not everyone passes through these stages in chronological order, but it is hoped each person will reach stage ten.

i. Stage One: State of Shock

During the first stage the grieving person experiences a state of temporary anesthesia that may last anywhere from a few minutes to a few days. Shock is a temporary escape from reality. As long as it is temporary, it is good. But, if the state of shock lasts over a week or two, if the person should prefer to remain in this dream world rather than face the reality of his loss, it is then, a sign of unhealthy grief and professional help should be offered before maladaptive behavior occurs. Caregivers should be near and available during this stage of grief but are advised not to take over tasks that the person can perform. Self-care is therapeutic and enables the person to proceed to the next stage.

活和工作，甚至导致心理疾病。

正常的悲伤时可见的情绪反应包括情绪麻木、震惊、不相信和/或否认，通常出现在亲人死亡后即刻，特别是在意外死亡的情况下。许多情感上的痛苦集中在与所爱的人分离的焦虑上，家属表现为对逝者的极度渴望以及频繁回忆以往片段。

这里介绍 Westberg 对丧亲者的悲伤的研究描述，他将丧亲者的悲伤概括为 10 个阶段。需要注意的是，并非每个人都要按照时间的先后顺序经历这些阶段，但每种情绪反应都是丧亲者预料中的正常反应。

（一）震惊

在第一阶段，悲伤的人们会经历短暂的感觉缺失。这种感觉缺失可能在任何地点持续几分钟至几天。如果震惊阶段的持续时间超过一周或两周，便预示着病理性悲伤的可能。例如，丧偶的老年人在灵堂内向前来吊唁的人们表示问候时表现得冷静、镇定。如果在 1 周或 2 周内没有机会释放其诸如疑虑、愤怒或者孤独的情感时，则意味着可能会有继发的适应不良行为。护理干预应在适应不良行为出现之前给予专业的帮助。在此阶段中，护士或社会工作者应时刻陪伴在悲痛者左右，倾听或鼓励其情感的发泄。需要注意的是，此阶段的护理中注意不要给予丧亲者不必要的生活辅助，应鼓励其完成力所能及的日常活动，鼓励自我关怀。自我关怀是一种治疗性措施，能够促使悲伤者向下一阶段的发展。

ii. Stage Two: Expressing Emotion

People are encouraged to express repressed emotion after a significant loss occurs. Westberg writes, "We have been given tear glands, and we are supposed to use them when we have good reason to use them." The feeling of loss and sad should be encouraged to release and the family members should not be ashamed to cry with the patients. Well, if not, the family member should know that they should let their grief take its natural course in any of a variety of ways.

iii. Stage Three: Depression and Loneliness

During the third stage, the person experiences feelings of utter depression and isolation. The caregiver is advised to "stand by" in quiet confidence and reassure the grieving person that loneliness and depression are normal reactions and eventually do pass.

iv. Stage Four: Physical Symptoms of Distress

Physical symptoms such as insomnia, chest pain, abdominal pain, and shortness of breath may occur when someone stops at one of the stages of the grief process. If no one helps the person to explore the reason for emotional and physical complaints associated with unresolved grief, an illness can develop. The classic example is the death of a widow or widower within a year of the spouse's death. Such persons are said to have died of "broken hearts" or they just gave up because they were unable to live without their mate. The physical consequences of distress resulted in death.

v. Stage Five: Panic

During the fifth stage the person is unable to think of anything except the loss. Concentration and productivity are impaired because of obsessive thoughts, causing the person to think she or he is "losing the mind." The helping person should encourage the grieving person in this stage to develop new and different interests and interpersonal relationships rather than to stay at home and prolong grief work.

vi. Stage Six: Guilt Feelings

Normal guilt is guilt that we feel when we have done something or neglected to do something for which we ought, by the standards of society, to feel guilty. On more than one occasion survivors of deceased persons have made comments such as "If only I had insisted he see a doctor" or "I should have realized she was sicker than she looked." Such statements express guilt feelings. Persons who say that they will "never forgive themselves" and continually berate themselves for their actions, out of proportion to the real situation, are exhibiting symptoms

（二）情感释放

丧失亲人是生活中的重大事件，释放压抑的悲痛情绪是正常的心理需求，应被接受和鼓励。Westberg 表示"我们被赋予了泪腺，因此我们应该适时的使用它们来释放情感"。安宁疗护成员应该理解并鼓励丧亲者释放情感。

（三）抑郁与孤独

在第三个阶段，丧亲者面临着彻底的沮丧与孤独，安宁疗护成员应给予默默地支持，告诉他孤独与抑郁是正常反应，最终都将会过去。

（四）悲伤的躯体表现

当丧亲者的悲伤停滞在某一阶段，失眠、胸痛、腹痛以及呼吸困难等症状便会伴随而来。如果任由这些躯体反应来表达丧亲者的负面情绪，便会产生与之相关的疾病。典型的例子是在配偶逝去的一年内寡妇或鳏夫也随之逝去。人们认为他们死于"伤心"，从医学心理学角度讲，是由于他们无法适应失去配偶的生活，由负面情绪诱发疾病而导致死亡。

（五）恐慌感

在第 5 个阶段，丧亲者陷入强烈的失落感。由于过度的思念，导致其过度关注逝者有关的事物，日常活动减少。安宁疗护人员应该鼓励丧亲者培养新的兴趣，建立和维护人际关系，而不是待在家中延长悲伤的时间。

（六）愧疚感

愧疚感是由于对那些我们已经做过的或者按照社会准则我们应该做却未做的事情感到内疚的情绪。许多丧亲者会有"如果我坚持要他去看医生"或者"我早应该想到她病得很重"的内疚想法。丧亲者很难宽恕自己，部分会长久的指责自身，但这些自责其实并不符合实际情况。安宁疗护人员应鼓励其表达自己的愧疚，从而帮助其有效地处理情绪。

of guilt. Such people should be encouraged to talk about guilt feelings so that they begin to handle them effectively and resume living

vii. Stage Seven: Anger and Resentment

Once the grieving person overcomes guilt feelings and is able to express emotions, stronger feelings such as anger and resentment may emerge. (Repressed or buried feelings of anger and resentment are unhealthy and can be very harmful to a person's personality.) During this stage the person may blame anyone or everyone for the loss. Most nurses have heard family members on at least one occasion question whether the attending physician did everything possible for the patient. "If only he had operated sooner. He waited too long," or "He should have called in a consultant when my husband didn't respond to treatment." These are examples of comments made by angry family members who resented the loss of a loved one. Such feelings are a normal part of grief and can be overcome in time.

viii. Stage Eight: Resistance

During this stage, grieving persons resist returning to normal daily living. They are intent on keeping the memory of a loved one or thing alive. Returning to normal activities may be too painful for some people because they experience emptiness in the world about them. Too many times grieving persons are forced to carry all the grief within themselves since they find it difficult to grieve in the presence of others. Society says "Okay, you had time to grieve. Now get back to work!" and expects the person to return to a normal state very shortly after a loss has occurred. Friends and relatives are encouraged to help keep the memory of the loss alive because this facilitates progress toward the stage of hope.

ix. Stage Nine: Hope

After a few weeks or many months of grief, hope generally emerges. Life does go on; opportunities do exist for change or improvement in one's life in spite of the recently experienced loss. New friends can gradually help one find meaning again in life.

x. Stage Ten: Affirming Reality

Grieving persons generally realize that life will never be the same again, but they begin to sense that there is much in life that can be appreciated and enjoyed. To affirm something is to say that it is good and worth living for. People who have a mature faith or belief in God often demonstrate an inner strength that helps them to face a serious loss without feeling that they have lost everything. Nurses must be aware of the religious beliefs and spiritual

（七）愤怒

在克服了愧疚感并且能够表达情感时，丧亲者又会陷入强烈的愤怒中。在这一阶段，人们可能因为亲人的离去而责怪其他人。护士常听到过家庭成员质疑医生是否对患者的治疗竭尽所能。家庭成员之间或对医务人员产生猜忌和愤恨。这种愤怒愤恨的感觉是悲伤的正常组成部分并且能够及时被克服。应注意的是，克制或者压抑愤怒的情绪是不健康的，如若不及时排解，会影响性格成长。

（八）抵制

在这个阶段，丧亲者拒绝回到正常的日常生活中，他们专注于钟爱之人的存活之物。回到日常活动中对一些人而言可能过于痛苦，因为他们在自己的世界中感到空虚，而同时，丧亲者少有机会彻底发泄自己的悲痛和思念之情。尽管人们全力劝说"你应该从悲伤中走出来，回到现实中！"但丧亲者的思念和悲痛无处发泄，因此会采用回避和隔离的方法，拒绝重现现实生活。此时应鼓励朋友和亲人帮助其保持逝者在世时的角色，以促进丧亲者回到正常的生活轨道。

（九）希望

在悲痛的几周或数月之后，希望渐渐出现，尽管最近经历了丧亲之痛，生活依然继续。新的朋友和社会关系能够帮助丧亲者再次找到生活的意义。

（十）接受现实

丧亲者渐渐意识到生活依旧，其实还有许多事情值得去欣赏与享受。对事物的肯定意味着生活下去的意义。

护士必须了解丧亲者的宗教信仰与精神需要，采取相应的护理干预和适当的帮助。调查显示，27% 的患者认为精神关怀与躯体关

needs of their patients so that nursing interventions can address these areas. 27% of those patients surveyed felt they had a need for spiritual care as well as physical care. Fifty-six percent did not feel nurses were aware of their spiritual needs during hospitalization.

II. Dysfunctional Grief

Generally speaking, when relatives die, family members and friends will have various emotional or psychological reactions. Dysfunctional grief or abnormal grief, often referred to as complicated grief, is found in only 3 to 25 percent of loss survivors. There are different types of dysfunctional grief:

i. Chronic Grief

Chronic grief reactions are prolonged and never reach a satisfactory conclusion. Because bereaved individuals are aware of their continuing grief, this reaction is fairly easy to recognize, a therapist can assess which tasks of grieving are not being resolved and why. The goal of intervention is to resolve these tasks.

ii. Delayed Grief

A pattern in which symptoms of distress, seeking, yearning, etc., occur at a much later time than is typical. At some future time the person may experience an intense grief reaction triggered by a subsequent smaller loss or by any other event that triggers sadness.

iii. Disenfranchised Grief

Disenfranchised grief often occurs when a grieving person's loss can't be openly acknowledged or is one that society does not accept as a real. This complicates the grieving process both because it cannot be expressed and because social support is not available. Doka described four major situations that cause disenfranchised grief: when a relationship is not recognized by others (e.g., cohabitation, same-sex partners); when a loss is not acknowledged (e.g., death of a pet); when the griever is excluded (e.g., very old adults, those with cognitive deficits), and when the circumstances of the death are disenfranchising (e.g., deaths caused by drunk driving or suicide).

iv. Exaggerated Grief

Exaggerated grief is intense reactions of grief that may include nightmares, phobias (abnormal fears), and thoughts of suicide. People with exaggerated grief may feel an overwhelming sense of being unable to live without the

怀对丧亲者同等重要，但是，56% 的患者在住院期间并未感觉到护士对他们精神需求给予的满足。

二、功能失调性悲伤

一般来说，亲人离世，家属和亲友会出现各种各样的情感或心理反应，悲伤是最为普遍和正常的心理反应。但是，长时间的悲伤会引起适应不良。功能失调性的悲伤是一种复杂的内心情绪体验，见于 3% ~ 25% 的丧亲者。功能失调性的悲伤可以分为以下几种类型：

（一）慢性悲伤

慢性悲伤反应会持续很长时间，永远不会得出令人满意的结论。丧亲者往往能够觉察出自己的悲伤反应，因此较容易判断。治疗师可以评估哪些悲伤的任务没有被解决以及原因。干预的目标是完成这些任务。

（二）迟发性悲伤

有意识的延迟悲伤情绪。迟发性悲伤与其他诱发悲伤的生活事件或悲伤过程中自我心理防御丧失有关。

（三）不被理解的悲伤

当一名悲伤者的行为不能被公开地接受时，称之为不被理解或接受的悲伤。

（四）过度悲伤

指悲伤反应强烈，如丧亲者出现持续的噩梦、惊恐发作和自杀的想法等。

deceased person. They may lose the sense that the acute grief is transient and may continue in this intense despair for a long time.

v. Sudden Grief

Sudden grief may take place when death takes place very suddenly without warning. Sudden grief can lead to exaggerated reactions and posttraumatic stress disorder (PTSD).

The cause of pathologic or dysfunctional grief is usually an actual or perceived loss of someone or something of great value to a person. Clinical features or characteristics include expressions of distress or denial of the loss; changes in eating and sleeping habits; mood disturbances, such as anger, hostility, or crying; and alterations in activity levels, including libido. The person experiencing dysfunctional grief idealizes the lost person or object, relives past experiences, loses the ability to concentrate, and is unable to work purposefully because of developmental regression. The grieving person may exhibit neurotic or psychotic symptoms in an attempt to cope with stress and anxiety owing to the actual or perceived loss. Examples of such behavior include development of physical symptoms similar to those experienced by the deceased person before death; progressive social isolation and interrupted interpersonal relationships with friends and relatives; extreme anger or hostility, directed at people associated with the lost person or object; agitated depression; or activities that are detrimental to one's social or economic existence. Nursing interventions include teaching about the stages of grief and encouraging verbalization of feelings as well as satisfying the needs of the bereavement family.

Box 21-2 Survivor's needs

1. To provide a quality of life for the dying person while preparing for a life without that loved person.

2. To be available to offer comfort and care even though the survivor feels like running away to escape the pain of death.

3. To hope that the loved one will somehow live in spite of obvious deterioration and inability to function. At this time, the survivor may pray for the peace of death.

4. To vent feelings of irritation and guilt over the dying person's demands and increased dependency needs.

5. To live and appreciate each day as one plans for a future without the loved one.

6. To reassure the dying person that the survivor will "continue in her or his footsteps" by holding the family together, raising the children, or managing the business, while knowing such talk about the future is painful to the dying person.

（五）突然的悲伤

如果逝者的死亡由于意外，丧亲者没有任何心理准备，则会出现突然的悲伤。突然的悲伤会导致一些夸张行为反应和创伤后应激障碍（PTSD）。

非正常（功能失调性的）悲伤的原因通常是由于没有充分的心理准备而突然失去亲人继而诱发强烈的失落感，具体表现为：否认丧失亲人的事实，表情抑郁，饮食和睡眠习惯改变或是情绪紊乱，如生气，憎恨或哭泣交替，以及日常活动的改变，如不修边幅、性欲减退等。功能失调性悲伤的丧亲者会把逝者理想化，沉迷于对逝者的回忆和思念中，注意力无法集中，无法恢复日常工作，这些心理和行为属于退化的防御机制。部分功能失调性悲伤的丧亲者可能会模仿逝者生前的行为，模仿其语言和体态，以此来表达对逝者的思念和悲痛。其他的表达方式有：脱离社会生活、中断与亲友的交往，沉迷于往事；对逝者发泄极度的愤恨；出现抑郁症的表现；出现反社会的行为。

Box 21-2 居丧者的需求

1. 要为临终者提供最好的生活质量，同时也要为丧偶者准备以后的生活。

2. 需要安慰和关怀，需要安全和依赖。

3. 希望尽可能延长将逝者的生命，并期望逝者离去时安详无痛苦。

4. 需要发泄内心的愤怒和内疚感。

5. 与家人一起，充实地过好每一天，以慰藉逝者。

6. 继续日常生活、工作，养育孩子，以慰藉逝者。

III. Care of the Bereaved Spouse

Widowhood is a major event in the lives of the elderly, which is a heavy blow to the elderly. Once encountering the death of spouse, the elderly often feels overwhelmed with grief and bewilderment. Continuing grief will lead to various mental disorders, including depression, aggravating the original physical diseases, and even leading to death. The number of deaths caused by psychological imbalance among the elderly who lost their spouses in the near future is seven times that of the general elderly.

The goal of nursing care for older persons who are grieving and mourning is not to "make them feel better" quickly, although nurses are often tempted to try to do so. Nurses should assist and support bereaved persons through the grieving process, recognizing that pain is a normal and healthy response to loss and allowing bereaved persons to accomplish the tasks of mourning in their own ways. Grief is deeply personal. The stage theory of grief remains a widely accepted model of bereavement adjustment. Although four phases and tasks of grief have been identified, everyone will move through them differently. The survived spouse may move through the phases quickly or slowly; she or he may move through them in a different order or may skip a phase or task altogether.

i. Psychological Adjustment of the Widowed

A four stages theory of grief for adjustment to bereavement that included: shock-numbness, yearning-searching, disorganization-despair, and reorganization.

1. Numbness It is the phase immediately following a loss. The grieving person feels numb, which is a defense mechanism that allows them to survive emotionally.

2. Searching and yearning It can also be referred to as pining and is characterized by the grieving person longing or yearning for the deceased to return. Many emotions are expressed during this time and may include weeping, anger, anxiety, and confusion.

三、丧偶老人的护理

丧偶是老年人生活中的重大事件，对老年人是沉重的打击。一旦遭遇老伴亡故，常会悲痛欲绝、不知所措，持续下去就会引发包括抑郁症在内的各种精神疾患，加重原有的躯体疾病，甚至导致死亡。在近期内失去配偶的老年人因心理失衡而导致死亡的人数是一般老年人死亡的 7 倍。

护士应协助和支持在悲伤过程中的死者家属，让其认识到痛苦和悲伤是正常的情绪反应，并允许丧亲者以自己的方式完成哀悼任务。尽管确定了悲伤的四个阶段和任务，但每个人的体验过程各有不同。

（一）丧偶老人的心理状态

老年人丧偶后，心理反应一般要经过 4 个阶段：

1. **麻木** 这是某些老年人在失去伴侣即刻就会出现的反应。很多老年人表现得麻木，面无表情。这种麻木并不意味着情感淡漠，而是情感休克的表现。麻木可以看作是对噩耗的排斥，是一种心理防御机制，避免丧偶老人经历剧烈的悲痛。这个阶段可能持续几个小时至数天。

2. **怀念** 居丧的老年人在强烈的悲哀情绪平息后，随着时间的流逝，会逐渐产生对逝者的深深怀念，感到失去他（她）之后，自己是多么的孤独。丧偶老人此时渴望逝者重生，以陪伴自己。这种状态可能持续几个星期甚至几年。老年人的情绪平静但充满思念和遗憾。

3. Disorganization and despair The grieving person now desired to withdraw and disengage from others and activities they regularly enjoyed. Feelings of pining and yearning become less intense while periods of apathy, meaning an absence of emotion, and despair increase.

4. Reorganization and recovery In this final phase, the grieving person begins to return to a new state of "normal". Weight loss experienced during intense grieving may be regained, energy levels increase, and an interest to return to activities of enjoyment returns. Grief never ends but thoughts of sadness and despair are diminished while positive memories of the deceased take over.

Because everyone grieves in their own way at their own pace, there is no timeline that these phases are supposed to be completed in. In Yale Bereavement Study (a longitudinal cohort study of 233 bereaved individuals living in Connecticut), the 5 grief indicators achieved their respective maximum values in the sequence (disbelief, yearning, anger, depression, and acceptance) predicted by the stage theory of grief. Nevertheless, receiving bereavement counseling and vent with other supporting members can help the grieving individual move through the phases fluidly.

ii. Fulfilment of Psychological Tasks

Through grieving and mourning people accomplished specific task. The concept of tasks implies that effort on the part of the individual is required. These tasks are:

1. Accept the reality of the loss Coming full face with the reality that the person is dead and will not return is the first task that needs to be completed. Without accomplishing this, the grieving person will not be able to continue through the mourning process.

2. Work through the pain Grief is painful, physically and emotionally. It is important to acknowledge the pain and not suppress it.

3. Adjust to the new environment in which the deceased is missing This may require adjusting to the roles that the deceased once carried out. If it is a spouse

3. **颓丧和绝望** 这阶段中人会觉得疲倦、无精打采，感到生活不再有目标。无法再感受到快乐和满足，即使是从那些以往可以获得满足感的事物中。

4. **恢复** 当居丧的老年人逐渐认识到"人的生老病死是无法抗拒的自然规律""对老伴最好的寄托和思念是保重身体、更好地生活下去"，理智战胜了感情，身心也就能逐渐恢复常态。悲伤期间下降的体重也恢复了，代谢水平也增加了，而且以前所喜欢参加的活动也重新拾起。虽然悲伤的感觉不会简单消失，但是悲伤和绝望的想法已经变少。虽然也常回忆起逝者，但此时的怀念多是希望逝者在"另一个世界"里平安、舒适。

老年丧偶者的悲伤因人而异，其程度、方式和持续时间都不尽相同，丧偶者在经历这些阶段所需要的时间有快有慢；有可能情绪变化出现的顺序会有所差异，或者是跳过其中一个阶段或者是各种表现都重叠在一起，因此没有一个固定的结束时间界限。但家人、朋友及社会的劝慰可以帮助丧偶老人更快地走出丧偶的重大打击，使其生活恢复常态。

（二）居丧老人的心理成长和成熟过程

丧亲之痛是个体在成长过程中必然经历的阶段。在此阶段，丧亲者需要经历成长的考验，做出努力，才能顺利完成心理的成长和成熟。这些心理成长的任务包括：

1. **接受丧亲的现实** 丧亲者首先要面对的就是亲人去世的现实，认识到人死不能复生。如果丧亲者采取否认或怀疑的态度，则不能继续完成心理成长任务达到成熟。

2. **经历伤痛的过程** 悲痛不仅是情感上而且是躯体经受的伤痛。护士应接受居丧者正在经历伤痛的事实，不要强求居丧者压抑其内心的感受，更不要忽视居丧者的身体不适反应。

3. **适应新环境和新角色** 居丧老人要逐渐接受独居生活和寡妇／鳏夫的身份。

that has died, it required the bereaved to accept their new identity as a widow.

4. Emotionally relocate the deceased and move on While the bereaved will never be compelled to totally give up on the relationship, the goal is to find an appropriate place in their emotional lives for the deceased. This requires a letting go of attachments so new relationships can begin to form.

Completing these tasks will help the bereaved come to terms with their loss and return to a new state of normalcy. Palliative care and hospice programs integrate bereavement care into their comprehensive approach to care. The goal of nursing care for older persons who are grieving and mourning is not to make them feel better quickly, although nurses are often tempted to try to do so. Nurses should assist and support bereaved persons through the grieving process, recognizing that pain is a normal and healthy response to loss and allowing bereaved persons to accomplish the tasks of mourning in their own ways.

IV. Grief Counseling

Over the past several decades, efforts to aid the bereaved have increasingly focused on the physical and psychological morbidity, and the spiritual suffering and social isolation associated with bereavement. Bereaved families are divided into three classes: well-functioning, intermediate and dysfunctional. Well-functioning families, which make up the majority, are equipped to handle the grieving process. Dysfunctional families, which make up 15%-20% of families of patients receiving palliative care, have high levels of conflict and poor communication. In between are the intermediate families, which are moderately cohesive but tend to break down under the stress of death and bereavement. Members of families that fall into the dysfunctional and intermediate classes are more prone to experience complicated grief, also known as pathological grief. Pathological grief leads to clinical depression, substance abuse, suicidal thoughts and other forms of impairment, which means that it is necessary to screen the families and determine which are in need of therapy.

Grief counseling is a form of psychotherapy that aims to help people cope with grief and mourning following the death of loved ones or with major life changes that trigger feelings of grief. Grief counseling is used to facilitate, successful progression through the grief

4. 发展新的关系 引导居丧老人适应新的生活环境、接受新的角色，也就意味着帮助其准备好开始建立新的关系，这并不是强迫老年人完全放弃与逝者的关系，其目的是在他们的感情生活中为逝者找出合适的位置。

经历丧亲之痛后，完成了以上的心理发展任务，有助于帮助丧亲者恢复正常的生活和心理状态。安宁疗护包含对丧亲者特别是对丧偶老人的帮助和照护。应注意的是，每个居丧者经历的心理过程不尽相同，护理目标不是让他们不要悲伤，而是向着健康积极的方向努力。社区护士和志愿者的任务就是帮助丧偶者顺利度过这个过程。悲伤本身就是一种正常的、健康的居丧方式，医护人员应允许悲伤者用他们自己的方式去表达情感。

四、哀伤辅导

对逝者亲属的援助主要集中在躯体不适、精神痛苦以及与社交隔离方面。逝者家庭功能的状态分为三类：功能良好、中等和功能失调。大多数功能良好的家庭有能力处理悲伤的过程。功能失调的家庭约占 15%～20%，成员关系冲突程度高，沟通差。介于两者之间的是中等家庭，这些家庭具有适度的凝聚力，但往往在丧亲后解体。后两者的家庭成员更容易经历复杂的悲伤，也称为病理性悲伤。病理性悲伤是导致抑郁、药物滥用、自杀的直接原因。护理人员有必要对这些家庭进行筛查，确定需要治疗的情况。

居丧者的护理用于帮助丧亲者成功度过丧失亲人后的居丧期，而心理治疗针对正在经受复杂悲伤情绪或功能失调性悲伤者。护士和其他医疗人员以及经过专业训练的志愿

process, whereas grief therapy is intended for those who are experiencing complicated mourning. It is natural that palliative care programs focus more on active patients than on the families of deceased patients. Hospices can use only so much of their limited resources on services for bereaved families, so those services are usually offered for limited periods. Nurses, other health professionals, and specially trained volunteers can provide grief counseling, whereas therapy should be conducted under the guidance of a skilled therapist.

Worden suggested four ways that grief counselors can assist grieving persons in the tasks of mourning. They are to increase the reality of the loss, help the counseled person deal with both expressed and latent effects, assist the consoled person in dealing with various impediments to readjustment after the loss, and encourage the counseled person to make a healthy emotional withdrawal from the deceased and to feel comfortable reinvesting that emotion in another relationship. Worden's grief counseling principles are as follows:

i. Help the Survivor Actualize the Loss

Nurses are often first to initiate this process, especially after the death of a client in a health care institution. Nurses are usually the professionals present to offer details and descriptions of the death or explanations of puzzling situations that family members may not understand. Having information about the death and the events preceding and following the death is important in helping to actualize the loss. Survivors may need to be encouraged to talk about the loss, to tell the story of events surrounding the death, and to relate memories of the deceased. This process takes time. Worden found that many survivors took up to 3 months before they began to accept the reality that their spouses were dead and not going to return.

ii. Help the Survivor Identify and Express His or Her Feelings

Because they are unpleasant, some feelings accompanying bereavement may not be expressed or recognized by the bereaved person. Nurses need to assess a bereaved person's feelings and ask specific questions that encourage expression. Feelings that often go unexpressed include anger, guilt, anxiety, and helplessness. Guilt and regret may be recognized and expressed through storytelling, writing in a journal, or writing a letter to the deceased. A ritual such as burying or burning the letter may assist the mourner in resolution. Sometimes, unpleasant emotions are displaced. For example, anger may be directed toward the deceased, toward God, or toward

者都可以进行居丧护理,而心理治疗需要在专业治疗师的指导下进行。

Worden 认为有 4 种方法可以帮助丧亲者应对悲伤情绪。这些方法使居丧者面对失去亲人的现实,帮助居丧者能够应对失去亲人所带来表面的和隐藏的影响,应对丧亲后的适应障碍,鼓励丧亲者以健康方式怀念逝者,走出悲伤,把感情投入到新的人际关系中。其具体方法和注意事项如下:

(一)帮助丧亲者面对现实

在医疗机构中,失去亲人的家属往往向护士询问逝者临终的细节以及临终期各种表现的解释。因此,护士全面掌握逝者信息以及临终的过程对帮助丧亲者面对现实有很大帮助。护士应鼓励丧亲的家属谈论或表达失去亲人的痛苦,逝者生前的故事及相关的丧亲者回忆。护士应认识到家属接受现实需要一定的时间,Worden 的研究提示,丧亲者一般需要 3 个月左右来接受配偶逝去的现实。

(二)帮助丧亲者宣泄情感

丧亲者情绪低落,他们自身可能没有意识到自身情绪的表达形式或没有恰当的表达。没有被表达出的情感通常包括气愤、内疚、焦虑和无助。讲述逝者生前的故事、写日记、写信可以帮助丧亲者认识和发泄内疚和后悔的情绪。传统仪式,例如烧信可以帮助丧亲者缓解悲伤情绪。有时丧亲者的悲伤情绪表现为愤怒,这种愤怒可能无法理解,但有助于宣泄丧亲者的强烈情绪。社会文化和年龄差异也会影响情感的宣泄。老年人的情感表

the physician or nurse who helped the family care for the loved one. Such anger may be difficult to understand, but it is helpful for the targets of the anger to detach themselves and not respond defensively. Socio-cultural and gender differences influence expression of emotions and need to be taken into account. Older persons may also express their emotions differently than younger ones, especially after dealing with multiple losses; for example, crying may be a less common indicator of sadness among older persons.

iii. Assist the Survivor in Living without the Deceased

The nurse needs to assess the survivor's daily living situation and identify any existing or potential problems. The roles played by the deceased must now be assumed by the survivor (or someone else) to accomplish tasks of daily living. Knowledge of community resources and teaching of practical skills are necessary to meet this need. In general, survivors should be advised to postpone making major decisions that involve life changes, such as selling property or moving. Calling on the survivor's social support system is also useful.

iv. Facilitate the Survivor's Emotional Withdrawal from the Deceased

The nurse needs to be especially sensitive to when the bereaved should emotionally withdraw from the deceased, while maintaining the bond to the deceased, and begin developing new relationships. This is especially difficult if the relationship lost was that of a spouse. Research has shown that older persons who lose a confidante are less likely than younger persons to replace the confidante. Perhaps they are unwilling to emotionally invest in another intimate relationship when the risk of repeated loss is so high. Other types of relationships such as close friendships may be encouraged to help meet an older person's needs for intimacy.

v. Provide the Survivor with Time to Grieve

It used to be believed that after the first anniversary of the death, grief should be resolved. This has been shown to be inaccurate; many factors influence the time for adjustment, as discussed previously. Two points in time seem to be especially critical: 3 months after the death and 1 year after the death. Older persons who have experienced multiple losses may need more time. For some, the losses may never be resolved; a person may simply learn to live with the feelings of grief.

达方式与年轻人不同，特别是那些经历多次家人去世的老年人，常见的悲伤表达不一定仅仅是哭泣。

（三）帮助丧亲者恢复日常生活

护士要评估丧亲者的生活现状，发现现存的和潜在的生活问题。死者生前的生活角色必须由丧亲者或其他人来承担，以继续日常生活。丧亲者能够认识并充分利用身边的社会资源，也有助于其恢复日常生活。居丧期间尽量避免生活中的重大变迁，如搬迁或变卖家产。

（四）协助丧亲者摆脱悲伤情绪

当丧亲者开始转移注意力，开始一段新的关系时，护士要密切关注丧亲者的状况。丧偶的老年人开始一段新的社会关系要比其他人难得多。调查显示，丧偶的老年人相比年轻人，一般较少开始一段新的关系。老年人内心担心再一次失去的痛苦，这种想法严重阻碍他们发展新的关系。一般这种丧偶的情感会由其他感情如友情来替代。

（五）给丧亲者悲伤的时间

过去常认为，在亲人逝去第一个周年纪念过去的时候，悲痛情绪通常就过去了。但这种说法不是很准确，许多因素影响悲痛的愈合。丧亲后有 2 个时间点对悲痛愈合很重要，分别是丧亲后的 3 个月和 1 年。经历多次失去亲人的老年人可能需要更长的时间。对一些人来说，悲痛可能终身难愈，他们可能渐渐习惯带着负面情绪继续生活。

vi. Interpret "Normal" Behavior for the Survivor

It is important that nurses, with a clear understanding of the range of normal grief responses, communicate acceptance and reassurance of the normalcy of a grieving person's responses. Grieving individuals can be reassured that they are not going crazy, that their physical and psychological responses are normal in the face of significant loss, that grief spasms may occur, and that they will feel better in time.

vii. Allow for Individual Survivor Differences

Just as nurses must be sensitive to individual differences in styles of grieving, family and friends need to accept differences among themselves in their grief responses. Nurses may need to explain the wide range of responses and assist mourners with allowing one another to grieve in their own ways.

viii. Provide Continuing Support for the Survivor

Although nurses' interactions with bereaved persons may be brief or intermittent, referrals can be made for outside support. This support may include community resources and support groups. Nurses can also encourage the bereaved to mobilize their own support system of family and friends.

ix. Examine the Survivor's Defenses and Coping Styles

Certain coping behaviors are healthy, whereas others are not. An older person has had a lifetime of experience coping with stressful situations and usually has well-established patterns of coping. Under normal circumstances these defenses and coping mechanisms can often be used successfully; however, they may not be effective in dealing with monumental or accumulated losses. Unhealthy coping mechanisms may lead to destructive behaviors such as alcoholism. Nurses can help the bereaved identify their coping mechanisms, evaluate their effectiveness, and either encourage their continued use or explore other ways of coping more positively.

x. Identify Pathologic Conditions for the Survivor and Make Appropriate Referrals

Assistance through grief counseling and professional guidance may not be sufficient if additional problems arise that require more intensive help. Nurses need to be particularly alert to serious depressive illness and should refer accordingly. Losing a spouse and living alone puts

（六）丧亲者要了解正常和异常居丧期的行为

护士理解丧亲后的正常行为和异常行为，掌握交流技巧，以便识别丧亲者的异常应对行为，及时提供帮助。面对巨大的生活变故，丧亲者需要了解生活习惯的改变只是暂时的。

（七）悲伤反应存在个体差异

护士及丧亲者都要了解个体的悲伤反应是存在差异的。护士需要向丧亲者解释悲痛的正常反应，协助丧亲者允许其他人以相同的或不同的方式表达情感。

（八）为丧亲者提供持续的支持

对丧亲者的护理不仅仅局限在医院内，院外的社会支持包括社区资源和支持群体；院内护士应与社区护士及安宁疗护的志愿者共同为丧亲者提供连续的帮助和心理支持。护士还可以鼓励丧亲者动员其家人朋友提供支持。

（九）丧亲者的心理防御机制

失去亲人是生活中的重大事件，对丧亲者而言是一种巨大的心理应激，此时，丧亲者可能采取各种心理防御机制，其中有些是健康的，如合理化、转移、升华等，有些则对心理健康不利，如退化行为。经历过很多次生活变故的老年人通常有健全的心理应对机制。而一些不健康的应对机制可能导致不利于身心健康的应对行为，如酗酒。护士可以帮助丧亲者识别他们的应对行为，并鼓励他们继续使用或寻找一些更有效的方式缓解强烈的情绪反应。

（十）警惕丧亲者的危险行为

护士要特别警惕严重抑郁症的发生，对丧亲者的情绪表达和情绪变化及时评估。丧偶老人有较高的自杀率，这提示抑郁可能是丧偶老人的主要心理问题。

older persons at risk for depression. Older white men have the highest suicide rate of any group, which may suggest that depression is a significant problem for this age group. Discussing with older men the meaning in their lives may give the nurse clues to problems in this area.

For the persons older than age 65, who is under more medication therapy than any other group, overuse of medications treating the symptoms of grief, such as anti-anxiety or sedation is a common problem. More types of drugs mean more interactions of different kinds of drugs. In addition, the risk of side effects and toxic reactions is increasing with aging.

A most recent systematic review shows that due to a paucity of nursing studies on controlled clinical trails, no rigorous evidence-based recommendation regarding the treatment of bereaved persons is currently possible except for the pharmacologic treatment of depression. The following five factors are suggested as impeding scientific progress regarding bereavement care interventions: excessive theoretical heterogeneity; stultifying between-study variation; inadequate reporting of intervention procedures; few published replication studies, and methodological flaws of study design. Thus, there will be a long way for nurses to solve the problem and much more systematic approach considering different culture background and the variety of individual response to this topic need further clinical research.

(GU Yanmei)

Key Points

1. 1Death, grief, and mourning are universal and natural aspects of the life process.

2. Nurses are supposed to offer professional help to the bereaved at any stages of grief.

3. As an ordinary person, the nurse has her own way of expressing grieving and coping to loss. Personal experiences impact a nurse's work more or less.

另外，一些丧偶老人可能使用镇静催眠或抗焦虑药来缓解悲伤带来的负面情绪和睡眠障碍，但65岁以上老年人在使用药物方面容易出现药物过量，其毒副作用更加危害老年人健康。另外，加上老年人原有疾病所使用的药物治疗，使药物之间的相互作用和相互影响更加复杂。

最新的系统评价表明，目前尚无严格的、基于证据的关于丧亲者服用抗抑郁药治疗的建议。临床护士可能会面对各种各样的丧亲者及各种丧亲后悲痛的表达方式。虽然护士能够识别他人的恰当或不恰当的心理防御和应对行为，但是，当护士自身面对类似事件时，自己并不一定能够意识到自身的心理和行为。另外，护士的个人经历也不可避免地影响护士对丧亲者的护理。一个经历过生活变故的护士对悲痛过程会有更深刻的理解，而一个正在经历丧亲悲痛的护士在工作中就可能有些力不从心。因此，护理管理者应意识到并注重评估临床护士对丧亲的应对心理和行为表现，以便及时调整工作安排和提供帮助。

（谷岩梅）

本章要点

1. 死亡、悲伤、悲哀是生命过程中普遍存在的自然现象。

2. 在悲伤的各个阶段护士都要为患者提供专业的护理。

3. 作为普通人，护士自身也存在对于悲伤和应对悲伤的问题。护士自身的经历影响其工作。

Critical Thinking Exercise

1. Please describe your own feels and impression of death and death issues with few words or in an essay.

2. Give the right nursing explanation to Do Not Resuscitate order, does it mean to the nurses that the life is ending and what we would do is waiting for the time?

3. What do the dying individuals suffer, from the time when he or she gets the bad news?

4. Have your ever experience grieving for any kind of loss in your life? How's the feeling? How did you come out of it? Anything helped you dealing with that?

批判性思维练习

1. 请用几句话或一篇文章来描述自己对死亡和死亡问题的感受。

2. 解释患者提出的不采取抢救措施的愿望,是否意味着生命结束了,医护人员只要等待患者死亡的时刻就行了?

3. 描述一下从患者得到坏消息到垂死时刻都可能经历哪些心理和情绪?

4. 回忆身边人的死亡?体会个人当时的感受?怎样走出丧亲之痛?是否得到某些帮助?

Appendix 1　Stanford Sleepiness Scale

This is a quick way to assess how alert you are feeling. If it is during the day when you go about your business, ideally you would want a rating of a one. Take into account that most people have two peak times of alertness daily, at about 9 a. m. and 9 p. m. Alertness wanes to its lowest point at around 3 p. m. ; after that it begins to build again. Rate your alertness at different times during the day. If you go below a three when you should be feeling alert, this is an indication that you have serious sleep debt and you need more sleep.

An Introspective Measure of Sleepiness

The Stanford Sleepiness Scale (SSS)

Degree of Sleepiness	Scale Rating
Feeling active, vital, alert, or wide awake	1
Functioning at high levels, but not at peak; able to concentrate	2
Awake, but relaxed; responsive but not fully alert	3
Somewhat foggy, let down	4
Foggy; losing interest in remaining awake; slowed down	5
Sleepy, woozy, fighting sleep; prefer to lie down	6
No longer fighting sleep, sleep onset soon; having dream-like thoughts	7
Asleep	X

Appendix 2　The Epworth Sleepiness Scale

老年护理学

How likely are you to doze off or fall asleep in the following situations, in contrast to feeling just tired? This refers to your usual way of life in recent times. Even if you have not done some of these things recently try to work out how they would have affected you. Use the following scale to choose the most appropriate number for each situation:

0 = no chance of dozing

1 = slight chance of dozing

2 = moderate chance of dozing

3 = high chance of dozing

Situation	Chance of Dozing
Sitting and reading	_____
Watching TV	_____
Sitting inactive in a public place (e. g a theater or a meeting)	_____
As a passenger in a car for an hour without a break	_____
Lying down to rest in the afternoon when circumstances permit	_____
Sitting and talking to someone	_____
Sitting quietly after a lunch without alcohol	_____
In a car, while stopped for a few minutes in traffic	_____

Appendix 3 Pittsburgh Sleep Quality Index (PSQI)

Name_____ ID_____ Date_____ Age_____

Instructions:

The following questions relate to your usual sleep habits during the past month ONLY. Your answers should indicate the most accurate reply for the majority of days and nights in the past month.

Please answer all questions.

1. During the past month, when have you usually gone to bed at night?

      USUAL BED TIME_____

2. During the past month, how long (in minutes) has it usually taken you to fall asleep each night?

      NUMBER OF MINUTES_____

3. During the past month, when have you usually gotten up in the morning?

      USUAL GETTING UP TIME_____

4. During the past month, how many hours of *actual sleep* did you get at night? (This may be different than the number of hours you spend in bed.)

      HOURS OF SLEEP PER NIGHT_____

For each of the remaining questions, check the one best response. Please answer *all* questions.

5. During the past month, how often have you had trouble sleeping because you …

(a) Cannot get to sleep within 30 minutes

Not during the   less than Once or   Three or more

Past month_____ once a week_____ twice a week_____ times a week_____

(b) Wake up in the middle of the night or early morning

Not during the   less than Once or   Three or more

Past month_____ once a week_____ twice a week_____ times a week_____

(c) Have to get up to use the bathroom.

Not during the   less than Once or   Three or more

Past month_____ once a week_____ twice a week_____ times a week_____

(d) Cannot breathe comfortably.

Not during the   less than Once or   Three or more

Past month_____ once a week_____ twice a week_____ times a week_____

(e) Cough or snore loudly.

Not during the   less than Once or   Three or more

Past month_____ once a week_____ twice a week_____ times a week_____

(f) Feel too cold.

Not during the   less than Once or   Three or more

Past month_____ once a week_____ twice a week_____ times a week_____

(g) Feel too hot.

Not during the   less than Once or   Three or more

Past month_____ once a week_____ twice a week_____ times a week_____

(h) Had bad dreams.

Not during the   less than Once or   Three or more

Past month_____ once a week_____ twice a week_____ times a week_____

(i) Have pain.

Not during the   less than Once or   Three or more

Past month_____ once a week_____ twice a week_____ times a week_____

(j) Other reason (s), please describe

_____

How often during the past month have you had trouble sleeping because of this?

Not during the less than Once or Three or more

Past month_____ once a week_____ twice a week_____ times a week_____

6. During the past month, how would you rate your sleep quality overall?

Very good _____

Fairly good _____

Fairly bad _____

Very bad _____

7. During the past month, how often have you taken medicine (Prescribed or "over the counter") to help you sleep?

Not during the less than Once or Three or more

Past month_____ once a week_____ twice a week_____ times a week_____

8. During the past month, how often have you had trouble staying awake while driving, eating meals, or engaging in social activity?

Not during the less than Once or Three or more

Past month_____ once a week_____ twice a week_____ times a week_____

9. During the past month, how much of a problem has it been for you to keep up enough enthusiasm to get things done?

No problem at all _____

Only a very slight problem _____

Somewhat of a problem _____

A very big problem _____

10. Do you have a bed partner or share a room?

No bed partner or do not share a room _____

Partner/ flatmate in other room _____

Partner in same room, but not same bed _____

Partner in same bed _____

11. If you have a bed partner or share a room, ask him/her how often in the past month you have had …

(a) Loud snoring.

Not during the less than Once or Three or more

Past month_____ once a week_____ twice a week_____ times a week_____

(b) Long pauses between breaths while asleep.

Not during the less than Once or Three or more

Past month_____ once a week_____ twice a week_____ times a week_____

(c) Legs twitching or jerking while you sleep.

Not during the less than Once or Three or more

Past month_____ once a week_____ twice a week_____ times a week_____

(d) Episodes of disorientation or confusion during sleep.

Not during the less than Once or Three or more

Past month_____ once a week_____ twice a week_____ times a week_____

(e) Other restlessness while you sleep: please describe

_____

Not during the less than Once or Three or more

Past month_____ once a week_____ twice a week_____ times a week_____

Appendix 4　Screening Instruments for Late-life Depression in Primary Care

Geriatric Depression Scale: Short Form (15-item)

Choose the best answer for how you have felt over

the past week:

1. Are you basically satisfied with your life? YES/NO
2. Have you dropped many of your activities and interests? YES/NO
3. Do you feel that your life is empty? YES/NO
4. Do you often get bored? YES/NO
5. Are you in good spirits most of the time? YES/NO
6. Are you afraid that something bad is going to happen to you? YES/NO
7. Do you feel happy most of the time? YES/NO
8. Do you often feel helpless? YES/NO
9. Do you prefer to stay at home, rather than going out and doing new things? YES/NO
10. Do you feel you have more problems with memory than most? YES/NO
11. Do you think it is wonderful to be alive now? YES/NO
12. Do you feel pretty worthless the way you are now? YES/NO
13. Do you feel full of energy? YES/NO
14. Do you feel that your situation is hopeless? YES/NO
15. Do you think that most people are better off than you are? YES/NO

Answers in bold indicate depression.

Score 1 point for each bolded answer.

A score > 5 points is suggestive of depression.

A score > 10 points is almost always indicative of depression.

A score > 5 points should warrant a follow-up comprehensive assessment.

The Geriatric Depression Scale-5

- Are you basically satisfied with your life? YES/NO
- Do you often get bored? YES/NO
- Do you often feel helpless? YES/NO
- Do you prefer to stay at home rather than going out and doing new things? YES/NO
- Do you feel pretty worthless the way you are now? YES/NO

Two out of five depressive responses ("no" to question 1 or "yes" to questions 2 through 5) suggests the diagnosis of depression.

PHQ-9 depression questionnaire

Name:			Date:	
Over the last two weeks, how often have you been bothered by any of the following problems?	Not at all	Several days	More than half the days	Nearly every day
Little interest or pleasure in doing things	0	1	2	3
Feeling down, depressed, or hopeless	0	1	2	3
Trouble falling or staying asleep, or sleeping too much	0	1	2	3
Feeling tired or having little energy	0	1	2	3
Poor appetite or overeating	0	1	2	3
Feeling bad about yourself, or that you are a failure, or that you have let yourself or your family down	0	1	2	3
Trouble concentrating on things, such as reading the newspaper or watching television	0	1	2	3
Moving or speaking so slowly that other people could have noticed? Or the opposite, being so fidgety or restless that you have been moving around a lot more than usual	0	1	2	3
Thoughts that you would be better off dead, or of hurting yourself in some way	0	1	2	3
Total ___ =	____	+ ___	+ ___	+ ___

PHQ-9 score ≥ 10: Likely major depression

Depression score ranges:

5 to 9: mild

10 to 14: moderate

15 to 19: moderately severe

≥ 20: severe

If you checked off any problems, how difficult have these problems made it for you to do your work, take care of things at home, or get along with other people?	Not difficult at all ____	Somewhat difficult ____	Very difficult ____	Extremely difficult ____

PHQ: Patient Health Questionnaire.

Short Patient Health Questionnaire (PHQ-2)

Over the last two weeks, how often have you been bothered by any of the following problems?	Not at all	Several days	More than half the days	Nearly every day
Little interest or pleasure in doing things	0	1	2	3
Feeling down, depressed, or hopeless	0	1	2	3

Two question screener

- "During the past month, have you been bothered by feeling down, depressed or hopeless?"
- "During the past month, have you been bothered by little interest or pleasure in doing things?"

Appendix 5 CDR Rating Guideline

	None 0	Questionable 0.5	Mild 1	Moderate 2	Severe 3
Memory	No memory loss or slight inconsistent forgetfulness	Consistent slight forgetfulness; partial recollection of events; "benign" forgetfulness	Moderate memory loss; more marked for recent events; defect interferes with everyday activities	Severe memory loss; only highly learned material retained; new material rapidly lost	Severe memory loss; only fragments remain
Orientation	Fully oriented	Fully oriented except for slight difficulty with time relationships	Moderate difficulty with time relationships; oriented for place at examination; may have geographic disorientation elsewhere	Severe difficulty with time relationships; usually disoriented to time, often to place	Oriented to person only
Judgment & Problem Solving	Solves everyday problems & handles business & financial affairs well; judgment good in relation to past performance	Slight impairment in solving problems, similarities, and differences	Moderate difficulty in handling problems, similarities, and differences; social judgment usually maintained	Severely impaired in handling problems, similarities, and differences; social judgment usually impaired	Unable to make judgments or solve problems
Community Affairs	Independent function at usual level in job, shopping, volunteer and social groups	Slight impairment in these activities	Unable to function independently at these activities although may still be engaged in some; appears normal to casual inspection	No pretense of independent function outside home. Appears well enough to be taken to functions outside a family home	Appears too ill to be taken to functions outside a family home
Home and Hobbies	Life at home, hobbies, and intellectual interests well maintained	Life at home, hobbies, and intellectual interests slightly impaired	Mild but definite impairment of function at home; more difficult chores abandoned; more complicated hobbies and interests abandoned	Only simple chores preserved; very restricted interests, poorly maintained	No significant function in home
Personal Care	Fully capable of self-care		Needs prompting	Requires assistance in dressing, hygiene, keeping of personal effects	Requires much help with personal care; frequent incontinence

Score only as decline from previous usual level due to cognitive loss, not impairment due to other factors.

Appendix 6 Management Strategies for Behavioral Problems

Behavioral Problems	Antecedents or Potential Causes	Management Strategies
Difficulty with personal care tasks	Task too difficulty or overwhelming	Divide task into small, successive steps
	Caregiver impatience, rushing	Be patient, allow ample time, or try again later
	Cannot remember task	Demonstrate action or task; allow patient to perform parts of the task that can still be accomplished
	Pain involved with movement	Treat underlying condition; consider pain medication or physiotherapy; modify or assist the movement needed
	Cannot understand or follow caregiver instructions	Repeat request simply; state instructions 1 step at a time
	Fear of tasks---cannot understand need for task or instructions	Reassure, comfort, distract from task with music or conversation; ask patient to help perform task
	Inertia, apraxia; difficulty initiating and completing a task	Set up task sequence by arranging materials (such as clothing) in the order to be used; help begin the task
Wandering	Stress-noise, clutter, crowding	Reduce excessive stimulation
	Lost-looking for someone or something familiar	Provide familiar objects, signs, pictures; offer to help find objects or place; reassure
	Restless, bored---no stimuli	Provide meaningful activity
	Medication side effect	Monitor, reduce, or discontinue medication
	Lifelong pattern of being active or usual coping style	Respond to underlying mood or motivation; provide safe area to move about (e. g. , secured circular path)
	Needing to use the toilet	Institute toileting schedule (such as every 2 hr); place signs or pictures on bathroom door
	Environmental stimuli---exit signs, people leaving	Remove or camouflage environmental stimuli; provide identification or alarm bracelets
Suspiciousness, paranoia	Forgot where objects were placed	Offer to help find; have more than one of same object available; have a list where objects should be placed; learn favorite hiding places
	Misinterpreting actions or words	Do not argue or try to reason; do not take personally; distract
	Misinterpreting who people are; suspicious of their intentions	Introduce self and role routinely; draw on old memory, connections; do not argue
	Change in environment or routine	Reassure, familiarize, set routine

Behavioral Problems	Antecedents or Potential Causes	Management Strategies
Suspiciousness, paranoia	Misinterpreting environment	Assess vision, hearing; modify environment as needed; explain misinterpretation simply; distract
	Physical illness	Evaluate medically
	Social isolation	Encourage and provide familiar social opportunities
	Someone actually taking something from the patient	Verify the situation
Agitation (also "sun downing", catastrophic reactions)	Discomfort, pain	Assess and manage sources of pain, constipation, infection, or full bladder; check clothing for comfort
	Physical illness (such as urinary tract infection)	Evaluate medically; eliminate caffeine and alcohol
	Fatigue	Schedule adequate rest; monitor activity
	Overstimulation---noise, overhead paging, people, radio, television, activities	Reduce noise, stress; remove from situation: use television sparingly; limit crowding (e. g. , dining hallways just before meals)
	Mirroring of caregiver's affect	Control affect; model calm with low tone and slow rate; use support system and groups for outlet
	Overextending capabilities (resulting in failure): caregiver expectations too high	Do not put in failure-oriented situations or tasks; understand losses and reduce expectations accordingly
	Patient is being "quizzed" (multiple questions that exceed abilities)	Avoid persistent testing of memory; pose 1 question at a time; eliminate questions that require abstract thought, insight, or reasoning
	Medication side effect	Assess, monitor, and reduce medication if possible; monitor health concerns
	Patient is thwarted from desired activity (e. g. , attempting to escape)	Redirect energy to similar activity; ask patient to help with meaningful activity; have diversionary tactics for outbursts; choose battles—assess whether behavior is merely irritating, rather than compromising patient safety or obstructing care
	Lowered stress threshold	Simplify tasks, create calm; lower expectations and demands; avoid arguments and reprimands
	Unfamiliar people or environment; change in schedule or routine	Be consistent; avoid changes, surprises; make change gradually
	Restless	Plan calming music, massage, or meaningful activities; assign tasks that provide exercise
Incontinence	Infection, prostate problem, chronic illness, medication side effect, stress or urge incontinence	Evaluate medically
	Difficulty in finding bathroom	Place signs, picture on door; ensure adequate lighting
	Lack of privacy	Provide for privacy
	Difficulty undressing	Simplify clothing, use elastic waistbands
	Difficulty in seeing toilet	Use contrasting colors on toilet and floor
	Impaired mobility	Evaluate medically, treat associated pain (include physiotherapy); provide a commode; reduce diuretics when possible

continued

Behavioral Problems	Antecedents or Potential Causes	Management Strategies
Incontinence	Dependence created by socialized reinforcement	Provide increased attention for continence rather than incontinence; allow independence when possible, even if time-consuming
	Cannot express need	Schedule toileting (such as every 2 hr while awake); reduce diuretics and bedtime liquids when possible
	Task overwhelming	Simplify; establish step-by-step routine
Sleep disturbance	Illness, pain, medication effect (e. g., causing daytime sleepiness or nocturnal awakening)	Evaluate medically
	Depression	Prescribe antidepressant (consider bedtime sedative such as trazodone)
	Less need for sleep	Schedule later bedtime; allow activities or tasks safely done at night; plan more daytime exercise
	Too hot, too cold	Adjust temperature
	Disorientation from darkness	Use night-lights
	Caffeine or alcohol effect	Reduce or eliminate alcohol; limit caffeine after noon
	Hunger	Provide nighttime snack
	Urge to void	Ensure clear, well-lit pathway to bathroom
	Normal age-and disease-related fragmentation of sleep (like that of an infant or toddler)	Accept; plan for safety
	Daytime sleeping	Eliminate or limit naps, provide activity and exercise instead; for naps, use recliner rather than bed
	Fear of darkness; restless	Provide soft music, massage, night-light
Inappropriate or impulsive sexual behavior	Dementia-related decreased judgment and social awareness	Do not overreact or confront; respond calmly and firmly; distract and redirect
	Misinterpreting caregivers interaction	Do not give mixed sexual message (double entendres and innuendos-even in jest); avoid nonverbal messages; distract while performing personal care, bathing
	Uncomfortable–too warm, clothing too tight; need to void; genital irritation	Check room temperature; assist with comfortable weather-appropriate clothing; ensure that elimination needs are met; examine for groin rash, perineal skin problems, stool impaction
	Need for attention, affection, intimacy	Increase or meet basic need for touch and warmth; model appropriate touch; offer soothing objects (such as stuffed animals); provide hand or back massage
	Self-stimulating, reacting to what feels good	Offer privacy; remove from inappropriate place

Appendix 7　Caring Techniques to Elderly with Dementia

Caring Techniques	Description	Examples	Working Mechanisms
Reminiscence	It is a structured process of reflection on significant life events rather than simply recalling the past	Biographical story of telling Activities that elicit pleasant memories by using pictures, photographs, music, foods, tools, or memorabilia	The ability to retrieve events from long-term memory can persist long after the capacity to recall newly learned information diminishes. Reminiscence may be effective in stimulating communication, promoting self-esteem, and decreasing depression in older adults with or without dementia
Art	Identify a medium that the person can manage, but is not childlike or demeaning	Painting and drawing under the guidance of a trained artistic facilitator Color with crayons	Exposure to art has been shown to reduce anxiety and depression, minimizing the negative effects of problem behaviors. Art may be an alternate form of communication for persons with dementia as the disease process makes language difficult or impossible. Sensory stimulation is provided
Music	Music creates emotions or interacts with the emotions we already feel. It is enjoyable and makes people "feel good"	Two types of music which are calming and individualized ones can be used	Calming music may mediate the release of stress hormones, altering the stress response, resulting in functionally adaptive behaviors. The individualized music chosen by personal preference can stimulate remote memory of patients. The elicitation of memories associated with positive feelings (e. g., happiness or love) has a soothing effect on the person with dementia, which in turn prevents or alleviates agitation

参考文献

1 ········• 郭桂芳.老年护理学：双语 [M].北京：人民卫生出版社，2012.

2 ········• 化前珍，胡秀英.老年护理学 [M].4 版.北京：人民卫生出版社，2017.

3 ········• 汪耀.实用老年病学 [M].北京：人民卫生出版社，2014.

4 ········• 黄金.老年病学 [M].2 版.北京：高等教育出版社，2009.

5 ········• 美国精神医学学会.精神障碍诊断与统计手册 [M].5 版.张道龙，译.北京：北京大学医学出版社，

2014.

6 ········• EPIOPOULOS C. Gerontological nursing[M]. Philadephia ：Lippincott-Raven Publisher，2014.